S0-BHU-825

Robbins and Cotran Atlas of Pathology

Robbins and Cotran
Atlas of Pathology

Edward C. Klatt, MD
Professor and Academic Administrator
Department of Biomedical Sciences
Year 2 Curriculum Director
Florida State University College of Medicine
Tallahassee, Florida

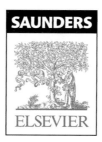
SAUNDERS
ELSEVIER

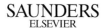

SAUNDERS
ELSEVIER

1600 John F. Kennedy Blvd.
Ste 1800
Philadelphia, PA 19103-2899

ROBBINS AND COTRAN ATLAS OF PATHOLOGY, 1/E

ISBN 13: 978-1-4160-0274-1
ISBN 10: 1-4160-0274-X
International Edition ISBN 13: 978-0-8089-2319-0
International Edition ISBN 10: 0-8089-2319-6

Copyright © 2006 by Saunders, Inc., an affiliate of Elsevier Inc.

All rights reserved. No part of this publication may be reproduced or transmitted in any form or by any means, electronic or mechanical, including photocopying, recording, or any information storage and retrieval system, without permission in writing from the publisher.

Permissions may be sought directly from Elsevier's Health Sciences Rights Department in Philadelphia, PA, USA: phone: (+1) 215 239 3804, fax: (+1) 215 239 3805, e-mail: healthpermissions@elsevier.com. You may also complete your request on-line via the Elsevier homepage (http://www.elsevier.com), by selecting Customer Support and then Obtaining Permissions.

Notice

Neither the Publisher nor the Authors assume any responsibility for any loss or injury and/or damage to persons or property arising out of or related to any use of the material contained in this book. It is the responsibility of the treating practitioner, relying on independent expertise and knowledge of the patient, to determine the best treatment and method of application for the patient.

The Publisher

Library of Congress Cataloging-in-Publication Data

Klatt, Edward C.,
    Robbins and Cotran atlas of pathology / Edward C. Klatt. — 1st ed.
       p.   cm.
    Includes index.
    ISBN 1-4160-0274-X
1. Pathology—Atlases. 2. Pathology. I. Robbins, Stanley L. (Stanley Leonard) II. Cotran, Ramzi S. III. Title. IV. Title: Atlas of pathology.
    RB33.K55   2006
    616.07—dc22

2006040877

Acquisitions Editor: William Schmitt
Managing Editor: Rebecca Gruliow
Design Direction: Ellen Zanolle

Working together to grow
libraries in developing countries

www.elsevier.com | www.bookaid.org | www.sabre.org

ELSEVIER   BOOK AID International   Sabre Foundation

Printed in Canada
Last digit is the print number: 9 8 7 6 5 4 3 2 1

Preface

This is the very first edition of an atlas in the Robbins series of texts. This atlas is organized into chapters that closely follow Unit II: Diseases of Organ Systems in the seventh edition of the "big" *Robbins and Cotran Pathologic Basis of Disease*. The atlas is designed to complement both the *Pathologic Basis of Disease* and *Basic Pathology* texts by providing even more examples of disease processes in a visual format. The majority of students are "visual" learners and readily take advantage of visual study materials. The gross, microscopic, and radiologic images utilized for the figures as presented in this atlas are designed to reinforce each other, as well as those present in other works in the Robbins series. In addition, there are examples of normal organs and tissues for review and orientation.

Each figure is accompanied by a brief description that provides the key points illustrated by the figure. For more complete study, the learner is directed to the Robbins texts. The labels

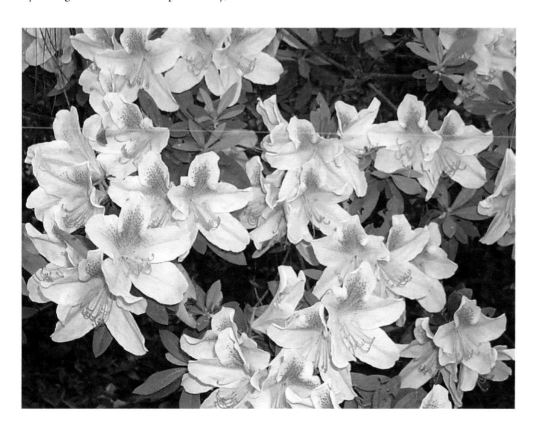

and descriptions provided for the figures will guide the learner in a discovery process while perusing these figures. Though concise, the figure descriptions cumulatively yield a considerable volume of reading. Correlations with findings from clinical history, physical examination, and clinical laboratory testing are included in many of the descriptions. The atlas author pursues an integrative approach to medical education, combining elements of basic science, clinical, and behavioral subjects into learning materials that promote a flowering of knowledge to benefit those in need of health care.

Acknowledgments

The author is indebted to the stalwart figures who fundamentally contributed to the development of the Robbins series, starting with the founding author Dr. Stanley Robbins, continuing with Dr. Ramzi Cotran, and ongoing with Dr. Vinay Kumar. These lead authors have set the standard of excellence that characterizes this series. In addition there have been and continue to be numerous contributing authors who have made the Robbins series into the valuable tool it remains for medical education. Just as no single monarch butterfly completes a migration, so too medical educators build upon the work of colleagues over many generations.

Persons associated with the publisher, Elsevier, require special thanks including the Production Editor, Ellen Sklar, and the Managing Editor, Rebecca Gruliow. Of course, none of this work would be possible without the support and vision provided by Mr. William Schmitt, Publishing Director of Medical Textbooks.

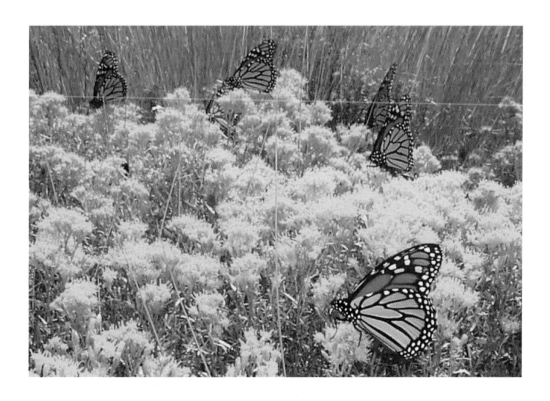

To all who strive for improving the health of everyone.

Contributors

Arthur J. Belanger, MHS
Autopsy Service Manager
Yale University School of Medicine
New Haven, Connecticut

Ofer Ben-Itzhak, MD
Associate Professor
Faculty of Medicine
Technion-Israel Institute of Technology
Haifa, Israel

Professor David Y. Cohen
Director of Pathology
Herzliyah Medical Center
Herzliyah-on-Sea, Israel

Richard M. Conran, MD, PhD, JD
Professor of Pathology
Uniformed Services University of the Health Sciences
Bethesda, Maryland

Todd Cameron Grey, MD
Chief Medical Examiner, State of Utah
Associate Clinical Professor of Pathology
University of Utah
Salt Lake City, Utah

Ilan Hammel
Professor of Pathology; Head, Graduate School; Chairman, Department of Pathology
Tel Aviv University
Tel Aviv, Israel

M. Elizabeth H. Hammond, MD
Professor of Pathology and Adjunct Professor of Internal Medicine
University of Utah School of Medicine
Salt Lake City, Utah

Sate Hamza, MD
Assistant Professor
University of Manitoba
Winnipeg, Manitoba, Canada

Walter H. Henricks, MD
Staff Pathologist and Director of Laboratory Information Services
The Cleveland Clinic Foundation
Cleveland, Ohio

Lauren C. Hughey, MD
Assistant Professor of Dermatology
University of Alabama at Birmingham
Birmingham, Alabama

Carl R. Kjeldsberg, MD
Professor of Pathology
University of Utah Health Sciences
Chief Executive Officer
ARUP Laboratories
Salt Lake City, Utah

Morton H. Levitt, MD, MHA
Associate Professor
Department of Biomedical Sciences
Florida State University
Tallahassee, Florida

Nick Mamalis, MD
Professor of Ophthalmology
John A. Moran Eye Center
University of Utah
Salt Lake City, Utah

Dr. John Nicholls
Associate Professor
Department of Pathology
The University of Hong Kong
Pok Fu Lam
Hong Kong, SAR

Sherrie L. Perkins, MD, PhD
Professor of Pathology
University of Utah Health Sciences and ARUP Laboratories
Salt Lake City, Utah

Mary Ann Sens, MD, PhD
Professor and Chair of Pathology
University of North Dakota School of Medicine and Health Sciences
Grand Forks, North Dakota

Hiroyuki Takahashi, MD, PhD
Assistant Professor
Department of Pathology
The Jikei University School of Medicine
Tokyo Japan

Amy Theos, MD
Assistant Professor of Dermatology
University of Alabama Medical Center
Birmingham, Alabama

Contents

CHAPTER 1

Blood Vessels

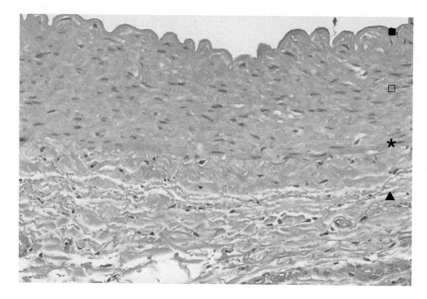

FIGURE 1–1 Normal artery, microscopic

Distally, major branches of the aorta bifurcate to small branches. This is a muscular artery in longitudinal section demonstrating a thin intima (■) on top of the internal elastic lamina. Below this is the thick media (□), with layers of circular smooth muscle and interspersed elastic fibers to withstand the arterial pressure load and dampen the pressure wave from left ventricular contraction. The media is bounded by the external elastic lamina (∗). Outside the media is the adventitia (▲), which merges with surrounding supporting connective tissue.

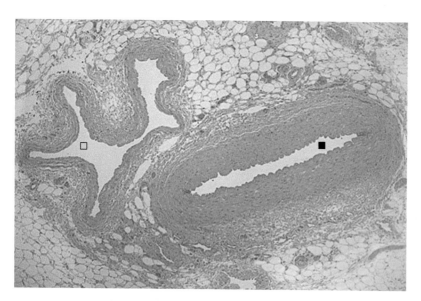

FIGURE 1–2 Normal artery and vein, microscopic

Seen here in cross-section is a normal artery (■) with a thick, smooth muscle wall alongside a normal vein (□) with a thin, smooth muscle wall, running in connective tissue in a fascial plane between muscle bundles of the lower leg. The larger arteries and veins are often grouped, along with a nerve, into a neurovascular bundle, to supply a body region. More distal areas of regional blood flow and the blood pressure are regulated by alternating vasoconstriction and dilation of small muscular arteries and arterioles.

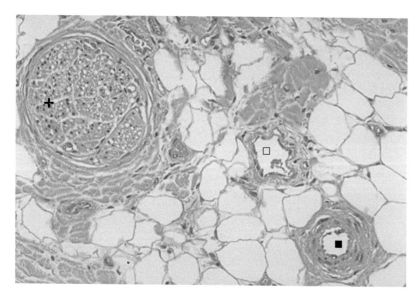

FIGURE 1–3 Normal arteriole and venule, microscopic

A normal arteriole (■) is alongside a normal venule (□) and a small peripheral nerve (+), all in cross-section, grouped into a loose neurovascular bundle. The major point of blood pressure regulation is at the arteriolar level. Exchange of solutes and gases with diffusion into tissues occurs at the capillary level. The diminished vascular pressure of the venules, along with the intravascular oncotic pressure exerted by plasma proteins, brings interstitial fluids back into the venules. Not seen here are the normally inconspicuous lymphatic channels that scavenge what little residual fluid is exuded from capillaries and not recovered into the venous system, thus preventing edema.

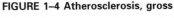

FIGURE 1–4 Atherosclerosis, gross

This is about as normal as an adult aorta in developed nations remains. The intimal surface is quite smooth, with only occasional small, pale yellow, fatty lipid streaks visible (*arrow*). Such fatty streaks may initially appear in children. (The faint reddish staining in this autopsy specimen comes from hemoglobin that leaked from red blood cells after death.) With a healthy lifestyle, there is unlikely to be a progression of these intimal fatty lesions without additional risk factors. The lipid streaks can serve as precursors for atheroma formation. Major risk factors advancing atheroma formation include increased serum LDL cholesterol, decreased HDL cholesterol, hypertriglyceridemia, diabetes mellitus, hypertension, and smoking.

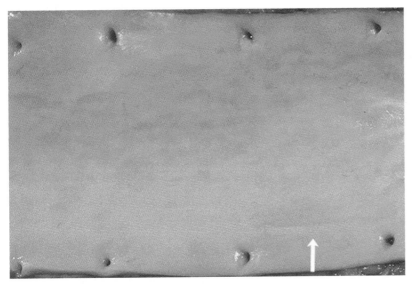

FIGURE 1–5 Atherosclerosis, gross

This coronary artery opened longitudinally shows yellowish atheromatous plaques over much of its intimal surface. There is focal hemorrhage into a plaque, a complication of atherosclerosis that can acutely narrow the lumen. Advanced atheromas can be complicated by erosion, ulceration, rupture, hemorrhage, aneurysmal dilation, calcification, and thrombosis. Arterial narrowing may lead to tissue ischemia. Marked or prolonged loss of blood supply may lead to infarction. In the heart, this may result in acute coronary syndromes. Endothelial dysfunction that impairs vasoreactivity or induces a thrombogenic surface or abnormally adhesive surface to inflammatory cells may initiate thrombus formation, atherosclerosis, and the vascular lesions of hypertension.

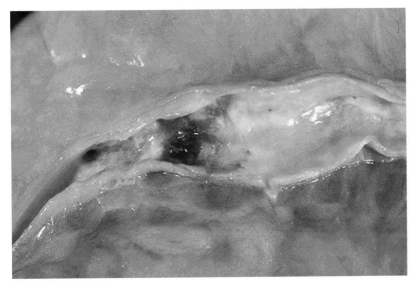

FIGURE 1–6 Atherosclerosis, gross

This is severe aortic atherosclerosis involving nearly the entire intimal surface, with ulceration of the atheromatous plaques along with formation of overlying mural thrombus. This marked degree of atherosclerosis may develop when atherogenesis proceeds over many years, or when there are significant risk factors driving atherosclerosis, such as aging, hyperlipidemia, diabetes mellitus, smoking, hypertension, and obesity. Treating or eliminating these risk factors through adoption of healthy lifestyles with increased exercise and reduced caloric intake can halt the progression of atherosclerosis, and atheromas can even regress over time, with reduced likelihood for complications!

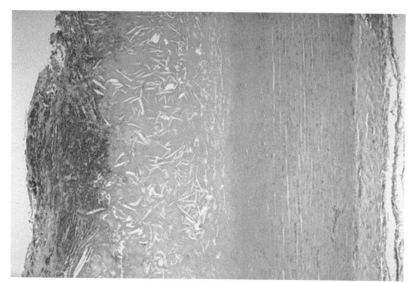

FIGURE 1–7 Atherosclerosis, microscopic

This cross-section of aorta shows a large overlying advanced atheroma containing numerous cholesterol clefts, from breakdown of lipid imbibed into foam cells. The luminal surface at the far left shows ulceration of its fibrous cap with hemorrhage. Despite this ulceration, which predisposes to mural thrombus formation, atheromatous emboli are rare (or at least, clinically significant complications from them are infrequent). Note that the thick medial layer is intact, and the adventitia appears normal at the right. As atheromas become larger, they can be complicated by ulceration, which promotes overlying thrombosis. Organization of the thrombus further increases the size of the plaque.

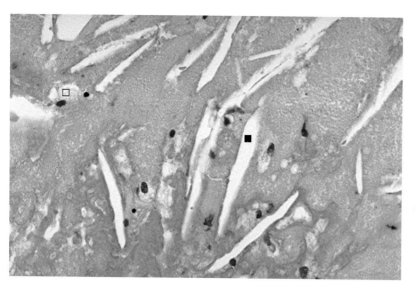

FIGURE 1–8 Atherosclerosis, microscopic

This high-magnification view of the necrotic center of an aortic atheroma demonstrates foam cells (□) and cholesterol clefts (■). In the process of atheroma formation, endothelial injury leads to increased permeability, leukocyte adhesion, and release of cytokines that attract blood monocytes, which become macrophages that accumulate lipids, becoming foam cells. Macrophages readily ingest oxidized LDL cholesterol through their scavenger receptors. Macrophages generate toxic oxygen species that oxidize LDL cholesterol. An increased serum LDL increases the oxidized LDL component, promoting this process. In contrast, HDL cholesterol tends to promote mobilization of lipid in an atheroma and transport to the liver.

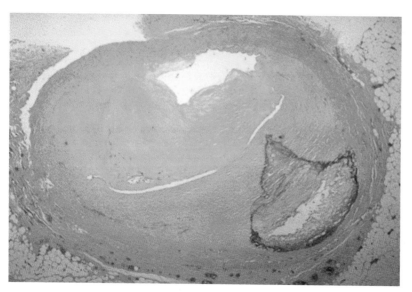

FIGURE 1–9 Atherosclerosis, microscopic

There is a severe degree of narrowing in this coronary artery. Smooth muscle cell migration and proliferation within the intima form an enlarging fibrofatty atheroma. This is a "complex" atheroma because of the large area of calcification at the lower right, which appears bluish with this H+E stain. Complex atheromas can have calcification, thrombosis, or hemorrhage. Such calcification would make coronary angioplasty to dilate the lumen more difficult. Reducing the radius of an artery by half increases the resistance to flow 16-fold. When the degree of narrowing is 70% or more, the clinical symptom of angina is often present. Such patients are at great risk for acute coronary syndromes, including myocardial infarction and sudden death from dysrhythmias.

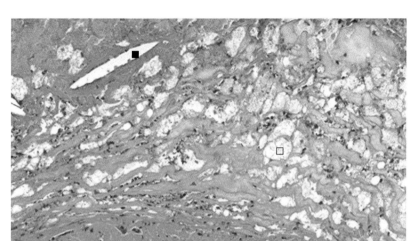

FIGURE 1–10 Atherosclerosis, microscopic

This coronary artery cross-section reveals residual smooth muscle in the media with overlying atheroma composed of extensive lipid deposition in lipophages (□), as well as a cholesterol cleft (■) from breakdown of those cells. Such plaques are prone to be complicated by rupture, hemorrhage, and thrombosis. Platelets become activated and adhere to sites of endothelial injury, then release cytokines such as platelet-derived growth factor that promote smooth muscle proliferation, and the adherent platelet mass increases the size of the plaque, while narrowing the residual arterial lumen. Use of antiplatelet agents such as aspirin helps reduce platelet "stickiness" and slows their participation in atheroma formation.

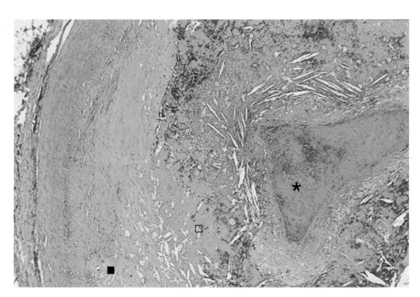

FIGURE 1–11 Atherosclerosis, microscopic

This coronary artery cross-section shows severe occlusive atherosclerosis. The atheromatous plaque is circumferential and markedly narrows the remaining lumen. Note the prominent cholesterol clefts within this atheroma. Note how this advanced atheromatous process involves both the arterial media (■) and the overlying intima (□). The remaining lumen has become occluded by a recent thrombus (*) that fills it. Thrombosis is often the basis for the acute coronary syndromes, including unstable angina, sudden death, and acute myocardial infarction.

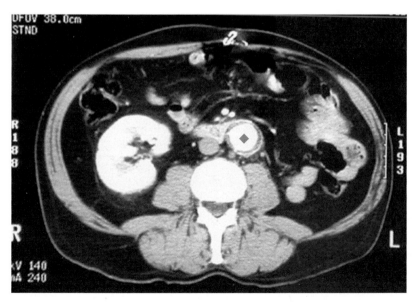

FIGURE 1–12 Atherosclerosis, CT image

This abdominal CT scan with contrast shows the abdominal aorta to be slightly dilated; the aortic lumen (◆) is highlighted by bright contrast material in the blood. Seen around the periphery of the lumen is darker gray mural thrombus in this patient with severe atherosclerosis. Mural thrombus can form atop advanced atheromas, and thrombus can organize and further narrow the lumen, or portions may break off and embolize distally to occlude smaller arterial branches in the systemic circulation. The aortic wall also has focal thin, bright areas of atheromatous calcification. (The left kidney is absent from prior nephrectomy. The right kidney is brightly attenuated as intravenous contrast filters through it.)

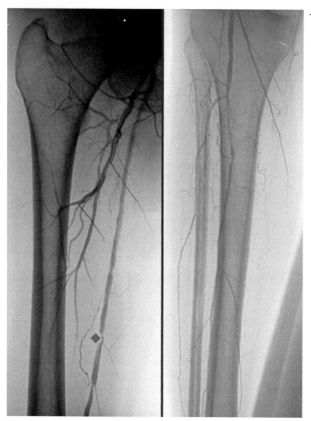

◀ **FIGURE 1–13 Atherosclerosis, angiogram**

This patient had poorly controlled type 1 diabetes mellitus for many years and developed claudication (pain with exercise) in the right lower extremity. This angiogram reveals multiple areas of atherosclerotic narrowing (◆) involving femoral arterial branches. The upper leg with femur is in the left panel and the lower leg with tibia and fibula in the right panel. The arterial lumens appear dark with the digital subtraction imaging technique shown here.

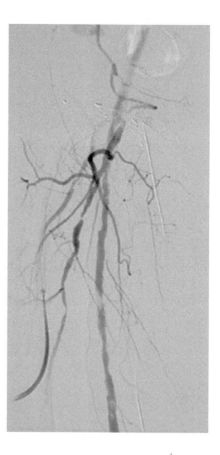

FIGURE 1–14 Atherosclerosis, angiogram ▶

There are multiple areas of atherosclerotic narrowing involving branches of the right femoral artery in this patient with poorly controlled diabetes mellitus who developed severe peripheral vascular disease with claudication. On physical examination, peripheral pulses are decreased or even absent with this degree of arterial occlusion.

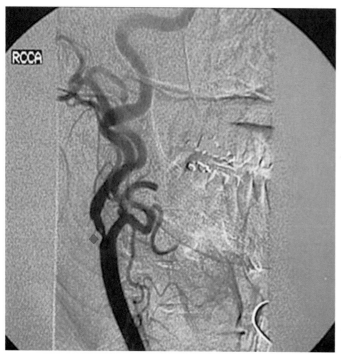

◀ **FIGURE 1–15 Atherosclerosis, angiogram**

The degree of atherosclerotic narrowing (◆) in this right internal carotid artery can produce mental status changes, including transient ischemic attacks, which could presage a "stroke" from ischemia to one or more areas of the brain. On physical examination, a bruit may be auscultated over such an area of large arterial narrowing, with faster turbulent flow of blood distal to the region of narrowing.

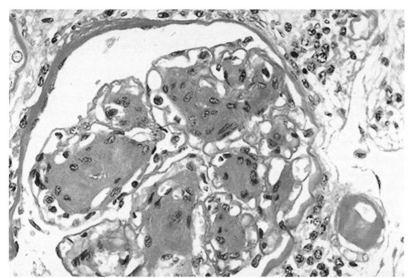

FIGURE 1–16 Hyaline arteriolosclerosis, microscopic

Two other forms of arteriosclerosis (hardening of the arteries) in addition to atherosclerosis are arteriolosclerosis and medial calcific sclerosis. Arteriolosclerosis is typically seen in kidneys and brain. One form, called hyaline arteriolosclerosis, is shown here involving the markedly thickened arteriole at the lower right of this glomerulus with PAS stain. This change often accompanies benign nephrosclerosis, leading to progressive loss of nephrons and renal atrophy. Hyaline arteriolosclerosis is also seen in elderly people, who are often normotensive. More advanced arteriosclerotic lesions are seen in people with diabetes mellitus or hypertension.

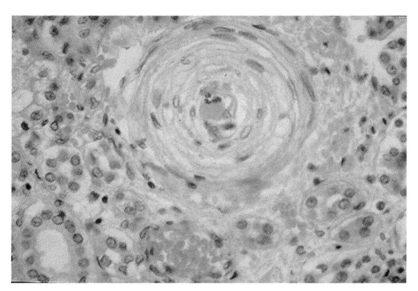

FIGURE 1–17 Hyperplastic arteriolosclerosis, microscopic

The hyperplastic form of arteriolosclerosis is prominent in this arteriole that has an "onion skin" appearance from concentric, laminated intimal and smooth muscle proliferation with marked narrowing of the arteriolar lumen. Affected arterioles may also undergo fibrinoid necrosis (necrotizing arteriolitis), and there may be local hemorrhage. Surrounding tissues may demonstrate focal ischemia or infarction. This lesion is most often associated with malignant hypertension, with diastolic blood pressure in excess of 120 mm Hg. Such malignant hypertension may occur *de novo* or may complicate long-standing hypertension.

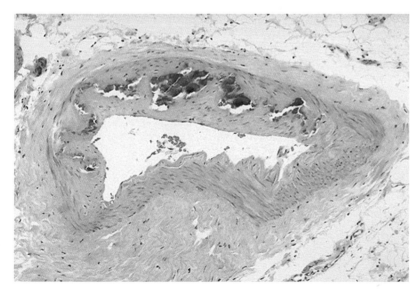

FIGURE 1–18 Medial calcific sclerosis, microscopic

Mönckeberg medial calcific sclerosis is the most insignificant form of arteriosclerosis (both atherosclerosis and arteriolosclerosis are definitely significant because of arterial luminal narrowing). It is more common in elderly people. Note the purplish blue calcifications involving just the media; note that the lumen appears unaffected by this process. Thus, no significant clinical consequences occur in most cases, and it is an incidental finding. Recall this process when you observe calcified muscular arteries on a radiograph of the pelvic region, although other regions such as the neck or breast may also be involved.

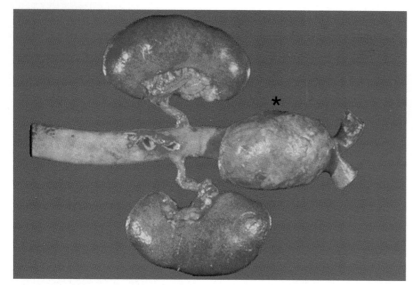

FIGURE 1–19 Aortic aneurysm, gross

Atherosclerosis involving the intima and media may focally weaken the wall of the aorta so that it bulges out to form an aneurysm. A classic atherosclerotic aortic aneurysm (AAA) typically occurs in the abdominal portion distal to the renal arteries, as shown here (*). Aortic aneurysms tend to enlarge over time, and those that get bigger than 5 to 7 cm are more likely to rupture. Aneurysms may also form in the larger arterial branches of the aorta, most often the iliac arteries. On physical examination, there may be a palpable pulsatile abdominal mass with an AAA. Increased expression of matrix metalloproteinases that degrade extracellular matrix components such as collagen is observed in aortic aneurysms.

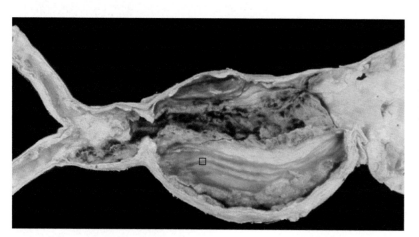

FIGURE 1–20 Aortic aneurysm, gross

The aorta has been sectioned longitudinally to reveal a large abdominal atherosclerotic aortic aneurysm distal to the renal arteries at the right and proximal to the iliac bifurcation at the left. This bulging aneurysm, 6 cm in diameter, is filled with abundant layered mural thrombus (□). Note the rough atheromatous surface of the aortic lumen.

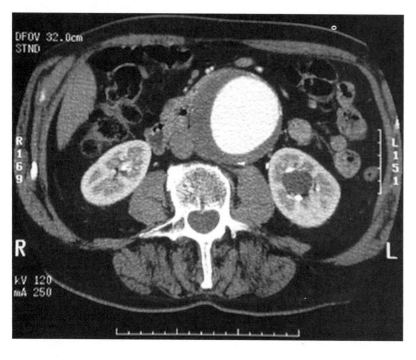

FIGURE 1–21 Aortic aneurysm, CT image

This abdominal CT scan with contrast reveals an abdominal atherosclerotic aortic aneurysm that extends distal to the level of the renal arteries past the takeoff of the inferior mesenteric artery. Note the bright contrast material in the blood filling the open aortic lumen, whereas the surrounding mural thrombus (◆) has decreased (darker) attenuation. The total aortic diameter here is about 7 to 8 cm in diameter, in great danger of rupture. A pulsatile abdominal mass was palpable in this patient. Although more common in the abdominal aorta, atherosclerotic aneurysms can be found in the thoracic aorta.

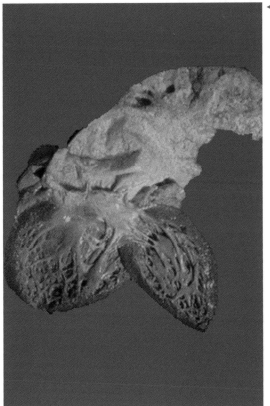

◀ **FIGURE 1–22 Syphilitic (luetic) aortitis, gross**

The aortic root is widened, and the commissures of the aortic valve cusps are pulled apart. The arch of the aorta shows peculiar irregular intimal wrinkling ("tree bark" pattern) that is typical of syphilitic aortitis. The widening of the root can cause aortic insufficiency and also aneurysmal dilation of the ascending aorta. Such dilation may also be seen with Marfan syndrome, but the intima would not show this wrinkling. Given the rarity of tertiary syphilis, atherosclerosis is now the most common cause of proximal aortic aneurysmal dilation.

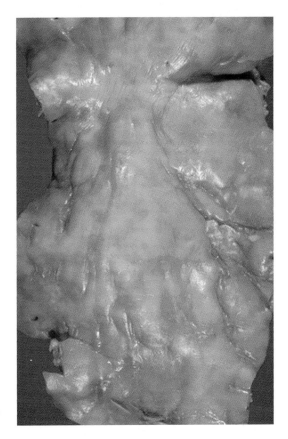

FIGURE 1–23 Syphilitic aortitis, gross ▶

The intimal surface of the aorta shows wrinkling or "tree-barking" that is typical of syphilitic aortitis. This aortitis is caused by infection with the spirochete *Treponema pallidum,* which involves the vasa vasorum (an "end aortitis") and leads to focal medial loss that produces the wrinkling. This is a complication of tertiary syphilis that manifests decades after the initial infection and typically is diagnosed with the appearance of a firm chancre on the genitalia.

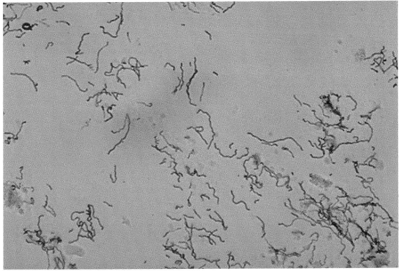

◀ **FIGURE 1–24 Spirochetes, microscopic**

These corkscrew-shaped organisms seen with Warthin-Starry silver staining are *Treponema pallidum* organisms, which cause syphilis. However, they are usually few in number in the tissue lesions of tertiary syphilis. The initial laboratory diagnosis of syphilis often starts with a screening test, the rapid plasma reagin (RPR) test, or the VDRL test, both of which detect anticardiolipin antibodies. More specific confirmatory tests detecting treponemal antigens include the fluorescent treponemal antibody absorption (FTA-abs) test and the microhemagglutinin assay for *T. pallidum* antibodies (MHATP). These tests may be negative in tertiary syphilis.

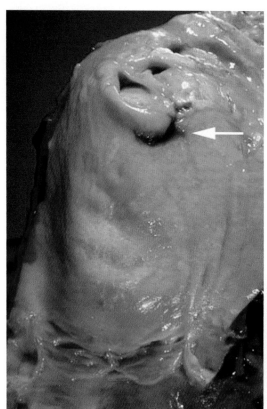

◄ FIGURE 1–25 Aortic dissection, gross

There is an intimal tear (*arrow*) located 7 cm above the aortic valve and proximal to the great vessels in this aorta with marked atherosclerosis. This is an aortic dissection. Risk factors include atherosclerosis, hypertension, and cystic medial degeneration. Once the tear occurs, the systemic arterial blood under pressure can begin to dissect into the aortic media. From there, the blood may reenter the aorta at a distal site through another tear, or it may dissect through the wall of the aorta and rupture into adjacent tissues or body cavities. Proximal ruptures may reach the pericardial cavity, with hemopericardium. There may be rupture into a pleural cavity, with hemothorax. With distal dissection, rupture into the abdominal cavity produces hemoperitoneum. Such an event is life-threatening.

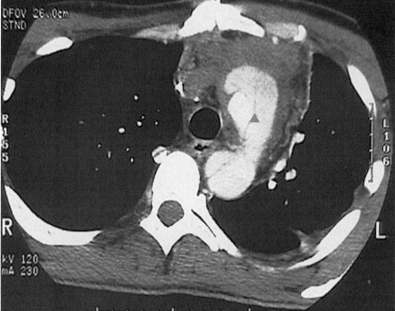

FIGURE 1–26 Aortic dissection, CT image ►

This chest CT scan with contrast demonstrates a dissection in the aortic arch. The thin, dark linear segments (▲) mark extension of blood into the aortic media. There is extension of this dissection to involve the left common carotid artery. Aortic dissections may be diagnosed with CT imaging, transesophageal echocardiography, MRI, or angiography. Angiography is preferred before surgical repair.

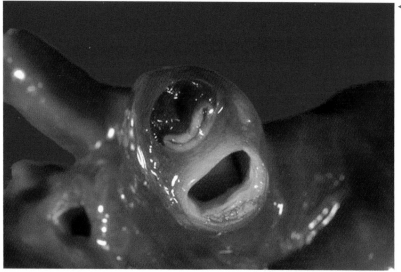

◄ FIGURE 1–27 Aortic dissection, gross

The right common carotid artery is compressed by blood dissecting upward from a tear with aortic dissection. Blood may also dissect to involve the coronary arteries. Thus, patients with aortic dissection may have symptoms of sudden, severe chest pain (for distal dissection) or may present with findings that suggest a stroke (with carotid compression from proximal dissection) or myocardial ischemia (with coronary arterial compression from proximal dissection). However, pain may be absent in proximal dissections.

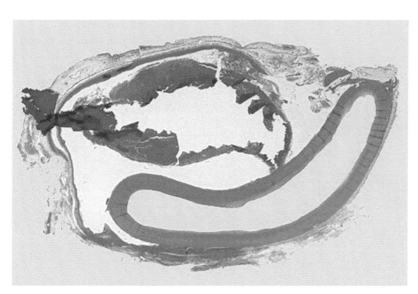

FIGURE 1–28 Aortic dissection, microscopic

This cross-section of the aorta demonstrates a red blood clot splitting the media and compressing the aortic lumen. This occurred as a result of aortic dissection in which there was a tear in the intima of the aortic arch, followed by dissection of blood at high pressure out into and through the muscular wall to the adventitia. This blood dissecting out can lead to sudden death from hemothorax, hemopericardium, or hemoperitoneum. Severe knifelike chest pain may be present.

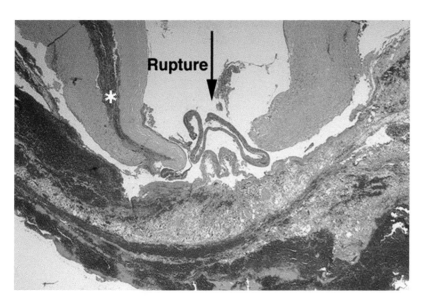

FIGURE 1–29 Aortic dissection, microscopic

The tear (*arrow*) in this aorta extends through the media, but blood also dissects along the media (*asterisk*). At surgery, the dissection can be repaired with closure of the tear and placement of a synthetic graft.

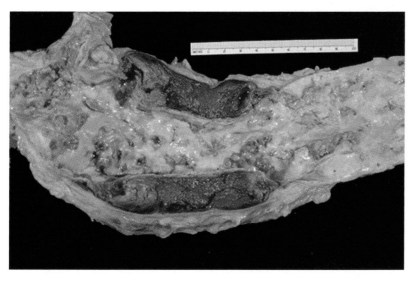

FIGURE 1–30 Aortic dissection, gross

This aorta has been opened longitudinally to reveal an area in the thoracic portion of fairly limited dissection that is organizing. The red-brown thrombus can be seen on both sides of the section as it extends around the aorta. The intimal tear would have been at the left. This creates a "double lumen" to the aorta. This aorta shows severe atherosclerosis, which was the major risk factor for dissection in this patient.

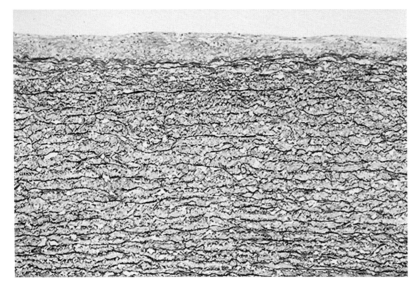

FIGURE 1–31 Normal aorta, microscopic

This is a longitudinal section through the normal aorta with an elastic tissue stain seen at low magnification. The intima is at the top, while the thick aortic media demonstrates parallel dark elastic fibers, here highlighted by the elastic stain. The smooth muscle fibers are between the elastic fibers. The smooth muscle and the elastic fibers give the aorta great strength and resiliency, allowing the pulse pressure of left ventricular systole to be transmitted distally.

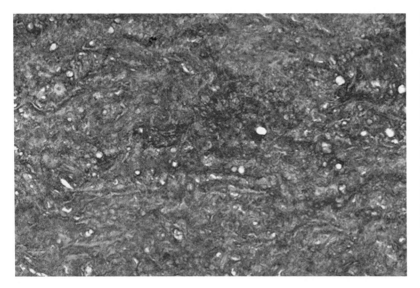

FIGURE 1–32 Cystic medial degeneration, microscopic

This mucin stain of the aortic media demonstrates cystic medial degeneration. Pink elastic fibers, instead of running in parallel arrays, are seen here to be disrupted by pools of blue mucinous ground substance. This is typical for Marfan syndrome affecting connective tissues containing elastin. This causes the connective tissue weakness that explains the propensity for aortic dissection, particularly when the aortic root dilates beyond 3 cm in diameter. Dilation of the aortic root can lead to aortic insufficiency. Patients with Marfan syndrome can undergo proximal aortic graft and aortic valve prosthesis placement to prevent aortic dissection.

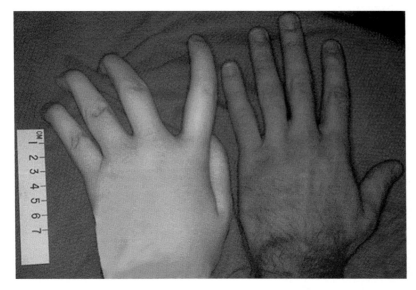

FIGURE 1–33 Arachnodactyly, gross

The hand at the left is that of a young woman with Marfan syndrome, while the hand at the right belongs to a normal man. Both people were of the same height, 188 cm. However, note that the woman's hand demonstrates arachnodactyly. Marfan syndrome is an autosomal dominant condition in which there is a mutation in the fibrillin-1 (*FBN1*) gene. The mutant product disrupts normal microfibril assembly, producing a "dominant negative" effect. As a consequence, there are abnormalities of connective tissues, particularly those with an elastic component, such as the aorta and the ligaments of the crystalline lens of the eye.

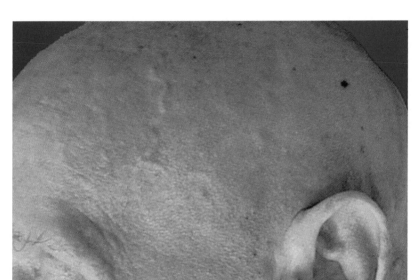

FIGURE 1–34 Giant cell (temporal) arteritis, gross

This form of arteritis is the most common of the vasculitides, and most often involves branches of the external carotid artery, most often the temporal artery, although the vertebral arteries, coronary arteries, and aorta may occasionally be involved. Patients with giant cell arteritis may have a visible firm, palpable, painful temporal artery that courses over the surface of the scalp. The inflammation tends to be focal. The involved arterial segment may be excised for diagnosis or therapy. Other branches of the external carotid artery provide collateral flow. A feared complication is occlusion of the ophthalmic arterial branch leading to blindness.

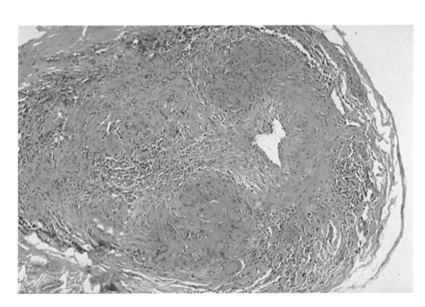

FIGURE 1–35 Temporal arteritis, microscopic

Temporal arteritis is one manifestation of giant cell arteritis, which can affect mainly branches of the external carotid artery but sometimes also the great vessels at the aortic arch and coronaries. Giant cell (temporal) arteritis is uncommon before 50 years of age. The erythrocyte sedimentation rate is often markedly elevated (100 mm/hr or more). Half of patients have polymyalgia rheumatica. The etiology is related to a cell-mediated immune response. The result is granulomatous inflammation of the media with narrowed arterial lumen, as seen here. There may be active inflammation with mononuclear infiltrates and giant cells, or fibrosis in more chronic lesions.

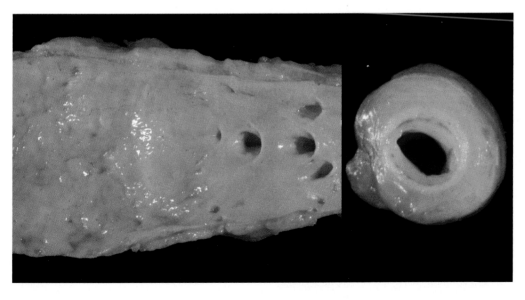

FIGURE 1–36 Takayasu arteritis, gross

This granulomatous arteritis typically involves the aortic arch but may involve the distal aorta, shown in the left panel, as well as renal and coronary arteries. There is marked luminal narrowing, mainly from intimal thickening, seen in cross-section of the carotid artery in the right panel. Luminal narrowing produces decreased pulses, often in the upper extremities and neck.

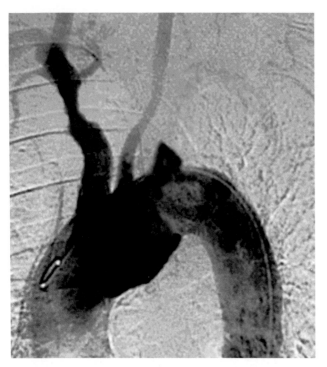

FIGURE 1–37 Takayasu arteritis, angiogram

The arch of the aorta, filled with dark-appearing intraluminal contrast media, demonstrates aneurysmal dilation. The left subclavian artery is completely occluded, appearing cut-off near its origin, and would be detectable from markedly reduced blood pressure in the left arm. The right innominate artery has irregular narrowing. Patients often have visual problems and neurologic changes. Less frequent involvement of the more distal aorta can lead to claudication of the lower extremities. If there is pulmonary arterial involvement, then pulmonary hypertension and cor pulmonale can occur. The disease course is variable. Most affected patients are younger than 50 years of age, typically women younger than 40 years. Microscopic findings are similar to those of giant cell arteritis, with more chronic changes, including fibrosis, giant cells, and lymphocytic infiltrates in the arterial walls.

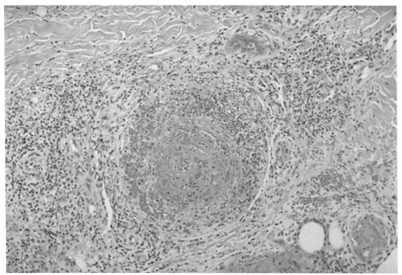

FIGURE 1–38 Polyarteritis nodosa (classic), microscopic

At low magnification, this muscular artery demonstrates a severe vasculitis with acute and chronic inflammatory cell infiltrates, along with necrosis of the vascular wall and occlusion of the lumen. This is a case of the classic form of polyarteritis nodosa (PAN), a vasculitis involving mainly small to medium-sized arteries anywhere in the body, but more often in the renal and mesenteric arteries. The serum antineutrophil cytoplasmic autoantibody (ANCA) test may be positive but is more likely to be positive with microscopic polyangiitis. Clinical manifestations include malaise, fever, weight loss, hypertension, abdominal pain, melena myalgias, arthralgias, and peripheral neuritis.

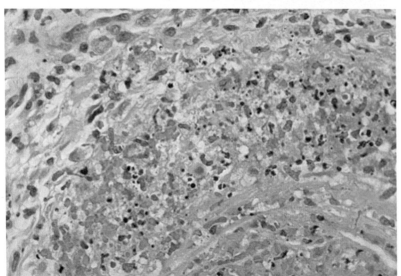

FIGURE 1–39 Polyarteritis nodosa (classic), microscopic

This is a higher magnification of the arterial wall with acute PAN in its classic form. In time, the lesion may heal with fibrosis and vascular luminal narrowing. The disease most often strikes young adults and may have an acute, subacute, or chronic course of exacerbations and remissions. Involvement of mesenteric arteries can lead to abdominal pain from bowel ischemia or infarction. Renal involvement can lead to renal failure. One third of patients with PAN are infected with hepatitis B virus. Therapy with corticosteroids and cyclophosphamide results in remissions or cures in 90% of cases, which would otherwise prove fatal.

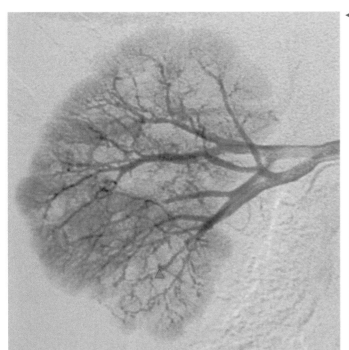

◄ **FIGURE 1–40 Polyarteritis nodosa (classic), angiogram**

In this angiogram of the right kidney can be seen arterial wall irregularity along with distal microaneurysm formation in vessels that demonstrate abrupt termination (▲). Classic PAN has a segmental distribution of transmural vascular inflammation that can acutely weaken arterial walls, leading to microaneurysm formation. As this vasculitis heals, there is vascular fibrosis with luminal narrowing and, possibly, obliteration, leading to areas of ischemic necrosis in affected organs. Various stages of inflammation are present at the same time, even in the same vessel.

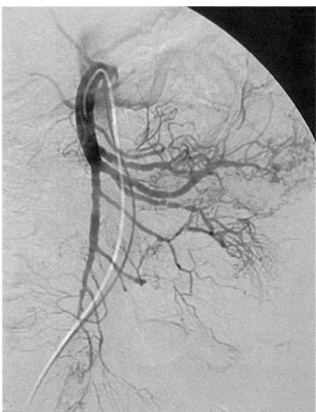

FIGURE 1–41 Polyarteritis nodosa (classic), angiogram ►

In this angiogram of the superior mesenteric artery can be seen arterial wall irregularity along with distal microaneurysm formation (▲) with abrupt termination in small distal arteries. Reduction in arterial flow can lead to ischemia and infarction of tissues. Both acute and chronic changes may coexist within the same arterial distribution. The ANCA is usually negative with classic PAN.

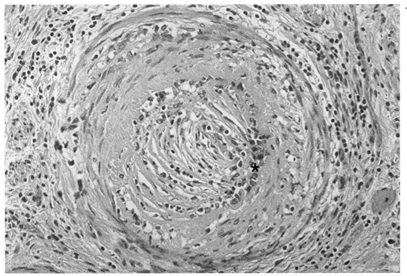

◄ **FIGURE 1–42 Vasculitis, chronic, microscopic**

This muscular artery demonstrates vasculitis with chronic inflammatory cell infiltrates. The endothelial cells (∗) have proliferated, and the lumen is absent. Often, vasculitis is a feature of an autoimmune disease, such as systemic lupus erythematosus, as was present in this patient. A more chronic form of classic PAN could appear very similar to this. In general, vasculitides are uncommon, and the various forms are confusing and difficult to diagnose and classify.

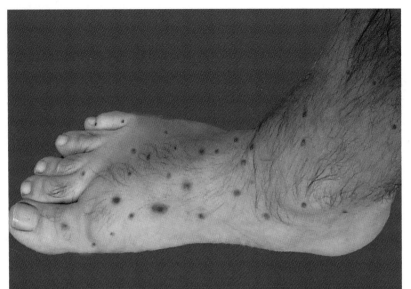

FIGURE 1–43 Microscopic polyangiitis, gross

Arterioles, capillaries, and venules are uniformly involved with microscopic polyangiitis (MPA), unlike larger vessels in classic PAN. MPA presents with palpable purpura, seen here on the foot. There is pulmonary capillaritis and necrotizing glomerulonephritis. Leukocytoclasis is often present. ANCA is positive in 70% of cases, but immune deposition is difficult to demonstrate ("pauci-immune injury"). Clinical findings include hemoptysis, arthralgia, abdominal pain, hematuria, proteinuria, and myalgia. A type III hypersensitivity reaction to drugs, infections, and neoplasms often precipitates MPA. A similar pattern of hypersensitivity angiitis is seen in Henoch-Schönlein purpura, vasculitis with autoimmune diseases, and essential mixed cryoglobulinemia.

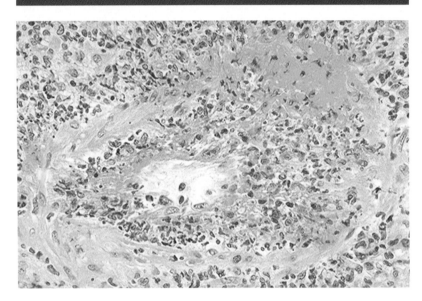

FIGURE 1–44 Wegener granulomatosis, microscopic

This vasculitis is seen to involve a renal artery branch. This is a necrotizing granulomatous vasculitis. In this case, the ANCA serology was positive, and a diagnosis of Wegener granulomatosis was made. Wegener granulomatosis most often involves the kidneys and the lungs.

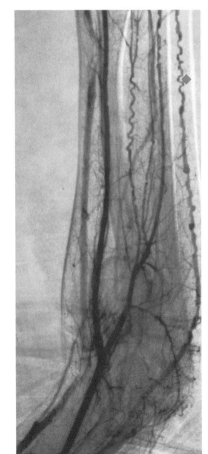

FIGURE 1–45 Thromboangiitis obliterans, angiogram

The angiogram of this extremity shows small muscular arterial branches with a corkscrew (◆) appearance, along with areas of narrowing, typical for changes from Buerger disease, a rare form of vasculitis with segmental, thrombosing, acute, and chronic inflammation of medium-sized and small arteries, principally the tibial and radial arteries. The inflammation can extend to adjacent veins and nerves. This condition is most often seen in young adults who are heavy cigarette smokers. There may be severe pain. Late complications include chronic ulcerations of the toes, feet, or fingers and frank gangrene.

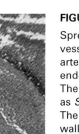

FIGURE 1–46 Infectious arteritis, microscopic

Spread of infection from parenchymal tissues to vessels, as in a pneumonia, can lead to infectious arteritis. Septicemia and septic emboli, as from endocarditis, may also lead to this complication. The infection is typically bacterial or fungal, such as *Staphylococcus aureus* or *Aspergillus* species. The infection can weaken or destroy the vascular wall and lead to aneurysm formation or hemorrhage. An aneurysm formed in such a manner is known as a *mycotic aneurysm*. The bacterial infection involving the muscular artery shown here is leading to necrosis, marked by an irregular luminal outline, along with inflammation and hemorrhage of the media and adventitia.

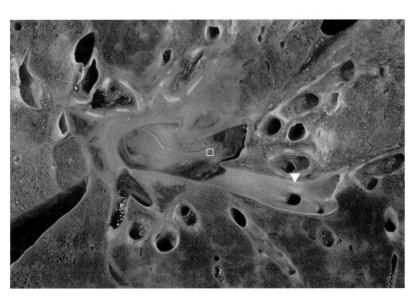

FIGURE 1–47 Invasive aspergillosis, gross

Aspergillus is a fungal organism that has a tendency to form thrombi (□) and invade vessels, even large pulmonary arterial branches as seen here. The thrombus is formed of fungal hyphae as well as thrombus, shown here filling the lumen of a pulmonary arterial branch. This can result in dissemination through the vascular system to other organs, as well as pulmonary infarction. Extensive pulmonary arterial occlusion with thrombi or emboli, or reduction in size of the pulmonary vascular bed from restrictive or obstructive lung diseases, can lead to pulmonary hypertension which, if chronic, can promote pulmonary arterial atheroma (▼) formation.

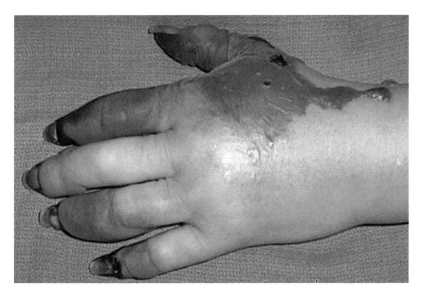

FIGURE 1–48 Raynaud phenomenon

A serious consequence of the "R" in the CREST syndrome (the form of systemic sclerosis known as *limited scleroderma*) is seen here. The fingertips are blackened and additional portions of the hand dark purplish with early gangrenous necrosis from vasospasm with Raynaud phenomenon. This is due to arterial narrowing, in contrast to Raynaud disease, which results from transient but intense vasospasm on exposure to a cold environment.

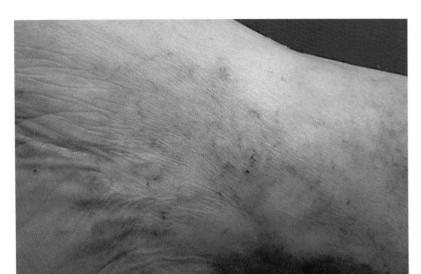

FIGURE 1–49 Varicose veins

The prominent superficial veins shown here on the lower leg are varicosities, which are a common problem, particularly with aging and in people whose occupations involve prolonged standing. The venous valves become incompetent over the years. Muscular atrophy with less muscle tone to provide a massage effect on the large superficial veins is a risk factor. Also, the skin becomes less elastic with time. Increased hydrostatic pressure from standing for long periods exacerbates the problem. Although there may be vascular stasis and thrombosis with local edema and pain, these superficial veins typically do not give rise to thromboemboli.

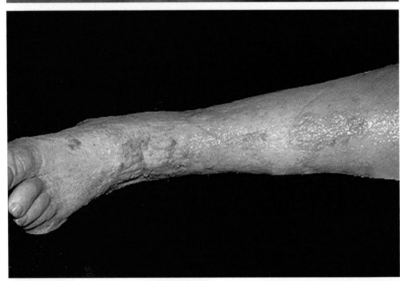

FIGURE 1–50 Stasis dermatitis, gross

Stasis dermatitis is seen here with brownish discoloration from hemosiderin deposition along with a thickened, rough appearance to the skin. Ulceration is possible as well. Years of poor circulation from poor cardiac function lead to chronic edema and venous stasis of blood with extravasation of red blood cells that leads to collection of dermal hemosiderin to give the skin this brown appearance.

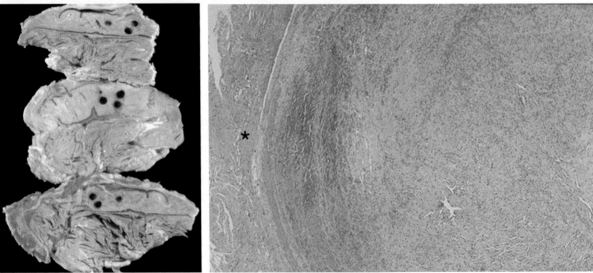

FIGURE 1–51 and 1–52 Phlebothrombosis, gross and microscopic

Large dark blue thrombi are seen in deep leg veins at the left. At the right is a large venous thrombus seen at low power. Note the thin muscular wall (*) typical of a vein. The thrombus displays varying degrees of organization, reflecting its propagation over time. Note the layering of the red blood cells and fibrin (lines of Zahn) at the periphery on the left, while there is organization of the thrombus on the right with granulation tissue and capillary proliferation, which result in the attachment of the thrombus to the vessel wall.

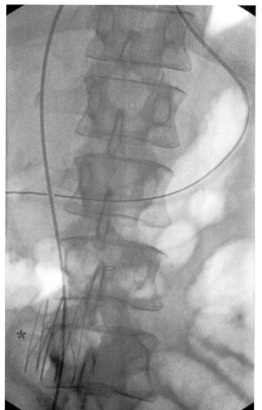

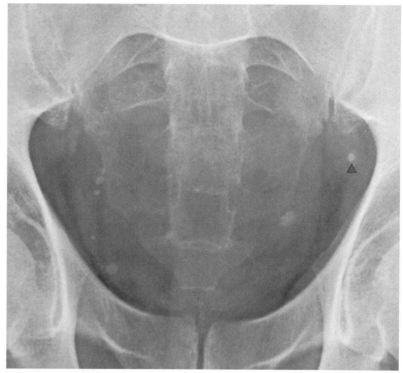

◀ **FIGURE 1–53 Inferior vena cava filter, radiograph**

This angiogram view in the lower abdominal region reveals the placement of an inferior vena cava filter (∗) in order to prevent massive and potentially fatal pulmonary thromboembolism in a patient who had a prior episode of thromboembolism and who had a Doppler ultrasound of the lower extremities that revealed thromboses in the larger leg veins, the usual source for such large, potentially fatal emboli. The metal struts of the filter extend to the venous intima and block passage of potentially life-threatening large thromboemboli to the pulmonary arteries.

FIGURE 1–54 Phleboliths, radiograph ▶

This abdominal plain film reveals multiple small, discrete bright densities (▲) in the pelvis. These are phleboliths, or small calcifications of veins that are a fairly common finding in middle-aged to older adults. Phleboliths have no significance, other than to distinguish them from other objects such as urinary tract calculi.

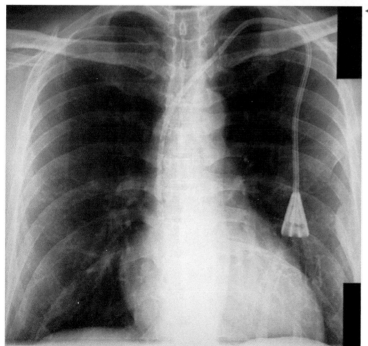

◀ **FIGURE 1–55 Central vascular catheter, radiograph**

This chest radiograph shows the proper position for a central line placed through the right subclavian vein that passes into the superior vena cava down to the right atrium. A central line can be used to monitor fluid status and cardiac function in the patient.

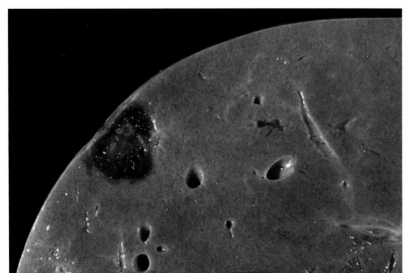

FIGURE 1–56 Hemangioma, gross

This benign hemangioma is just beneath the capsule of the liver. About 1 person in 50 has such a neoplasm in the liver, which is typically just an incidental finding because most are 1 cm or less in diameter. They can sometimes be multiple. Hemangiomas are common pediatric neoplasms and may manifest at birth. One third of all hemangiomas occur in the liver. It is unlikely that malignant transformation will occur in such a hemangioma.

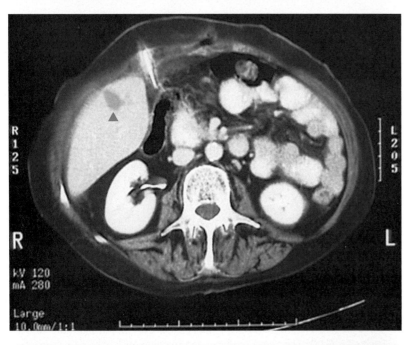

FIGURE 1–57 Hemangioma, CT image

Seen in the lower right lobe of the liver in this CT of the abdomen is a small lesion (▲) with rounded margins and decreased attenuation, compared with the adjacent hepatic parenchyma, consistent with a hemangioma. A small hemangioma is an incidental finding that is unlikely to be clinically significant.

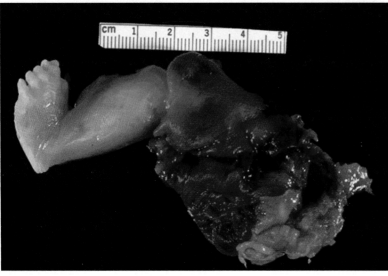

FIGURE 1–58 Congenital hemangioma, gross

The left lower extremity is shown here at 19 weeks' gestation. Also seen is a mass lesion in the fetus' pelvic region. A large irregular red mass lesion extends down the extremity from the pelvis. This is a congenital hemangioma. Although histologically benign, the large size of this neoplasm with increased vascular flow through the blood vessels resulted in congestive heart failure and fetal demise.

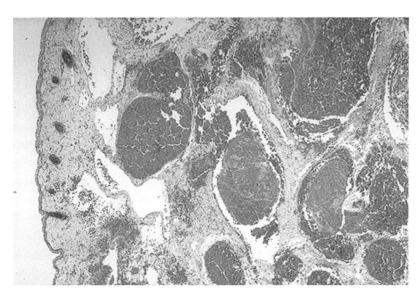

FIGURE 1–59 Hemangioma, microscopic

Beneath the skin surface at the left are many large vascular channels filled with numerous red blood cells. This is a cavernous hemangioma with large, dilated vascular spaces that extend to the underlying adipose tissue. A reddish "mole" on the skin that is small and round and raised may also represent a hemangioma. The vascular channels, which may vary in size and shape, are lined by flattened endothelial cells. These lesions on physical examination appear to change slowly over time, if at all, and seem to have been present as long as the patient can remember. A capillary hemangioma will have smaller vascular channels; it is most common on the skin and may grow rapidly in infancy before regressing.

FIGURE 1–60 Congenital lymphangioma, gross

There is a large mass involving the left upper arm and left chest of this fetus at 18 weeks' gestation. This congenital neoplasm is composed of irregular vascular channels resembling lymphatics—a lymphangioma. Smaller lymphangiomas are incidental findings, but larger ones may produce a mass effect, and they may be difficult to remove because, although histologically benign, they do not have distinct borders and may infiltrate into surrounding soft tissues.

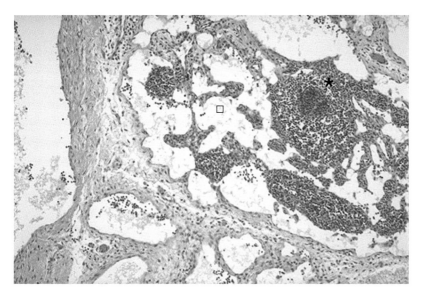

FIGURE 1–61 Lymphangioma, microscopic

These large, irregular lymphatic spaces (□) are lined by a thin endothelium. Note the absence of red blood cells within these vascular channels. The adjacent stroma has lymphoid nodules (*). Lymphangiomas appearing in children tend to involve the head, neck, and chest regions. A cystic hygroma composed of cavernous lymphatic channels is a pediatric head, neck, or upper chest lesion; a variant of cystic hygroma is present with monosomy X (Turner syndrome).

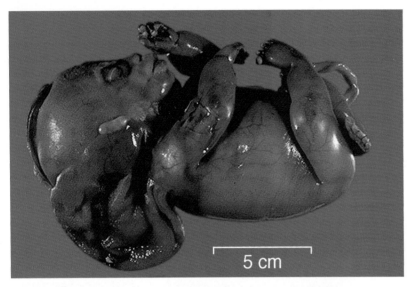

FIGURE 1–62 Cystic hygroma, gross

One very characteristic feature of a fetus with monosomy X (Turner syndrome, with 45, X gonadal dysgenesis karyotype) is the "cystic hygroma" of the posterior neck region. This lesion is not a true neoplasm, but represents developmental failure of lymphatics to form and drain properly. It is this structure that eventually forms the "web neck" feature of women with Turner syndrome. Note the gray coloration seen here from prolonged intrauterine fetal demise in this 18-week fetus. Microscopically, the cystic hygroma consists of irregularly dilated lymphatic spaces in the soft tissues of the posterior neck.

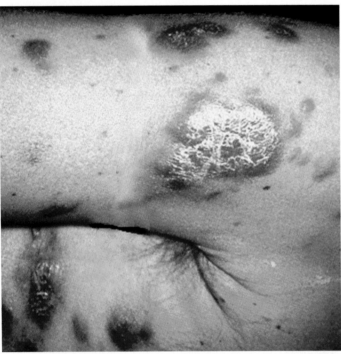

FIGURE 1–63 Kaposi sarcoma, gross

There were endemic forms of Kaposi sarcoma (KS) seen before the AIDS epidemic, but they were uncommon. The epidemic form of KS seen with AIDS usually appears in men who have sex with men and is rare in other risk groups for HIV infection. The risk factor for KS is infection with human herpesvirus 8 (HHV-8), known as the Kaposi sarcoma–associated herpes virus (KSHV), which can be sexually transmitted. The seroprevalence of HHV-8 is 5% to 10% of the general population but 20% to 70% of homosexual populations.

The lesions can start as small reddish to red-purple plaques or patches on one or more areas of the skin. Over time, the lesions may become nodular, larger, and more numerous. In patients testing positive for HIV, KS is diagnostic of AIDS. The use of highly active antiretroviral therapy (HAART) markedly decreases the incidence of KS.

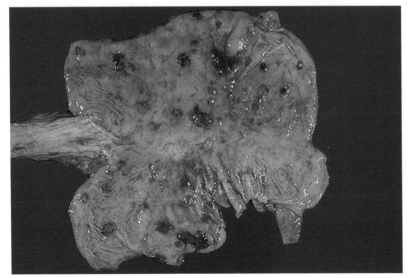

FIGURE 1–64 Kaposi sarcoma, gross

Visceral involvement with KS in AIDS is common. Here are multiple reddish nodules seen over the gastric mucosa. The lesions are rarely large enough to cause gastrointestinal tract obstruction, but they may bleed. Lung involvement with KS may lead to restrictive lung disease.

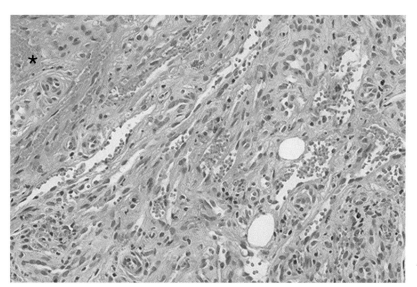

FIGURE 1–65 Kaposi sarcoma, microscopic

KS consists of an ill-defined area of irregular slitlike vascular spaces lined by pleomorphic spindle cells. Areas of hemorrhage (∗) are seen within the neoplasm, accounting for the grossly red to purplish color. In patients with AIDS, KS has a high probability (75%) of also involving visceral organs such as lung or gastrointestinal tract.

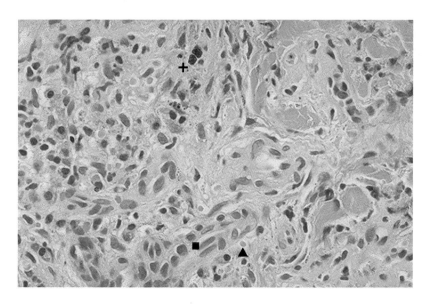

FIGURE 1–66 Kaposi sarcoma, microscopic

The atypical endothelial cells (■) of KS that line the irregular vascular spaces are shown here. The lesions characteristically have deposits of hemosiderin granules (+) and faint, pale pink hyaline globules (▲).

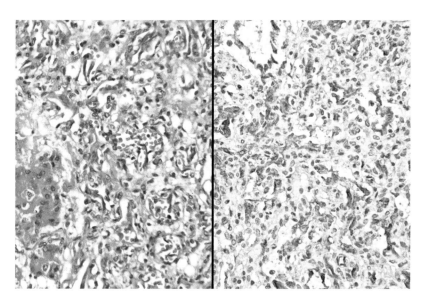

FIGURE 1–67 Hemangioendothelioma, microscopic

In infants, this tumor can appear in skin and viscera as single or multiple lesions with well-formed, thin vascular channels supported by a fibrous stroma. Immunohistochemical staining for factor VIII–related antigen, seen in the right panel, is typical of endothelium lining vascular channels. Thrombosis, calcification, fibrosis, and myxoid change may also be present. Complications include congestive heart failure, failure to thrive, jaundice, and liver failure. In adults, these soft tissue tumors most often involve medium-sized and large veins. Although most are localized and behave in a benign fashion, up to 40% recur, and up to 30% eventually metastasize.

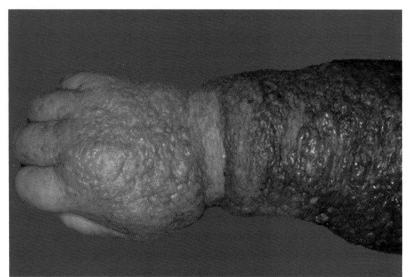

FIGURE 1–68 Angiosarcoma, gross

This angiosarcoma involving the skin and soft tissue of the arm doubled in size in 3 months. Sarcomas are often quite aggressive. Angiosarcomas are derived from endothelial cells. They are rare. They may arise *de novo* or in the setting of chronic lymphedema. Rare hepatic angiosarcomas may be related to environmental exposure to polyvinyl chloride.

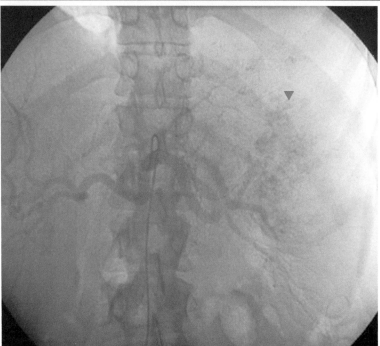

FIGURE 1–69 Angiosarcoma, angiogram

After injection of contrast into the celiac axis from the aorta, this angiographic view demonstrates a vascularized mass (▼) involving the spleen.

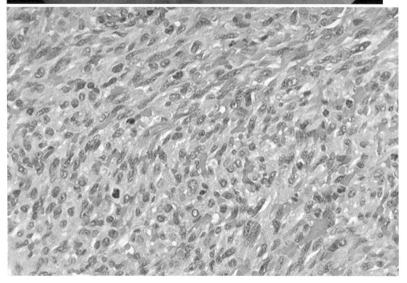

FIGURE 1–70 Angiosarcoma, microscopic

The atypical cells of angiosarcoma are plump and oblong to spindle-shaped. Occasional mitoses are seen. There are many small, irregular vascular spaces filled with blood. The overall prognosis for these neoplasms is poor.

CHAPTER 2

The Heart

FSU COLLEGE OF MEDICINE
MEDICAL LIBRARY

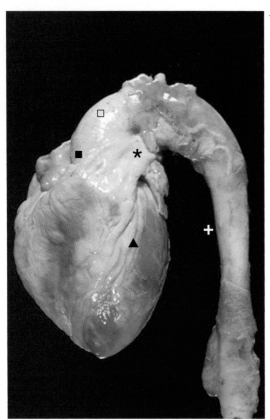

◄ **FIGURE 2–1 Normal heart and aorta, gross**

From this anterior view can be seen the aortic root (■), aortic arch (□), and thoracic aorta (+). The pulmonic trunk (*) is present. On the anterior surface of the heart is the anterior descending coronary artery (▲). Note the smooth epicardial surface with yellowish epicardial adipose tissue.

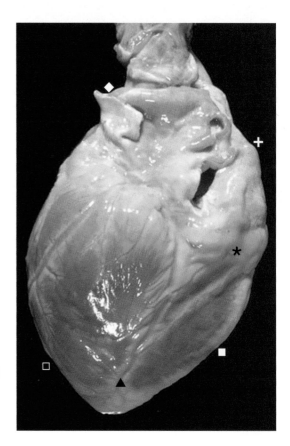

FIGURE 2–2 Normal heart, gross ▶

The posterior surface of the heart has the right coronary artery (*), which becomes the posterior descending artery (▲). Note the right ventricle (■) and the left ventricle (□), as well as the right atrium (+) and the left atrium (◆).

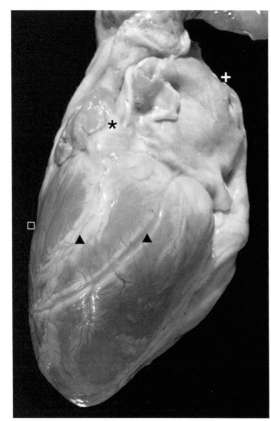

◄ **FIGURE 2–3 Normal heart, gross**

This is the appearance of the left lateral aspect of the heart with the left atrial appendage (+) and left ventricle (□). The circumflex artery (*) gives off marginal branches (▲). The normal adult heart weighs about 250 to 300 gm in women and 300 to 350 gm in men. The left ventricle, averaging 1.3 to 1.5 cm in thickness, produces the cardiac output that serves the systemic circulation. The right ventricle, from 0.3 to 0.5 cm in thickness, works under a lower pressure to supply the pulmonary circulation.

The ejection fraction (EF) is the amount of blood ejected from the left ventricle (LV) with each heart beat and is normally more than 55%. An EF can be calculated with an echocardiogram, a left ventriculogram done during a cardiac catheterization, or a nuclear study called a MUGA. The method of calculating the EF involves tracing the dimensions of the LV at the end of its contraction period (systole) and at the end of its relaxation period (diastole).

Cardiac output = (stroke volume) × (heart rate)

Cardiac index = (cardiac output) / (body surface area)

Stroke volume = (chamber volume at end diastole) − (chamber volume at end systole)

Ejection fraction = ([stroke volume] / [chamber volume at end diastole]) × 100

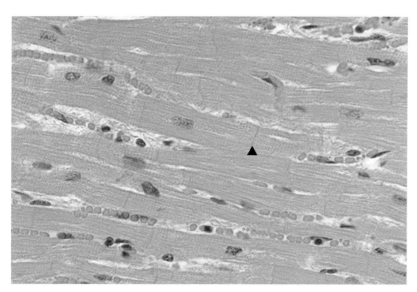

FIGURE 2–4 Normal myocardium, microscopic

Normal cardiac muscle in longitudinal section shows a syncytium of myocardial fibers (cardiac myocytes) with centrally located nuclei. Cardiac muscle is a form of striated muscle, with contractile units called *sarcomeres* that contain the contractile proteins myosin and actin. Faint dark pink intercalated discs (▲), forming mechanical and electrical couplings through gap junctions, cross some of the fibers. Red blood cells are seen in single file in the numerous capillaries between the myocardial fibers.

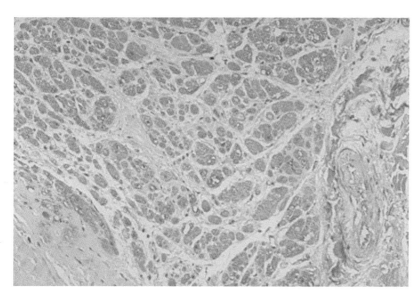

FIGURE 2–5 Normal conduction system, microscopic

The cardiac conduction system, difficult to observe histologically in humans, consists of specialized myocardial fibers that conduct electrical impulses more readily than surrounding myocardial fibers. The neural features of these fibers are brought out by this S100 immunohistochemical stain, which highlights the atrioventricular (AV) node in cross-section here. The initial pacemaker of the heart is the sinoatrial (SA) node in the right atrium, and the specialized conducting myocytes spread excitation pulses, leading to a wave of depolarization through the atria, which is then conducted through the AV node and down the bundle of His into the ventricles.

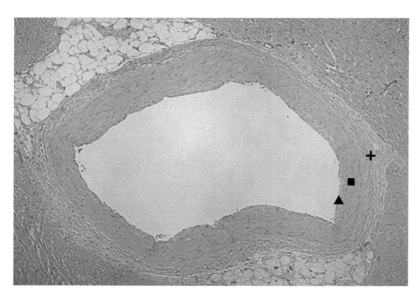

FIGURE 2–6 Normal coronary artery, gross

The three major coronary branches (left anterior descending, left circumflex, and right coronary) supply blood to the heart. The intima (▲) is normally so thin that it is indistinct. The media (■) with smooth muscle forms the bulk of the artery. The adventitia (+) is outside the media and merges with surrounding epicardial adipose and connective tissue. Distally, major branches of the coronary artery bifurcate to smaller branches. Here is a distal coronary artery branch with a prominent lumen that is adjacent to the myocardium. Such arteries anchored in the myocardium are less likely to have turbulent blood flow and less likely to develop atherosclerosis. Atherosclerosis tends to develop in the proximal portions of major coronary arteries.

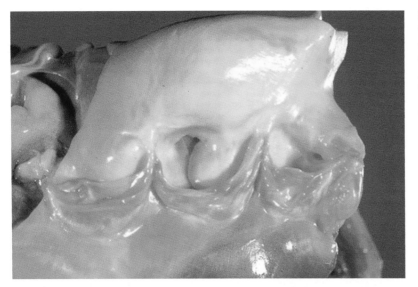

FIGURE 2–7 Normal aortic valve, gross

The aortic valve, like the other semilunar valve—the pulmonic valve—has three thin and delicate cusps. The coronary artery orifices can be seen just above the cusps. The endocardium is smooth, beneath which can be seen the red-brown myocardium. The aorta above this valve displays a smooth intimal surface with no atherosclerosis.

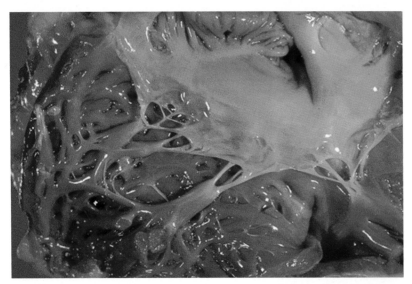

FIGURE 2–8 Normal tricuspid valve, gross

The leaflets of the atrioventricular valves (mitral and tricuspid) are thin and delicate. Just like the mitral valve, the leaflets shown here have thin chordae tendineae that attach the leaflet margins to the papillary muscles of the ventricular wall below the valve. The right atrium is seen above the valve.

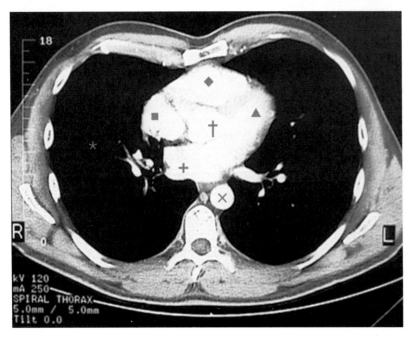

FIGURE 2–9 Normal heart, CT image

This normal chest CT scan in "bone window" demonstrates the right lung (∗), left lung (□), right atrium (■), right ventricle (◆), left atrium (+), left ventricle (▲), aortic root (†), and descending aorta (×) in the upper chest. The lungs, filled with air, have greatly decreased attenuation (brightness) consistent with "air density" for x-rays. The chest wall is normal.

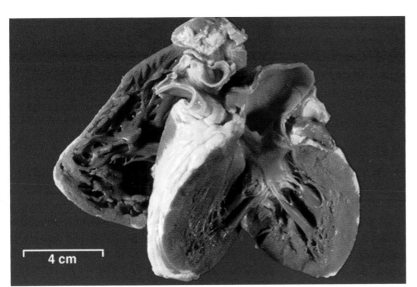

FIGURE 2–10 Brown atrophy, gross

Virtually all cardiac diseases lead to an enlarged heart. Here is a rare example of "brown atrophy," in which the heart is small, with chocolate-brown myocardium. In this condition, there is excessive lipochrome (lipofuscin) deposition within the myocardial fibers. Aging and malnutrition may favor this process, which results from cellular autophagocytosis. Additional microscopic changes with aging include basophilic degeneration of myocytes. In the normal aging process, the amount of lipofuscin increases within myocardial fiber cytoplasm, but not to the degree seen here.

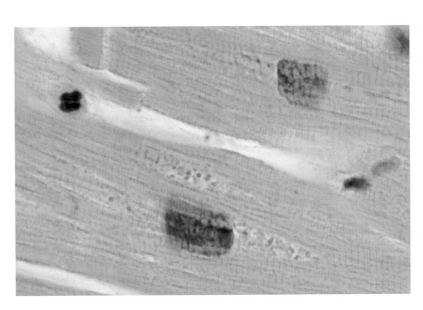

FIGURE 2–11 Lipofuscin, microscopic

The stippled, finely granular, intracytoplasmic, golden-brown pigment that lies primarily in a perinuclear location within these myocardial fibers is lipofuscin (lipochrome) pigment. This is a "wear-and-tear" pigment representing remnants of long-term autophagocytosis and cell remodeling accompanying free radical formation and lipid peroxidation. In the small amounts seen here, which increase with aging, there is no significant pathologic effect.

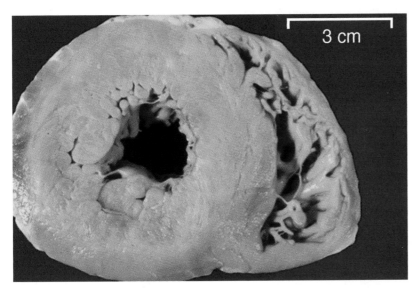

FIGURE 2–12 Cardiac hypertrophy, gross

There is prominent concentric left ventricular hypertrophy. The number of myocardial fibers does not increase, but their size can increase in response to an increased workload, leading to the marked thickening of the left ventricle. Increased pressure load from systemic hypertension is the most common cause for left ventricular hypertrophy. An increased volume load from aortic regurgitation can also lead to hypertrophy. Some degree of cardiac chamber dilation also accompanies ventricular failure. There is decreased capillary density and increased fibrous tissue and synthesis of abnormal proteins that predispose to heart failure.

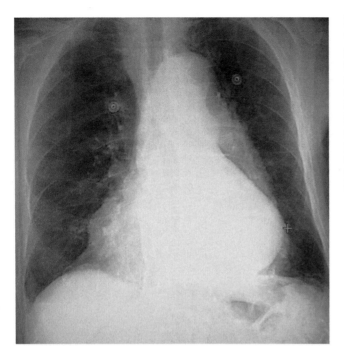

FIGURE 2–13 Cardiomegaly, x-ray

This chest radiograph demonstrates marked cardiomegaly, with the left heart edge (+) appearing far into the left chest. Ordinarily, the cardiac shadow occupies about half the distance across the chest from one rib margin to the other. An enlarged heart may occur from a variety of causes. The most common cause is ischemic heart disease. However, systemic hypertension is also a frequent cause. Intrinsic disease of the myocardium may produce a cardiomyopathy. Pulmonary hypertension can lead to cor pulmonale with initial right-sided enlargement. Eventually, failure of left or right ventricle leads to failure of the opposite ventricle, and there is more likely to be global cardiac enlargement with long-standing disease.

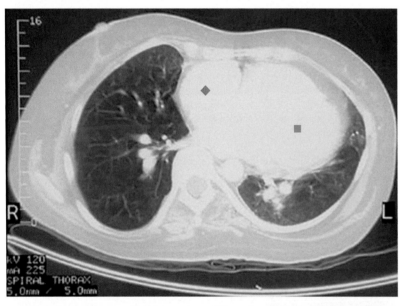

FIGURE 2–14 Cardiomegaly, CT image

Note the large size of the heart, with the left heart filling much of the chest cavity, in this patient with cardiomegaly. Both right (◆) and left (■) ventricles are dilated. In this "lung window" the interstitial markings within the lungs appear more prominent.

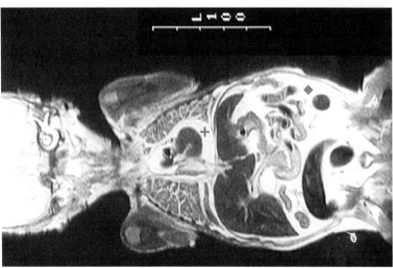

FIGURE 2–15 Heart failure and effusions, MRI

This T2-weighted MRI of a neonate in coronal view demonstrates a bright pericardial effusion (+) around the heart. There is also ascites with bright fluid (◆) around the organs in the peritoneal cavity. Such effusions can occur with hydrops, as well as heart failure from anemia, infection, and congenital cardiac anomalies.

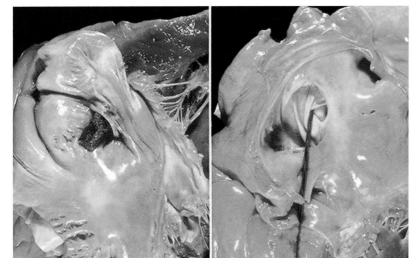

FIGURE 2–16 Patent foramen ovale, gross

At the right is a probe patent foramen ovale in an adult. A metal probe lifts the septum secundum and reveals the abnormal opening. Normally, the left atrial pressure keeps the foramen closed, but if right atrial pressures rise with pulmonary hypertension (as with pulmonary embolus), the foramen may open and even allow a thrombus to go from right to left. This is a *paradoxical embolus*, which is rare (seen in the left panel), and so called because a thromboembolus arising from the venous circulation can travel to the systemic circulation.

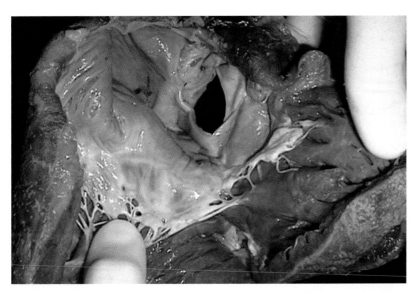

FIGURE 2–17 Atrial septal defect, gross

This large atrial septal defect (ASD) with left-to-right shunt resulted in pulmonary hypertension with increased pulmonary arterial pressures that eventually caused reversal and right-to-left shunt, resulting in marked right ventricular hypertrophy. This result from a cardiac septal defect is known as Eisenmenger complex. The examiner's finger at the lower left is holding a markedly thickened right ventricular free wall below the tricuspid valve, and the finger at the right is holding the interventricular septum below the mitral valve. About 90% of ASDs such as this one are secundum defects. Primum defects account for 5% of ASDs and are often associated with an anterior mitral leaflet cleft. The remainder are sinus venosus defects near the entrance of the superior vena cava.

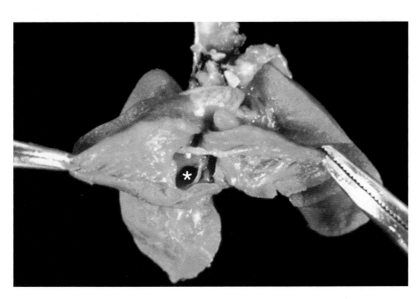

FIGURE 2–18 Ventricular septal defect, gross

This heart from autopsy of a premature stillborn with a chromosomal abnormality and multiple congenital anomalies shows a large ventricular septal defect (VSD) (*). However, one third of VSDs occur as isolated defects without accompanying anomalies. This VSD is located in the membranous septum, as are 90% of VSDs, whereas 10% occur in the muscular interventricular septum. About half of small VSDs may eventually close. A large VSD can produce a significant left-to-right shunt that leads to cardiac failure. VSDs increase the risk for endocarditis. If a large VSD is not corrected surgically, the shunt leads to pulmonary hypertension with cor pulmonale and eventual reversal to a right-to-left shunt (Eisenmenger complex).

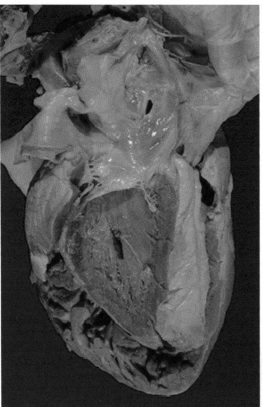

◄ **FIGURE 2–19 Atrial septal defect and ventricular septal defect, gross**

Here is a heart with both an ASD and a muscular VSD. The heart is opened on the left side with the left ventricular free wall reflected superiorly. Such small VSDs do not produce significant left-to-right shunting, but they do increase the risk for infective endocarditis, and a holosystolic murmur is often audible on auscultation.

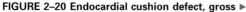

FIGURE 2–20 Endocardial cushion defect, gross ►

Here is a severe form of endocardial cushion defect in which there is only a single large atrioventricular valve, as seen from above, that separates a single ventricle from a single atrium. This patient was able to survive with this two-chambered heart because a small amount of residual interventricular septum provided some direction to flow of oxygenated and unoxygenated blood, and also because of pulmonic stenosis, which protected the lungs from the shunting. (This is an explanted heart from a cardiac transplantation procedure, so most of the atria are not present.)

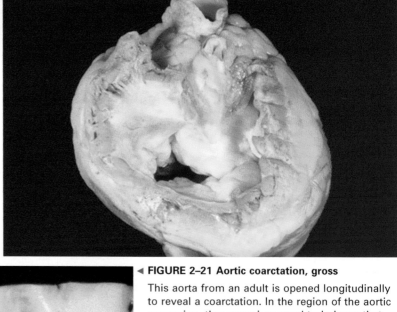

◄ **FIGURE 2–21 Aortic coarctation, gross**

This aorta from an adult is opened longitudinally to reveal a coarctation. In the region of the aortic narrowing, there was increased turbulence that led to increased atherosclerosis. Males are affected twice as often as females. However, coarctation is a common feature of monosomy X (Turner syndrome). The classification of coarctation concerns position in relation to the ductus arteriosus. The preductal form with proximal aortic tubular hypoplasia is also known as the *infantile* form because of symptoms appearing in early childhood. The postductal form becomes symptomatic later in life, with findings related to diminished blood flow to lower extremities but hypertension in the upper body.

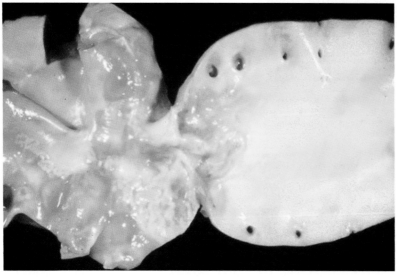

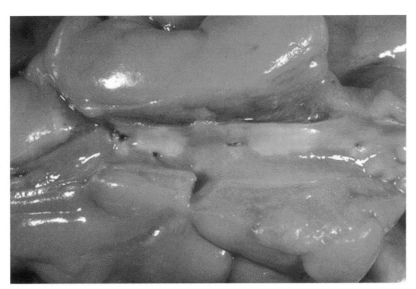

FIGURE 2–22 Coronary atherosclerosis, gross

This is a minimal amount of coronary atherosclerosis, with a few scattered yellow lipid plaques seen on the intimal surface of the opened coronary artery traversing the epicardial surface of a heart. The degree of atherosclerosis here is not great enough to cause significant luminal narrowing but could be the harbinger of worse atherosclerosis to come, if the plaques continue to enlarge. Atherosclerosis is initiated with endothelial damage and inflammation with leukocyte elaboration of cytokines such as tumor necrosis factor, interleukin-6, and interferon-γ. This process is promoted by uptake of increased circulating oxidized LDL cholesterol into macrophages.

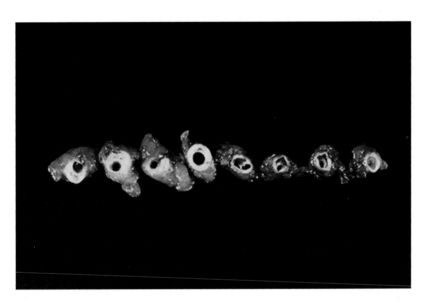

FIGURE 2–23 Coronary atherosclerosis, gross

These cross-sections of the left anterior descending coronary artery demonstrate atherosclerosis with more pronounced narrowing at the left, which is the more proximal portion of this artery. Atherosclerosis is generally worse at the beginning of a coronary artery, in the first few centimeters, where turbulent blood flow is greater. The turbulent flow over many years promotes endothelial damage that favors inflammation with insudation of lipids to promote formation of atheromas.

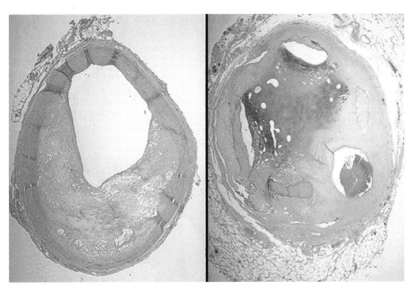

FIGURE 2–24 Coronary atherosclerosis, microscopic

Here is occlusive coronary atherosclerosis. The coronary artery in the left panel is narrowed by 60% to 70%, on the verge of producing angina, which could be precipitated by transient vasoconstriction. Acute coronary syndromes from marked ischemia are more likely to occur when luminal narrowing reaches 70%. The coronary artery seen in the right panel has even more severe occlusion, with evidence for previous thrombosis and organization of the thrombus leading to recanalization, such that there are three small lumens remaining.

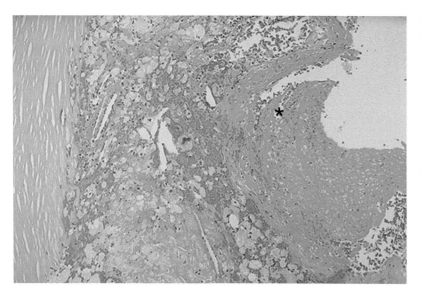

FIGURE 2–25 Coronary atherosclerosis, microscopic

This atheromatous plaque in a coronary artery shows endothelial denudation with plaque disruption and overlying thrombus (∗) formation from platelet aggregation. Note the composition of the plaque with foam cells, cholesterol clefts, and areas of hemorrhage. Such a plaque with rapid overlying thrombus formation can lead to an acute coronary syndrome resulting in an ischemic event. The first sign of ischemic heart disease may be angina pectoris, a symptom complex characterized by recurrent acute episodes of substernal or precordial chest pain. Occlusive coronary atherosclerosis increases the risk for myocardial infarction.

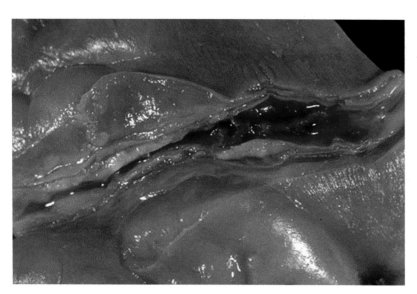

FIGURE 2–26 Coronary thrombosis, gross

This coronary thrombosis is one of the severe complications of atherosclerosis, shown here with thickened arterial walls with yellow-tan plaques that narrow the arterial lumen. The dark-red thrombus is seen in this anterior descending coronary artery opened longitudinally. The thrombus occludes the lumen to produce ischemia or infarction of the myocardium supplied by the artery. One possible outcome of coronary thrombosis is sudden death. Other complications include arrhythmias and congestive heart failure.

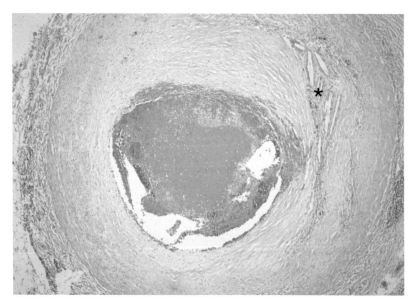

FIGURE 2–27 Coronary thrombosis, microscopic

A coronary thrombosis is seen here nearly occluding the remaining small lumen of this coronary artery already involved with severe atherosclerosis. Note the fibrointimal proliferation (∗) with cholesterol clefts. Endothelial damage with platelet activation promotes thrombosis. A small amount of aspirin taken each day helps reduce platelet function, making the platelets less "sticky" and less prone to participate in thrombotic events.

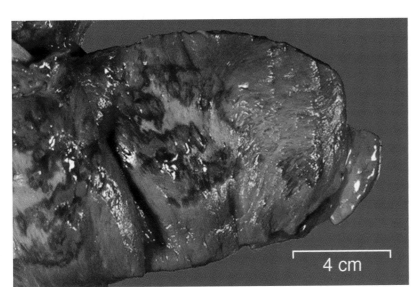

FIGURE 2–28 Myocardial infarction, gross

The interventricular septum of the heart has been sectioned at autopsy to reveal an extensive acute myocardial infarction. The dead muscle is tan-yellow, with a surrounding hyperemic border. This appearance is characteristic of an infarction that is 3 to 7 days old. Serum creatinine kinase (CK), specifically the isozyme from heart, CK-MB, and troponin I are released from damaged myofibers and start to rise 3 to 4 hours after the initial ischemic event. The CK-MB peaks about a day later, then declines to negligible levels by 3 days. However, the troponin I level will remain increased for 10 to 14 days. Serum myoglobin can be increased starting 3 hours after myocardial infarction, but it is not specific for myocardium.

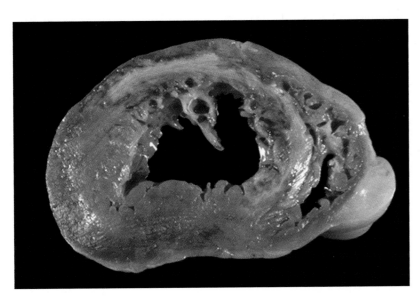

FIGURE 2–29 Myocardial infarction, gross

This axial section through the heart reveals a large myocardial infarction involving the anterior left ventricular wall and interventricular septum in the distribution of the left anterior descending coronary artery. Note the yellowish area of necrosis with the hyperemic border that is nearly transmural. Radionuclide imaging would show decreased uptake into this region. Echocardiography would show diminished ventricular wall motion with such a large infarction, and the ejection fraction would be decreased.

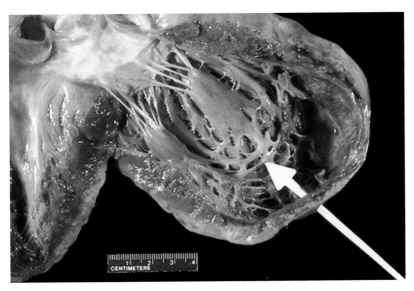

FIGURE 2–30 Myocardial infarction, gross

In cross-section, the point of rupture of the left ventricular free wall myocardium is shown at the arrow. In this case, there was a previous myocardial infarction 3 weeks before, accounting for the thinning of the ventricular wall seen here, and a subsequent myocardial infarction occurred, rupturing through the already thinned ventricular wall 3 days later. The mitral valve with chordae tendineae and the papillary muscles appear normal. Rupture is most likely to occur 3 to 7 days after a transmural infarction, when the necrotic muscle is soft, and before any significant amount of organization with ingrowth of capillaries and fibroblasts has occurred.

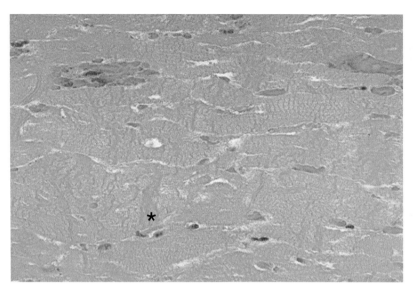

FIGURE 2–31 Myocardial infarction, microscopic

The earliest change histologically seen with acute myocardial infarction during the first 24 hours is contraction band necrosis. The myocardial fibers are beginning to lose cross-striations, and the nuclei are not clearly visible in most of the cells seen here. Note the many irregular, darker-pink, wavy contraction bands (∗) extending across the fibers. Serologic markers for infarction include nonspecific myoglobin and the more specific markers of cardiac muscle injury, including CK-MB and troponin I. Use of thrombolytic agents, percutaneous transluminal coronary angioplasty, and coronary arterial bypass grafting are methods to help restore blood flow and prevent further damage.

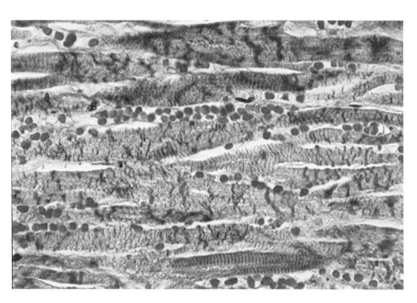

FIGURE 2–32 Myocardial infarction, microscopic

This section of myocardium with trichrome stain shows the appearance of an early acute myocardial infarction (MI), less than 1 day old, with prominent contraction band necrosis. Karyolysis has led to loss of the nuclei. If the area of infarction remains small, the MI may be "silent" without signs or symptoms and detectable only by electrocardiography or by serum cardiac muscle enzyme elevation. The myocardial irritability following an MI leads to electrical conduction disturbances with arrhythmias such as sinus bradycardia, heart block, asystole, and ventricular fibrillation.

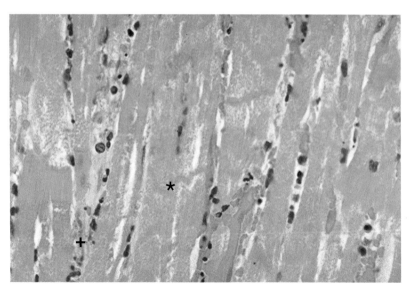

FIGURE 2–33 Myocardial infarction, microscopic

This is an early acute MI about 1 to 2 days old. There is increasing loss of cross-striations, and some contraction bands (∗) are also seen. The cardiac fiber nuclei have undergone karyolysis and are no longer visible. Some neutrophils (+) are beginning to infiltrate into this necrotic myocardium. The loss of the nuclei represents an irreversible form of cellular injury. Reperfusion of such damaged muscle may lead to increased production of toxic free radicals that can potentiate further myocardial damage. Thus, thrombolytic therapy to treat acute coronary thrombosis is most beneficial within 30 minutes of the initial arterial occlusion.

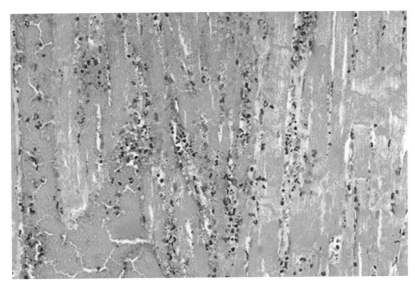

FIGURE 2–34 Myocardial infarction, microscopic

There is extensive acute inflammation with neutrophils infiltrating into these myocardial fibers undergoing coagulative necrosis. This MI is about 3 to 4 days old. There is an extensive acute inflammatory cell infiltrate, and the myocardial fibers are so necrotic that the outlines of them are only barely visible. Clinically, such an acute MI is marked by changes in the electrocardiogram such as ST-segment elevation and T-wave inversion, and by a rise in the CK-MB fraction. In addition to chest pain, patients with MI may have a rapid, weak pulse, hypotension, diaphoresis, and shortness of breath from acute left-sided congestive heart failure.

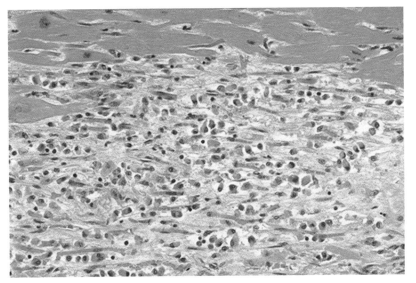

FIGURE 2–35 Myocardial infarction, microscopic

Toward the end of the first week after the ischemic event that triggered infarction, healing of the MI becomes more prominent, with numerous capillaries, fibroblasts, and macrophages filled with hemosiderin. The granulation tissue seen here becomes most prominent 2 to 3 weeks after onset of infarction. This area of granulation tissue is nonfunctional and noncontractile, reducing the ejection fraction, but it is unlikely to rupture.

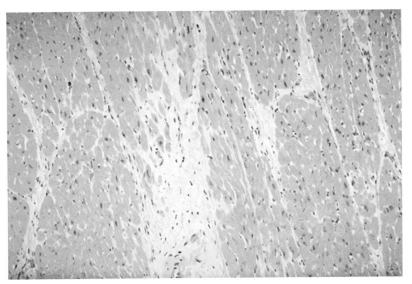

FIGURE 2–36 Myocardial infarction, microscopic

Two to 3 weeks after the onset of infarction, healing at the site of myocardial necrosis is well under way, and there is more extensive collagen deposition. The remote MI is evidenced by a dense collagenous scar after 2 months, seen here as irregular pale areas within surrounding surviving myocardial fibers. The size of the MI determines the clinical findings. As expected, larger MIs are more likely to become complicated by heart failure and arrhythmias.

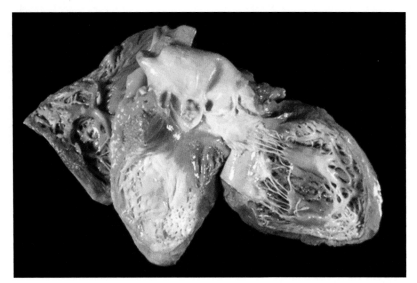

FIGURE 2–37 Myocardial infarction, gross

This heart is opened to reveal the left ventricular free wall on the right and the interventricular septum at the center, with the right ventricle at the left. There has been a remote MI that extensively involved the anterior left ventricular free wall and septum. Involvement of the right ventricle is uncommon. The white appearance of the endocardial surface indicates the extensive scarring. This scarred area is noncontractile, and the ejection fraction and cardiac output will be reduced. The papillary muscles appear to be spared.

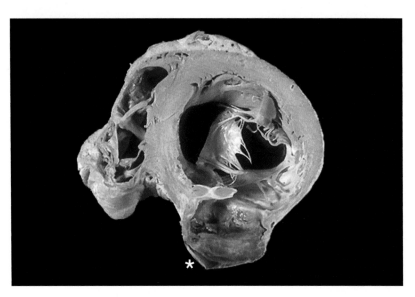

FIGURE 2–38 Myocardial infarction, gross

A previous extensive transmural MI involving the free wall of the left ventricle has reduced the thickness of the myocardial wall. The infarction was so extensive that, after healing, the ventricular wall was replaced by a thin band of collagen, forming an aneurysm (∗). Such an aneurysm represents noncontractile tissue that reduces stroke volume and strains the remaining myocardium. The stasis of blood in the aneurysm predisposes to mural thrombosis. This cross-section through the heart reveals a ventricular aneurysm with a very thin wall. Note how the aneurysm bulges out. The stasis in this aneurysm allows mural thrombus, which is present here, to form within the aneurysm.

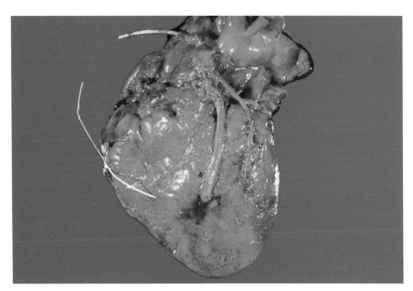

FIGURE 2–39 Myocardial infarction, microscopic

This patient underwent myocardial revascularization for ischemic heart disease. This is coronary artery bypass grafting with autogenous vein (saphenous vein) grafts seen here. The largest graft runs down the center of the heart to anastomose with the left anterior descending artery distally. Another graft extends in a Y fashion just to the right of this to marginal branches of the circumflex artery. A white temporary pacing wire to treat arrhythmias extends from the mid left surface, and a Swan-Ganz catheter that extended to a peripheral pulmonary artery to measure wedge pressure, equivalent to left atrial pressure, emerges from the right atrium.

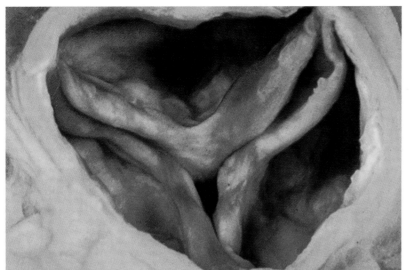

FIGURE 2–40 Calcific aortic stenosis, gross

An aortic valve need not be bicuspid to calcify. Sometimes in older adults, a normal tricuspid aortic valve will undergo slowly progressive dystrophic calcification over many years, a so-called *senile calcific aortic stenosis.* Nodules of calcification are seen on these cusps, as viewed from the aortic outflow tract. The deposition of calcium interferes with valvular motion and leads to progressive stenosis. This increased pressure load leads to left ventricular hypertrophy. The pulse pressure is subsequently diminished. As the cross-sectional area of the remaining valve outlet approaches 1 cm^2, sudden left ventricular failure may occur.

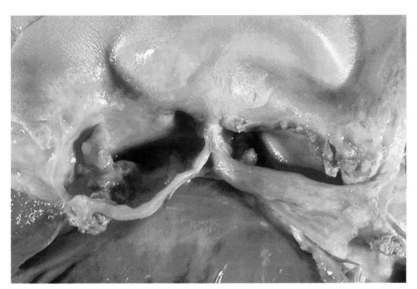

FIGURE 2–41 Bicuspid aortic valve, gross

One of the most common congenital cardiac defects is bicuspid aortic valve, seen in 1% of the population. Most bicuspid valves are prone to undergo calcification, but patients can remain relatively asymptomatic until middle age, when the stenosis reaches a critical point at which congestive heart failure rapidly ensues. The dense white nodules of calcification shown are present on both valve surfaces. The valve here has been opened with the aortic outflow above and the left ventricular myocardium below. The increasing pressure gradient leads to left ventricular hypertrophy and eventually to left-sided congestive heart failure marked by pulmonary congestion and edema.

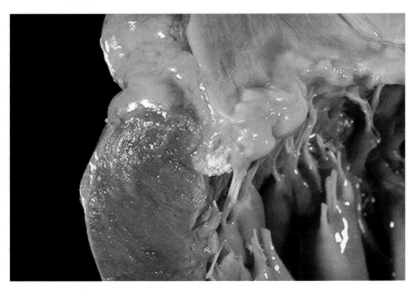

FIGURE 2–42 Mitral annular calcification, gross

A relatively benign and not too common condition that may appear on radiographic studies is mitral valve ring calcification. It is most common in older adults, particularly women older than 60 years. This process produces a doughnut-shaped ring of calcification around the mitral valve annulus. In severe cases, there may be valvular regurgitation with a murmur on auscultation of the chest. The white circular deposit shown here represents just such a ring that has been sectioned as the heart was opened at autopsy. The red-brown myocardium of the left ventricular wall is completely normal.

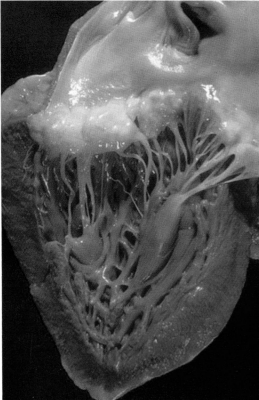

FIGURE 2–43 and 2–44 Myxomatous degeneration with floppy mitral valve, gross

The leaflets of the mitral valve are redundant and ballooned upward (*). This is characteristic of floppy mitral valve with mitral valve prolapse. The chordae tendineae that anchor the leaflets to the ventricle become elongated and thin. This condition can occur sporadically and affects up to 3% of the population. It can be seen with Marfan syndrome. There is microscopic myxomatous degeneration of the valve, which weakens the connective tissue. Most patients are asymptomatic. There may be an audible heart murmur in the form of a midsystolic "click." In more severe cases, mitral regurgitation can occur, with a late systolic or holosystolic murmur.

Seen below is another example of mitral valve prolapse. Rupture of the chordae is possible, leading to appearance of acute valvular insufficiency.

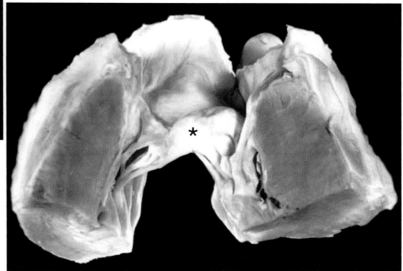

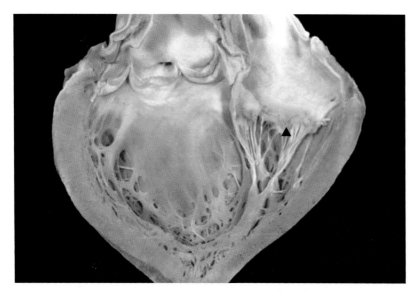

FIGURE 2–45 Rheumatic heart disease, gross

Acute rheumatic fever can produce pancarditis, but shown here are the characteristic small verrucous vegetations (▲) of rheumatic endocarditis. These vegetations are located over areas of fibrinoid degeneration on the valve cusp margins and are composed mainly of fibrin. These vegetations, composed of platelets and fibrin and located at the valve closure line, are usually no more than 2 mm in size but may produce an audible murmur. These lesions are not likely to embolize and do not produce significant valvular deformity at this early stage of rheumatic valvulitis.

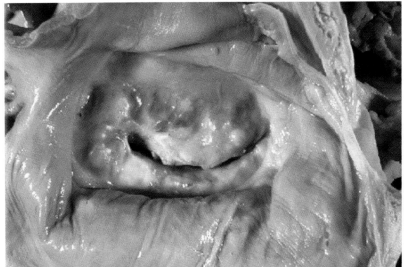

This mitral valve is seen from the inflow from the left atrium and demonstrates the typical fish mouth shape following chronic rheumatic valvulitis with scarring. The mitral valve is most often affected with rheumatic heart disease, followed by mitral and aortic together, then aortic alone, then mitral, aortic, and tricuspid together.

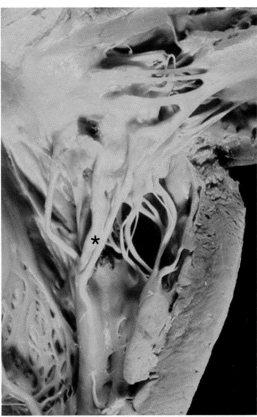

FIGURE 2–47 and 2–48 Rheumatic heart disease, gross ►

In time, chronic rheumatic valvulitis may develop by organization of the acute endocardial inflammation along with fibrosis, as shown here affecting the mitral valve. Note the shortened and thickened (∗) chordae tendineae. This complication can take decades to become symptomatic. Valvular stenosis can lead to prominent left atrial enlargement, which predisposes to mural thrombus (■) formation, as shown in the lower panel at the right.

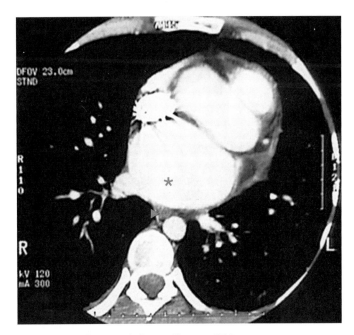

FIGURE 2–49 Rheumatic heart disease, CT image ▲

Chronic rheumatic valvulitis can produce either valvular insufficiency or stenosis, and an element of both may be present simultaneously, but stenosis usually predominates. Since the mitral valve is most often involved, a common finding is marked left atrial enlargement. The enlarged left atrium (∗) may displace the adjacent esophagus (►) and lead to dysphagia.

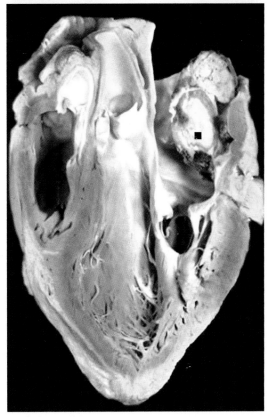

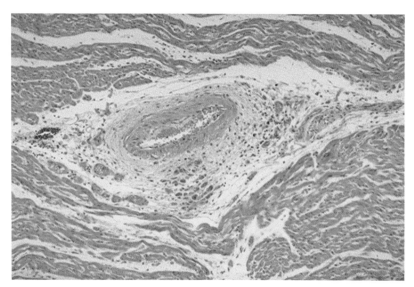

FIGURE 2–50 Rheumatic heart disease, microscopic

A characteristic microscopic feature is the Aschoff nodule, which typically occurs in the myocardial interstitium. It is a nodular collection of inflammatory cells, mainly mononuclear. It is a manifestation of acute rheumatic fever, which occurs 10 days to 6 weeks after group A streptococcal pharyngitis. This carditis results from an immunologic cross-reaction with the streptococcal capsular M protein and can affect endocardium, myocardium, and epicardium, producing a pancarditis. Serologic markers of rheumatic fever may include antistreptolysin O, antihyaluronidase, and anti-DNAse B.

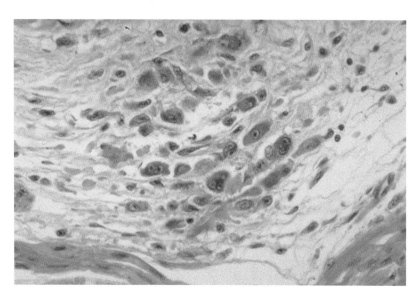

FIGURE 2–51 Rheumatic heart disease, microscopic

Here is an Aschoff nodule at high magnification. The most characteristic cellular component is the Aschoff giant cell. Several of these appear here as large cells with two or more nuclei that have prominent nucleoli. Scattered inflammatory cells accompany them and can be mononuclear cells or occasionally neutrophils. Such inflammation can occur not only in the myocardium but also in the endocardium (including valves) and the epicardium. Involvement of all three cardiac layers is termed *pancarditis*. Myocardial involvement leads to death in about 1% of patients with acute rheumatic fever.

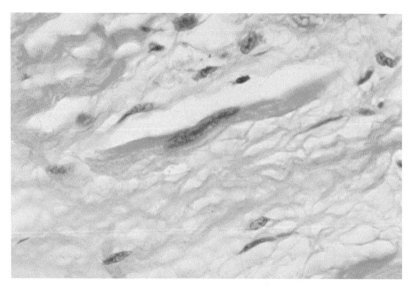

FIGURE 2–52 Rheumatic heart disease, microscopic

Another peculiar cell seen with acute rheumatic carditis is the Anitschkow myocyte. This is a long, thin cell with an elongated nucleus. Signs and symptoms of acute rheumatic fever (RF) are most likely to appear in children. Extracardiac manifestations may include "major" Jones criteria: subcutaneous nodules, erythema marginatum, fever, and polyarthritis. "Minor" criteria include arthralgia, fever, previous RF, leukocytosis, elevated sedimentation rate, and C-reactive protein. There is a propensity for reactivation of RF with subsequent episodes of group A streptococcal pharyngitis. Thus, chronic rheumatic disease is usually the result of multiple recurrent episodes of acute RF.

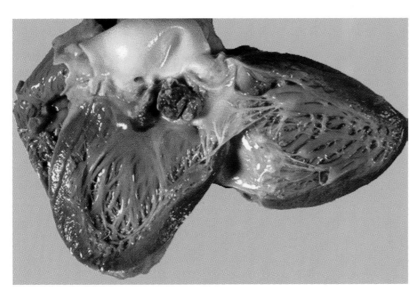

FIGURE 2–53 Infective endocarditis, gross

The aortic valve demonstrates a large, irregular, reddish tan vegetation. Virulent organisms, such as *Staphylococcus aureus*, produce an "acute" bacterial endocarditis similar to the lesion shown here, whereas some organisms, such as the viridans group of *Streptococcus,* produce a "subacute" bacterial endocarditis. Endocarditis is marked by fever with heart murmur. Predisposing risks for endocarditis include bacteremia and previously damaged or deformed valves. However, endocarditis can involve anatomically normal valves.

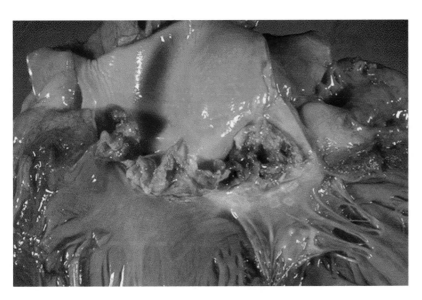

FIGURE 2–54 Infective endocarditis, gross

The more virulent bacteria causing the acute bacterial form of infective endocarditis can lead to serious valvular destruction, as shown here involving the aortic valve. Irregular reddish tan vegetations overlie valve cusps that are being destroyed by the action of the proliferating bacteria. Portions of the vegetation can break off and become septic emboli that travel to other organs, leading to foci of infarction or infection.

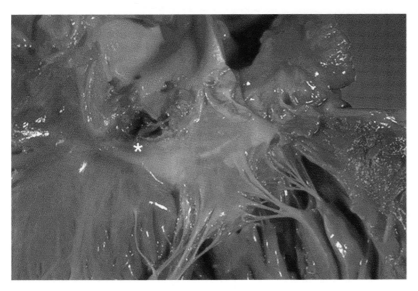

FIGURE 2–55 Infective endocarditis, gross

In this case of the subacute form of endocarditis with the pyogenes group of streptococci, the infective endocarditis is not as florid, but it is persistent and demonstrates how the infection tends to spread from the valve surface. Here, vegetations can be seen involving the endocardial surfaces, and the infection is extending into the underlying myocardium (∗). Blood culture is required to diagnose the causative organism, which is most often a bacterium, but in 10% of cases, no organism may be found.

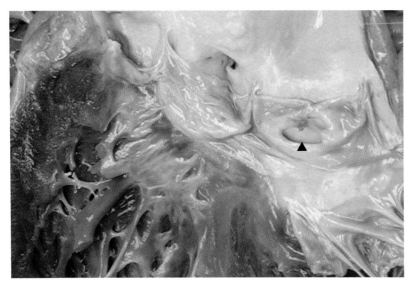

FIGURE 2–56 Infective endocarditis, gross

Healing of infective endocarditis may leave residual valve damage. Seen here are a smaller fenestration and a larger fenestration (▲) of an aortic valve cusp as a consequence of healed infective endocarditis with partial destruction of another cusp. The result of this valvular damage is aortic insufficiency and a "jet lesion" with adjacent focal endocardial fibrosis of the left ventricular myocardium. A murmur may be audible. Larger fenestrations may cause valvular insufficiency.

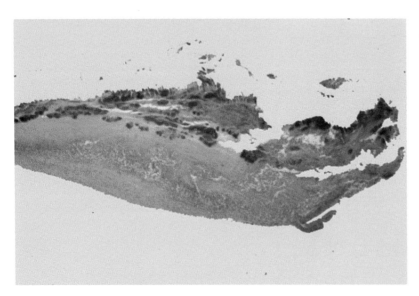

FIGURE 2–57 Infective endocarditis, microscopic

This valve demonstrates friable vegetations composed of fibrin and platelets (pink) mixed with inflammatory cells and bacterial colonies (blue). The friability of the vegetation explains how portions of the vegetation can break off and embolize. Left-sided endocarditis can be complicated by embolization to the systemic circulation, whereas right-sided embolization affects the lungs. Cardiac valves are relatively avascular, so that high-dose, prolonged antibiotic therapy is needed to eradicate the infection.

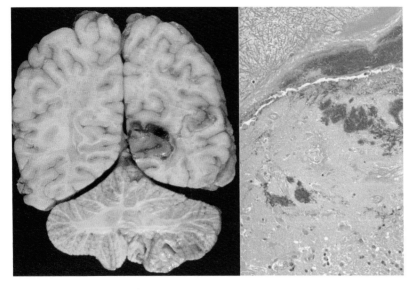

FIGURE 2–58 Mycotic aneurysm, gross and microscopic

Embolization from infective endocarditis spreads the infection to other parts of the body. Left-sided valvular lesions shower emboli to the systemic circulation, and embolic lesions can subsequently lodge in organs such as the brain, spleen, and kidneys. Seen here is an embolic infarct involving a cerebral hemisphere in the left panel, which microscopically demonstrates features of a mycotic aneurysm in the right panel, with destruction of an arterial wall by the inflammation, characterized here by fuzzy blue areas representing the proliferating bacterial colonies.

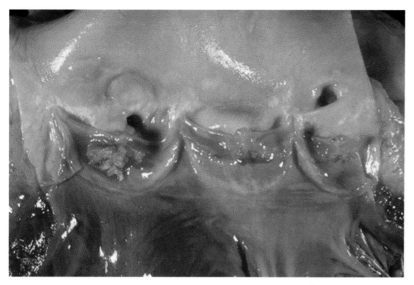

FIGURE 2–59 Nonbacterial thrombotic endocarditis, gross

The small pink vegetation on the leftmost aortic cusp margin represents the typical finding with nonbacterial thrombotic endocarditis (NBTE), or so-called *marantic endocarditis*. This is one form of noninfective endocarditis. NBTE tends to occur in people with a hypercoagulable state (such as Trousseau syndrome, a paraneoplastic syndrome associated with malignancies) and in very ill patients. These vegetations are rarely larger than 0.5 cm. However, they are very prone to embolize. Patients with NBTE often have concomitant venous thromboembolic disease. Note the normal right and left coronary artery orifices above the valve cusps.

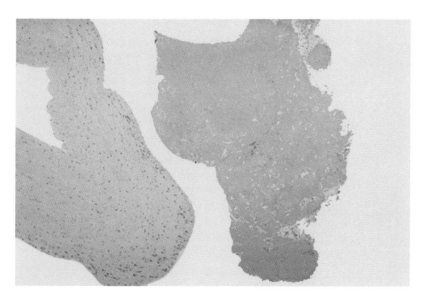

FIGURE 2–60 Nonbacterial endocarditis, microscopic

The valve is seen on the left, and a bland vegetation is seen to the right. It appears pink because it is sterile and composed of fibrin and platelets. It displays about as much morphologic variation as a brown paper bag. Such bland vegetations are typical of the noninfective forms of endocarditis. The vegetations of NBTE, although small, are friable and prone to embolize.

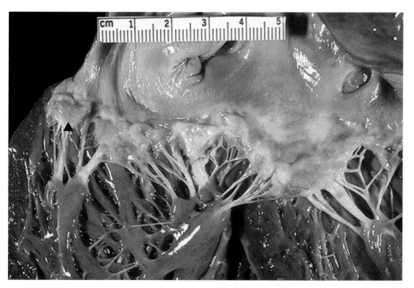

FIGURE 2–61 Libman-Sacks endocarditis, gross

Here are flat, pale tan, spreading vegetations (▲) over the mitral valve surface. They even spread onto the adjacent chordae tendineae. This patient has systemic lupus erythematosus (SLE). These vegetations can be on any valve or even on endocardial surfaces and are consistent with Libman-Sacks endocarditis. These vegetations appear in about 4% of SLE patients and rarely cause problems because they are not large and rarely embolize. Note also the thickened, shortened, and fused chordae tendineae that represent remote rheumatic heart disease.

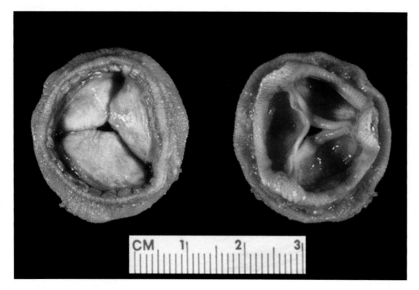

FIGURE 2–62 Porcine bioprosthesis, gross

A porcine bioprosthesis is shown with the undersurface at the left and the outflow side at the right. Note there are three cusps sewn into a synthetic ring. The main advantage of this bioprosthesis is the lack of need for continued anticoagulation. The drawback of this type of prosthetic heart valve is the limited life span of the prosthetic cusps, on average 5 to 10 years (but sometimes shorter), because of wear and subsequent calcification that reduces cusp motion and leads to stenosis.

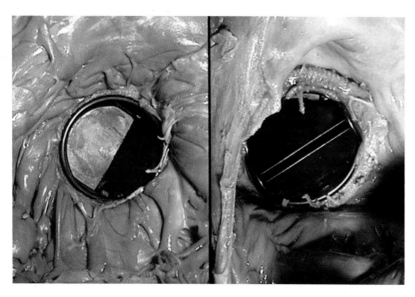

FIGURE 2–63 Mechanical valve prosthesis, gross

This is a mechanical valve prosthesis of the more modern tilting disc variety replacing the native mitral valve. Such mechanical prostheses will last indefinitely from a structural standpoint, but the patient with such a prosthesis requires continuing anticoagulation because the exposed nonbiologic surfaces are prone to thrombosis. The inferior aspect is seen in the left panel with the left ventricular chamber below. The outflow tract from this prosthesis is seen in the right panel, with the two leaflets tilted outward toward the left atrium. Another complication is infective endocarditis, which is most prone to involve the ring.

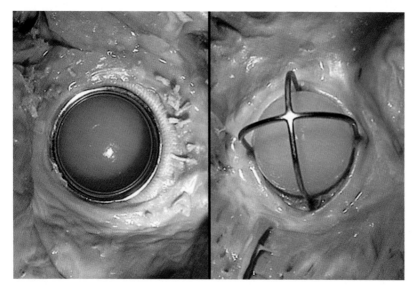

FIGURE 2–64 Mechanical prosthesis, gross

This is a mitral mechanical valve prosthesis of the older ball-and-cage variety. Such mechanical prostheses will last indefinitely from a structural standpoint, but the patient requires continuing anticoagulation because of the exposed nonbiologic surfaces. The superior aspect (here the left atrium) is seen in the left panel, whereas the inflow into the left ventricle is seen in the right panel.

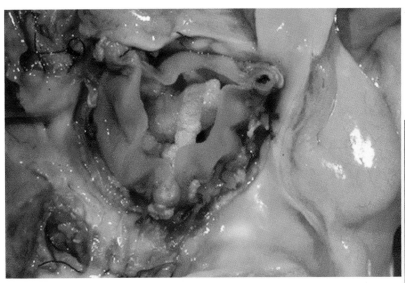

◀ **FIGURE 2–65 Porcine bioprosthesis, gross**

This bioprosthesis, a porcine artificial heart valve, is sutured in place with blue-green sutures around the valve ring. The valve cusps are still pliable, but the valve has become infected, with a large vegetation filling the valve orifice. This is an uncommon complication of valve prostheses.

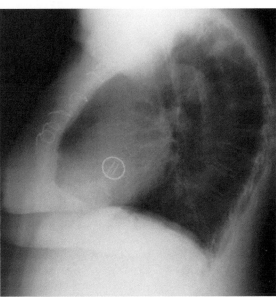

FIGURE 2–67 Mechanical prosthesis, x-ray ▶

This chest radiograph in lateral view reveals the presence of a bileaflet, tilting disc, mechanical aortic valve prosthesis. Note that the two leaflets are open and seen on edge.

◀ **FIGURE 2–67 Pacemaker, gross**

The right ventricle and atrium are opened to reveal a pacemaker wire that extends to the apex to embed on the septum. Pacemakers aid in maintaining a rhythm in hearts prone to arrhythmias.

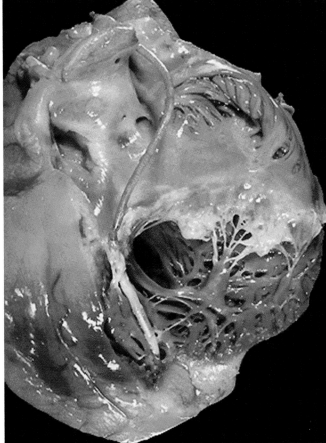

FIGURE 2–68 Pacemaker, x-ray ▶

This chest radiograph demonstrates the presence of a cardiac pacemaker battery implanted under the skin on the right chest wall. The leads from the battery extend down to the right atrium and the apex of the right ventricle.

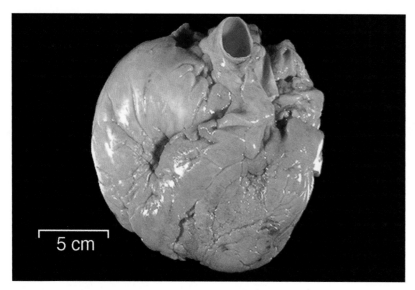

FIGURE 2–69 Dilated cardiomyopathy, gross

This very large heart has a globoid shape because all the chambers are dilated. It felt very flabby at autopsy, and the myocardium in life was poorly contractile. This is a *cardiomyopathy*, a term used to denote conditions in which the myocardium functions poorly and the heart is typically large and dilated, but there is often no characteristic histologic finding. Many cases are idiopathic. One fourth to one third of cases of dilated cardiomyopathy are familial. Some cases may occur after myocarditis, whereas others may appear in the peripartum period with pregnancy. Some cases occur as a consequence of chronic alcohol abuse.

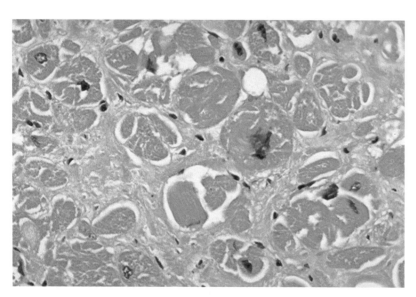

FIGURE 2–70 Cardiomyopathy, microscopic

The myocardium in many cases of cardiomyopathy demonstrates hypertrophy of myocardial fibers, which have prominent dark enlarged nuclei as seen here, along with interstitial fibrosis. This same appearance could follow ischemic injury, in which case the term *ischemic cardiomyopathy* could be applied. However, in most cases of idiopathic dilated cardiomyopathy, the coronary arteries show little or no atherosclerosis.

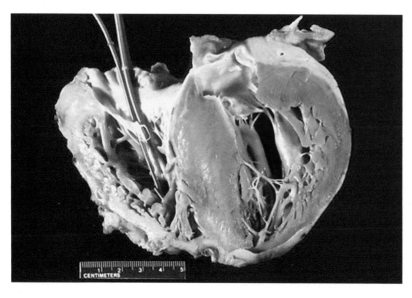

FIGURE 2–71 Hypertrophic cardiomyopathy, gross

There is marked left ventricular hypertrophy, with asymmetric bulging of a very large interventricular septum into the left ventricular chamber. This is hypertrophic cardiomyopathy. About half of these cases are familial, although a variety of different gene mutations may be responsible for this disease. Both children and adults can be affected, and sudden death can occur, typically from an arrhythmia. Seen here is an explanted heart, explaining the absence of atria. Pacemaker wires enter the right ventricle. The atria with venous connections, along with great vessels, remained behind to connect to the transplanted heart (provided by someone who cared enough to make transplantation possible).

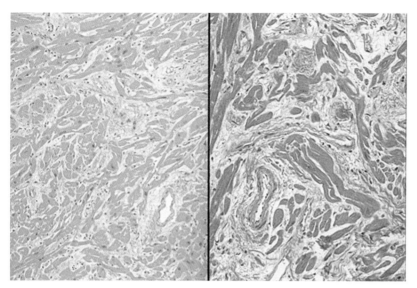

FIGURE 2–72 Hypertrophic cardiomyopathy, microscopic

The myocardium demonstrates "myofiber disarray" with a hypertrophic cardiomyopathy, typically within the interventricular septum. In the left panel with H+E stain and in the right panel with trichrome stain are sections of myocardium demonstrating these irregular myofibers with surrounding collagen. Such abnormal areas predispose to arrhythmias. Many cases are due to mutations in genes encoding for sarcomeric proteins, such as ß-myosin heavy chain, troponin T, myosin-binding protein C, and α-tropomyosin. Clinical findings are related to reduced ventricular compliance with impaired left ventricular diastolic filling. Functional left ventricular outflow obstruction may also occur.

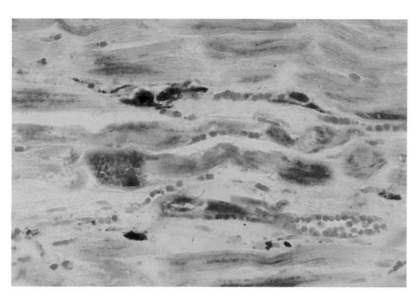

FIGURE 2–73 Restrictive cardiomyopathy, microscopic

Restrictive forms of cardiomyopathy lead to decreased ventricular compliance with impaired ventricular filling during diastole. It may be idiopathic or due to an identifiable cause, like hemochromatosis, with excessive iron deposition, shown here with Prussian blue iron stain. The deposition of iron leads to myocardial dysfunction with cardiac heart enlargement and failure. Much rarer causes of restrictive cardiomyopathy include endomyocardial fibrosis with dense collagen deposition in endocardium and subendocardium, and endocardial fibroelastosis with fibroelastic thickening of the left ventricle in children younger than 2 years.

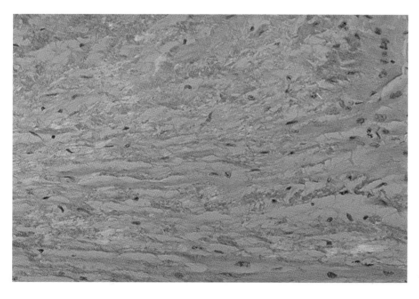

FIGURE 2–74 Restrictive cardiomyopathy, microscopic

Amorphous deposits of pale pink material between myocardial fibers seen with H+E staining have a characteristic "apple green" birefringence with Congo red stain under polarized light microscopy, as shown here. The amyloid stains orange-red with Congo red stain under routine light microscopy. Amyloidosis is a nightmare for anesthesiologists when intractable arrhythmias occur during surgery. Underlying causes can include AL amyloid deposition with multiple myeloma, AA amyloid infiltration with chronic inflammatory conditions, and "senile" cardiac amyloid derived from serum transthyretin protein.

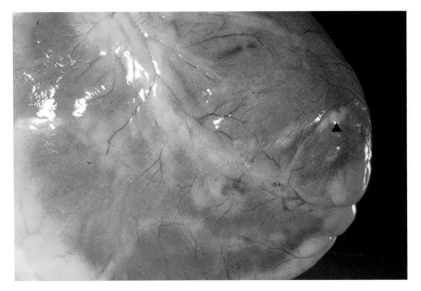

FIGURE 2–75 Myocarditis, gross

The epicardial surface of the heart shows small yellowish microabscesses (▲). Microabscesses may appear in patients who are septic and have hematogenous spread of infection. They may also represent emboli from an infective endocarditis in which small portions of cardiac vegetation have embolized into the coronary arteries. Myocarditis caused by other microorganisms can give a similar pattern of focal inflammation with necrosis. Patients with myocarditis can have fever, chest pain, dyspnea from left-sided heart failure, and peripheral edema from right-sided heart failure. Arrhythmias may lead to sudden death.

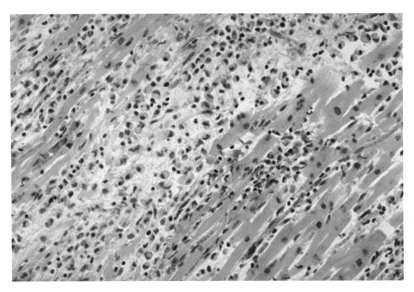

FIGURE 2–76 Myocarditis, microscopic

Here is an example of a florid myocarditis, which is defined by the presence of myofiber inflammation with necrosis. This myocarditis consists mainly of mononuclear cells but is mixed with some scattered neutrophils as well. The pattern is that of a patchy myocarditis. This is consistent with *Toxoplasma gondii* infection, which occurs in immunocompromised patients, although no free tachyzoites or pseudocysts with bradyzoites are seen here. Immune suppression also increases the risk for cytomegalovirus infection and other opportunistic infections.

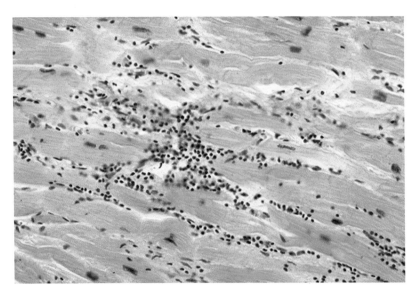

FIGURE 2–77 Myocarditis, microscopic

The interstitial lymphocytic infiltrates shown are characteristic for a viral myocarditis, which is probably the most common type of myocarditis. There is usually little accompanying myofiber necrosis. Many of these cases are probably subclinical, but findings may include fever and chest pain. In severe cases, cardiac failure leads to dyspnea and fatigue. The first manifestation may be arrhythmia, which can be a cause for sudden death in young people. A late sequela may be dilated cardiomyopathy. The most common viral agents are coxsackieviruses A and B. People infected with HIV can have similar findings. About 5% of people with Lyme disease develop myocarditis.

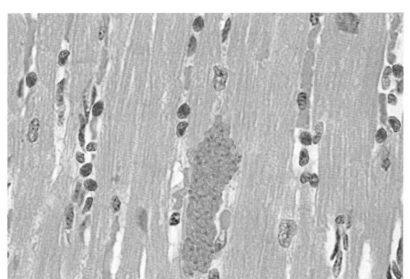

FIGURE 2–78 Chagasic myocarditis, microscopic

A pseudocyst in the myocardium contains many intracellular amastigotes of *Trypanosoma cruzi*, along with interstitial lymphocytic infiltrates; an acute myocarditis rarely occurs. Most deaths in acute Chagas disease are due to heart failure. The acute symptoms resolve spontaneously in virtually all patients, who then enter the asymptomatic or indeterminate phase. Chronic Chagas disease becomes apparent years or even decades later, when there is heart failure from dilation of several cardiac chambers, fibrosis, thinning of the ventricular wall, aneurysm formation (especially at the left ventricular apex), and mural thrombosis.

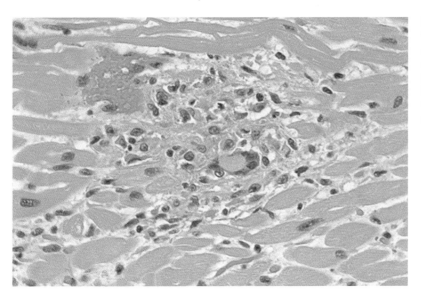

FIGURE 2–79 Myocarditis, microscopic

There is a granuloma with a giant cell seen here, along with myocyte necrosis. No infectious organisms can be found, so the term applied here is simply *giant cell myocarditis*. This is a rare, idiopathic form of myocarditis seen mostly in young to middle-aged adults. It has a poor prognosis.

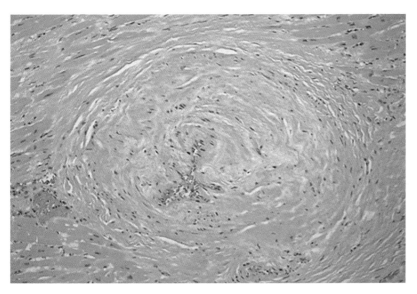

FIGURE 2–80 Arteriopathy, microscopic

The peripheral coronary arteries may undergo sclerosis, as seen here in an artery branch with a very small lumen, with chronic hypertension. Similar findings may be seen with cocaine-induced cardiomyopathy. The acute effects of cocaine, including sudden death, may be related to catecholamine effect with focal myocyte necrosis, including contraction bands. Arteriopathy occurs with chronic heart transplant rejection. In fact, virtually every transplanted heart has some degree of arteriopathy, which becomes the rate-limiting step to long-term survival.

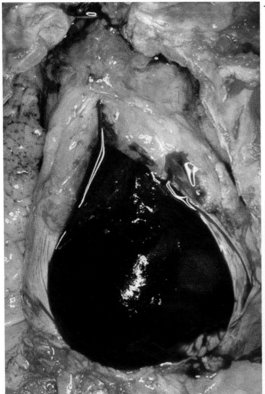

◄ **FIGURE 2–81 Hemopericardium, gross**

Note the dark blood in the pericardial sac opened at autopsy. Massive blunt force trauma to the chest (often from rapid deceleration with impact on the steering wheel in a vehicular crash) causes a rupture of the myocardium or coronary arteries with bleeding into the pericardial cavity. The extensive collection of blood in this closed space leads to cardiac tamponade from impaired ventricular filling. An aortic dissection proximally may also result in hemopericardium, as the blood dissects into the pericardial space.

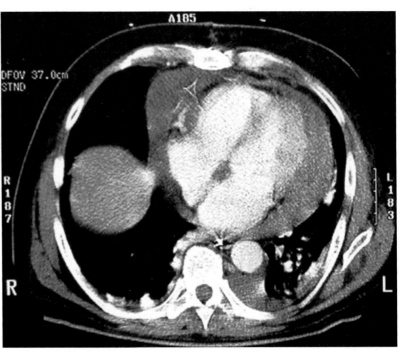

FIGURE 2–82 Pericardial effusion, CT image ►

This chest CT scan shows a large effusion (+) within the pericardial sac around the heart. The dome of the liver appears at the right. An acute serous pericarditis, with minimal inflammatory exudate but significant transudation of fluid, could produce a similar finding.

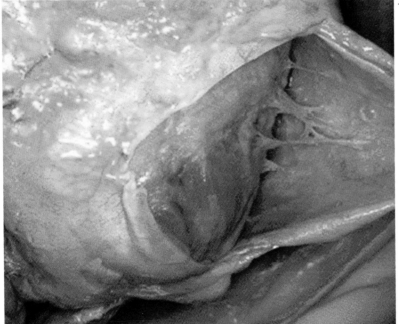

◄ **FIGURE 2–83 Fibrinous pericarditis, gross**

A window of adherent pericardium has been reflected to reveal the epicardial surface of the heart. The thin strands of fibrinous exudate extend from the epicardial surface to the pericardium. This is a typical appearance of a fibrinous pericarditis. A key clinical finding is a friction rub (heard by the student on the night of admission to hospital but disappearing with increasing serous fluid collection by the time the attending physician examines the patient on morning rounds, by which time the term *serofibrinous pericarditis* is more appropriate). Diffuse fibrinous pericarditis is more typical of systemic conditions such as uremia or SLE, whereas focal pericarditis may overlie a transmural MI (Dressler syndrome).

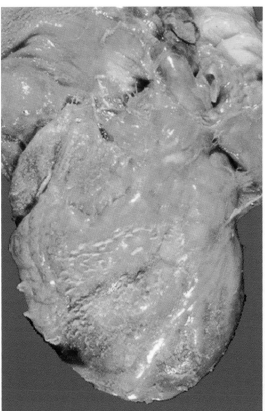

◄ **FIGURE 2–84 Fibrinous pericarditis, gross**

The epicardial surface of the heart shows a shaggy fibrinous exudate. This is another example of fibrinous pericarditis. These surfaces appear roughened with shaggy exudate formed by the organizing strands of fibrin, described as "bread-and-butter" pericarditis, although the appearance is more reminiscent of buttered bread dropped onto a carpet. The fibrin can result in an audible "friction rub" on auscultation, as the strands of fibrin on epicardium and pericardium rub against each other. In general, some degree of serous effusion also accompanies fibrinous exudation. However, the volume of fluid is usually not large enough to produce cardiac tamponade. Most cases resolve without significant collagenization, so there is no significant interference with ventricular wall motion.

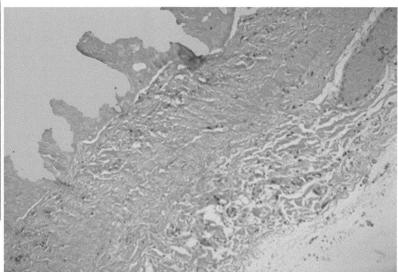

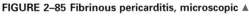

FIGURE 2–85 Fibrinous pericarditis, microscopic ▲

The pericardial surface here shows strands of pink fibrin extending outward. There is underlying inflammation. Eventually, the fibrin can be organized and cleared, although sometimes adhesions may remain. Fibrinous pericarditis results from inflammation or vascular injury that leads to exudation of fibrin, typically with fluid. Causes include an underlying myocardial infarction, uremia, rheumatic carditis, autoimmune diseases (although these are most often mostly serous), radiation to the chest, and trauma.

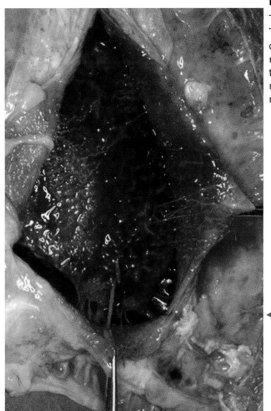

◄ **FIGURE 2–86 Hemorrhagic pericarditis, gross**

The pericardium is opened and reflected to reveal a pericarditis that has not only fibrin strands but also hemorrhage. Thus, this is termed *hemorrhagic pericarditis*. It is really just fibrinous pericarditis with hemorrhage. Without inflammation, blood in the pericardial sac would be called *hemopericardium*. This is the result of more severe inflammation or vascular injury, but it is not so acute as to be merely termed a hemopericardium. Causes include epicardial metastases, tuberculosis, bleeding diatheses, and cardiac surgery.

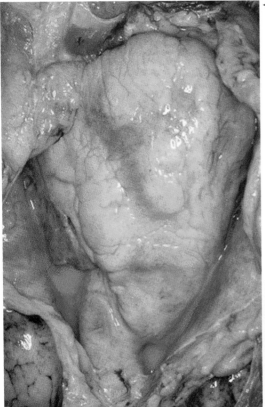

◄ **FIGURE 2–87 Purulent pericarditis, gross**

The pericardial sac has been opened and reflected. Note the yellowish exudate that has pooled in the lower pericardial sac seen here. A bacterial organism is usually implicated in this process, and the infection typically spreads from the adjacent lungs. A purulent pericarditis can have variable components of fibrinous exudate and serous effusion. If the inflammation is severe, it could even become hemorrhagic.

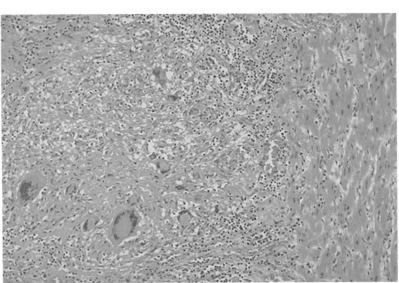

**FIGURE 2–88 Tuberculous pericarditis, ►
microscopic**

A pericarditis from *Mycobacterium tuberculosis* infection can produce extensive granulomatous inflammation with resultant calcification that can severely restrict cardiac motion (so-called *constrictive pericarditis*). Seen here is granulomatous inflammation over the surface of the heart. This is a chronic process.

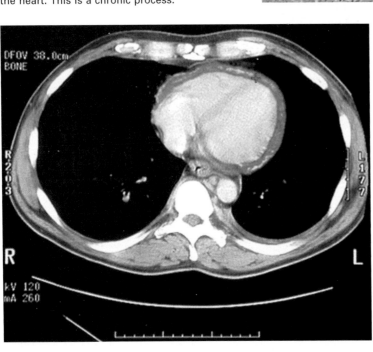

◄ **FIGURE 2–89 Constrictive pericarditis, CT image**

In this chest CT scan, there is a thickened pericardium encasing the heart. Within the thickened pericardium can be seen areas of brighter calcification (+). This proved to be a tuberculous pericarditis. The thickening and calcification constrict cardiac movement, resulting in a so-called *constrictive pericarditis* with a clinical finding of "pulsus paradoxus" with an exaggerated decrease (>10 mm Hg) in the amplitude of the arterial pulsation during inspiration and an increased pulse amplitude during expiration. Constrictive pericarditis is not common because most forms of pericarditis heal without significant scarring. However, a tuberculous pericarditis or severe purulent pericarditis may lead to this complication.

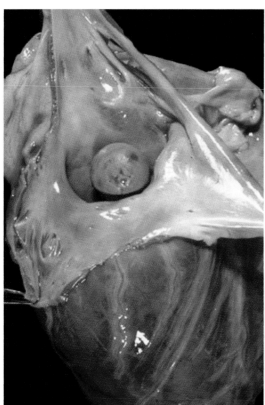

◀ **FIGURE 2–90 Cardiac myxoma, gross**

The left atrium has been opened to reveal the most common primary cardiac neoplasm—an atrial myxoma. These benign masses are attached to an atrial wall in more than 90% of cases, but they can also arise on a valve surface or on a ventricular wall. Myxomas can produce a ball–valve effect by intermittently occluding an atrioventricular valve orifice to produce clinical findings resembling a transient ischemic attack. Elaboration of interleukin-6 by the tumor may produce fever and malaise. Embolization of fragments of the tumor may also occur. Myxomas are easily diagnosed by echocardiography. Surgical removal is easily accomplished.

FIGURE 2–91 Cardiac myxoma, CT image ▶

This chest CT scan reveals a faint circumscribed left atrial myxoma (+) in a patient with a history of syncope. Although they are uncommon, myxomas are the most common primary cardiac tumor, and most are found in the atria, where larger ones may cause focal outflow obstruction. Portions of the myxoma may break off and embolize, often to the brain to produce clinical findings of a "stroke."

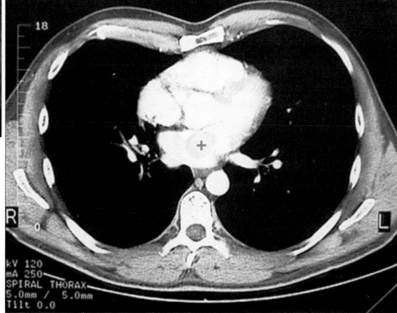

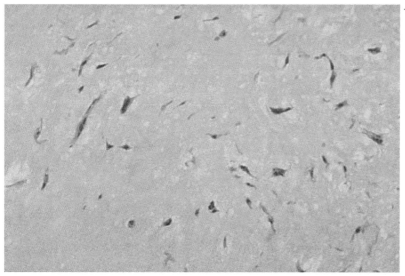

◀ **FIGURE 2–92 Cardiac myxoma, microscopic**

This high-power microscopic appearance of a cardiac myxoma shows minimal cellularity. Only scattered spindle cells with scant pink cytoplasm are present within a loose myxoid stroma. Although most myxomas occur sporadically, about 10% of cases are associated with the familial autosomal dominant Carney syndrome, half of which have a mutated *PRKA1* gene. This syndrome is suggested by the presence of multiple cardiac or extracardiac myxomas.

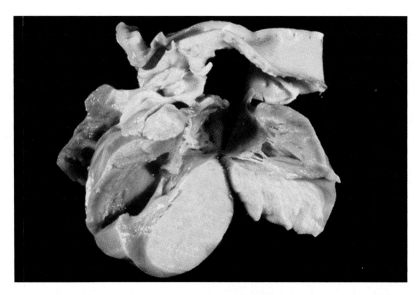

FIGURE 2–93 Cardiac rhabdomyoma, gross

This two-year-old child died suddenly. At autopsy, a large, firm, white tumor mass is shown filling much of the left ventricle, which obstructed the flow of blood. Such primary tumors of the heart are rare, and they are seen mainly in children. This lesion is thought to be a hamartoma or malformation, rather than a true neoplasm. Cardiac rhabdomyomas, although rare, are the most common primary cardiac tumor in infants and children. They can also be seen in association with tuberous sclerosis. Microscopically, the cells have prominent processes, giving them a spider-like appearance. The malignant counterpart, a rhabdomyosarcoma, is a very rare neoplasm in adults.

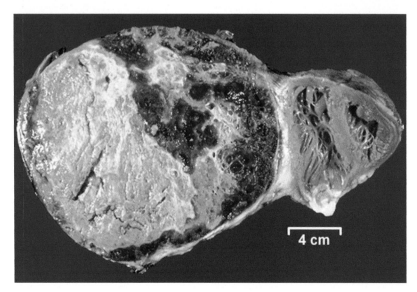

FIGURE 2–94 Cardiac angiosarcoma, gross

This malignant neoplasm arises in the epicardium in the groove between the right atrium and right ventricle. Although rare, it is one of the most common primary malignancies in the heart. Grossly, it is a variegated, hemorrhagic mass. The neoplastic cells are oblong to spindle-shaped, form ill-defined vascular spaces, and are positive for vimentin and CD-34, but negative for cytokeratin. In the differential diagnosis is Kaposi sarcoma, which usually is manifested by multiple nodules that rarely exceed 2 cm in size. Mesotheliomas tend to encase the heart and are CD-34 negative. In this case, complete resection, along with orthotopic cardiac transplantation, was performed. However, there is a great tendency for cardiac sarcomas to recur locally.

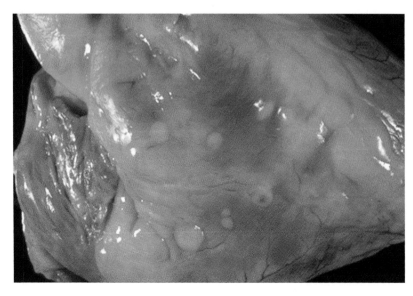

FIGURE 2–95 Cardiac metastases, gross

Primary tumors of the heart are uncommon. Metastases to the heart are more common, but rare overall (only about 5% to 10% of all malignancies have cardiac metastases, usually when widespread metastases are present). Seen over the surface of the epicardium are pale white-tan nodules of metastatic tumor. Metastases may lead to pericardial inflammation with effusions, including hemorrhagic pericarditis. Another pattern of cardiac involvement can be seen with bronchogenic carcinomas with contiguous spread to the heart.

CHAPTER 3

Red Blood Cell Disorders

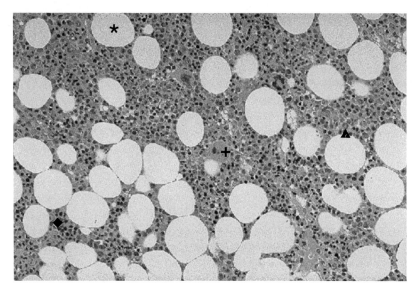

FIGURE 3–1 Normal bone marrow, microscopic

At medium-power magnification, normal marrow is seen to be a mixture of hematopoietic elements and adipose tissue. This marrow is taken from the posterior iliac crest of a middle-aged person, so it is about 50% cellular at age 50, declining by 10% per decade thereafter. In very elderly people, most remaining hematopoiesis is concentrated in vertebrae, sternum, and ribs. The erythroid islands (♦) and granulocytic precursors (▲) form the bulk of the hematopoietic components, admixed with steatocytes (*). The large multinucleated cells are megakaryocytes (+). Small numbers of lymphocytes, mainly memory B cells, and plasma cells secreting immunoglobulins are present.

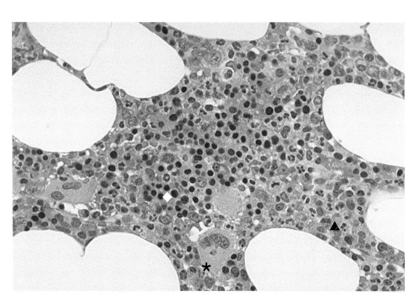

FIGURE 3–2 Normal bone marrow, microscopic

At higher magnification, note the presence of megakaryocytes (*), erythroid islands (♦), and granulocytic precursors (▲). The normal myeloid to erythroid ratio is about 2 : 1 to 3 : 1. A high proliferation rate from CD34+ stem cells differentiating into various colony-forming units (CFUs) under the influence of c-*KIT* ligand is needed because granulocytes last less than a day in circulation, platelets less than a week, and red blood cells (RBCs) about 120 days. Erythropoietin stimulates RBC production, thrombopoietin platelet formation, granulocyte-macrophage colony-stimulating factor (GM-CSF), granulocyte and monocyte-macrophage proliferation, and granulocyte colony-stimulating factor (G-CSF) neutrophil production.

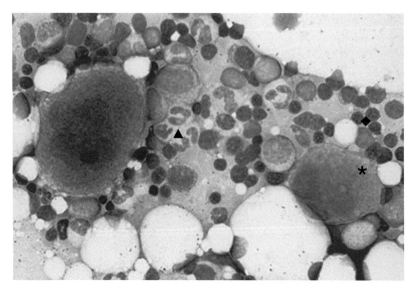

FIGURE 3–3 Normal bone marrow smear, microscopic

In this normal bone marrow smear at high magnification, note the presence of megakaryocytes (*), erythroid precursors (♦), and granulocytic precursors (▲). Erythroid precursors are nucleated, but the nucleus is normally lost before mature RBCs are released into the circulation. Newly released RBCs, called reticulocytes, have a slightly increased mean corpuscular volume and increased RNA content that imparts a slightly basophilic appearance, and this RNA can be precipitated by supravital staining for identification and enumeration (the "retic" count). Platelets are formed by budding off megakaryocyte cytoplasm.

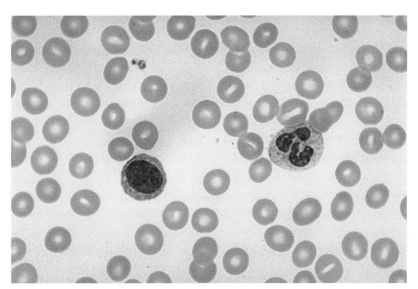

FIGURE 3–4 Normal peripheral blood smear, microscopic

These are happy, normal RBCs with a zone of central pallor about one third the size of the RBC diameter. These RBCs demonstrate minimal variation in both size (anisocytosis) and shape (poikilocytosis). A small blue-staining platelet is present. A normal mature lymphocyte on the left can be compared with a segmented neutrophil (polymorphonuclear leukocyte, or PMN) on the right. An RBC is about two thirds the size of a normal lymphocyte. The hemoglobin in RBCs supplies most of the oxygen carrying capacity:

$$O_2 \text{ content} = 1.34 \times \text{Hgb} \times \text{saturation} + (0.0031 \times \text{PO}_2)$$

With Hgb 15 g/dL, PaO_2 100 mm Hg, and O_2 saturation 96%, the O_2 content of the blood is 19.6 mL O_2/dL upon leaving the pulmonary capillaries.

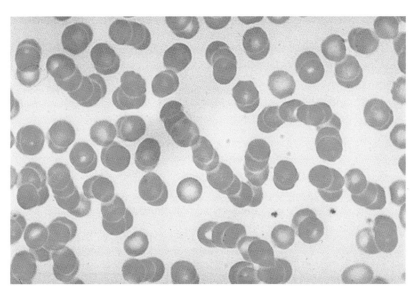

FIGURE 3–5 Rouleaux formation, microscopic

The RBCs here have stacked together in long chains, known as "rouleaux formation." This phenomenon occurs with an increase in serum proteins, particularly fibrinogen, C-reactive protein, and globulins. Such long chains of RBCs sediment more readily when left to stand in a column. This is the mechanism for measuring the erythrocyte sedimentation rate (ESR), or "sed rate," which increases nonspecifically when inflammation is present and there is an increase in the "acute-phase" serum proteins. Thus, the "sed rate" is a nonspecific indicator of an inflammatory process.

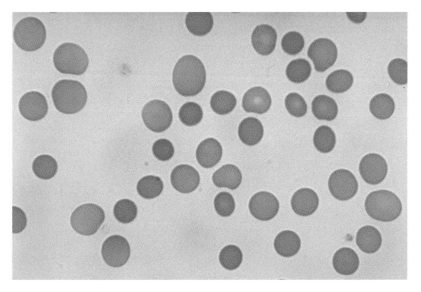

FIGURE 3–6 Hemolytic anemia, microscopic

This peripheral blood smear shows many smaller RBCs lacking central pallor—spherocytes. There are some larger bluish-staining reticulocytes from increased release from the marrow to compensate for RBC loss. This patient had an autoimmune hemolytic anemia from antibody coating the RBC surface membranes. Subsequently, portions of RBC membranes are removed, mostly in the spleen, decreasing RBC size (microcytosis). Reduction in size or number of RBCs results in anemia. The bone marrow can respond to anemia with increased erythropoiesis, indicated by an elevated reticulocyte count. The increased RBC turnover with rapid recycling leads to unconjugated (indirect) hyperbilirubinemia.

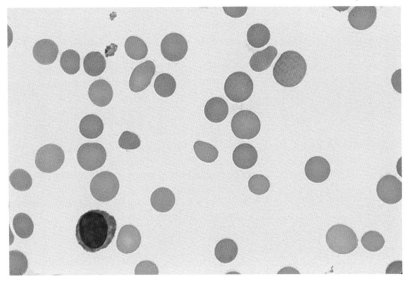

FIGURE 3–7 Hereditary spherocytosis, microscopic

The size of many of these RBCs is quite small, with lack of the central zone of pallor and loss of the biconcave shape. These RBCs are known as spherocytes. In hereditary spherocytosis, an autosomal dominant condition most frequent in northern Europeans, there is a lack of key RBC cytoskeletal membrane proteins such as spectrin or ankyrin. This produces membrane instability that forces the cell to take the smallest volume possible—a sphere. In the laboratory, this is demonstrated by increased osmotic fragility. The spherocytes do not survive in circulation for as long as normal RBCs. Note the reticulocyte from increased bone marrow production of RBCs.

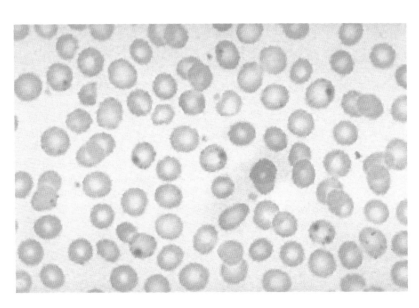

FIGURE 3–8 Glucose-6-phosphate dehydrogenase deficiency, microscopic

This peripheral blood smear with methylene blue stain shows RBC Heinz body inclusions in glucose-6-phosphate dehydrogenase (G6PD) deficiency. The defect is in the HMP shunt, which helps protect RBCs from oxidation. This X-linked disorder, found in 12% of African American males, is also seen in people from the Mediterranean region, including Italy, Greece, and Turkey. Older RBCs exposed to oxidizing agents such as primaquine, sulfa, the nitrofurantoin family, aspirin, and phenacetin undergo hemolysis. Foods such as fava beans may have a similar effect. G6PD deficiency is asymptomatic until stress occurs from infection or ingestion of an oxidizing drug. Laboratory findings may include anemia, reticulocytosis, indirect hyperbilirubinemia, and decreased haptoglobin.

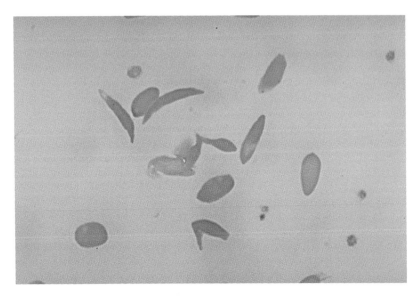

FIGURE 3–9 Sickle cell anemia, microscopic

This is sickle cell anemia in sickle cell crisis. The abnormal hemoglobin S is prone to polymerization with tactoid formation when oxygen tension is low, and the RBCs change shape to long, thin sickle forms that do not exchange oxygen well. The sickled cells are prone to stick together, plugging smaller vessels and leading to decreased blood flow with ischemia from decreased oxygen delivery to tissues, with clinical findings such as acute abdominal pain, chest pain, and back pain. Hemoglobin electrophoresis in sickle cell disease will demonstrate 90% to 95% Hgb S, 1% to 3% Hgb A2, and 5% to 10% Hgb F. In sickle cell trait, there is 40% to 45% Hgb S, 55% to 60% Hgb A1, and normal amounts (1% to 3%) of Hgb A2, and the RBCs have minimal sickling.

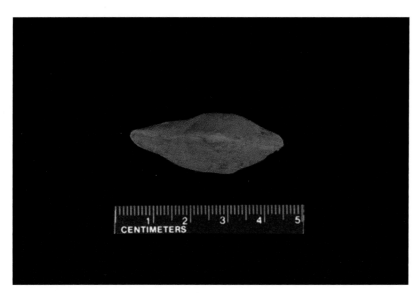

FIGURE 3–10 Sickle cell anemia, gross

The genetic defect with Hgb S is a single point mutation with glu → val substitution. Although in early childhood the spleen may be enlarged with sickle cell anemia, continual stasis and trapping of abnormal RBCs in the spleen leads to extensive infarctions that eventually reduce the size of the spleen tremendously by adolescence. This is called "*autosplenectomy*." Seen here is the small remnant of spleen in a teenage patient with sickle cell anemia. Lack of a spleen predisposes the patient to infections, particularly with encapsulated bacterial organisms such as pneumococcus. In the United States, the gene frequency for Hgb S is about 1 in 25 in African Americans, with a carrier rate of 1 in 12, and thus a 1 in 625 chance for sickle cell disease.

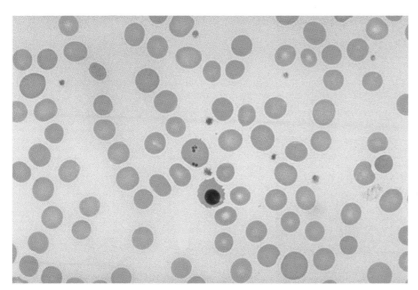

FIGURE 3–11 Howell-Jolly bodies, microscopic

The RBC in the center of this peripheral blood smear field contains two dark blue Howell-Jolly bodies, or inclusions of nuclear chromatin remnants. There is also a nucleated RBC just beneath this RBC. Abnormal RBCs and aged RBCs approaching their 120-day life span are typically removed by the spleen. The appearance of increased poikilocytosis, anisocytosis, and RBC inclusions on a peripheral blood smear suggests that the patient's spleen is not present. The presence of a nucleated RBC is typical for hemolysis with increased red cell turnover, so that the bone marrow is stressed to release not only reticulocytes, but also RBC precursors.

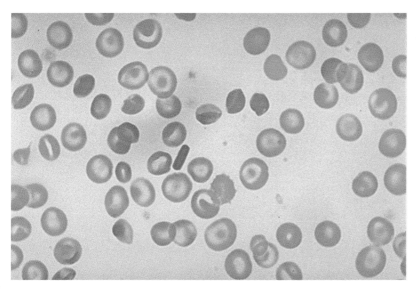

FIGURE 3–12 Hemoglobin SC disease, microscopic

This patient has both Hgb S and Hgb C present within RBCs. With SC disease, the RBCs may sickle, but not as commonly as with Hgb SS disease (sickle cell anemia). The Hgb C leads to the formation of "target" cells—RBCs that have a central reddish dot within the zone of pallor, as shown in this peripheral blood smear. In the center of the field is a rectangular RBC that is indicative of an Hgb C crystal, which is also characteristic of Hgb C disease.

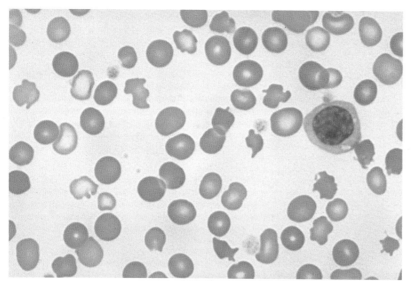

FIGURE 3–13 β-Thalassemia major, microscopic

This peripheral blood smear demonstrates marked poikilocytosis (abnormally shaped RBCs) as well as some anisocytosis (variation in RBC size), although many are small (microcytosis). This patient has β-thalassemia, a hereditary disorder with deficient β-globin chain synthesis that leads to ineffective erythropoiesis and a chronic, microcytic anemia. Increased but insufficient production of Hgb F and Hgb A2 compensate. Some of these RBCs resemble jigsaw puzzle pieces. Patients severely affected (β-thalassemia major) have increased iron absorption, leading to hemochromatosis. Iron overload is worsened if multiple transfusions of RBCs are given to treat chronic anemia. Each unit of packed RBCs contains 250 mg of iron.

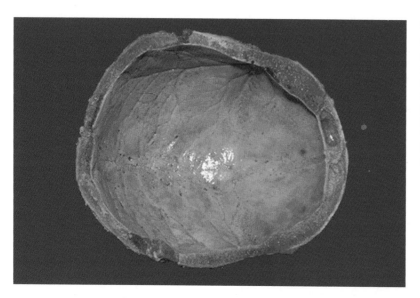

FIGURE 3–14 β-Thalassemia major, gross

Severe, chronic anemias (such as thalassemias and sickle cell anemia) can increase the bone marrow response to produce RBCs. This drive for erythropoiesis may increase the mass of marrow and lead to increase in marrow in places, such as the skull seen here, that it is not normally found. Such an increase in marrow in skull may lead to "frontal bossing" or forehead prominence because of the skull shape change. Bone deformity with fracture may occur elsewhere.

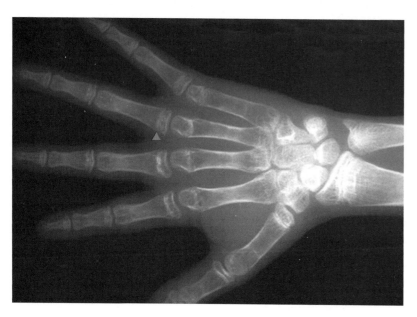

FIGURE 3–15 β-Thalassemia major, x-ray

This patient has β-thalassemia major, an inherited disorder of β-globin chain synthesis leading to ineffective erythropoiesis with marked expansion of marrow spaces to compensate. The result can be bony prominence with prominent epiphyseal regions (▲), as seen in this 20-year-old man. The hemochromatosis can lead to cardiomyopathy, hepatic failure, and "bronze" diabetes mellitus from iron deposition in islets of Langerhans.

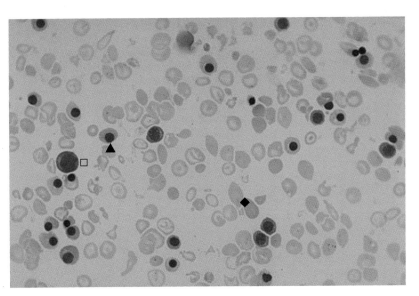

FIGURE 3–16 α-Thalassemia major, microscopic

A severely hydropic stillborn fetus with α-thalassemia major has the appearance on peripheral blood smear shown here. Note that predominantly hemoglobin Barts production from lack of α-globin chain synthesis results in marked anisocytosis and poikilocytosis of RBCs, with expansion of erythropoiesis and the presence of many immature RBCs in the peripheral blood, as evidenced by polychromasia (◆), nucleated RBCs (▲) and even erythroblasts (□). α-Thalassemia major occurs when all four α-globin chain genes have a mutation. α-Thalassemia minor, which leads to a mild microcytic anemia, results from the presence of mutations involving only two α-globin chains.

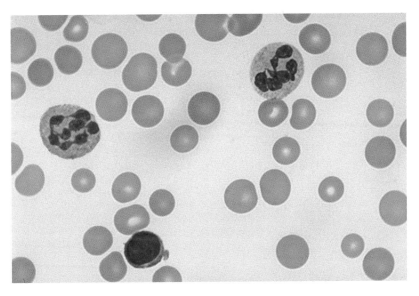

FIGURE 3–17 Megaloblastic anemia, microscopic

Hypersegmented neutrophils are present along with macro-ovalocytes in a case of pernicious anemia. The neutrophil at the left has eight lobes instead of the usual three or four. Such anemias can be due to folate or vitamin B_{12} deficiency. The increased size of the RBCs (macrocytosis) is hard to appreciate in a blood smear. Compare the RBCs to the lymphocyte at the lower left center. The CBC shows a markedly increased mean corpuscular volume. The mean corpuscular volume can be mildly increased in people recovering from blood loss or hemolytic anemia because the newly released RBCs, the reticulocytes, are increased in size over normal RBCs, which decrease in size slightly with aging.

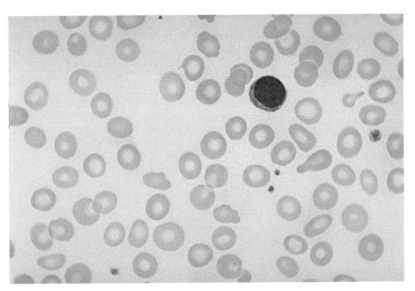

FIGURE 3–18 Hypochromic anemia, microscopic

The RBCs here are smaller than normal and have an increased zone of central pallor. This is indicative of a hypochromic (less hemoglobin in each RBC) and microcytic (smaller size of each RBC) anemia. There is also increased anisocytosis (variation in size) and poikilocytosis (variation in shape). The most common cause of hypochromic microcytic anemia is iron deficiency. The most common nutritional deficiency is lack of dietary iron. Thus, iron deficiency anemia is common, and people at greatest risk are children and women in their reproductive years (from menstrual blood loss and from pregnancy).

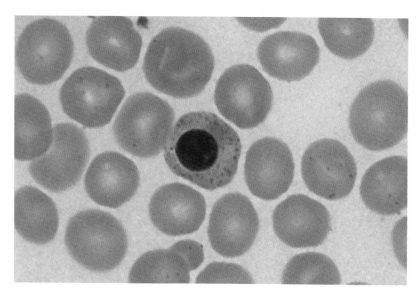

FIGURE 3–19 Basophilic stippling, microscopic

This peripheral blood smear demonstrates a nucleated RBC in the center that contains basophilic stippling of the cytoplasm. This suggests a toxic injury to the bone marrow, such as lead poisoning. Such stippling may also appear with severe anemia, such as a megaloblastic anemia.

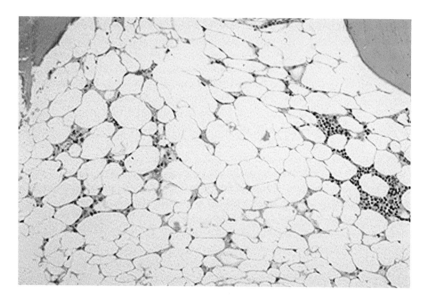

FIGURE 3–20 Aplastic anemia

The reduction of hematopoietic elements in the bone marrow shown here, with mainly adipocytes remaining, leads to pancytopenia (anemia, neutropenia, thrombocytopenia). The most common cause is pharmacologic therapy, often with drugs known to be toxic to bone marrow, such as chemotherapy agents. Such agents may damage or suppress stem cells from which the erythroid, myeloid, and megakaryocytic cells are derived. Exposure to radiation may damage the marrow. Exposure to a drug such as a sulfonamide or to toxic substances such as benzene may precede development of an aplastic marrow. Some cases are idiopathic. If CD34+ stem cells remain, then the marrow can become repopulated.

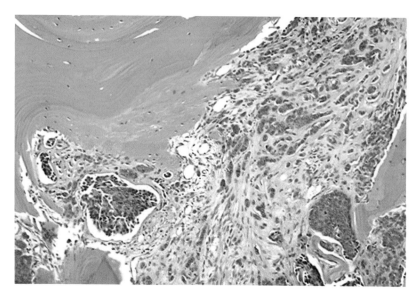

FIGURE 3–21 Myelophthisic anemia, microscopic

The marrow spaces between the trabecular bone are filled with metastatic carcinoma replacing normal hematopoietic cells. The primary site in this case was breast. A bone scan can help to identify metastases. A bone marrow biopsy can confirm the diagnosis. This process is typical for a space-occupying process that destroys substantial marrow and reduces the ability of the marrow to produce hematopoietic cells—a myelophthisic process. Metastases, leukemias, and lymphomas, as well as infections, can produce this effect. As a consequence, the peripheral blood shows a leukoerythroblastic appearance with both immature white blood cells and nucleated RBCs.

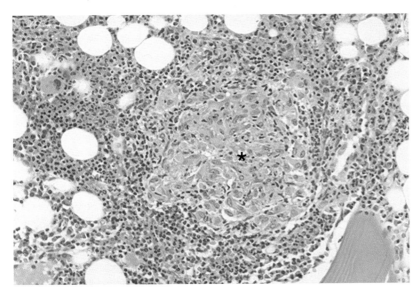

FIGURE 3–22 Marrow granuloma, microscopic

This granuloma (∗) in a bone marrow biopsy can be part of a potential myelophthisic (space-occupying) process. Such granulomas tend to be small and poorly formed. This one consists mainly of epithelioid macrophages. Multiple cultures and special stains are done to determine whether there is an infectious etiology, such as a mycobacterial or fungal infection. In this case, no organism was demonstrated, and the clinical features fit with sarcoidosis. Patients with a "fever of unknown origin" may have such a finding. A myelophthisic process may lead to release of hematopoietic precursors, giving the peripheral blood a "leukoerythroblastic" picture with metamyelocytes, myelocytes, and nucleated RBCs.

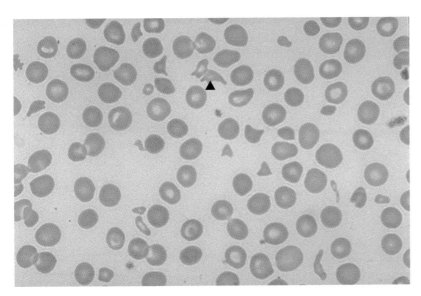

FIGURE 3–23 Microangiopathic hemolytic anemia, microscopic

The numerous fragmented RBCs seen in this peripheral blood smear include irregular shapes such as "helmet" cells (▲). These fragmented RBCs known as "*schistocytes*" are indicative of a microangiopathic hemolytic anemia or other cause such as trauma for intravascular hemolysis. Schistocytes can appear with thrombotic thrombocytopenic purpura and with disseminated intravascular coagulopathy (DIC). In DIC, consumption of platelets and coagulation factors leads to hemorrhage. Thus, in DIC, the prothrombin time and the partial thromboplastin time are increased, whereas the D-dimer (indicative of fibrin degradation product formation) is increased.

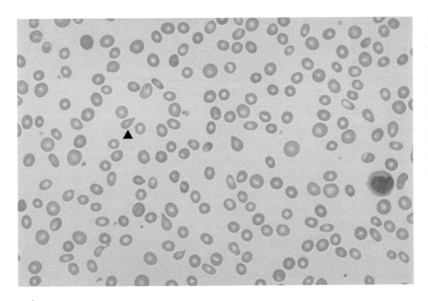

FIGURE 3–24 Myelofibrosis with tear drop cells, microscopic

This peripheral blood smear demonstrates "tear drop" cells (▲). These characteristically shaped RBCs can be seen in patients with myelofibrosis. Myelofibrosis can be the end result of a chronic myeloproliferative process, with reticulin fibrosis filling the marrow spaces, reduction in hematopoiesis, and peripheral pancytopenia. A reticulocyte is present here, but the reticulocyte count would not be as increased as it should, given that the marrow reserve is gone.

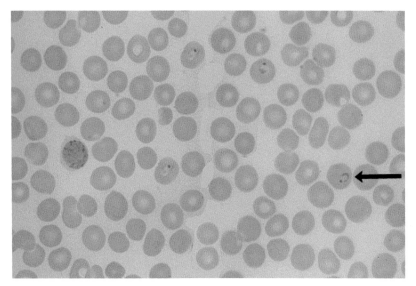

FIGURE 3–25 Malaria, microscopic

Malaria is a parasitic disease caused by the parasitic genus *Plasmodium*, of which there are four species that affect humans (*Plasmodium vivax, falciparum, ovale,* and *malariae*). Shown here are "ring forms" of *P. vivax* in red blood cells. A gametocyte is present at the left. This disorder can produce fever with hemolysis and anemia.

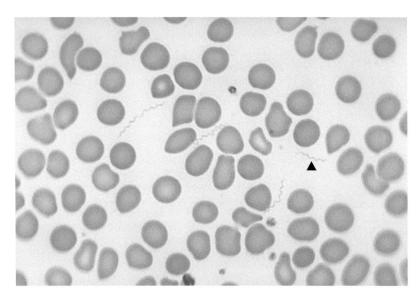

FIGURE 3–26 Borreliosis, microscopic

This peripheral blood smear demonstrates multiple *Borrelia recurrentis* organisms (▲) among the RBCs of a peripheral blood smear. This organism produces the clinical picture of "relapsing fever."

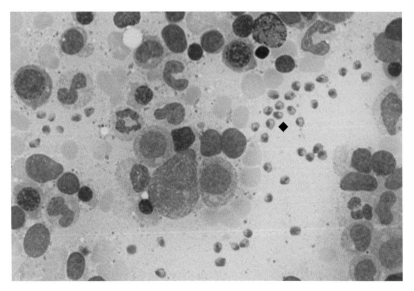

FIGURE 3–27 Leishmaniasis, microscopic

A myelophthisic anemia may result from infections involving the marrow, including fungal, mycobacterial, and parasitic infections. Seen here are multiple (◆) amastigotes of *Leishmania donovani infantum* in a bone marrow smear. The infiltrative process does not have to fill up much of the marrow to produce a characteristic peripheral blood leukoerythroblastic pattern.

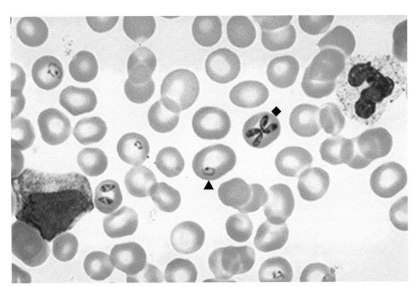

FIGURE 3–28 Babesiosis, microscopic

Babesiosis caused by infection with *Babesia microti* is a rare disease endemic to the northeastern United States and parts of Europe. The organism proliferates within RBCs and can produce a hemolytic anemia. Seen here is a characteristic "tetrad" (◆) as well as ring forms (▲).

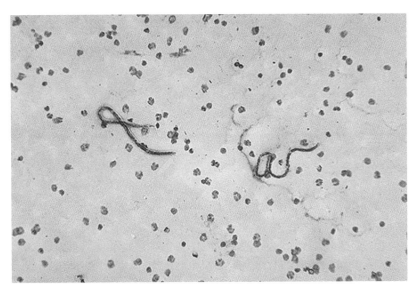

FIGURE 3–29 Filariasis, microscopic

Two microfilaria seen here are in lymph node aspirate fluid from a patient with peripheral eosinophilia. Infective larvae transmitted by mosquito bite migrate either to lymphatics (*Wuchereria bancrofti*, *Brugia malayi*) or to subcutaneous connective tissues (*Onchocerca volvulus*). There they mature into adult worms that mate, and females release microfilaria. Varying host responses and repeated infections account for the manifestations. In lymphatic filariasis, the worms cause lymphedema of lower extremities, external genitalia, and sometimes upper extremities, called "*elephantiasis*" because of marked enlargement. Onchocerciasis can cause blindness, dermatitis with pruritus, depigmentation or hyperpigmentation, and fibrosis with nodularity.

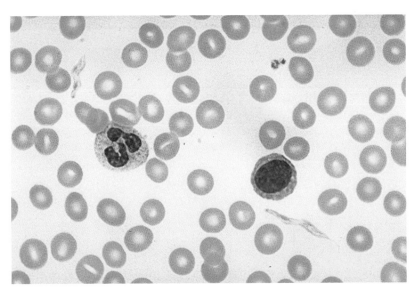

FIGURE 3–30 Trypanosomiasis, microscopic

Two trypomastigotes of *Trypanosoma brucei rhodesiense*, about 2 to 3 times as long and up to half as wide as an RBC, are present in this peripheral blood smear. The bite of the tsetse fly introduces infective trypomastigotes into the circulation, where they divide and multiply and also spread to lymph nodes and spleen. Eventually they reach the central nervous system and proliferate in cerebrospinal fluid. Systemic manifestations include fever, lymphadenopathy, headache, and arthralgias. Central nervous system involvement follows and can manifest with convulsions, behavioral changes, and coma (hence the disease may be termed "*sleeping sickness*").

CHAPTER 4

Hematopathology

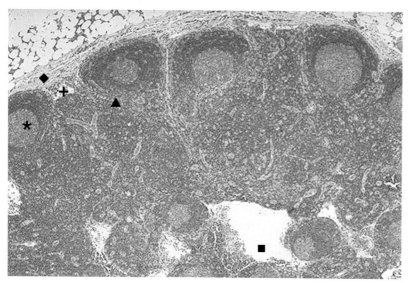

FIGURE 4–1 Normal lymph node, microscopic

This benign reactive lymph node has a well-defined connective tissue capsule (◆), and beneath that a subcapsular sinus (+) where afferent lymphatics drain lymph fluid from tissues peripheral to the node. The lymph may contain macrophages and dendritic cells, both forms of antigen-presenting cells, carrying antigens to the node. Beneath the subcapsular sinus is the paracortical zone (▲) with lymphoid follicles having pale germinal centers with a predominance of B lymphocytes. In the germinal centers (∗), immune responses to antigens are generated, assisted by a darker mantle zone of mainly T lymphocytes. Central to the follicles are sinusoids extending to the hilum of the node. The efferent lymphatics drain out the hilum (■).

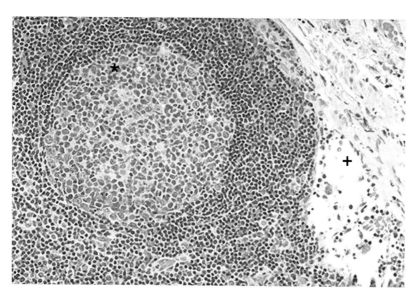

FIGURE 4–2 Normal lymph node, microscopic

At high magnification, a lymph node follicle with a germinal center (∗) contains larger lymphocytes undergoing cytokine activation. At the lower right is the subcapsular sinus (+). The center of the lymphoid follicle—the germinal center—is where CD4 helper lymphocytes and antigen-presenting cells (macrophages and follicular dendritic cells) interact with B lymphocytes, leading to an antibody-mediated immune response.

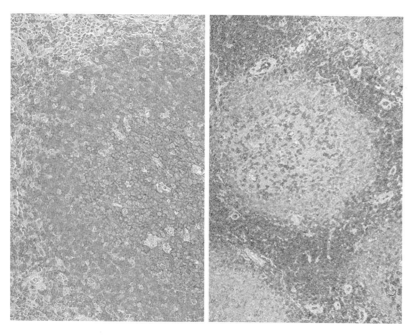

FIGURE 4–3 Normal lymph node, microscopic

The nature of the cell population and function of a lymph node are shown in the left panel with an immunohistochemical stain for CD20, a B-cell marker. Note the larger number of B cells staining with the red-brown reaction product within the germinal center of a lymph node follicle, with additional B cells scattered in the interfollicular zone. The node in the right panel has been stained for CD3, a T-cell marker. Note the larger number of T cells around the germinal center of a follicle, with additional T cells extending into the paracortex.

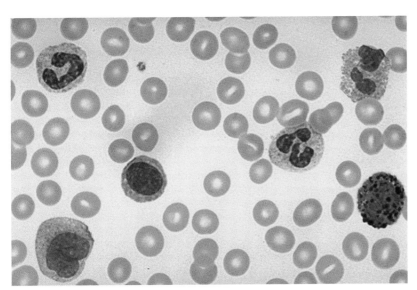

FIGURE 4–4 Normal white blood cells, microscopic

The normal types of leukocytes that are routinely observed on the peripheral blood smear are shown here, including a segmented neutrophil, band neutrophil, eosinophil, basophil, lymphocyte, and monocyte. The red blood cells (RBCs) appear normal, and there is a normal platelet present. A complete blood count includes a total white blood cell (WBC) count. The types of leukocytes may be enumerated by a machine that measures size and chemical characteristics. A manual WBC differential count is performed by observing the peripheral blood smear with Wright-Giemsa stain by light microscopy.

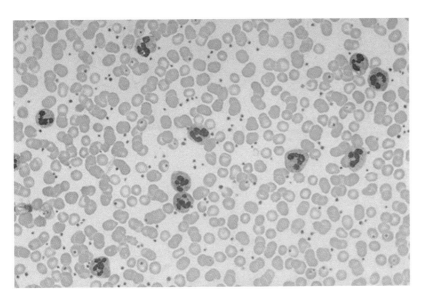

FIGURE 4–5 Leukocytosis, microscopic

Note the presence of many granulocytes, both segmented neutrophils and band neutrophils, in this peripheral blood smear. An elevated WBC count with neutrophilia suggests inflammation or infection. A very high WBC count (>50,000) that is not a leukemia is known as a "leukemoid reaction." This leukemoid reaction is more pronounced than just the "left shift" with bandemia and the occasional metamyelocyte with acute inflammation. An acute inflammatory reaction is also accompanied by a rise in "acute-phase reactants" in the plasma such as C-reactive protein (CRP). Inflammatory cytokines such as tumor necrosis factor (TNF) and interleukin-1 (IL-1) stimulate proliferation and differentiation of marrow granulocytic cells.

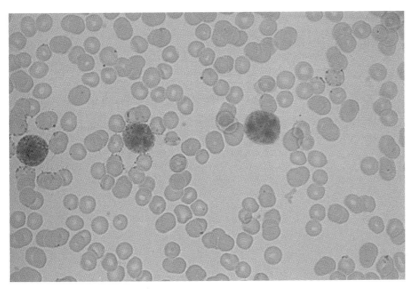

FIGURE 4–6 Leukocyte alkaline phosphatase test, microscopic

Distinguishing a leukemoid reaction from chronic myelogenous leukemia (CML) may be done with the leukocyte alkaline phosphatase (LAP) stain. Seen here are neutrophils with red granular cytoplasmic staining for LAP. Counting granulocytic cells that are staining with LAP yields a score. A high LAP score is seen with a leukemoid reaction, whereas a low LAP score suggests CML. The myeloid cells in CML are not as differentiated as the normal myeloid cells. A leukemoid reaction is typically a transient but exaggerated bone marrow response to inflammatory cytokines such as IL-1 and TNF, which stimulate bone marrow progenitor cells.

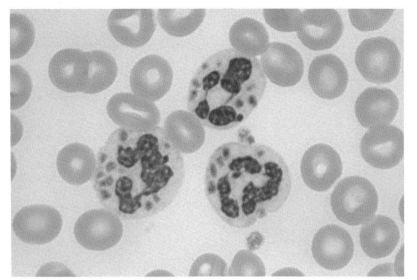

FIGURE 4–7 Chediak-Higashi syndrome, microscopic

A history of recurrent bacterial infections and giant granules seen in peripheral blood leukocytes is characteristic for Chediak-Higashi syndrome. This disorder results from a mutation in the LYST gene on chromosome 1q42 that encodes a protein involved in intracellular trafficking of proteins. Microtubules fail to form properly, and the neutrophils do not respond to chemotactic stimuli. Giant lysosomal granules fail to function. Soft tissue abscesses with *Staphylococcus aureus* are common. Other cells affected by this disorder include platelets (bleeding), melanocytes (albinism), Schwann cells (neuropathy), natural killer cells, and cytotoxic T cells (aggressive lymphoproliferative disorder).

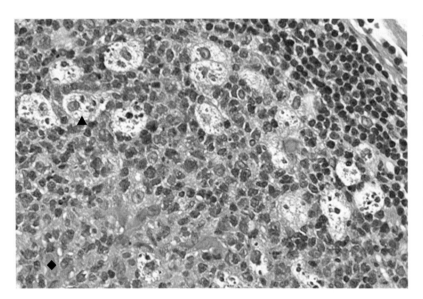

FIGURE 4–8 Lymphadenitis, microscopic

This is a pronounced reactive change in a lymph node, with a large follicle and germinal center demonstrating prominent macrophages (▲) with irregular cytoplasmic debris (so-called tingible body macrophages). Blood vessels (♦) are also more prominent. Note that multiple types of leukocytes are present, indicative of a polymorphous population of cells, or polyclonal immune response, typical for a benign process reacting to multiple antigenic stimulants. In general, lymph nodes in a benign reactive process are more likely to enlarge quickly, they are often tender on palpation during physical examination, and they diminish in size after the infection.

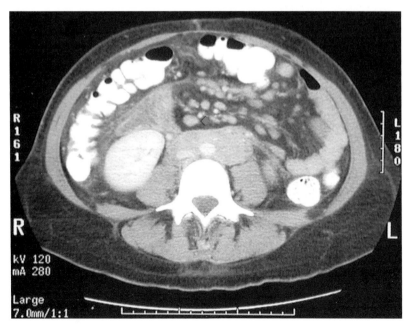

FIGURE 4–9 Lymphadenopathy, CT image

Note the prominent mesenteric lymph nodes (♦) in this patient with mesenteric lymphadenitis. Both benign and malignant processes can lead to lymph node enlargement. Infections are a common cause for lymphadenopathy. Lymph fluid draining from the site of infection reaches regional lymph nodes. The lymph fluid carries antigens and antigen-presenting cells to the node. Antigens may also circulate out of the regional node and be carried around the body by the bloodstream, reaching other lymphoid tissues in which clones of memory lymphocytes may be present that can react to specific antigens. After the infection or inflammatory process has subsided, the stimulated nodes diminish in size.

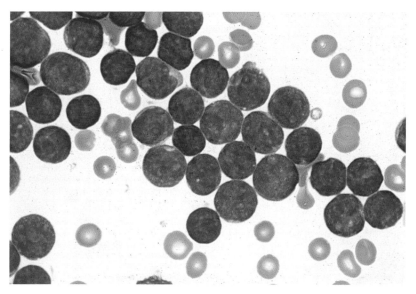

FIGURE 4–10 Acute lymphoblastic leukemia, microscopic

The WBCs seen here are leukemic blasts—very immature leukocytes with large nuclei that contain multiple nucleoli. These abnormal lymphocytes are indicative of acute lymphoblastic leukemia (ALL). These cells have the B-cell markers CD10, CD19, and CD22. About 85% of ALLs are precursor B-cell neoplasms. The cells of ALL originate in the marrow but often circulate to produce leukocytosis. Patients with ALL often have generalized lymphadenopathy along with splenomegaly and hepatomegaly. Bone pain is common. ALL is more common in children than adults. Many cases of ALL in children respond well to treatment, and many are curable.

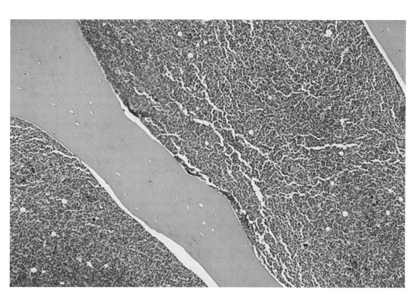

FIGURE 4–11 Leukemia, microscopic

Leukemia results in a highly cellular marrow. The marrow between the pink bone trabeculae seen here is nearly 100% cellular, and it consists of the leukemic cells of ALL that have virtually replaced or suppressed normal hematopoiesis. There is a near absence of adipocytes. The bone spicules are unlikely to become affected by the leukemic process. Although the marrow is quite cellular, there can be peripheral blood cytopenias. This explains the usual leukemic complications of infection (lack of normal leukocytes), hemorrhage (lack of platelets), and anemia (lack of RBCs) that often appear in the clinical course of leukemia.

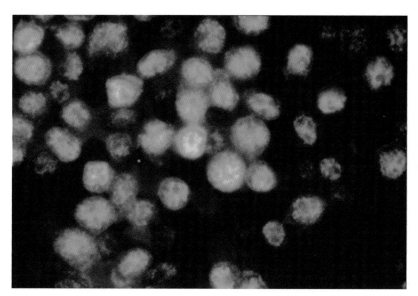

FIGURE 4–12 Lymphoblastic leukemia, microscopic

Terminal deoxyribonucleotidyl transferase (TdT) is a specialized DNA polymerase expressed only by pre-B and pre-T lymphoblasts. Seen here is immunofluorescence staining of a pre-B-cell ALL with TdT. TdT is expressed in more than 95% of ALL cases. Cytogenetic abnormalities in ALL can include hyperploidy (>50 chromosomes), polyploidy, and translocations including t(12;21), t(9;22), and t(4;11), which may correlate with the immunophenotype and sometimes predict prognosis.

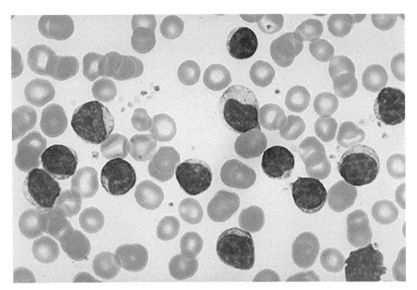

FIGURE 4–13 Chronic lymphocytic leukemia, microscopic

These mature-appearing lymphocytes in the peripheral blood are markedly increased in number. This form of leukocytosis is indicative of chronic lymphocytic leukemia (CLL), a disease most often seen in older adults, with a male-to-female ratio of 2:1. The cells often mark with CD19, CD20, CD23, and CD5 (a T-cell marker). Monoclonal immunoglobulin is displayed on cell surfaces, but there is unlikely to be a marked increase in circulating immunoglobulin. The peripheral leukocytosis is highly variable. CLL responds poorly to treatment, but it is indolent. In 15% to 30% of cases, there is transformation to a more aggressive lymphoid proliferation.

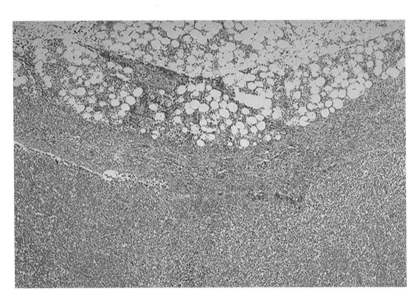

FIGURE 4–14 Small lymphocytic lymphoma, microscopic

This pattern of malignant lymphoma is diffuse, and no lymphoid follicles are identified. At low power, note that the normal architecture of this lymph node is obliterated. The lymph node is replaced by an infiltrate of small (mature-appearing) neoplastic lymphocytes, and the infiltrate extends through the capsule of the node and into the surrounding adipose tissue. The diagnosis is small lymphocytic lymphoma (SLL), which is the tissue phase of chronic lymphocytic leukemia (CLL). The molecular and biochemical characteristics of these SLL cells are identical to those of CLL. About 10% of cases transform to a diffuse large B-cell lymphoma.

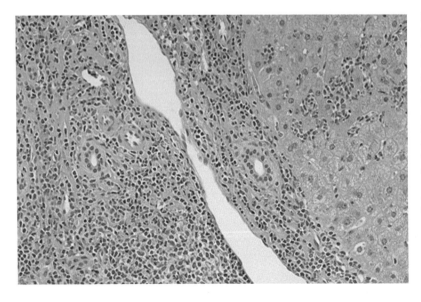

FIGURE 4–15 Small lymphocytic lymphoma, microscopic

These infiltrates within the liver are composed of small lymphocytes. The involvement of tissues in cases of CLL is SLL. Liver, spleen, and lymph nodes may become enlarged, although organ function is often not markedly diminished. This disease, CLL/SLL, has an indolent course. Chromosomal translocations are rare in CLL/SLL, although the immunoglobulin genes of some CLL/SLL patients are somatically hypermutated, and there may be a small immunoglobulin "spike" in the serum. An autoimmune hemolytic anemia appears in about one sixth of CLL/SLL cases.

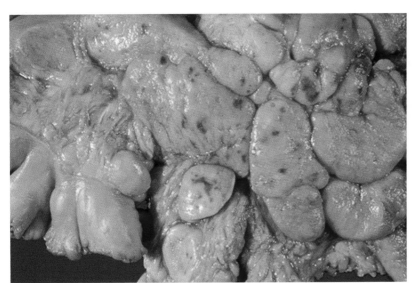

FIGURE 4–16 Non-Hodgkin follicular lymphoma, gross

This is a cross-section through the mesentery to reveal multiple enlarged lymph nodes that abut each other and are nearly confluent. Unlike metastases, lymph nodes involved by lymphoma tend to have little necrosis and only focal hemorrhage. They grossly maintain a solid, fleshy tan appearance on sectioning. High-grade non-Hodgkin lymphoma (NHL) may involve a single lymph node, a localized group of lymph nodes, or an extranodal site. Low-grade NHL tends to involve multiple lymph nodes at multiple sites, whereas high-grade NHLs tend to be more localized.

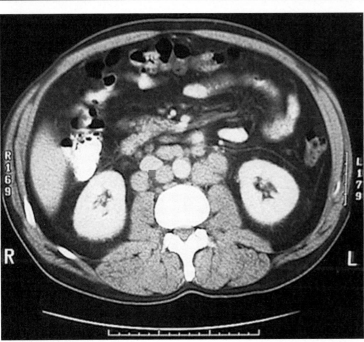

FIGURE 4–17 Follicular lymphoma, CT image

This abdominal CT with contrast demonstrates prominent periaortic lymphadenopathy (■) involving multiple nodes in a patient with low-grade non-Hodgkin follicular lymphoma. However, this appearance could represent any lymphoid neoplasm. Lymphadenopathy is the hallmark of many lymphoid neoplasms. Leukemia describes neoplasms with extensive bone marrow involvement and often peripheral leukocytosis. Lymphoma describes proliferations arising as discrete tissue masses either in lymph nodes or at extranodal sites. Hodgkin lymphoma (HL) is clinically and histologically distinct from the NHLs, is treated in a unique fashion, and is important to distinguish. All HLs and two thirds of NHLs present with nontender nodal enlargement. Plasma cell neoplasms are composed of terminally differentiated B cells and most commonly arise in the bone marrow, rarely involve lymph nodes, and rarely have a leukemic phase.

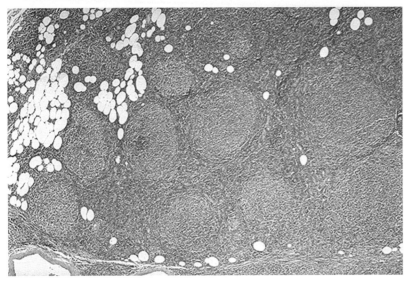

FIGURE 4–18 Follicular lymphoma, microscopic

Here is a lymph node involved by follicular lymphoma. The capsule of the node has been invaded, and the lymphoma cells extend into the surrounding adipose tissue. Note that the follicles are numerous and irregularly shaped, giving the nodular appearance seen here at low magnification. This is another form of B-cell lymphoma. The markers CD19, CD20, and CD10 (CALLA) are often present. In 90% of cases, a karyotype shows the t(14;18) translocation, which brings the immunoglobulin H (IgH) gene locus into juxtaposition with the *BCL2* gene, leading to overexpression of the BCL2 protein that inhibits apoptosis and promotes survival and accumulation of the abnormal lymphocytic cells. One third to one half of cases may transform to diffuse large B-cell lymphoma.

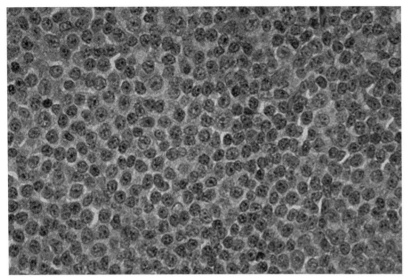

FIGURE 4–19 Diffuse large B-cell lymphoma, microscopic

Many NHLs in adults are large cell lymphomas such as the one here at medium power. Most are sporadic and most often of B-cell origin. The cells seen here are large, with large nuclei having prominent nucleoli and moderate amounts of cytoplasm. The cells often mark with CD10, CD19, and CD20 but are negative for TdT. The *BCL2* gene may be activated. Dysregulation of *BCL6*, a DNA-binding zinc-finger transcriptional regulator required for the formation of normal germinal centers, is often present. This disease tends to be localized (low stage), but with more rapid nodal enlargement and a greater propensity to be extranodal than the low-grade NHL.

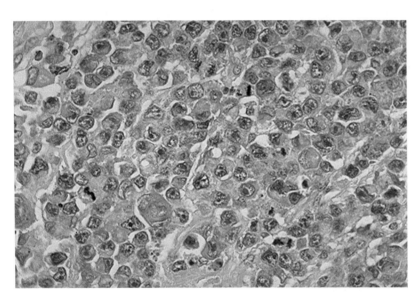

FIGURE 4–20 Diffuse large B-cell lymphoma, microscopic

The tumor cells have a round or oval vesicular nucleus with either multiple nucleoli located adjacent to the nuclear membrane or a single nucleolus centrally placed. The moderately abundant cytoplasm may be pale or basophilic. Mitoses are frequent. More anaplastic tumors may contain multinucleated cells with large, inclusion-like nucleoli, and these may be termed immunoblastic lymphoma. The major differential diagnosis in this case would be a metastatic carcinoma. The presence of cell surface monoclonal immunoglobulin as demonstrated by immunohistochemical staining would help to confirm this lesion as a malignant lymphoma.

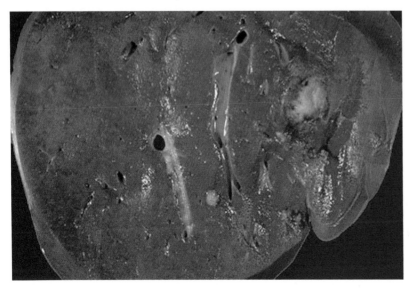

FIGURE 4–21 Diffuse large B-cell lymphoma, gross

Large cell NHLs have a propensity to involve extranodal locations. The Waldeyer ring of oropharyngeal lymphoid tissues, including tonsils and adenoids, is often involved, as are extranodal sites such as liver, spleen, gastrointestinal tract, skin, bone, and brain. Bone marrow involvement occurs late in the course, and leukemia is rare. Seen here on the cut surface of the liver are two rounded mass lesions. The color can range from white to tan to red, often intermixed. Diffuse large B-cell lymphoma can be associated with immunosuppressed states such as AIDS from HIV infection, whereas another subset arises with Kaposi sarcoma herpesvirus (KSHV) infection and leads to body cavity involvement marked by malignant pleural or peritoneal effusions. These aggressive neoplasms may respond to chemotherapy.

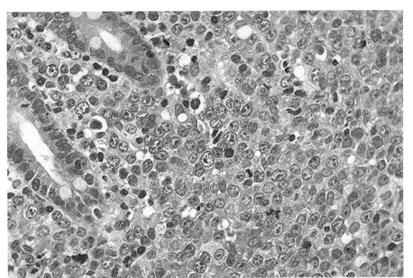

FIGURE 4–22 Burkitt lymphoma, microscopic

Seen here in small intestinal mucosa are large infiltrating cells of a Burkitt lymphoma, one of the most common lymphomas in Africa that most often appears in children and young adults and involves extranodal sites, particularly the mandible or the abdomen. In the United States, abdominal involvement is the most common presentation. The cells mark for CD10, CD19, and CD20. Mitoses and apoptosis with cellular debris cleared by large macrophages producing a "starry sky" pattern are prominent features. All forms of Burkitt lymphoma are associated with t(8;14) of the c-*MYC* gene on chromosome 8 to the IgH locus. Latent Epstein-Barr virus (EBV) infection occurs in essentially all endemic tumors, about 25% of HIV-associated tumors, and 15% to 20% of sporadic cases.

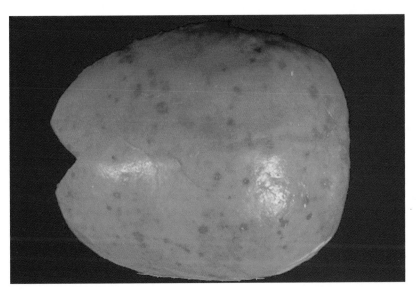

FIGURE 4–23 Multiple myeloma, gross

This skull removed at autopsy demonstrates the characteristic rounded "punched-out" lesions of multiple myeloma. The focal areas of plasma cell proliferation result in bone lysis to produce these lytic lesions. Such lesions can produce bone pain. A solitary lesion is termed plasmacytoma. Myeloma results from a monoclonal proliferation of relatively well-differentiated plasma cells often capable of producing light-chain and heavy-chain immunoglobulins. Proliferation and survival of these cells is dependent on elaboration of IL-6 by plasma cells and marrow stromal cells. Cytogenetic abnormalities may include t(4;14), which juxtaposes the IgH locus with the fibroblast growth factor receptor 3 (*FGFR3*) gene.

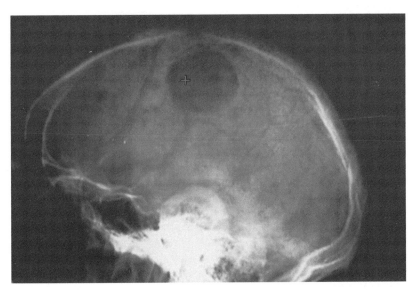

FIGURE 4–24 Multiple myeloma, x-ray

The "punched-out" circular lytic lesions (+) in the skull seen here are the result of multiple myeloma in an older adult. These lesions consist of a neoplastic proliferation of plasma cells that can produce laboratory findings, including hypercalcemia and an elevated serum alkaline phosphatase. A serum monoclonal globulin spike is typical. Increased production of immunoglobulin light chains can lead to excretion of the light chains in the urine, termed Bence-Jones proteinuria. The diminished amount of normal circulating immunoglobulin increases the risk for infections, particularly with bacterial organisms such as *Streptococcus pneumoniae*, *Haemophilus influenzae*, *Staphylococcus aureus*, and *Escherichia coli*.

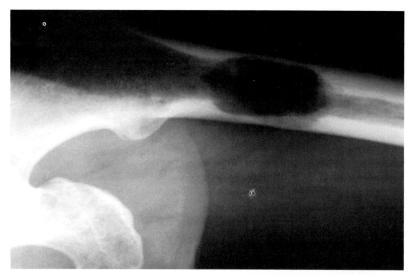

FIGURE 4–25 Plasmacytoma, x-ray

The rounded lucency seen here in the upper diaphysis of the femur is a plasmacytoma, a collection of plasma cells producing this lytic femoral lesion. About 3% to 5% of plasma cell neoplasms are solitary, but many progress to myeloma. Because this patient had other bone lesions, this is not a solitary plasmacytoma, but multiple myeloma. Cytokines produced by the tumor cells include MIP1a and the receptor activator of NF-*kB* ligand (RANKL) that serves as an osteoclast-activating factor. Chromosome analysis may show deletions of 13q and translocations involving the IgH locus on 14q32 with *FGFR3* on chromosome 4p16.

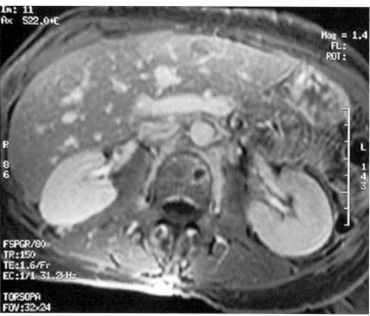

FIGURE 4–26 Multiple myeloma, MRI

The rounded lucency (▲) seen here in a vertebral body on T2-weighted MRI is one focus of plasma cells in a case of multiple myeloma. This patient had lesions in multiple sites. The lesions can produce bone pain. The total serum immunoglobulin level is often increased, with an immunoglobulin "spike" (of "M protein") seen on serum protein electrophoresis, and monoclonal bands of a single heavy-chain or light-chain class on immunoelectrophoresis of serum. Half of myelomas produce IgG and a fourth IgM. In 60% to 70% of cases, increased light chains (either kappa or lambda), known as Bence-Jones proteins, are produced and excreted in the urine, are toxic to renal tubules, and can lead to tubular injury with renal failure. The excessive light chain production may lead to the AL form of amyloidosis, with deposition of amyloid in many organs.

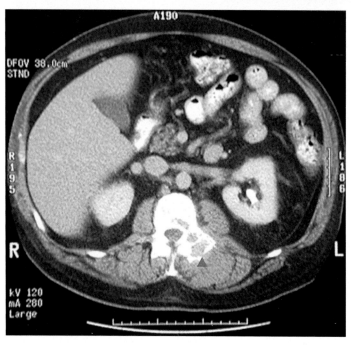

FIGURE 4–27 Plasmacytoma, CT image

The destructive, expansile lytic lesion (▲) seen here involving the L2 vertebral pedicle on the left with an abdominal CT scan is a solitary plasmacytoma. Bones in the axial skeleton are most often involved with plasma cell neoplasms: vertebral column, 66%; ribs, 44%; skull, 41%; pelvis, 28%; femur, 24%; clavicle, 10%; and scapula, 10%. The focal lesions typically begin in the medullary cavity, erode cancellous bone, and progressively destroy the bony cortex, leading to pathologic fractures, typically vertebral compressed fractures. The bone lesions appear radiographically as punched-out defects, usually 1 to 4 cm in diameter. Most cases of solitary plasmacytoma involving bone evolve into multiple myeloma.

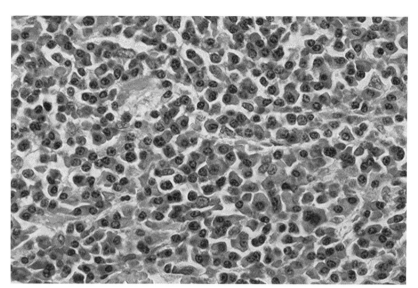

FIGURE 4–28 Multiple myeloma, microscopic

In this bone marrow biopsy section at medium power, there are sheets of plasma cells that are very similar to normal plasma cells, with eccentric nuclei and abundant pale purple cytoplasm. In some cases, the myeloma cells may also be poorly differentiated. Usually, the plasma cells are differentiated enough to retain the function of immunoglobulin production, but in less than 1% of cases, there is no increase in circulating immunoglobulin. Thus, myelomas are typically detected by an immunoglobulin "spike" on protein electrophoresis or by the presence of Bence-Jones proteins (light chains) in the urine. Immunoelectrophoresis characterizes the type of monoclonal immunoglobulin being produced.

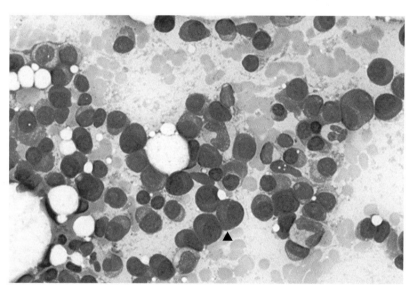

FIGURE 4–29 Multiple myeloma, microscopic

Here is a smear of bone marrow aspirate from a patient with multiple myeloma. The neoplastic plasma cells (▲) usually constitute more than 30% of the cellularity. Note that there are numerous well-differentiated plasma cells with eccentric nuclei and a perinuclear halo of clearer cytoplasm (representing the Golgi apparatus). Clear cytoplasmic droplets contain immunoglobulin. There is also an abnormal plasma cell with a double nucleus. However, this neoplasm is typically well differentiated, with easily recognizable plasma cells, most of which are hardly distinguishable from normal plasma cells, except by their increased numbers. Plasma cell leukemia is rare.

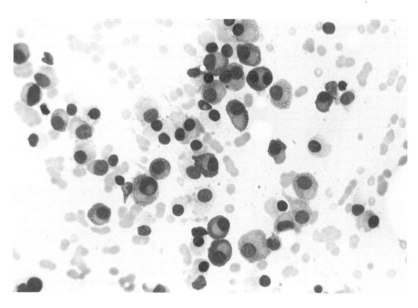

FIGURE 4–30 Waldenström macroglobulinemia, microscopic

This form of B-cell lymphoma, illustrated here in a bone marrow smear, is seen in older adults and is widely distributed, but it has plasmacytoid differentiation so that many cells resemble plasma cells and can secrete immunoglobulin. There are characteristic PAS-positive cytoplasmic inclusions known as Dutcher bodies. Many of these neoplasms secrete substantial amounts of monoclonal IgM, leading to a hyperviscosity syndrome with clinical findings of reduced vision, headaches, dizziness, coagulopathy, and cryoglobulinemia with cold agglutinins and hemolytic anemia.

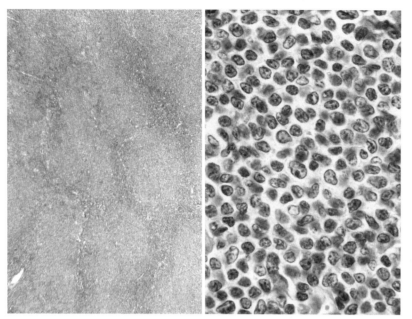

FIGURE 4–31 Mantle cell lymphoma, microscopic

At low power, there is a vaguely nodular pattern, and at high power, the slightly large lymphocytes have folded (cleaved) nuclei. In addition to pan-B markers CD19 and CD20, these cells mark with CD5 and CD22, but not CD23. Most cases involve the bone marrow, but about 20% are associated with leukemia. Mantle cell lymphoma has a tendency to involve the GI tract with submucosal polypoid nodules. The characteristic karyotypic abnormality is t(11;14) with fusion of the cyclin D1 gene on chromosome 11 to the immunoglobulin heavy-chain promoter/enhancer region on chromosome 14, leading to increased cyclin D1 expression with loss of cell cycle regulation.

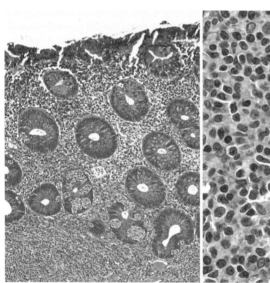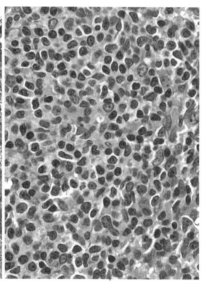

FIGURE 4–32 Marginal zone lymphoma, microscopic

The extranodal lymphoma seen here involving gastric mucosa is known as a mucosa-associated lymphoid tissue (MALT) lesion and is composed of small round to irregular lymphocytes resembling those seen in the marginal zone of lymphoid follicles. Some of the cells may be plasmacytoid. The cells tend to invade epithelium as small nests. MALT lesions often arise in areas of chronic inflammation, such as gastritis with *Helicobacter pylori* infection, sialadenitis with Sjögren syndrome, and Hashimoto thyroiditis. MALT lesions are indolent and may regress after elimination of a predisposing inflammatory stimulus or by local excision.

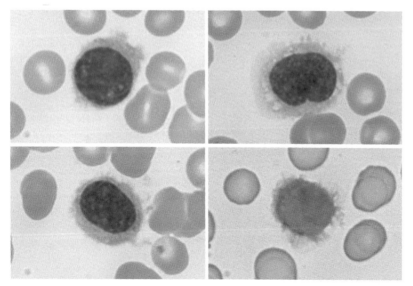

FIGURE 4–33 Hairy cell leukemia, microscopic

This collage of peripheral blood smears depicts abnormal lymphocytes with indistinct cytoplasmic borders and projections, giving the cells a "hairy" appearance. The red cytoplasmic staining is from tartrate-resistant acid phosphatase (TRAP) positivity. Hairy cell leukemia (HCL) is an uncommon B-cell proliferation seen mostly in older males. Hairy cells usually express pan-B-cell markers CD19 and CD20, surface IgH, CD11c, CD25, and CD103. Clinical manifestations include splenomegaly, often massive. Hepatomegaly is less common and not marked; lymphadenopathy is rare. Pancytopenia occurs in more than half of cases. HCL often has an indolent course, and chemotherapy often produces long-lasting remission.

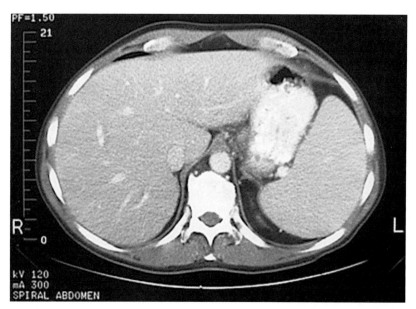

FIGURE 4–34 Hairy cell leukemia, CT image

This abdominal CT with contrast demonstrates marked splenomegaly in a 55-year-old man with HCL. The liver is only slightly increased in size. Both liver and spleen have uniform attenuation, typical for lymphoid neoplasms, which are often diffusely infiltrative and rarely necrotic or hemorrhagic. The clinical findings of HCL most often result from splenic and bone marrow involvement, with pancytopenia from decreased marrow function as well as increased splenic sequestration of peripheral blood cells (secondary hypersplenism). Thus, unlike many other leukemias, a peripheral leukocytosis is the exception and not the rule in HCL.

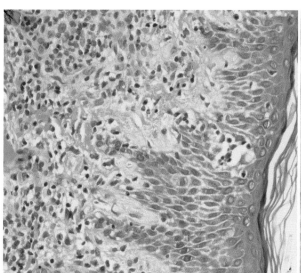
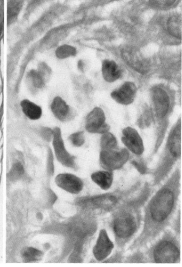

FIGURE 4–35 Mycosis fungoides, microscopic

This is the most common form of cutaneous lymphoma, a local or generalized T-cell neoplasm of CD4 helper cells. Note the small cells with convoluted nuclei infiltrating the dermis and extending into epidermis as Pautrier microabscesses. An inflammatory premycotic phase progresses through a plaque phase to a tumor phase on the skin. The course of the disease tends to be indolent.

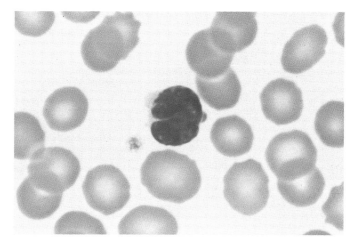

FIGURE 4–36 Sézary syndrome, microscopic

Disease progression of mycosis fungoides is characterized by extracutaneous spread, most commonly to lymph nodes and bone marrow. Sézary syndrome occurs when skin involvement is manifested by generalized exfoliative erythroderma and an associated leukemia of "Sézary" cells with characteristic cerebriform nuclei. Note the appearance of the deep-clefted, cerebriform nucleus in this circulating lymphocyte. Late in the course of this disease, transformation to a large T-cell lymphoma often occurs.

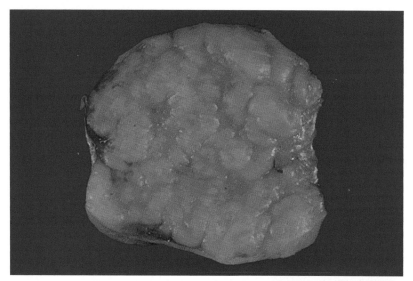

FIGURE 4–37 Hodgkin lymphoma, gross

Here is an enlarged 5-cm lymph node (obviously from a patient with lymphadenopathy). A lymph node should normally be soft and pink and less than 1 cm in size. This lymph node is involved with HL. This gross appearance could pass for NHL as well, with a slightly lobulated, tan to pink cut surface and no or minimal necrosis and hemorrhage. On physical examination, nodes involved with a neoplasm are usually nontender. HL, just like NHL, can involve a single node, a group of nodes, or multiple lymph node sites. HL (previously termed Hodgkin disease) may also be extranodal and involve bone marrow, spleen, and liver.

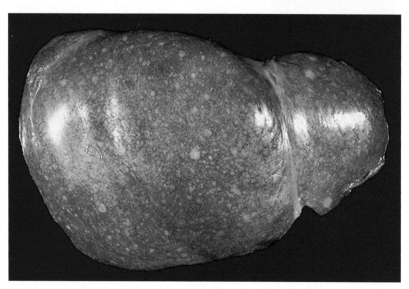

FIGURE 4–38 Hodgkin lymphoma, gross

This is a liver that is involved with HL. The staging of HL is very important in determining therapy. Thus, it is important to determine whether the patient has only a single lymph node region involved, multiple node regions, or extranodal involvement. HL typically occurs with contiguous spread. Grossly and radiographically, mass lesions are often present. This picture could probably suffice for extranodal NHL hepatic disease as well.

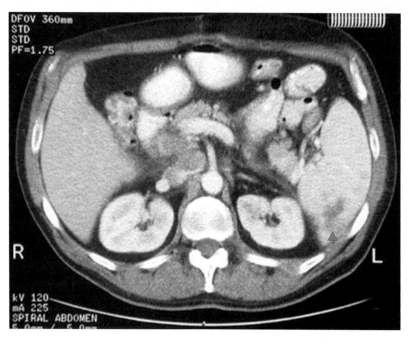

FIGURE 4–39 Hodgkin lymphoma, CT image

This abdominal CT reveals one larger (▲) and several smaller more darkly attenuated splenic mass lesions representing extranodal involvement by HL. There is also prominent lymphadenopathy (◆). Staging of HL is important to determine therapy and the prognosis. Staging is often done by radiographic means, with CT scans used to determine where lymphadenopathy or extranodal lesions are located, ultrasonography to determine size and lesions of liver and spleen, and chest radiograph. Staging laparotomy is not commonly used because radiographic procedures yield excellent results. Many patients respond to chemotherapy, particularly those at a younger age, with lower stage of disease, and with absence of constitutional symptoms. After therapy, about 5% of patients develop myelodysplastic syndromes, acute myelogenous leukemia or carcinomas, particularly of the lung.

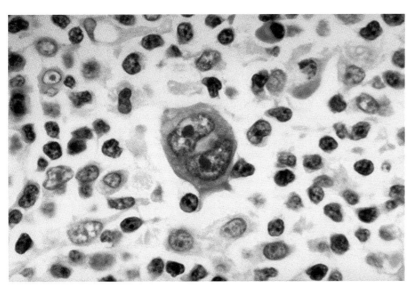

FIGURE 4–40 Hodgkin lymphoma, microscopic

The classic microscopic finding with HL is the Reed-Sternberg cell. This multinucleated cell typically comprises only 1% to 5% of the cellular mass of the neoplasm, with the remainder composed of reactive cells and connective tissue. The prototypical Reed-Sternberg cell is bilobed with mirror-image halves, and the large nuclei have an "owl eye" appearance from prominent nucleoli. These cells can be multinucleated. Clinical findings in about 40% of cases may include constitutional ("B") symptoms, such as fever, night sweats, and weight loss. Some patients have pruritus. Ingestion of alcohol may cause pain at involved sites.

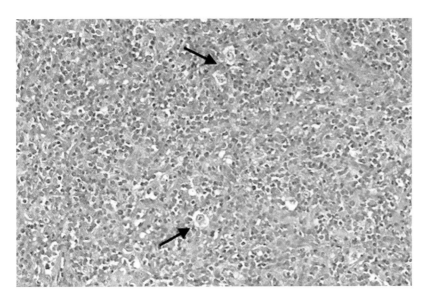

FIGURE 4–41 Hodgkin lymphoma, microscopic

There are scattered large cells with a surrounding prominent clear space, an artefact of formalin fixation. These are lacunar cells, a mononuclear variant of the Reed-Sternberg cell, which are often seen in HL, and they are most characteristic of the nodular sclerosis type of HL. Note the background of reactive cells that compose most of the cellular mass of HL, which accumulate as a consequence of cytokine release by Reed-Sternberg cells, including IL-5, IL-6, IL-13, TNF, and granulocyte-macrophage colony-stimulating factor. EBV DNA is found in some cases. Laboratory findings may include anemia, leukocytosis, and an elevated erythrocyte sedimentation rate.

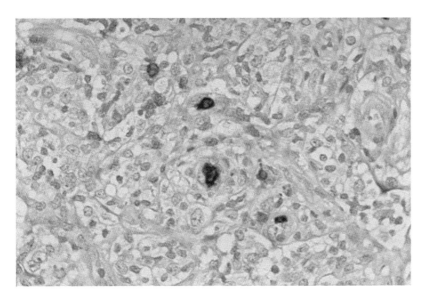

FIGURE 4–42 Hodgkin lymphoma, microscopic

Reed-Sternberg and lacunar cells can be identified in HL, marking with CD15 and CD30, but not CD20 or CD45. Note that these cells compose only a fraction of the volume of the cellular proliferation, as shown here marked with CD-15. Cytokines released by Reed-Sternberg cells and their variants lead to the accumulation of the multitude of reactive cells, including lymphocytes, granulocytes, macrophages, and fibroblasts. Cell-mediated immunity is often reduced, as evidenced by anergy with skin testing.

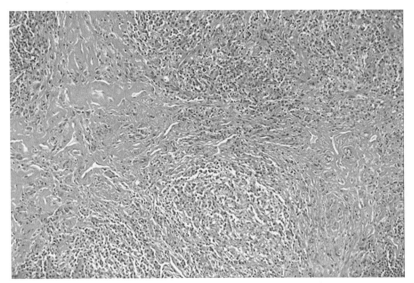

FIGURE 4–43 Hodgkin lymphoma, nodular sclerosis, microscopic

Note the bands of pink collagenous tissue dividing the low-power field in this lymph node. Nodular sclerosing HL is the most common form of HL, constituting about two thirds of HL cases. It is most common in young adults. It is characterized by prominent bands of fibrosis. The background has lymphocytes, plasma cells, eosinophils, and macrophages. There can be scattered Reed-Sternberg cells, as well as lacunar cells that are common in this type of HL. Histologic diagnosis is typically made from biopsy of an involved lymph node. A bone marrow biopsy is usually performed as well. Most nodular sclerosis cases are the lower stage I or II.

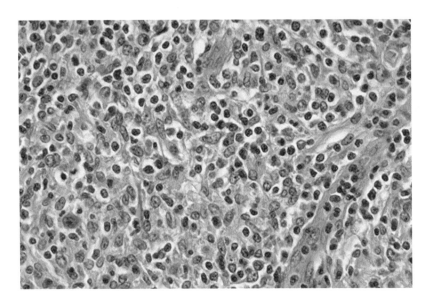

FIGURE 4–44 Hodgkin lymphoma, mixed cellularity, microscopic

Note the many different cell types, including small lymphocytes, eosinophils, and macrophages. There are often many lacunar cells and Reed-Sternberg cells. It is more common in males and strongly associated with EBV. Compared with the lymphocyte predominance and nodular sclerosis subtypes, mixed cellularity subtype is more likely to be associated with older age, systemic symptoms such as night sweats, and weight loss. Although more than half of cases of HL of this histologic type are the higher stage III or IV, the prognosis is still good.

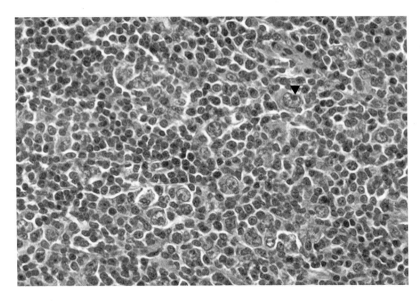

FIGURE 4–45 Hodgkin lymphoma, lymphocyte predominance, microscopic

The background of lymphocytes and paucity of Reed-Sternberg cells make this type of HL sometimes difficult to distinguish from small cell lymphomas. Variant Reed-Sternberg cells with multilobulated or large nuclei (▼) are seen here. In the lymphocyte-rich form of HL, reactive lymphocytes make up most of the cellular infiltrate. In most cases, lymph nodes are diffusely effaced, but vague nodularity due to the presence of residual B-cell follicles can sometimes be seen. This form is distinguished from the lymphocyte predominance type by the presence of frequent Reed-Sternberg cells. It is associated with EBV in about 40% of cases and also has a very good to excellent prognosis.

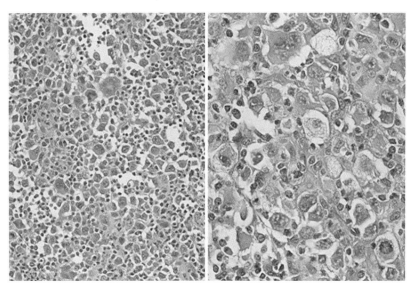

FIGURE 4–46 Hodgkin disease, lymphocyte depletion, microscopic

Many Reed-Sternberg variants are present here. Few lymphocytes or other reactive cells are found. The lymphocyte depletion type of HL is the least common form. They may resemble large cell NHLs. Lymphocyte depletion HL most often occurs in older patients, particularly men, or in association with HIV infection. It is often EBV associated. Advanced stage and systemic symptoms are frequent, and the overall outcome is somewhat less favorable than with other subtypes.

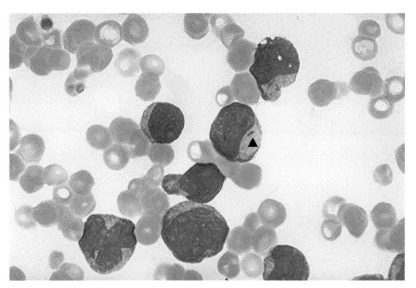

FIGURE 4–47 Acute myelogenous leukemia, microscopic

Acute myelogenous leukemias (AMLs) arise when acquired genetic alterations inhibit terminal myeloid differentiation, leading to replacement of normal marrow elements by relatively undifferentiated blasts exhibiting one or more types of early myeloid differentiation. On this peripheral blood smear are large, immature myeloblasts with nuclei that have fine chromatin and multiple nucleoli. A distinctive feature of these blasts is the linear red "Auer rod" (▲) composed of crystallized azurophilic granules. AML is most prevalent in young adults. Subclassifications of AML are based on cellular morphology. The M2 type seen here, the most common type, has prominent Auer rods with a range of immature to mature myeloid cells present.

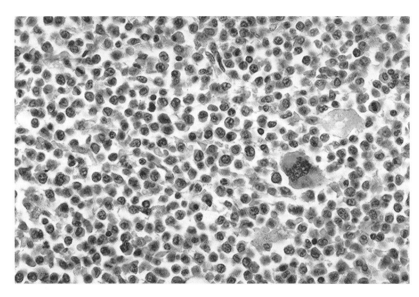

FIGURE 4–48 Acute myelogenous leukemia, microscopic

This bone marrow of a patient with AML has one lone megakaryocyte, and the remaining cells are mainly immature myeloid precursors. Leukemias typically fill the marrow, displacing normal hematopoiesis. The marrow here is essentially 100% cellular but composed almost exclusively of leukemic cells. Normal hematopoiesis is reduced by replacement (a "myelophthisic" process) or by suppressed stem cell division. Thus, leukemic patients are prone to anemia, thrombocytopenia, and granulocytopenia and all the complications that ensue, particularly complications of bleeding and infection.

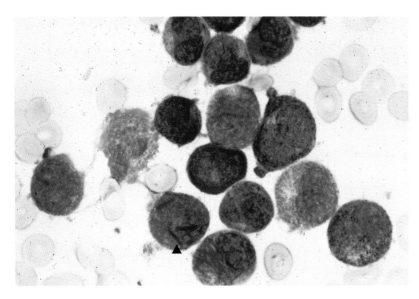

FIGURE 4–49 Acute promyelocytic leukemia, microscopic

This M3 variant of AML, with cells resembling promyelocytes, shows numerous coarse azurophilic cytoplasmic granules as well as Auer rods (▲). The characteristic t(15;17) karyotypic abnormality with M3 results in fusion of the retinoic acid receptor α-gene on chromosome 17 with the PML gene on chromosome 15, leading to blockage of myeloid differentiation at the promyelocytic stage. For this reason, treatment with retinoic acid, a vitamin A analog, overcomes the block. Cell death with release of granules into the peripheral blood can cause disseminated intravascular coagulation.

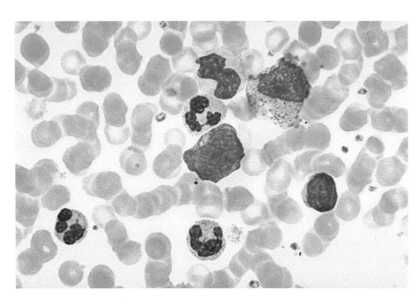

FIGURE 4–50 Chronic myelogenous leukemia, microscopic

On this peripheral blood smear are immature myeloid cells and band neutrophils. CML is one of the myeloproliferative disorders, and unlike AML, there are less than 10% circulating blasts. CML is most prevalent in middle-aged adults. A useful test to help distinguish CML from leukemoid reaction is the LAP score, which should be low with CML and high with a leukemoid reaction. CML may also involve the spleen, liver, and lymph nodes. Since some cases arise from malignant transformation in a pleuripotential cell line, there may also be erythroid and megakaryocytic involvement.

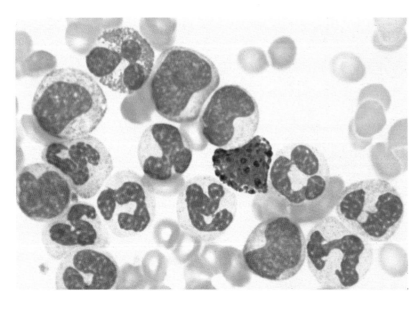

FIGURE 4–51 Chronic myelogenous leukemia, microscopic

Often in CML, the numbers of basophils and eosinophils, as well as bands and immature myeloid cells (metamyelocytes and myelocytes), are increased. Myeloid cells of CML also have the Philadelphia chromosome (Ph1) on karyotyping from a translocation of a portion of the q arm of chromosome 22 to the q arm of chromosome 9, designated t(9:22). This translocation brings the C-*ABL* proto-oncogene on chromosome 9 in approximation with the *BCR* (breakpoint cluster) gene on chromosome 22. The hybrid BCR-ABL fusion gene encodes a tyrosine kinase that has growth-promoting effects through nuclear stimulation.

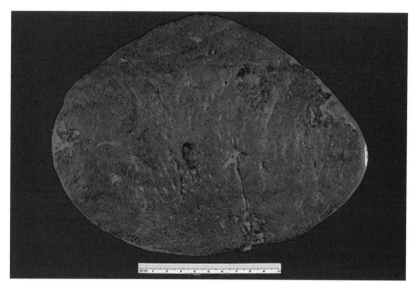

FIGURE 4–52 Myeloproliferative disorder, gross

This large spleen (the ruler is 15 cm long) has subcapsular yellow-tan infarcts. Massive splenomegaly is usually indicative of myeloproliferative disorders including CML, polycythemia vera, essential thrombocytosis, and primary myelofibrosis. They may "blast out" to an acute leukemia. They often terminate in marrow fibrosis, with pancytopenia, extramedullary hematopoiesis, and splenomegaly. Although congestive splenomegaly is unlikely to exceed 1000 gm, a spleen larger than 1000 gm suggests underlying myeloproliferative, lymphoproliferative, or hematopoietic disorders. Chronic infections such as malaria or leishmaniasis may also produce marked splenomegaly. Secondary hypersplenism follows.

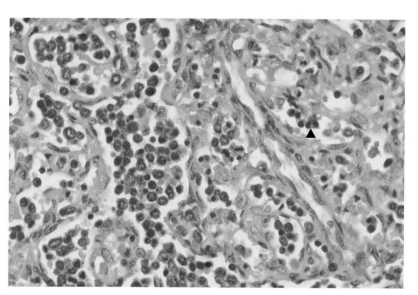

FIGURE 4–53 Myeloproliferative disorder, microscopic

This spleen shows extramedullary hematopoiesis, a proliferation of RBC and other hematopoietic precursors (▲), usually in the organs of the mononuclear phagocyte system, that often accompanies a myeloproliferative disorder involving bone marrow. Peripheral blood findings in myeloproliferative disorders include leukoerythroblastosis and giant platelets. As the disease progresses to myelofibrosis from secretion of cytokines such as transforming growth factor-β and platelet-derived growth factor, there is pancytopenia, and the patient is at risk for infection, bleeding, and high-output congestive heart failure. Some myeloproliferative disorders evolve to AML.

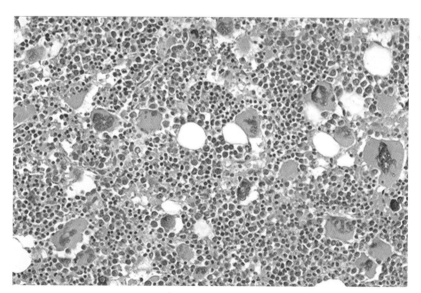

FIGURE 4–54 Essential thrombocytosis, microscopic

Seen here in bone marrow are numerous megakaryocytes in an uncommon process called essential thrombocytosis in which peripheral platelet counts can exceed 1,000,000/μm. A myeloproliferative process can involve the marrow, filling it up with abnormal cellular proliferations. There can be a proliferation of predominantly myeloid elements to produce findings of CML, erythroid elements to produce polycythemia vera, or megakaryocytic elements to yield essential thrombocytosis. The chronic myeloproliferative process may continue for years or "blast out" into a leukemia or "burn out" into a myelofibrosis.

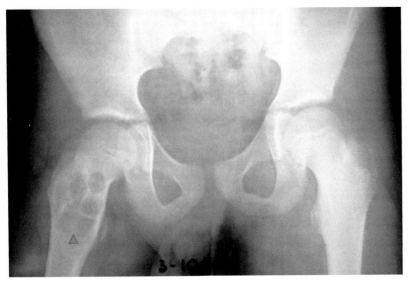

FIGURE 4–55 Langerhans cell histiocytosis, CT image

There are several forms of Langerhans cell histiocytosis, a proliferative disorder of immature dendritic cells with features of macrophages. The acute disseminated form known as Letterer-Siwe disease is seen before 2 years of age with mainly cutaneous lesions and visceral involvement. There is a unifocal to multifocal form called eosinophilic granuloma that mainly involves bones in children and young adults. Seen here in the right upper femur is a multilocular eosinophilic granuloma of bone (▲). Such lesions can be unilocular as well as multilocular. If the pituitary stalk is involved, there is a Hand-Schüller-Christian triad of skull lesions with diabetes insipidus and exophthalmos.

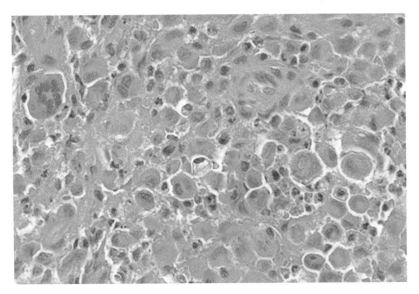

FIGURE 4–56 Langerhans cell histiocytosis, microscopic

The eosinophilic granuloma of bone is one of the Langerhans cell histiocytoses. The characteristic cell is an oval to round macrophage-like cell, interspersed with inflammatory cells, including eosinophils. Eosinophilic granuloma is most common in children and young adults. This lesion forms within the marrow cavity and can expand to cause erosion of bone that produces pain or pathologic fracture. Some lesions heal spontaneously by fibrosis, whereas others may require curettement. Sites of involvement with more disseminated forms of Langerhans cell histiocytosis include skin, lymph nodes, spleen, liver, lungs, and bone marrow.

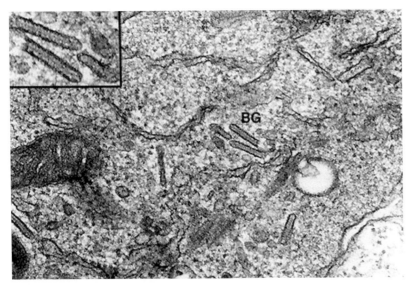

FIGURE 4–57 Langerhans cell histiocytosis, EM

Birbeck granules (inset shows several at higher magnification) are seen here in a Langerhans cell from a case of histiocytosis X, one of the forms of peculiar neoplastic proliferations known as the Langerhans cell histiocytoses. The cells express HLA-DR, S-100, and CD1a. They have abundant, often vacuolated cytoplasm and vesicular nuclei containing linear grooves or folds. Pulmonary Langerhans cell histiocytosis is most often seen in adult smokers, can regress spontaneously on cessation of smoking, and usually comprises a polyclonal population of Langerhans cells, suggesting it is a reactive hyperplasia rather than a true neoplasm.

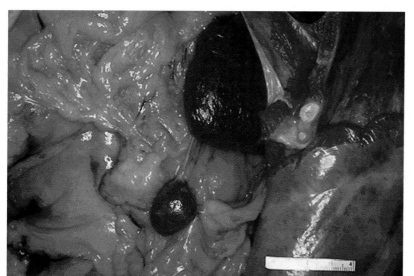

FIGURE 4–58 Normal spleen with accessory spleen, gross

The normal spleen in the left upper quadrant seen here at autopsy is accompanied by a smaller accessory spleen. An accessory spleen is not that uncommon and is usually just an incidental finding. Remember, though, that the accessory spleen can undergo all the changes that the larger spleen can. There is also an uncommon condition known as "splenosis" that occurs when portions of a disrupted spleen (usually from blunt abdominal trauma) implant on peritoneal surfaces and grow and continue to function, even after the damaged spleen is removed ("born again" spleen).

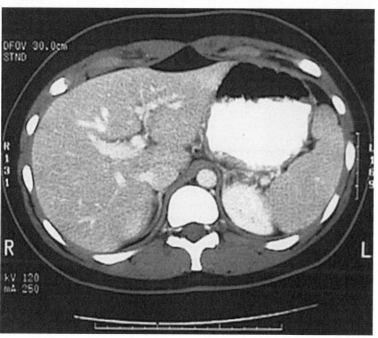

FIGURE 4–59 Normal spleen, CT image

The normal size and position of the spleen in an abdominal CT with intravenous contrast (and oral contrast in the stomach) is shown. The attenuation (brightness) of the normal spleen and liver are similar. The spleen acts as a filter, removing old RBCs and RBC inclusions, such as Heinz bodies and Howell-Jolly bodies, as RBCs move through sinusoids. Splenic phagocytes also actively remove other particulate matter from the blood, such as bacteria, cell debris, and WBCs. The spleen also acts as a storage area for about one third of all circulating platelets. Abnormal macromolecules produced with some inborn errors of metabolism, such as Gaucher disease and Niemann-Pick disease, may accumulate in splenic phagocytes and lead to splenomegaly.

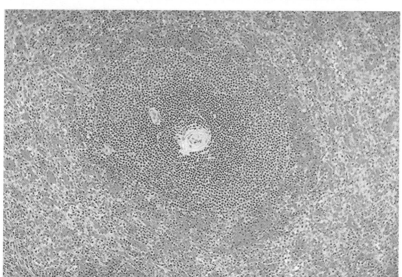

FIGURE 4–60 Normal spleen, microscopic

Note the small lymphocytes centered on the splenic arteriole at the center, forming the white pulp. Around this is the red pulp composed of many splenic sinusoids. The spleen, a key part of the immune system, has dendritic cells in periarterial lymphatic sheaths that trap antigens and present them to T lymphocytes, where T and B cells interact at the edges of white pulp follicles, generating antibody-secreting plasma cells found mainly within the sinuses of red pulp. The lack of splenic function from splenectomy or with autoinfarction (sickle cell disease) leads to susceptibility to disseminated infection with encapsulated bacteria such as pneumococcus, meningococcus, and *Haemophilus influenzae*.

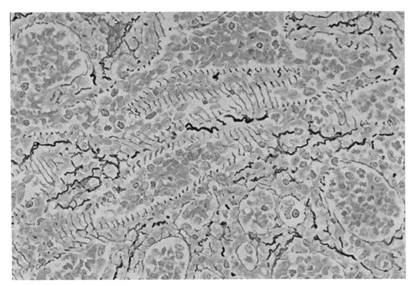

FIGURE 4–61 Normal spleen, microscopic

The normal structure of splenic red pulp in normal spleen is demonstrated here with a reticulin stain. The "barrel ribs" of reticulin fibers outline longitudinal sinusoids in the red pulp through which the blood flows. RBCs must squeeze through slit pores in the sinusoids, and in so doing must deform. RBCs with abnormal shape or size, such as spherocytes or elliptocytes or sickled cells, cannot do so and may be removed from circulation. RBCs with immunoglobulin or complement bound to their surfaces are more likely to be removed in the spleen, a process called extravascular hemolysis.

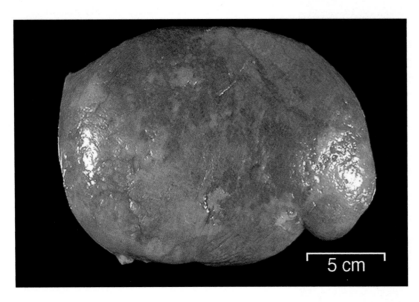

FIGURE 4–62 Congestive splenomegaly, gross

One of the most common causes of splenomegaly is portal hypertension with hepatic cirrhosis. It may also result from right-sided cardiac failure with cor pulmonale. Either micronodular cirrhosis from chronic alcohol abuse or macronodular cirrhosis after hepatitis B or C infection may lead to portal hypertension. Note that this spleen also shows irregular tan-white fibrous plaques over the purple capsular surface. This "sugar icing" has the name hyaline perisplenitis. The increased portal venous pressure causes dilation of sinusoids, with slowing of blood flow from the cords to the sinusoids that prolongs the exposure of the blood cells to the cordal macrophages, resulting in excessive trapping and destruction (hypersplenism).

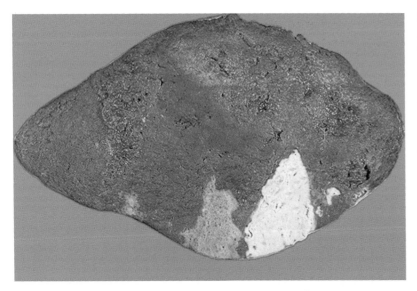

FIGURE 4–63 Splenic infarcts, gross

Here are splenic infarcts as a consequence of systemic arterial embolization in a patient with an infective endocarditis involving either aortic or mitral valve. Portions of the friable vegetations have embolized to the spleen through the splenic artery branch from the celiac axis and then to the peripheral splenic artery branches. Most splenic infarcts are due to emboli that arise from thrombi in the heart, either vegetations on valves or mural thrombi. These infarcts are typical of ischemic infarcts: they are based on the capsule, pale, and wedge-shaped. The remaining splenic parenchyma appears dark red. Clinical findings of left upper quadrant pain and splenic enlargement may occur.

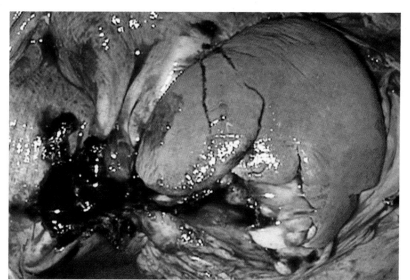

FIGURE 4–64 Splenic trauma, gross

Splenic rupture results most often from blunt force injury with abdominal trauma. Seen here are two large capsular lacerations in a patient who was involved in a motor vehicle crash. Note the hematoma formation resulting from the splenic rupture. The hemorrhage can extend into the peritoneal cavity to produce hemoperitoneum. Enlargement of the spleen from predisposing conditions that render the spleen prone to rupture even with minor trauma include infectious mononucleosis, malaria, typhoid fever, and lymphoid neoplasms.

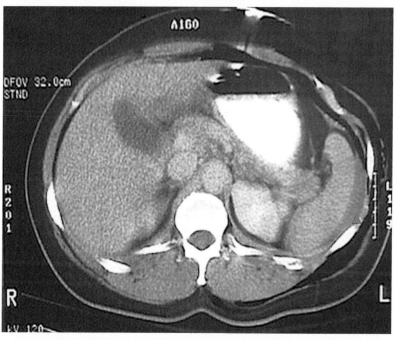

FIGURE 4–65 Splenic trauma, CT image

This abdominal CT with contrast demonstrates a hematoma (▲) lateral to a ruptured spleen from blunt force abdominal trauma. The peritoneal lavage performed on this patient yielded bloody fluid, a clue to the diagnosis. The spleen needs to be surgically removed after such injury with splenic capsular rupture since the capsule cannot be repaired.

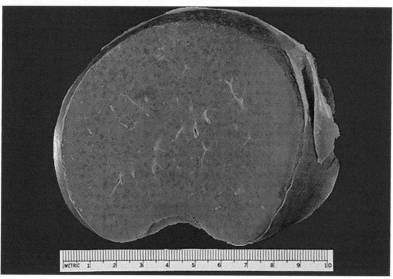

FIGURE 4–66 Splenic amyloidosis, gross

This enlarged spleen has the gross appearance and feel of wax. This is amyloidosis of the spleen, which can have either the diffuse "lardaceous" pattern seen here, or the nodular "sago" pattern with amyloid deposited mainly in the white pulp. This amyloid proved to be of the immunologic AL type (primary amyloidosis) because the patient had multiple myeloma. The AA type of amyloid from reactive systemic processes (secondary amyloidosis) can produce similar findings.

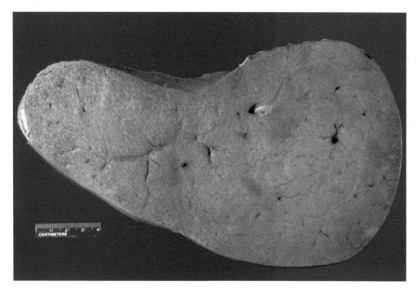

FIGURE 4–67 Gaucher disease, gross

This enlarged spleen is pale and has a firm feel. This young patient had an inborn error of metabolism with lack of the enzyme glucocerebrosidase, resulting in accumulation of storage product in cells of the mononuclear phagocyte system. There are three types of Gaucher disease. The most common, type 1 (99% of cases), is the non-neurologic form in which the affected person has normal intelligence and lives into adulthood. Type 2 is the neuronopathic form lethal in infancy, whereas type 3 has a course intermediate between the other types.

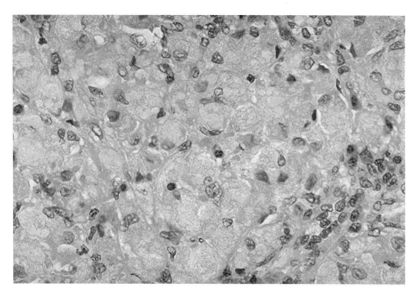

FIGURE 4–68 Gaucher disease, microscopic

This is a type of lysosomal storage disease with accumulation of the nonmetabolized storage product mainly in macrophages. Note the large pale pink macrophages here. Numerous clusters of these macrophages are present in an enlarged spleen, an appearance typical of a storage disease. The accumulation of these cells in marrow may produce a mass effect with bone pain, deformity, and fracture. Other tissues of the mononuclear phagocyte system, including lymphoid tissues and liver, may also be involved. Perivascular accumulation of macrophages in type 2 Gaucher disease leads to neuronal loss.

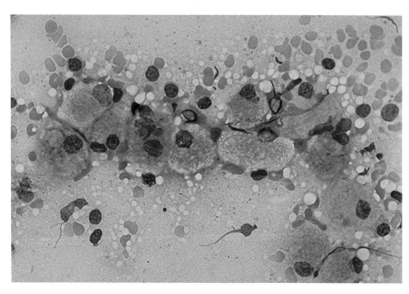

FIGURE 4–69 Gaucher disease, microscopic

The delicate cytoplasm of Gaucher cells in a bone marrow smear resembles crinkled tissue paper from the abundance of accumulated cytoplasmic lipid. As in many genetic diseases resulting from enzymic abnormalities, measurement of enzyme activity, in this case glucocerebrosidase activity, in peripheral blood leukocytes or skin fibroblasts can be performed to confirm the diagnosis. As in many genetic diseases, multiple allelic mutations in Gaucher disease complicate detection, for there is often no single genetic test to detect all cases. Different alleles may lead to different enzymic activities, with variable severity of the disease.

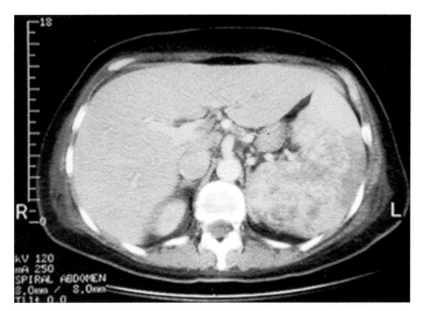

FIGURE 4–70 Splenic angiosarcoma, CT image

Considering its size and blood flow, the spleen is an uncommon site of either primary hematologic or metastatic neoplasms, probably because of its role in immunologic surveillance. If the spleen is the site of a neoplastic process, it is most often involved by leukemias, but may also be the site of extranodal involvement with NHL or HL. Seen here in on abdominal CT scan is a large heterogenous mass that expands the spleen and that proved to be an angiosarcoma, a malignant proliferation of primitive mesenchymal cells with vascular differentiation.

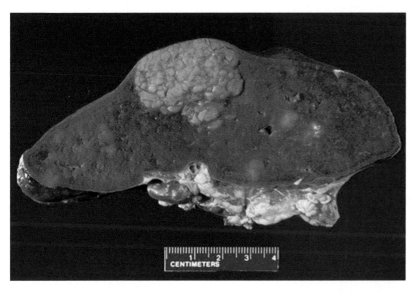

FIGURE 4–71 Splenic Hodgkin lymphoma, gross

The large pale nodule and several smaller nodules seen in this section are the result of splenic involvement by HL. Splenic masses are more likely to be due to hematopoietic diseases rather than metastases.

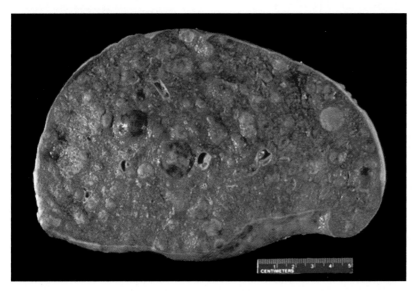

FIGURE 4–72 Splenic metastases, gross

Despite its size, the spleen is a rare site of metastases from nonhematologic malignancies. Seen here are metastases from a malignant melanoma of the skin. Note that most of these masses are tan, but some have brown-black pigmentation from the melanin elaborated by the neoplastic cells. Melanomas are aggressive neoplasms that can often be widely metastatic.

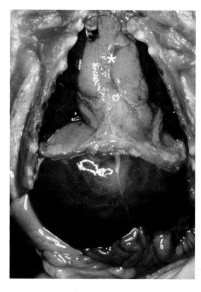
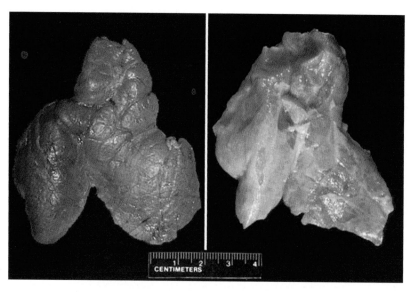

FIGURE 4–73 Normal infant in situ, gross and 4–74 Comparison of normal fetal and adult thymus, gross

The thymus (∗) in the anterior mediastinum of the chest is prominent in late fetal life, as seen on the far left, in infancy, as well as in childhood. On the left is the normal pink thymus of a term infant, compared with the somewhat smaller adult thymus on the right. In development of the immune system, the thymus is an important place to which marrow stem cells migrate and give rise to T-lymphocytes. In adults, the thymus is almost completely replaced by adipose tissue.

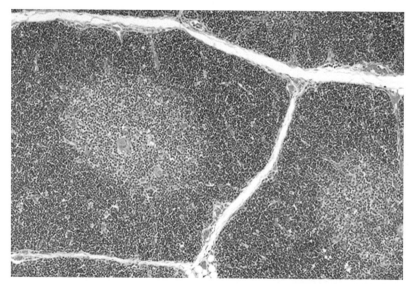

FIGURE 4–75 Normal thymus, microscopic

The normal third-trimester thymus of a fetus seen here at low magnification is well populated with T lymphocytes. There is a well-defined cortex and medulla. There are Hassall corpuscles composed of epithelial cells in the center of the medullary regions. In embryonic development of the immune system, progenitor cells of marrow origin migrate to the thymus and give rise to mature T cells that are exported to the periphery. The thymic production of T cells slowly declines during adulthood as the organ atrophies. In addition to the thymocytes and epithelial cells, macrophages, dendritic cells, few B lymphocytes, rare neutrophils and eosinophils, and scattered myoid (muscle-like) cells are found within the thymus.

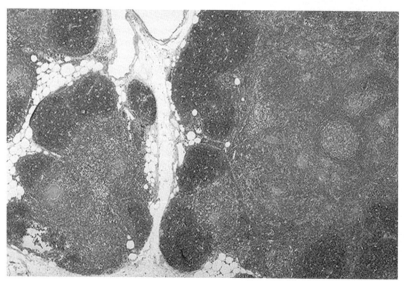

FIGURE 4–76 Thymic hyperplasia, microscopic

About two thirds to three fourths of patients diagnosed with myasthenia gravis (MG) have thymic hyperplasia, as seen here at low magnification. Ordinarily, the thymus in an adult is composed mostly of adipose tissue, with a few clusters of lymphocytes and residual Hassall corpuscles. Here the lymphoid tissue is abundant, with lymphoid follicles present. The follicular hyperplasia seen in this case of thymic hyperplasia with MG is associated with autoantibody production. It is the acetylcholine receptor antibodies that diminish the receptor function in the skeletal muscle motor end plates, leading to the onset of muscular weakness, particularly with repetitive muscular contraction.

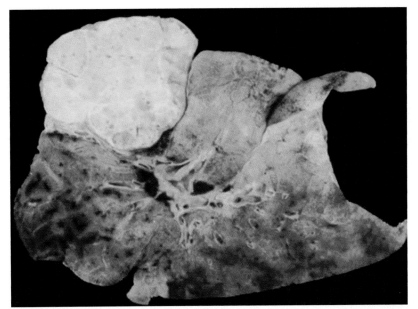

FIGURE 4–77 Thymoma, gross

Thymomas arising in the anterior mediastinum can compress adjacent structures as they enlarge. Seen here at autopsy anterior to the lung is a discrete but lobulated tan-white mass that proved to be a thymoma. Both benign and malignant thymomas usually arise in adults older than 40 years of age. Most are found in the anterior superior mediastinum, but sometimes they occur in the neck, thyroid, pulmonary hilus, or elsewhere. They account for only 20% to 30% of tumors in the anterosuperior mediastinum because this is also a common location for the nodular sclerosis type of HL and certain forms of NHL, such as T-cell lymphoblastic lymphoma.

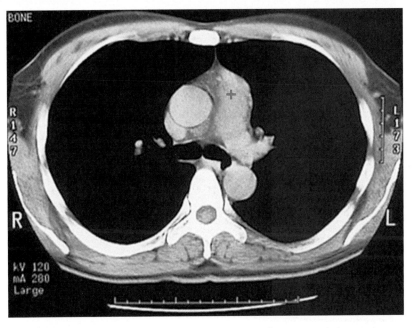

FIGURE 4–78 Thymoma, CT image

Here is a thymoma (+) of the anterior superior mediastinum seen with this chest CT scan. It is arising in the left aspect of the thymus anterior and to the left of the aortic arch. Thymomas can be slow growing and act in a benign fashion. Malignant thymomas, however, can be locally invasive. Those that are cytologically malignant are termed thymic carcinoma. About 40% of thymomas are found when symptoms occur from impingement on mediastinal structures, and another 30% to 45% are present with MG. The remainder are discovered incidentally during imaging studies or during cardiothoracic surgery.

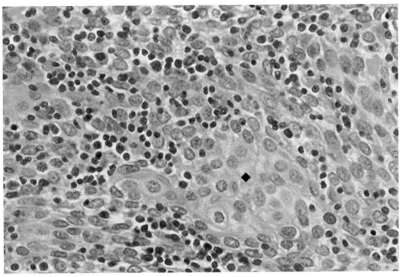

FIGURE 4–79 Thymoma, microscopic

A thymoma contains epithelial elements (◆), with a background of small round lymphocytes that are not neoplastic themselves. One third to one half of all thymomas occur in association with MG. The neoplastic epithelial elements of this thymoma display minimal pleomorphism, but this tumor was locally invasive and, therefore, a malignant thymoma. About 10% of thymomas are associated with systemic paraneoplastic syndromes other than myasthenia gravis, including Graves disease, pure red cell aplasia, polymyositis, Cushing syndrome, and pernicious anemia.

CHAPTER 5

The Lung

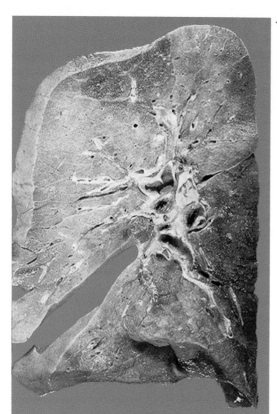

◀ **FIGURE 5–1 Normal lung, gross**

This is a cross-section of normal lung (with only minimal posterior congestion at the lower right). The hilar lymph nodes are small and have enough anthracotic pigment (from dusts in the air breathed in, scavenged by pulmonary macrophages, transferred to lymphatics, and collected in lymph nodes) to make them appear grayish black.

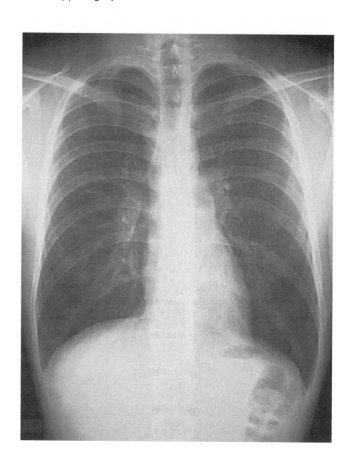

FIGURE 5–2 Normal lung, radiograph ▶

This chest radiograph reveals the normal PA projection appearance of the lungs in a normal adult male. The darker air density represents the parenchyma, with soft tissue of the chest wall and hilum brighter. Note that the normal heart shadow is about the width of the left lung.

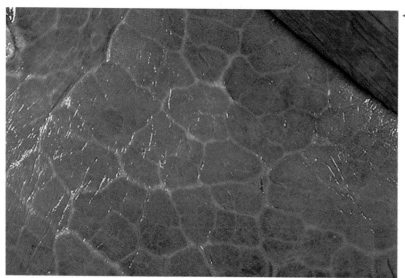

◀ **FIGURE 5–3 Normal lung, gross**

The smooth, glistening pleural surface of a lung is shown here. This patient had marked pulmonary edema, which increased the amount of fluid in the lymphatics that run between lung lobules. Thus, the lung lobules are outlined here by the white markings. Anthracotic pigmentation derived from inhaled carbonaceous dusts is also carried by the lymphatics to the pleural surfaces as well as to hilar lymph nodes. Small amounts of anthracotic pigment are present in every adult lung. Smokers have more anthracosis.

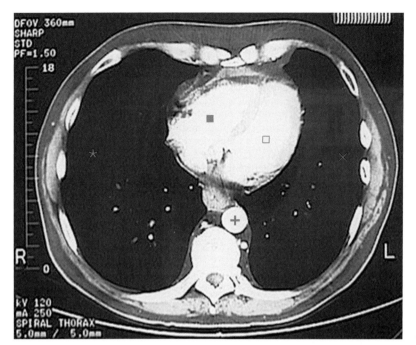

FIGURE 5–4 Normal lung, CT image

This chest CT scan at soft tissue density reveals the normal appearance of the right (*) and left (×) lungs—essentially black from air density—in a normal adult male. Contrast material in the bloodstream gives the right (■) and left (□) chambers of the heart, as well as the aorta (+), a bright appearance. Bone of the vertebral body and ribs also appears bright. The AP diameter is normal.

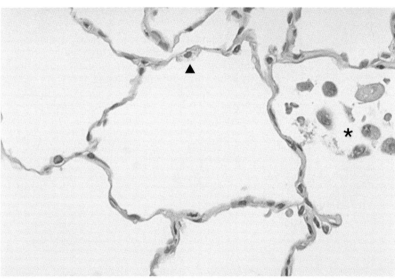

FIGURE 5–5 Normal adult lung, microscopic

The delicate alveolar walls of the lung are seen here at high magnification. The attenuated cytoplasm of the alveolar type I epithelial cells cannot easily be distinguished from the endothelial cells of the capillaries that are present within the alveolar walls. These thin alveolar walls provide for efficient gas exchange so that the alveolar-arterial (A-a) oxygen gradient is typically less than 15 mm Hg in young, healthy people, although the A-a gradient may increase beyond 20 mm Hg in elderly people. Within the alveoli can be found occasional alveolar macrophages (*). The type II pneumocytes (▲) produce surfactant that lowers surface tension to increase lung compliance and help keep the alveoli expanded.

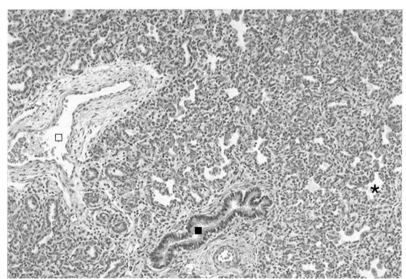

FIGURE 5–6 Normal fetal lung, microscopic

Normal fetal lung appears much more cellular than the adult lung. The alveoli have not developed completely, and the interstitium is more prominent. In this view of the canalicular phase in the late second trimester, the bronchioles (*) are forming sacculations that will become the alveoli. There are developing bronchi (■) and pulmonary artery branches (□). In the first part of the second trimester, the fetal lung is in the glandular phase (tubular phase) of development. There are only primitive rounded bronchioles, and no alveoli have yet formed. In the third trimester, the saccular phase is marked by increasing alveolar development.

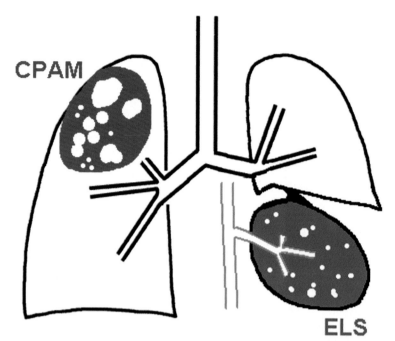

FIGURE 5–7 Congenital anomalies, diagram

This diagram illustrates the appearance of pulmonary extralobar sequestration (ELS) and congenital pulmonary airway malformation (CPAM). With CPAM, a rare anomaly appearing in about 1 in 5000 live births, there is a mass lesion with cystic and solid components. The ELS, which typically lacks a bronchial connection, also acts as a mass lesion, but is a portion of lung that typically has a blood supply from the aorta, not the pulmonary arterial tree. In contrast, an intralobar sequestration occurs entirely within the lung parenchyma. Although some intralobar sequestrations are congenital, many are thought to develop with recurrent pneumonic episodes.

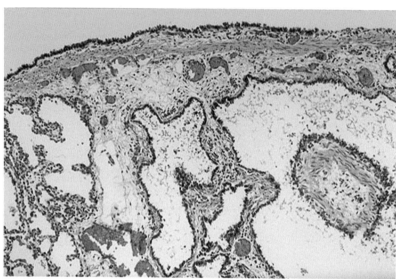

FIGURE 5–8 Congenital pulmonary airway malformation, microscopic

The irregular cystic spaces lined by bronchial epithelium seen here in fetal lung are part of a lung mass known as CPAM. Although the lesion is benign microscopically (much like a hamartoma), it can enlarge and act as a space-occupying lesion, resulting in hypoplasia of remaining functional lung parenchyma, producing respiratory difficulties from birth. Grossly, a CPAM can be composed of large cysts (type I), small cysts (type II), or mainly a solid mass (type III).

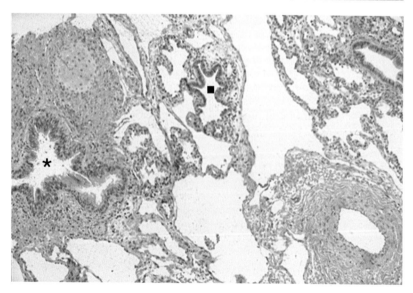

FIGURE 5–9 Extralobar sequestration, microscopic

Seen here are irregular bronchi (∗) as well as dilated distal airspaces, some of which are lined by bronchial epithelium (■) in this mass separate from remaining normal lung. The vascular arterial supply here is systemic, not from a pulmonary artery, and so this portion of lung does not function in normal oxygenation. When such a sequestered segment lies within surrounding normal lung, it is called an *intralobar sequestration*. In either case, the sequestered lung acts as a mass lesion, and it may become infected.

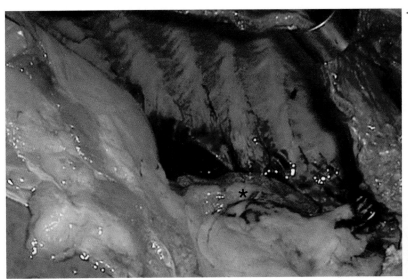

◀ **FIGURE 5–10 Atelectasis, gross**

This right lung (∗) seen at autopsy is collapsed. In this case, blood filled the pleural cavity (hemothorax) after chest wall trauma. Such a compression atelectasis can also result from filling the potential pleural space of the chest with air (pneumothorax), transudate (hydrothorax), lymph (chylothorax), or purulent exudate (empyema). The collapsed lung is not aerated, creating a ventilation/perfusion (V/Q) mismatch, acting as a shunt similar to a cardiac right-to-left shunt that bypasses the lungs, with blood gas parameters similar to the mixed venous blood entering the right heart.

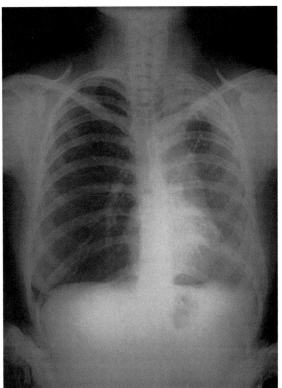

FIGURE 5–11 Atelectasis, x-ray ▶

This chest radiograph reveals decreased attenuation on the right—a right pneumothorax. Note the expansion of the right chest cavity with displacement of the heart to the left. A pneumothorax occurs with a penetrating chest injury, inflammation with rupture of a bronchus to the pleura, rupture of an emphysematous bulla, or barotrauma from positive pressure mechanical ventilation. The escape of air into the pleural space eliminates the negative pressure of the thoracic cavity and collapses the lung. The example seen here is a "tension" pneumothorax shifting the mediastinum, because a ball–valve air leak is increasing the amount of air in the right chest cavity. A chest tube can be placed through the chest wall to reexpand the lung. In contrast, a resorption atelectasis from airway obstruction and resorption of air in the lung parenchyma leads to collapse with a shift of the mediastinum toward the involved lung.

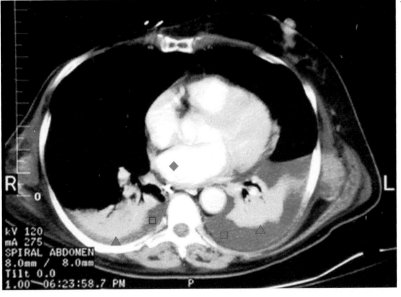

◀ **FIGURE 5–12 Atelectasis, CT image**

This chest CT scan demonstrates a large right pleural effusion (■) and a smaller left pleural effusion (□). The pleural effusions seen here resulted from right heart failure as a consequence of rheumatic mitral stenosis with chronic pulmonary congestion and subsequent pulmonary hypertension. Note the enlargement of the right atrium (◆). Note also that this large effusion has produced bilateral atelectasis of the lower lobes, characterized by a small dense crescent of lung tissue in the region of the effusion on each side (▲).

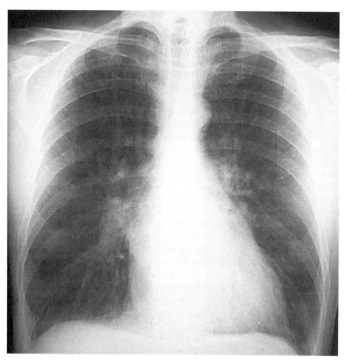
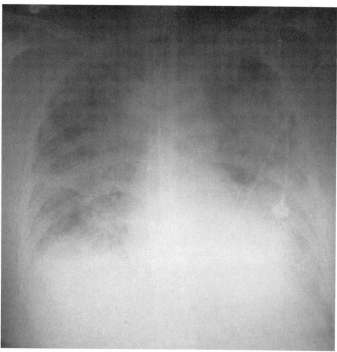

FIGURES 5–13 and 5–14 Pulmonary edema, x-rays

Passive congestion increases pulmonary interstitial markings, and edema fluid spills into alveoli, creating infiltrates. The PA chest radiograph at the left demonstrates pulmonary congestion and edema throughout all lung fields. The pulmonary veins are distended near the hilum. The left heart border is prominent because of left atrial enlargement. This patient had mitral stenosis. The PA chest radiograph at the right shows extensive congestion and edema throughout all lung fields from severe congestive heart failure from cardiomyopathy, and the edema obscures the cardiac silhouette.

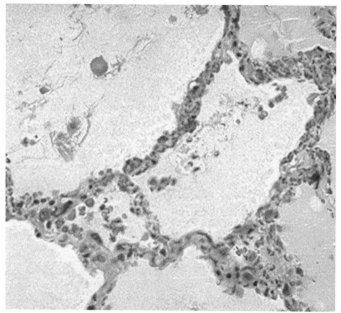
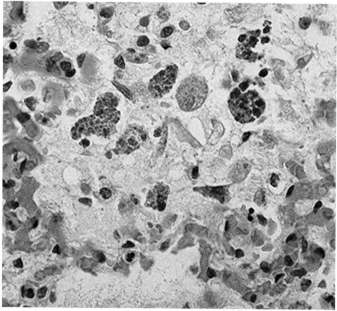

FIGURES 5–15 and 5–16 Pulmonary edema, microscopic

The alveoli at the left are filled with a smooth to slightly floccular pink material characteristic of pulmonary edema. Note also that capillaries within alveolar walls are congested, filled with many red blood cells (RBCs). Pulmonary congestion with edema is common in patients with heart failure and in areas of inflammation of the lung. At the right is more marked pulmonary congestion with dilated capillaries and leakage of blood into alveolar spaces, leading to the appearance of hemosiderin-laden macrophages ("heart failure cells") containing brown cytoplasmic hemosiderin granules from breakdown of RBCs.

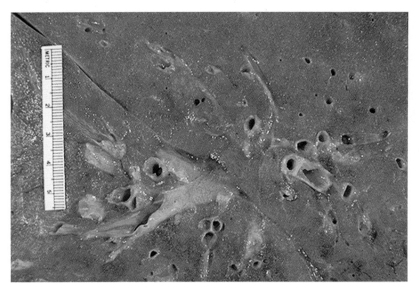

FIGURE 5–17 Diffuse alveolar damage, gross

This lung is virtually airless, diffusely firm, and rubbery with a glistening appearance on cut section. Clinically, this is known as adult respiratory distress syndrome (ARDS). Diffuse alveolar damage (DAD) is a form of acute restrictive lung disease resulting from capillary wall endothelial injury from multiple causes, including pulmonary infections, sepsis, inhaled noxious gases, microangiopathic hemolytic anemias, trauma, oxygen toxicity, aspiration, fat embolism, or opiate overdose. DAD causes severe hypoxemia. The lung diffusing capacity for carbon monoxide (D_{LCO}) is reduced. Diseases that affect the alveolar walls (DAD or emphysema) or the pulmonary capillary bed (thromboembolism or vasculitis) will decrease the D_{LCO}.

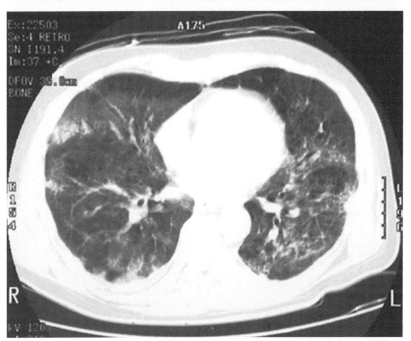

FIGURE 5–18 Diffuse alveolar damage, CT image

The chest CT shown here with the "lung window" setting reveals extensive bilateral ground-glass opacifications of the lung parenchyma consistent with DAD. The acute phase of DAD can develop within hours of capillary injury, with increased vascular permeability and leakage of interstitial fluid into alveoli, forming diffuse ground-glass infiltrates. The exuded blood proteins can then form hyaline membranes. Injury to type II pneumocytes diminishes surfactant production and reduces lung compliance. Release of interleukin-1 (IL-1), IL-8, and tumor necrosis factor (TNF) promotes neutrophil chemotaxis and activation that further potentiates parenchymal injury.

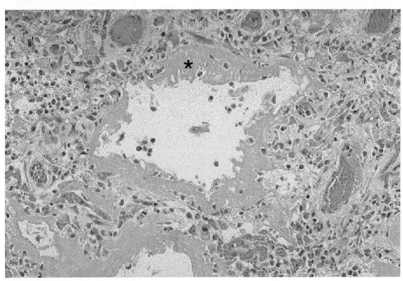

FIGURE 5–19 Diffuse alveolar damage, microscopic

DAD is simply the final common pathway for a variety of severe lung injuries. In early DAD, there are hyaline membranes (*), as seen here, lining the alveoli. Later in the first week after lung injury the hyaline membranes resolve, and macrophage proliferation occurs. If the patient survives more than a week, interstitial inflammation and fibrosis become increasingly prominent, and lung compliance decreases. There are V/Q mismatches. High oxygen tension is needed to treat the hypoxia resulting from DAD, and the oxygen toxicity from this therapy further exacerbates the DAD.

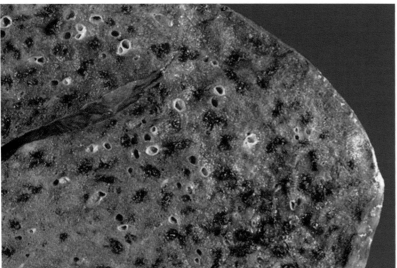

FIGURE 5–20 Pulmonary emphysema, gross

There are two major types of emphysema: centrilobular (centriacinar) and panlobular (panacinar). The former involves primarily the upper lobes, while the latter involves all lung fields, particularly the bases. The central lobular loss of lung tissue with intense black anthracotic pigmentation is apparent here. Unlike the risk for lung cancer, which diminishes when a smoker stops smoking, the lung tissue loss with emphysema is permanent. Centrilobular emphysema occurs with loss of the respiratory bronchioles in the proximal portion of the acinus, with sparing of distal alveoli. This pattern of emphysema is most typical for cigarette smokers.

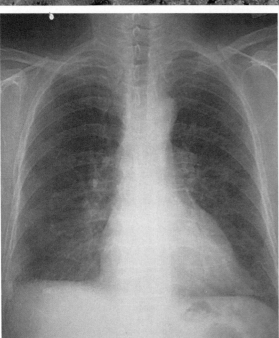

FIGURE 5–21 Pulmonary emphysema, radiograph

The PA chest radiograph seen here shows increased interstitial markings with an irregular architecture, an increase in total lung volume, along with bilateral flattening of the diaphragmatic leaves, consistent with centrilobular emphysema. The flattening of the diaphragm reduces the efficiency of muscular contraction and lung excursion, increasing the work of breathing, As the severity of emphysema increases, affected persons begin to use accessory muscles of respiration, such as intercostal muscles and sternocleidomastoids. Affected persons may also exhibit "pursed lip" breathing to increase central airway pressure to keep distal airways from collapsing as a consequence of the increased compliance. Most of the increase in total lung capacity seen with emphysema results from an increase in residual volume.

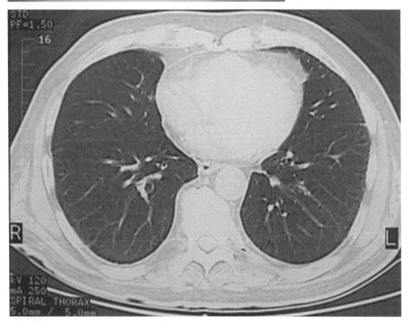

FIGURE 5–22 Pulmonary hypertension, chest CT

The CT of the chest seen here in the lung window reveals an increase in bright vascular lung markings from pulmonary hypertension. There are parenchymal lucencies consistent with a pattern of centrilobular emphysema. The AP diameter of the chest is increased, as a consequence of increased total lung volume, mainly the result of increased residual volume.

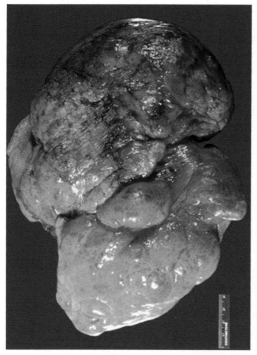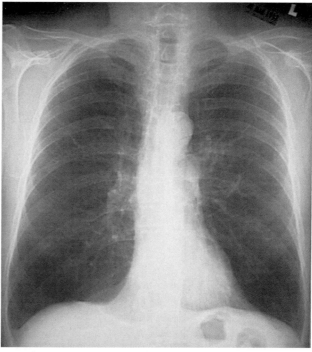

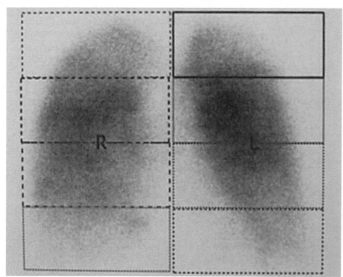

▲ **FIGURES 5–23 and 5–24 Pulmonary panacinar emphysema, gross and chest x-ray**

Panacinar emphysema occurs with loss of all portions of the acinus from the respiratory bronchiole to the alveoli. This pattern is typical for α_1-antitrypsin (AAT) deficiency. Note that the bullae seen here are most prominent in the lower lobe at the left. The typical chest radiographic appearance of panlobular emphysema, with increased lung volume and diaphragmatic flattening, is shown above at the right.

◄ **FIGURE 5–25 Pulmonary emphysema, ventilation scan**

There are areas of abnormal ventilation, with decreased (pale) areas of radionuclide emission, most marked in the lung bases, consistent with panlobular emphysema.

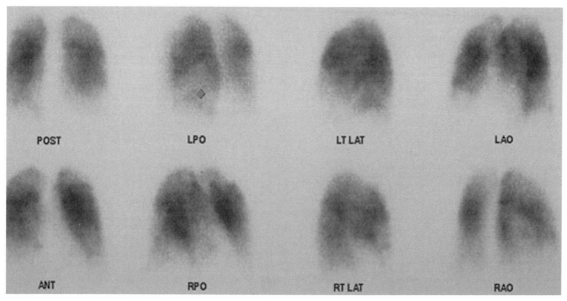

◄ **FIGURE 5–26 Pulmonary emphysema, perfusion scan**

There are areas of decreased perfusion (◆) from reduction in pulmonary alveoli with loss of capillary beds, most marked in the lung bases, consistent with bullous panacinar emphysema.

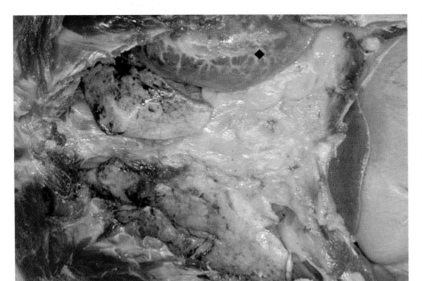

FIGURE 5–27 Pulmonary emphysema, gross

The chest cavity is opened anteriorly at autopsy to reveal a large bulla (◆) of the left lung in a patient dying from pulmonary emphysema. Bullae are large dilated airspaces that bulge out from beneath the pleura. Large bullae can act as space-occupying lesions that further reduce pulmonary function. Emphysema is characterized by a loss of lung parenchyma from destruction of alveoli so that there is permanent dilation of remaining airspaces. As emphysema progresses, there is a loss in diffusing capacity (decreased DLCO), hypoxemia, and hypercapnia leading to respiratory acidosis.

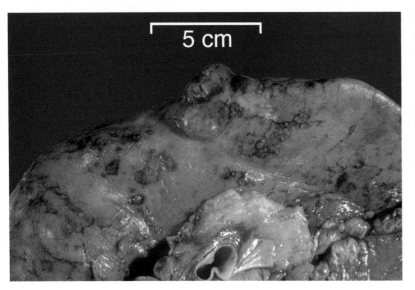

FIGURE 5–28 Paraseptal emphysema, gross

A more localized form of emphysema is known as *paraseptal*, or *distal acinar, emphysema*, which can follow focal scarring of the peripheral lung parenchyma. Paraseptal emphysema is not related to smoking. Since this process is focal, pulmonary function is not seriously affected, but the peripheral location of the bullae, which are up to 2 cm in size, along septae may lead to rupture into the pleural space, causing spontaneous pneumothorax. This is most likely to occur in young adults, with sudden onset of dyspnea. Seen here are two small bullae just beneath the pleural surface.

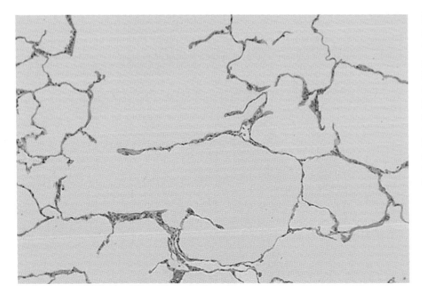

FIGURE 5–29 Pulmonary emphysema, microscopic

There is loss of alveolar ducts and alveoli with emphysema, and the remaining airspaces become dilated. There is less surface area for gas exchange. Emphysema leads to loss of lung parenchyma, loss of elastic recoil, increased lung compliance, and increased pulmonary residual volume with increased total lung capacity, mainly from an increased residual capacity. There is decreased diaphragmatic excursion and increased use of accessory muscles for breathing. Over time, the PaO_2 decreases and the $PaCO_2$ increases.

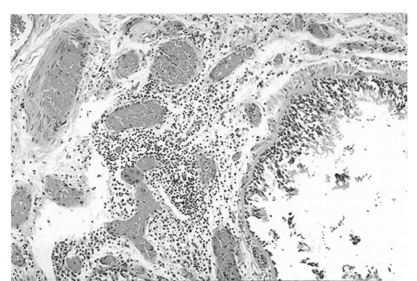

FIGURE 5–30 Chronic bronchitis, microscopic

This bronchus has increased numbers of chronic inflammatory cells in the submucosal region. Chronic bronchitis does not have characteristic pathologic findings, but is defined clinically as a persistent productive cough for at least 3 consecutive months in at least 2 consecutive years. Most patients are smokers, but inhaled pollutants such as sulfur dioxide can exacerbate chronic bronchitis. Often, there is parenchymal destruction with features of emphysema as well, and the two conditions overlap clinically. Secondary infections are common and further worsen pulmonary function. There is often overlap between pulmonary emphysema and chronic bronchitis, with patients having elements of both.

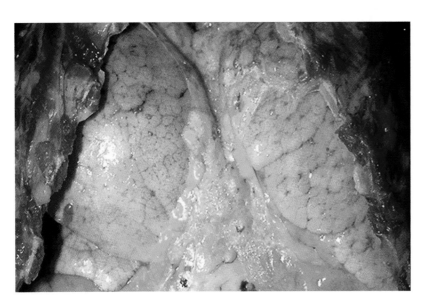

FIGURE 5–31 Bronchial asthma, gross

These lungs appear essentially normal, but are the hyperinflated lungs of a patient who died with status asthmaticus. There are two major clinical forms of asthma that can overlap:
Atopic (extrinsic) asthma: There is typically an association with atopy (allergies) that is mediated by type 1 hypersensitivity, and asthmatic attacks are precipitated by contact with inhaled allergens. This form occurs most often in childhood.
Nonatopic (intrinsic) asthma: Asthmatic attacks are precipitated by respiratory infections, exposure to cold, exercise, stress, inhaled irritants, and drugs such as aspirin. Adults are most often affected.

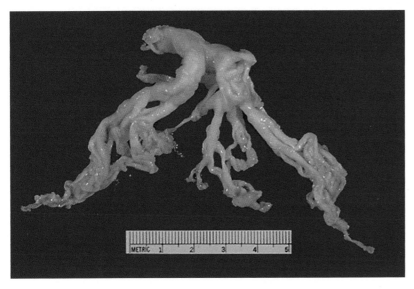

FIGURE 5–32 Bronchial asthma, gross

This cast of the bronchial tree is formed from inspissated mucus secretions and was coughed up by a patient during an acute asthmatic attack. The outpouring of mucus from hypertrophied bronchial submucosal glands along with the bronchoconstriction and dehydration all contribute to the formation of mucus plugs that can block airways in asthmatic patients. The result is sudden, severe dyspnea with wheezing and hypoxemia. A severe attack, known as *status asthmaticus*, can be life-threatening.

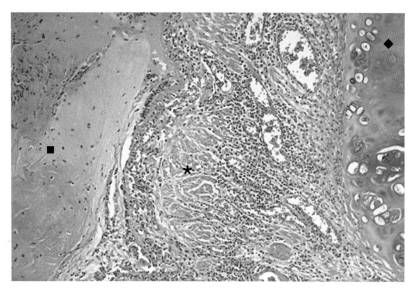

FIGURE 5–33 Bronchial asthma, microscopic

Between the bronchial cartilage (♦) at the right and the bronchial lumen (■) filled with mucus at the left is a submucosa widened by smooth muscle hypertrophy (∗), edema, and an inflammatory infiltrate with many eosinophils. These are changes of bronchial asthma, more specifically atopic asthma from type I hypersensitivity to allergens. Sensitization to inhaled allergens promotes a subtype 2 helper T-cell (TH2) immune response with release of IL-4 and IL-5 promoting B-cell immunoglobulin E (IgE) production and eosinophil infiltration and activation. The peripheral blood eosinophil count or the sputum eosinophils can be increased during an asthmatic attack.

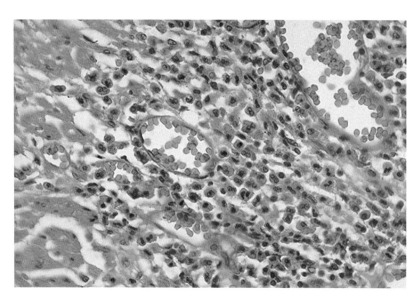

FIGURE 5–34 Bronchial asthma, microscopic

At high magnification, the numerous eosinophils are prominent from their bright red cytoplasmic granules in this case of bronchial asthma. The two major clinical forms of asthma, atopic and nonatopic, can overlap in both symptomatology and pathologic findings. In the early phase of an acute atopic asthmatic attack, there is cross-linking by allergens of IgE bound to mast cells, causing degranulation with release of biogenic amines and cytokines producing an immediate response in minutes with bronchoconstriction, edema, and mucus production. A late phase develops over hours from leukocyte infiltration with continued edema and mucus production.

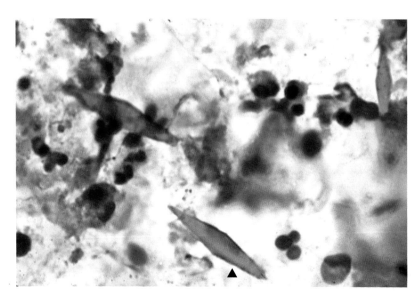

FIGURE 5–35 Bronchial asthma, microscopic

Analysis of the sputum from a patient with an acute asthmatic episode may reveal numerous eosinophils and also Charcot-Leiden crystals (▲) derived from breakdown of eosinophil granules. Pharmacologic therapies used emergently to treat asthma include short-acting β-adrenergic agonists such as epinephrine and isoproterenol. Theophylline, a methylxanthine, promotes bronchodilation by increasing cyclic adenosine monophosphate (cAMP), while anticholinergics such as atropine sulfate also produce bronchodilation. Long-term asthma control includes use of glucocorticoids, leukotriene inhibitors such as zileuton, receptor antagonists such as montelukast, and mast cell-stabilizing agents such as cromolyn sodium.

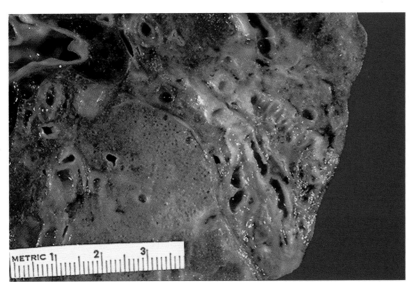

FIGURE 5–36 Bronchiectasis, gross

This focal area of dilated bronchi is typical of a less common form of obstructive lung disease known as *bronchiectasis*. Bronchiectasis tends to be a localized process with diseases such as pulmonary neoplasms and aspirated foreign bodies that block a portion of the airways, leading to obstruction with distal airway distention mediated by inflammation and airway destruction. Widespread bronchiectasis is more typical in patients with cystic fibrosis who have recurrent infections and obstruction of airways by mucus plugs throughout the lungs. A rare cause is primary ciliary dyskinesia, seen with Kartagener syndrome, with loss of ciliary activity.

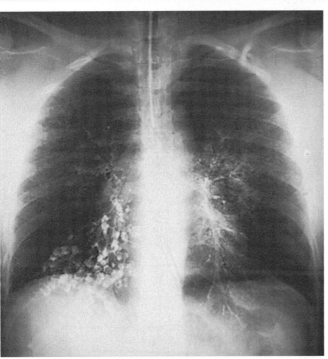

FIGURE 5–37 Bronchiectasis, chest radiograph

This bronchogram demonstrates saccular bronchiectasis involving the right lower lobe. The contrast medium fills dilated bronchi, giving them a saccular outline. Bronchiectasis occurs when there is obstruction or infection with inflammation and destruction of bronchi so that there is permanent bronchial dilation. Once these dilated bronchi are present, the patient is then predisposed to recurrent infections because of the stasis in these airways. Copious purulent sputum production with cough is a common clinical manifestation. There is a risk for sepsis and dissemination of the infection elsewhere. In cases of severe, widespread bronchiectasis, cor pulmonale can occur.

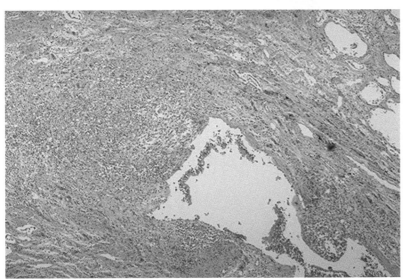

FIGURE 5–38 Bronchiectasis, microscopic

The mid lower portion of this photomicrograph demonstrates a dilated bronchus in which the mucosa and bronchial wall are not clearly seen because of the necrotizing inflammation with tissue destruction. Bronchiectasis is not a specific disease, but a consequence of another disease process that destroys airways.

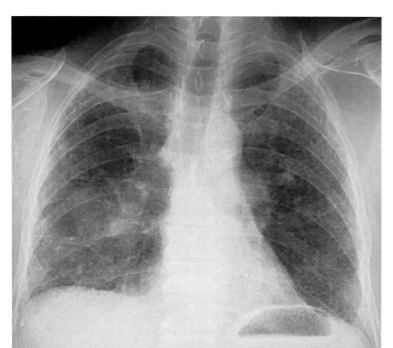

FIGURE 5–39 Idiopathic pulmonary fibrosis, radiograph

There are increased interstitial markings in all lung fields as a consequence of idiopathic pulmonary fibrosis (usual interstitial pneumonitis, or UIP). Affected patients will have continuing loss of lung volumes so that pulmonary function studies show that the forced vital capacity (FVC) is reduced, and the forced expiratory volume at 1 second (FEV_1) is reduced as well, so the FVC/FEV_1 ratio generally remains unchanged. These reductions are typically proportional with restrictive lung diseases such as idiopathic pulmonary fibrosis (IPF). This disease is probably mediated by an inflammatory response to alveolar wall injury, but the inciting event in IPF is not known. Patients may survive weeks to years, depending on the severity, with eventual end-stage honeycomb fibrosis.

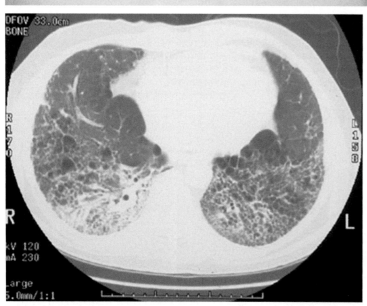

FIGURE 5–40 Idiopathic pulmonary fibrosis, CT image

This chest CT scan in the lung window mode shows very prominent interstitial markings, particularly in the posterior lung bases. There are also smaller lucent areas that represent honeycomb change, a characteristic feature of UIP, an idiopathic and progressive restrictive lung disease that can affect middle-aged people with progressive dyspnea, hypoxemia, and cyanosis. Patients develop pulmonary hypertension and cor pulmonale as a result. *UIP* is a descriptive term, not an etiologic diagnosis.

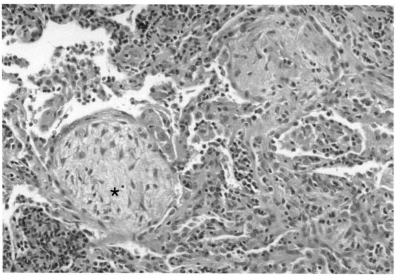

FIGURE 5–41 Cryptogenic organizing pneumonia, microscopic

Cryptogenic organizing pneumonia (COP), also termed *bronchiolitis obliterans organizing pneumonia* (BOOP), involves distal airways with plugs (*) of organizing exudate in response to inflammation or infection. The effect is similar to an acute interstitial lung disease. By treating the underlying condition, such as an infection or a transplant rejection, along with use of corticosteroid therapy, most patients improve.

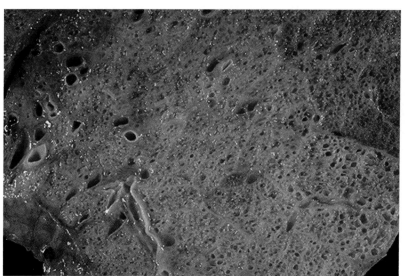

FIGURE 5–42 Honeycomb change, gross

Regardless of the etiology of restrictive lung diseases, many eventually lead to extensive pulmonary interstitial fibrosis. The gross appearance shown here in a patient with organizing diffuse alveolar damage is known as *honeycomb lung* because of the appearance of the irregular residual dilated airspaces between bands of dense fibrous interstitial connective tissue. The lung compliance is markedly diminished so that patients receiving mechanical ventilation require increasing positive end-expiratory pressure (PEEP), predisposing them to airway rupture and development of interstitial emphysema.

FIGURE 5–43 Interstitial fibrosis, microscopic

A trichrome stain highlights in blue the collagenous interstitial connective tissue of pulmonary fibrosis. The extent of the fibrosis determines the severity of disease, which is marked by progressively worsening dyspnea. The alveolitis that produces fibroblast proliferation and collagen deposition is progressive over time. Remaining airspaces may become dilated and may become lined by metaplastic bronchiolar epithelium. If such patients are intubated and given mechanical ventilation, just as in the case of severe chronic obstructive pulmonary disease, it is unlikely that they can be extubated. Thus, determining patient advance directives for medical care is crucial.

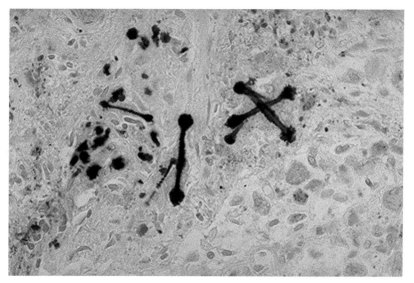

FIGURE 5–44 Ferruginous bodies, microscopic

Sometimes the etiology for interstitial lung disease is known. The causative agent for asbestosis is a long, thin object known as an *asbestos fiber*. Some houses, business locations, and ships still contain building products with asbestos, particularly insulation materials, so care must be taken to prevent inhalation of asbestos when doing remodeling or reconstruction. *In vivo*, the inhaled asbestos fiber becomes coated with iron and calcium, which is why it is often called a *ferruginous body*, as seen here with a Prussian blue iron stain. Ingestion of these fibers by macrophages sets off a fibrogenic response through release of cytokine growth factors that promote continued collagen deposition by fibroblasts.

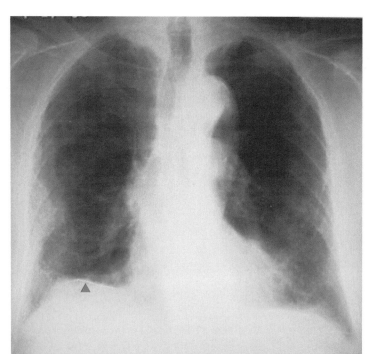

FIGURE 5–45 Pneumoconiosis, radiograph

This PA chest radiograph demonstrates interstitial fibrosis with irregular infiltrates. There is a right pleural plaque (▲) with calcification as well as a left pleural plaque. This patient had significant exposure to asbestos. Inhaled dusts are phagocytized by macrophages, which then secrete cytokines such as transforming growth factor-β that can activate fibroblasts that produce collagenous fibrosis that increases over time. The amount of dust inhaled and the length of exposure determine the severity of the disease. Patients may remain asymptomatic for years until progressive massive fibrosis reduces vital capacity and there is onset of dyspnea. The most common pneumoconiosis is silicosis. There is an interstitial pattern of disease with eventual development of larger silicotic nodules. The nodules can become confluent.

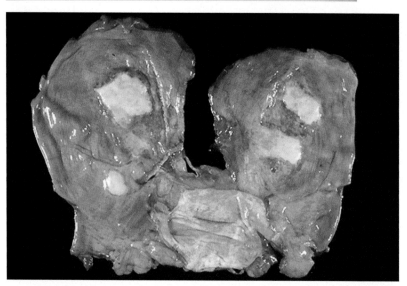

FIGURE 5–46 Pleural fibrous plaques, gross

Seen here on the pleural aspects of the diaphragmatic leaves are several tan-white pleural plaques typical of pneumoconioses and of asbestosis in particular. Chronic inflammation induced by the inhaled dust particles results in fibrogenesis.

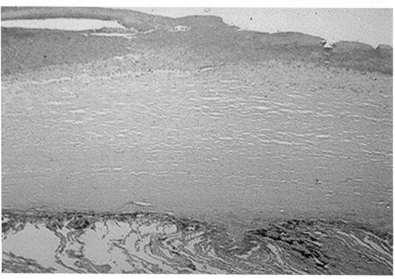

FIGURE 5–47 Pleural fibrous plaque, microscopic

This fibrous pleural plaque is composed of dense layers of collagen that give a pink appearance with H+E staining and a white to tan appearance grossly. Progressive pulmonary fibrosis leads to restrictive lung disease. Reduction in pulmonary vasculature leads to pulmonary hypertension and cor pulmonale with subsequent right-sided congestive heart failure manifested by peripheral dependent edema, hepatic congestion, and body cavity effusions.

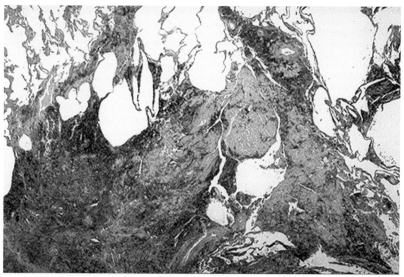

FIGURE 5–48 Coal worker's pneumoconiosis, microscopic

Anthracotic pigment deposition in the lung is quite common, but ordinarily is not fibrogenic because the amount of inhaled carbonaceous dusts from environmental air pollution is not large. Smokers have more anthracotic pigmentation due to the tars in tobacco smoke, but still do not have significant disease from the carbonaceous material. With massive amounts of inhaled particles (as in "black lung disease" in coal miners) a fibrogenic response can be elicited to produce the coal worker's pneumoconiosis with the coal macule seen here. This results in progressive massive fibrosis. There is no increased risk for lung cancer.

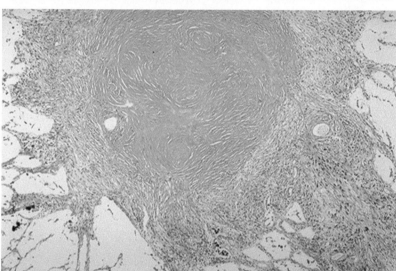

FIGURE 5–49 Silicosis, microscopic

The silicotic nodule in lung seen here is composed mainly of bundles of interlacing pink collagen, and there is a minimal inflammatory reaction. Macrophages that phagocytize the silica crystals release cytokines such as TNF that promote fibrogenesis. The greater the degree of exposure to silica and an increasing length of exposure determine the amount of silicotic nodule formation and the degree of restrictive lung disease, which is progressive and irreversible. Silicosis increases the risk for lung carcinoma only about two-fold.

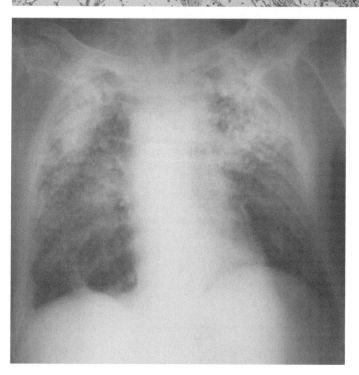

FIGURE 5–50 Pneumoconiosis, radiograph

This chest radiograph demonstrates so many bright, irregularly shaped silicotic nodules that they have become confluent (progressive massive fibrosis) and have resulted in severe restrictive lung disease. This patient became severely dyspneic. All lung volumes are diminished.

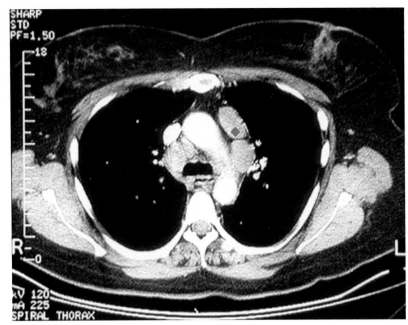

◀ **FIGURE 5–51 Sarcoidosis, CT image**

Sarcoidosis is an idiopathic granulomatous disease that can affect many organs, but lymph node involvement is present in 100% of cases, and the hilar lymph nodes are most often involved. The chest CT image seen here with the bone window setting shows prominent hilar lymphadenopathy (◆) in a middle-aged woman with sarcoidosis. Patients often have fever, nonproductive cough, dyspnea, chest pain, night sweats, and weight loss.

FIGURE 5–52 Sarcoidosis, radiograph ▶

One cause of pulmonary interstitial fibrosis is sarcoidosis. In addition to increased interstitial markings, the chest radiograph may display prominent hilar lymphadenopathy (from noncaseating granulomatous inflammation) as shown here (◀). Most patients have a benign course with minimal pulmonary disease that often resolves with corticosteroid therapy. Some patients have a relapsing and remitting course. About one fifth of patients, typically those in whom pulmonary parenchymal involvement is greater than lymph node involvement, go on to develop progressive restrictive lung disease.

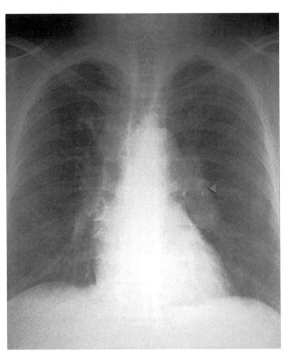

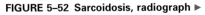

◀ **FIGURE 5–53 Sarcoidosis, microscopic**

The interstitial granulomas can produce a restrictive lung disease. The granulomas tend to have a bronchovascular distribution. The small sarcoid granulomas are typically noncaseating, but larger granulomas may have central caseation. The inflammation is characterized by collections of epithelioid macrophages, Langhans giant cells, lymphocytes (particularly CD4 cells), and fibroblasts. The CD4 cells participate in a T_H1 immune response. Not seen here are inclusions such as asteroid bodies and Schaumann bodies that can be seen with sarcoidosis.

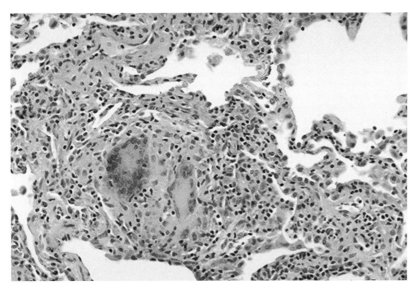

FIGURE 5–54 Hypersensitivity pneumonitis, microscopic

This type of interstitial pneumonitis is known as extrinsic allergic alveolitis because it occurs when inhaled organic dusts produce a localized form of type III hypersensitivity (Arthus) reaction from antigen–antibody complex formation. Symptoms of dyspnea, cough, and fever abate when the affected patient leaves the environment with the offending antigen. The disease shown here has become a more chronic, granulomatous type of inflammation, indicative of type IV hypersensitivity. The diagnosis and the offending antigen are often difficult to determine. Radiographic imaging reveals reticulonodular infiltrates. Progression to fibrosis, however, is not common.

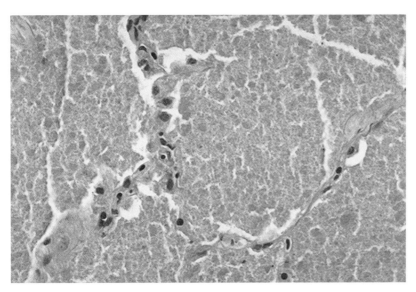

FIGURE 5–55 Pulmonary alveolar proteinosis, microscopic

This is a rare disease known as *pulmonary alveolar proteinosis*. The alveolar walls are normal histologically, but the alveoli become filled with a PAS-positive granular exudate containing abundant lipid and lamellar bodies (by electron microscopy). Patients may cough up copious amounts of gelatinous sputum. Patients are treated with lung lavage to try to remove the proteinaceous fluid. The disease results from a deficiency of granulocyte-macrophage colony-stimulating factor receptor involving alveolar macrophages.

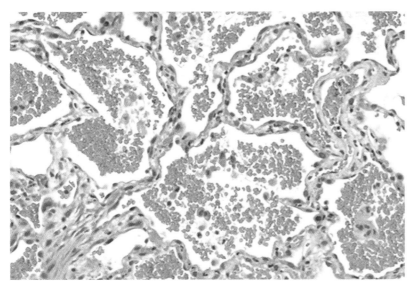

FIGURE 5–56 Diffuse pulmonary hemorrhage, microscopic

The acute intra-alveolar hemorrhage seen here is a consequence of capillary injury from basement membrane antibody in a patient with Goodpasture syndrome. The glomerular capillaries are targeted as well, leading to a rapidly progressive glomerulonephritis. The target antigen in Goodpasture syndrome is a component of the noncollagenous (NCl) domain of the α_3 chain of type IV collagen, the α_3 chain being preferentially expressed in glomerular and pulmonary alveolar basement membrane. Circulating antiglomerular basement membrane antibody can be detected. Plasmapheresis can be used as treatment.

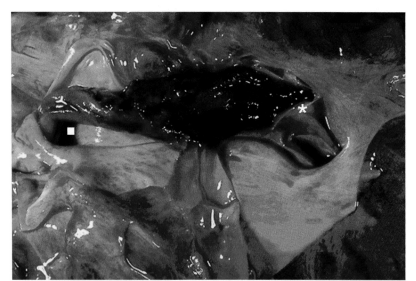

FIGURE 5–57 Pulmonary embolism, gross

Here is a "saddle embolus" that bridges the pulmonary artery trunk from the heart as it divides into right (■) and left (∗) main pulmonary arteries. Such a saddle embolus can be a cause of sudden death from acute cor pulmonale. This thromboembolus displays a somewhat irregular surface, and there are pale tan areas admixed with dark red areas. The embolus often has the outlines of the vein in which it originally formed as a thrombus. Most large pulmonary thromboemboli originate within large veins of the lower extremities.

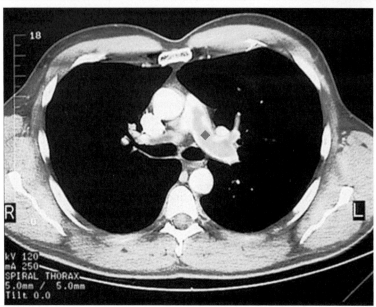

FIGURE 5–58 Pulmonary embolism, CT image

In most cases of suspected pulmonary embolism, the most definitive, readily available study in hospitalized patients is a chest CT scan. A saddle pulmonary embolus (♦) with extension into the right pulmonary artery is seen here. A common laboratory finding is an increased plasma D-dimer, although this test is more useful as a negative predictor of pulmonary embolism when it is not elevated. Risks for pulmonary thromboembolism include prolonged immobilization, advanced age, and hypercoagulable states.

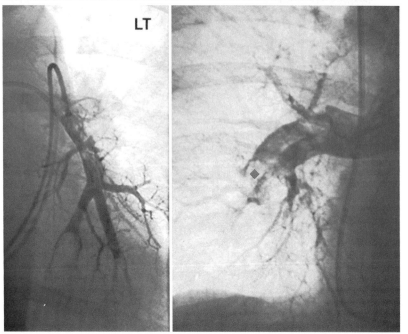

FIGURE 5–59 Pulmonary embolism, angiogram

These views from a thoracic CT angiogram demonstrate multiple pulmonary thromboemboli (♦). There should be contrast filling pulmonary arteries into the periphery. This patient's risk factors included older age, history of smoking, and immobilization during prolonged hospitalization for bowel obstruction. Although the angiogram is the gold standard for demonstration of pulmonary thromboemboli, a standard CT scan has a high sensitivity for diagnosis. Clinical findings include dyspnea, tachypnea, cough, fever, and chest pain.

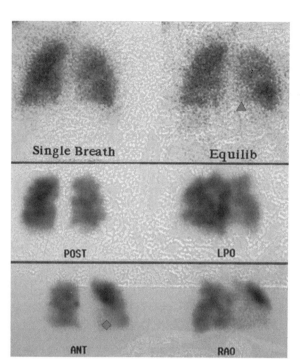

Single Breath   Equilib

POST   LPO

ANT   RAO

FIGURE 5–60 Pulmonary embolism, V/Q scan

This is a V/Q scan. In the top panel, ventilation is assessed as the patient inhales a radiolabeled compound that becomes distributed throughout the lung. In this case, distribution appears relatively uniform, except for a portion of the left lower lobe in which there is lack of ventilation (▲). Perfusion is assessed after injection of a radiolabeled compound that is distributed through the pulmonary vasculature. In the bottom two panels, various views indicate multiple areas in which perfusion is diminished (◆), and these areas are different from the area of decreased ventilation. Thus, there is a V/Q mismatch that gives a high probability for pulmonary embolism. Since the lung is ventilated, but not perfused, giving an affected patient oxygen therapy will increase the PaO_2 minimally.

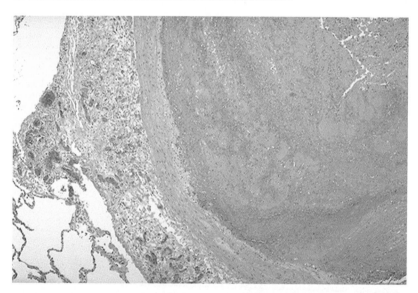

FIGURE 5–61 Pulmonary embolism, microscopic

Within this pulmonary artery are interdigitating areas of pale pink and red that form the lines of Zahn characteristic of a thrombus. These lines represent layers of red cells, platelets, and fibrin that are laid down as the thrombus forms in a vein. Here the thrombus has become a thromboembolus that has traveled through the vena cava and the right heart to become packed into a pulmonary artery branch. Over time, if the patient survives, the thromboembolus can undergo organization and dissolution.

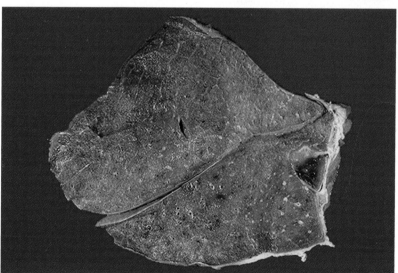

FIGURE 5–62 Pulmonary infarct, gross

Medium-sized thromboemboli (blocking a pulmonary artery to a lobule or set of lobules) can produce a hemorrhagic pulmonary infarction because the patient survives. The infarct is wedge shaped and based on the pleura. These infarcts are hemorrhagic because, although the pulmonary artery carrying most of the blood and oxygen is cut off, the bronchial arteries from the systemic circulation (supplying about 1% of the blood to the lungs) are not cut off. It is also possible to have multiple small pulmonary thromboemboli that do not cause sudden death and do not occlude a large enough branch of pulmonary artery to cause infarction. Clinical findings include chest pain and hemoptysis.

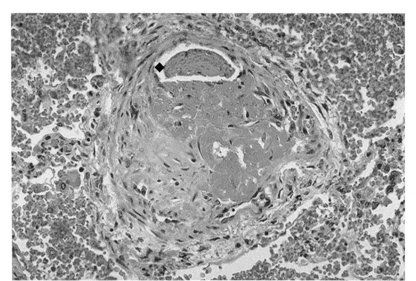

FIGURE 5–63 Pulmonary embolism, microscopic

Here is a small peripheral pulmonary artery thromboembolus in the region of a hemorrhagic infarct, marked by many RBCs within alveolar spaces. There is partial recanalization (◆) of this blocked artery. Such a small embolus would probably not cause dyspnea or pain unless there were many emboli and they were showered into the lungs over a period of time. They could collectively block enough small arteries to produce secondary pulmonary hypertension with cor pulmonale.

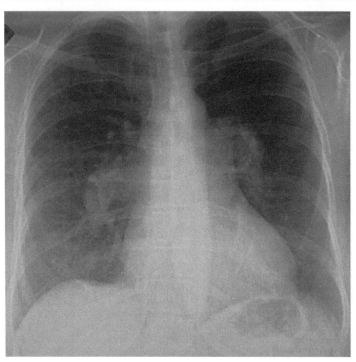

FIGURE 5–64 Pulmonary hypertension, radiograph

This PA chest radiograph shows prominent dilated pulmonary arteries that are branching from the hilar regions. The lung fields are clear. This patient had the rare condition of primary pulmonary hypertension, without an underlying restrictive or obstructive lung disease to account for the pulmonary hypertension. The result is a reduction of the pulmonary vascular bed with an increased pulmonary arterial pressure. The pulmonary capillary wedge pressure tends to remain normal until late in the disease, when right heart failure leads to left heart failure and impaired left ventricular filling. This familial form of pulmonary hypertension results from mutations in the bone morphogenetic protein receptor type 2 (*BMPR2*) gene. *BMPR2* signaling inhibits smooth muscle proliferation. Additional genetic and environmental factors also contribute.

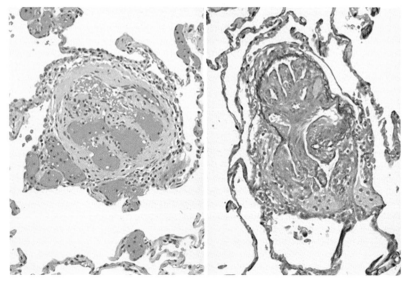

FIGURE 5–65 Pulmonary hypertension, microscopic

Both restrictive and obstructive lung diseases can affect the pulmonary arterial circulation. The loss of normal lung parenchyma leads to pulmonary hypertension, resulting in thickening of the small arteries along with reduplication to form a plexiform lesion, as seen here in a peripheral pulmonary artery, in the left panel with H+E stain and in the right panel with elastic tissue stain.

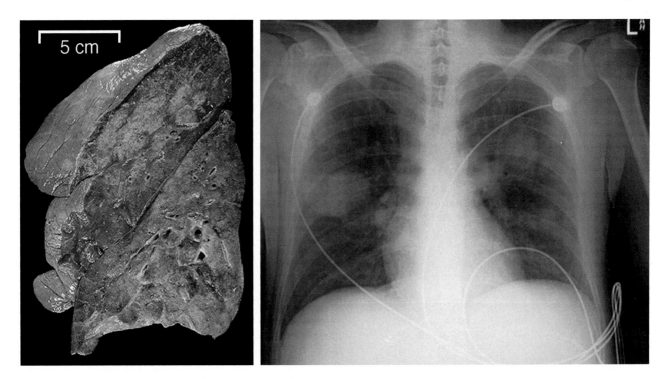

FIGURES 5–66 and 5–67 Bacterial pneumonia, gross and radiograph

At the left are lighter areas that appear to be raised on cut surface from the surrounding lung. Bronchopneumonia (lobular pneumonia) is characterized by patchy areas of pulmonary consolidation. The PA chest radiograph at the right demonstrates extensive bilateral patchy infiltrates that are composed primarily of alveolar exudates. The infiltrates seen here are made even more dense through hemorrhage from vascular damage by infection with *Pseudomonas aeruginosa*.

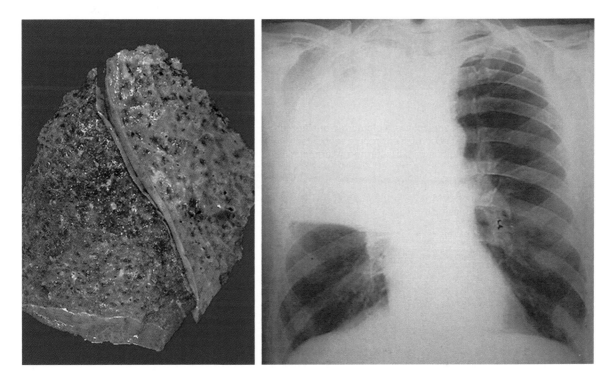

FIGURES 5–68 and 5–69 Bacterial pneumonia, gross and radiograph

This is a lobar pneumonia with consolidation of the entire left upper lobe as seen at the left. This pattern is much less common than the bronchopneumonia pattern. Most are due to *Streptococcus pneumoniae* (pneumococcus) infection. The PA chest radiograph at the right shows complete right upper lobe consolidation, consistent with a lobar pneumonia. The mediastinal and right heart borders are obscured by this process.

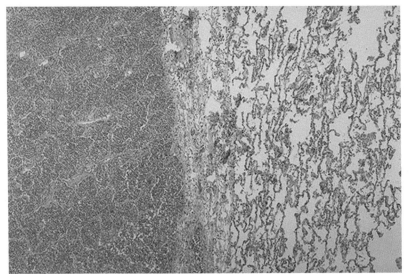

FIGURE 5–70 Bacterial pneumonia, microscopic

At the left the alveoli are filled with a neutrophilic exudate that corresponds to the areas of grossly apparent consolidation with bronchopneumonia. This contrasts with the aerated lung on the right. The pattern matches the patchy radiographic distribution of bronchopneumonia. The consolidated areas may match the distribution pattern of lung lobules (hence the term *lobular pneumonia*). A bronchopneumonia is classically a hospital-acquired pneumonia seen in patients already ill from another disease process. Typical causative bacterial organisms include *Staphylococcus aureus*, *Klebsiella pneumoniae*, *Haemophilus influenzae*, *Escherichia coli*, and *Pseudomonas aeruginosa*.

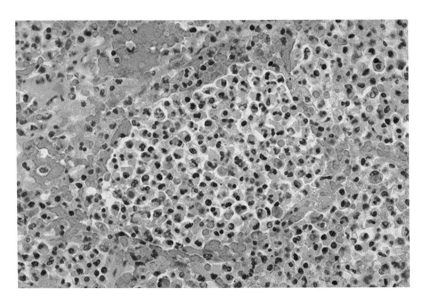

FIGURE 5–71 Bacterial pneumonia, microscopic

These alveolar exudates are composed mainly of neutrophils. The surrounding alveolar walls have capillaries that are congested (dilated and filled with RBCs). Such an exudative process is typical of bacterial infection. This exudate gives rise to the productive cough of purulent yellow sputum seen with bacterial pneumonias. The alveolar structure is still maintained, which is why even an extensive pneumonia often resolves with minimal residual destruction or damage to the pulmonary parenchyma. However, in patients with compromised lung function from underlying obstructive or restrictive lung disease, or cardiac disease, even limited pneumonic consolidation can be life-threatening.

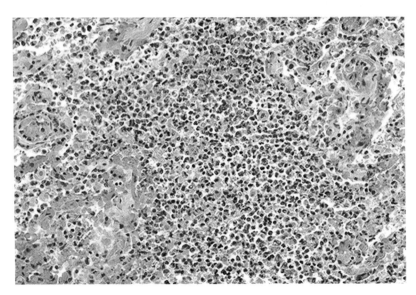

FIGURE 5–72 Bacterial pneumonia, microscopic

More virulent bacterial organisms or more severe inflammation with pneumonia can be associated with destruction of lung tissue and hemorrhage. Here, alveolar walls are no longer visible because there is early abscess formation with sheets of neutrophils, and also hemorrhage. Many bronchopneumonias follow an earlier viral pneumonia, particularly in older people in the colder months when infection with viral agents such as influenza is more common.

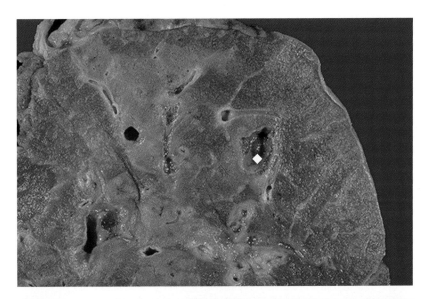

FIGURE 5–73 Lung abscesses, gross

This is an abscessing bronchopneumonia in which several abscesses (◆) with irregular, rough-surfaced walls are seen within areas of tan consolidation. Lung abscesses, if large enough, will contain liquefied necrotic material and purulent exudate that often results in an air-fluid level on chest radiograph or CT scan. An abscess is typically a complication of severe pneumonia, most often from virulent organisms such as *Staphylococcus aureus*. Abscesses often complicate aspiration, particularly in obtunded patients and those with neurologic diseases, in whom they appear more frequently in the right posterior lung. Abscesses can continue to be a source of septicemia and are difficult to treat.

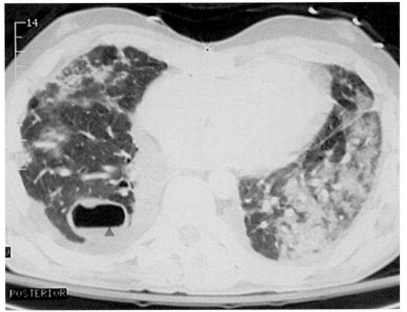

FIGURE 5–74 Lung abscess, CT image

The chest CT in the lung window setting demonstrates an air-fluid level (▲) within an abscess involving the right lower lobe. Note the adjacent areas of bright, patchy pneumonic infiltrates, which are bilateral and extensive. Also note the indentation of the anterior chest in the midline, a variation known as *pectus excavatum*. Abscesses may develop after aspiration, from antecedent bacterial infections, with septic embolization from venous sources or from right-sided infective endocarditis, and after bronchial obstruction. Affected patients can have fever with cough productive of copious purulent sputum. Spread of the infection with sepsis and septic emboli to other organs can complicate pulmonary abscesses.

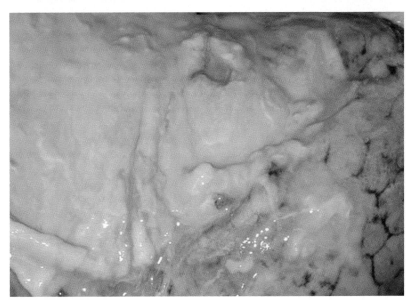

FIGURE 5–75 Empyema, gross

This pleural surface demonstrates a thick yellow-tan purulent exudate, and the pleural cavity is filled with purulent exudate. This is a collection of pus in the pleural space—an empyema. Pneumonia may spread within the lung and may be complicated by pleuritis. Initially, there may just be an effusion with a transudate into the pleural space. There may also be exudation of blood proteins to form a fibrinous pleuritis. However, bacterial infections in the lung can spread to the pleura to produce a purulent pleuritis. A thoracentesis will yield fluid characteristic of an exudate, with a high protein and a high white blood cell count, mainly neutrophils.

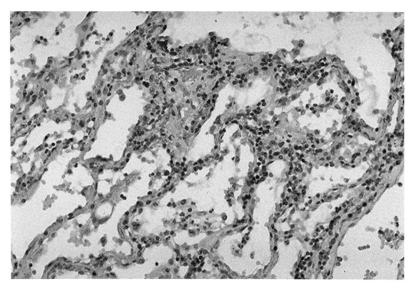

FIGURE 5–76 Viral pneumonia, microscopic

A viral pneumonia is characterized by interstitial lymphocytic infiltrates. Note that an alveolar exudate is absent. Thus, a patient with this type of pneumonia will probably have a nonproductive cough. The most common causes of viral pneumonia are influenza virus types A and B, parainfluenza virus, adenovirus, and respiratory syncytial virus (RSV), which appears mostly in children. Cytomegalovirus infection is most common in immunocompromised hosts. Viral cultures of sputum or bronchoalveolar lavage fluid may be performed. Alternatively, serologic testing may reveal the causative agent. Some strains of coronavirus can cause severe acute respiratory syndrome.

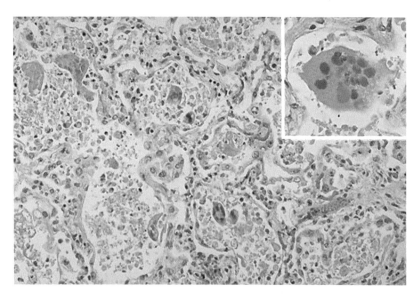

FIGURE 5–77 Respiratory syncytial virus (RSV) pneumonia, microscopic

This is RSV pneumonia in a child. Note the giant cells, which are a consequence of the viral cytopathic effect. The inset demonstrates a typical multinucleated giant cell with a prominent round, pink intracytoplasmic inclusion. RSV accounts for many cases of pneumonia in children younger than 2 years and can be a cause of death in infants 1 to 6 months of age or older.

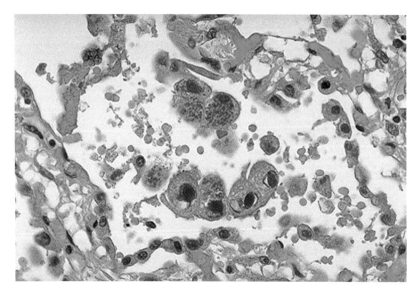

FIGURE 5–78 Cytomegalovirus pneumonia, microscopic

Note the very large cells that have large violet intranuclear inclusions surrounded by a small clear halo. Basophilic stippling can be seen in the cytoplasm of these cytomegalic cells. This is an infection typically seen in immunocompromised patients, such as those with HIV infection. Both endothelial and epithelial cells can become infected. There are no characteristic gross or microscopic features of cytomegalovirus pneumonia.

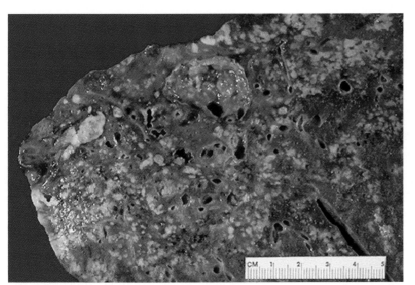

FIGURE 5–79 Secondary tuberculosis, gross

These scattered tan granulomas are present mostly in upper lung fields. Granulomatous lung disease grossly appears as irregularly sized, rounded nodules. Larger nodules may have central caseous necrosis that includes elements of both liquefactive and coagulative necrosis. This upper lobe pattern of involvement is most characteristic of secondary (reactivation or reinfection) tuberculosis, typically seen in adults. However, fungal granulomas (histoplasmosis, cryptococcosis, coccidioidomycosis) can mimic this pattern as well. This propensity of granulomas to involve upper lobes is typical and helps distinguish this infection from metastatic disease with radiographic imaging studies.

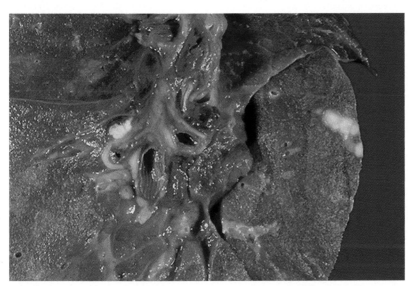

FIGURE 5–80 Primary tuberculosis, gross

There is a small tan-yellow subpleural granuloma in the mid-lung field. In the hilum is a small yellow-tan granuloma in a hilar lymph node next to a large bronchus. This is the Ghon complex that is the characteristic gross appearance with primary tuberculosis. In most people, this granulomatous disease is subclinical and does not progress further. Over time, the granulomas decrease in size and can calcify, leaving a focal calcified spot on a chest radiograph that suggests remote granulomatous disease. Primary tuberculosis is the pattern seen with initial infection, most often in children.

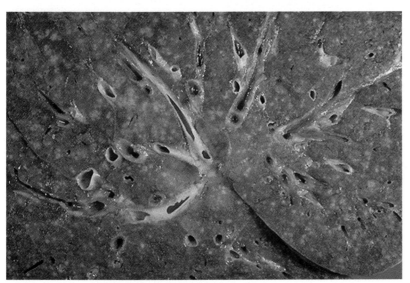

FIGURE 5–81 Miliary tuberculosis, gross

When the immune response is poor or is overwhelmed by an extensive infection, then it is possible to see the gross pattern of granulomatous disease known as a *miliary* pattern because there are a multitude of small, tan granulomas, averaging 2 to 4 mm in size, scattered throughout the lung parenchyma. The miliary pattern gets its name from the resemblance of the granulomas to millet seeds. Dissemination of the causative infectious agent (*Mycobacterium tuberculosis*, or fungi) may produce a similar miliary pattern in other organs.

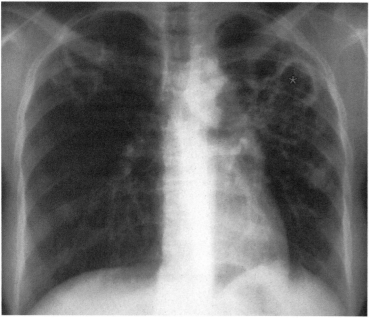
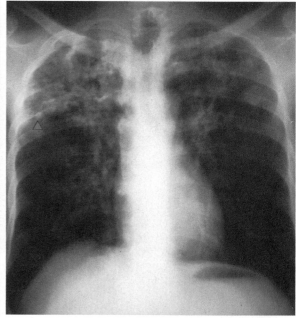

FIGURES 5–82 and 5–83 Secondary tuberculosis, radiographs

The PA chest radiograph at the left reveals upper lobe granulomatous disease marked by irregular reticular and nodular densities and upper lobe cavitation (∗) due to the central caseous necrosis typical for tuberculosis. The PA chest radiograph at the right reveals extensive granulomatous disease of both lungs. Note the focal brighter calcifications that are typical of healed tuberculosis. Other small white calcifications (▲) are scattered, mainly in mid to upper lung fields, seen here more prominently on the right. There can be reactivation or reinfection to produce this pattern for secondary tuberculosis.

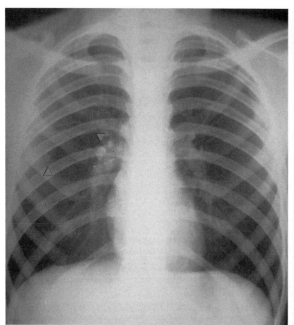
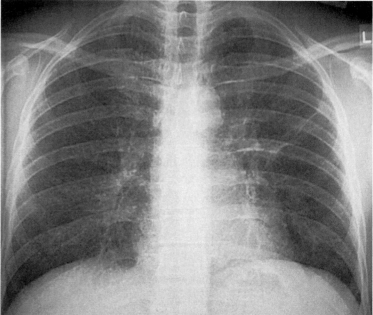

FIGURES 5–84 and 5–85 Primary and miliary tuberculosis, radiographs

The PA chest radiograph at the left is characteristic of primary tuberculosis with a subpleural granuloma (▲) and marked hilar lymphadenopathy (▼). These two findings together constitute the Ghon complex. Most cases of primary tuberculosis are asymptomatic. The PA chest radiograph at the right reveals a miliary pattern in all lung fields. Note the stippled appearance throughout, an effect reminiscent of the pointillist style of art.

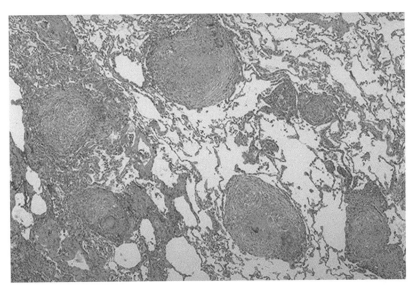

FIGURE 5–86 Tuberculosis, microscopic

Well-defined granulomas have rounded outlines with discrete borders. Granulomas are composed of transformed macrophages called epithelioid cells, along with lymphocytes, occasional polymorphonuclear leukocytes, plasma cells, and fibroblasts. The macrophages that are stimulated by cytokines, such as interferon-γ secreted from nearby T lymphocytes, may group together to form Langhans giant cells. The localized, small appearance of these granulomas suggests that the immune response is fairly good and the infection is being contained. This would produce a reticulonodular radiographic pattern in the lungs.

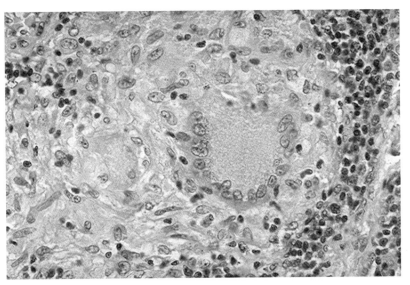

FIGURE 5–87 Tuberculosis, microscopic

A granulomatous inflammatory response to tuberculosis includes mainly epithelioid cells, lymphocytes, and fibroblasts. The granuloma demonstrates that the epithelioid macrophages are elongated with long, pale nuclei and pink cytoplasm. The macrophages organize into committees called *giant cells*. The typical giant cell for infectious granulomas is called a *Langhans giant cell* and has the nuclei lined up along one edge of the cell. The process of granulomatous inflammation takes place over months to years (did you ever hear of a committee action that was completed in a short time?).

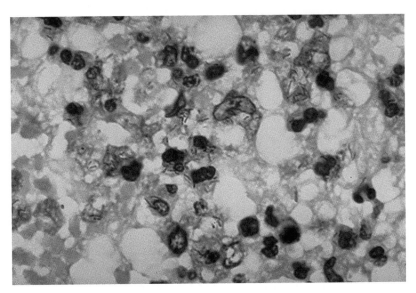

FIGURE 5–88 Acid-fast bacilli, microscopic

To identify the mycobacteria in a tissue section, a stain for acid-fast bacilli is performed. The mycobacteria stain as red rods, seen here at high magnification. The large amount of lipid in the form of mycolic acid imparts this acid-fast property to the mycobacteria and accounts for their resistance to immune cell destruction. Their destruction depends upon a T_H1 immune response with CD4 cell elaboration of interferon-γ that recruits monocytes and transforms them into epithelioid macrophages, then stimulates up-regulation of nitric oxide synthase within epithelioid cell and giant cell phagosomes.

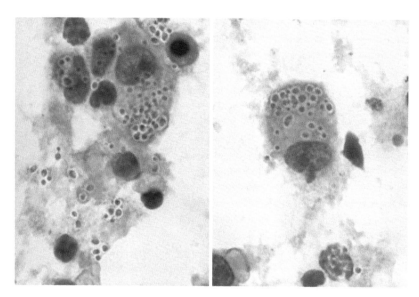

FIGURE 5–89 Histoplasmosis, microscopic

Inhalation of aerosols from soil with bird or bat droppings contaminated with spores of *Histoplasma capsulatum* can produce pulmonary granulomatous inflammation. Pulmonary infection can spread to other organs, particularly in immunocompromised people. Macrophages ingest the organisms, as shown here filled with numerous small 2- to 4-μm organisms. The macrophages elaborate interferon-γ to activate and recruit more macrophages to destroy these yeasts. The organisms have a clear zone around a central blue nucleus, which gives the cell membrane the appearance of a capsule; hence, the name of the organism.

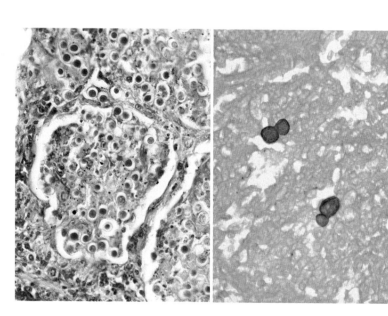

FIGURE 5–90 Blastomycosis, microscopic

Soil contaminated with the mycelial form of *Blastomyces dermatitidis* may be inhaled, producing pulmonary granulomatous inflammation. The pulmonary infection may become disseminated to other organs. A rare cutaneous form of disease occurs with direct skin inoculation. The 5- to 15-μm organisms exist in the yeast phase at body temperature. Note the broad-based budding, highlighted by the GMS stain in the right panel. This organism has a fairly broad distribution in temperate to semitropical areas of North America, Africa, and India.

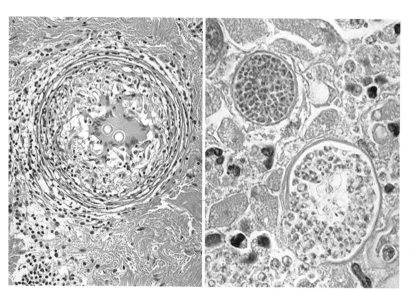

FIGURE 5–91 Coccidioidomycosis, microscopic

The well-formed granuloma seen in the left panel has a large Langhans giant cell at the center containing two small spherules of *Coccidioides immitis*. At higher magnification in the right panel, with a disseminated infection to liver, the thick walls of two *C. immitis* spherules are seen. Note how one spherule is bursting to expel its endospores, which grow and continue the infection. In the United States, *C. immitis* is endemic to the desert Southwest, but it can be found inhabiting dry plains of North and South America. In nature, *C. immitis* exists in a hyphal form with characteristic alternating arthrospores.

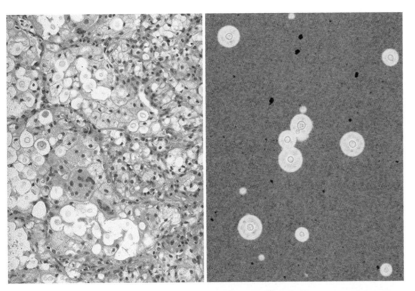

FIGURE 5–92 Cryptococcosis, microscopic

In the left panel are numerous *Cryptococcus neoformans* organisms that have a large polysaccharide capsule, giving the appearance of a clear zone around a faint, central round nucleus. The India ink preparation in the right panel highlights the clear capsule around the nucleus. This capsule inhibits inflammatory cell recruitment and macrophage phagocytosis. Cryptococcal infection with pneumonia can occur after inhalation of aerosols from soils contaminated with bird droppings. These 5- to 10-μm yeasts can become disseminated to other organs, particularly the CNS, often producing meningitis in immunocompromised people. The inflammatory reaction can range from suppurative to granulomatous.

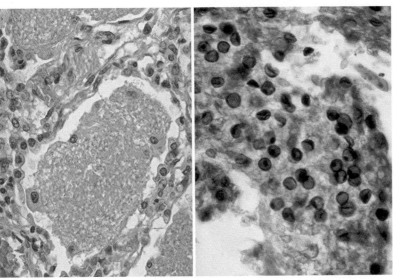

FIGURE 5–93 Pneumocystis, microscopic

In the left panel, the granular pink alveolar exudate of *Pneumocystis carinii (jirovecii)* pneumonia is seen. The exudate consists of edema fluid, protein, *Pneumocystis* organisms, and dead inflammatory cells. In the right panel, a Gomori methenamine silver stain on bronchoalveolar lavage fluid shows the 4- to 8-μm dark cyst walls, with the organisms appearing as crushed ping-pong balls. This infection occurs in immunocompromised people and is uncommonly disseminated. Patients typically present with fever, nonproductive cough, and dyspnea. Radiographic studies show bilateral diffuse infiltrates, most pronounced in perihilar regions.

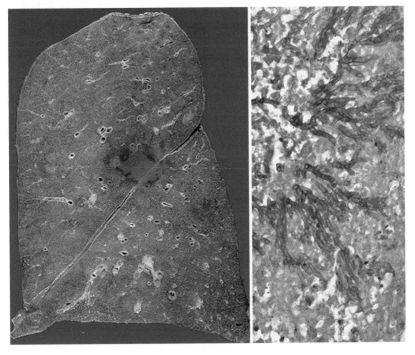

FIGURE 5–94 Aspergillosis, microscopic

In the left panel, a sagittal section of left lung shows a necrotizing fungal "target lesion" with a hemorrhagic border invading across the major fissure and into vessels. In the right panel, the 5- to 10-μm thick branching septate hyphae of *Aspergillus* are seen. Inhalation of airborne conidia of *Aspergillus* species may produce pulmonary infection, particularly in immunocompromised people, especially those with neutropenia or receiving corticosteroid therapy. Hematogenous dissemination to other organs can occur. *Aspergillus* may colonize preexisting cavitary lesions caused by tuberculosis, bronchiectasis, abscess, or infarct. An allergic reaction to this fungus with a T$_H$2 cell-mediated immune response can lead to allergic bronchopulmonary aspergillosis with acute features similar to those of asthma and chronic changes of obstructive lung disease.

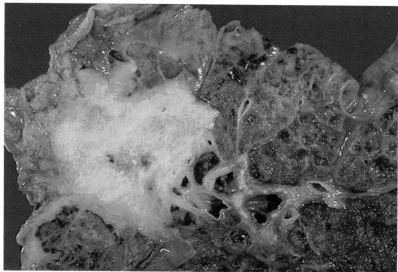

◀ **FIGURE 5–95 Squamous cell carcinoma, gross**

This carcinoma is arising centrally in the lung (as most squamous cell carcinomas do) and is obstructing the right main bronchus. This neoplasm is very firm and has a pale white to tan cut surface. This is one of the most common primary malignancies of lung and is most often seen in smokers; emphysema is also seen here. The black areas represent anthracotic pigment trapped in the tumor and hilar lymph nodes.

FIGURES 5–96 and 5–97 Squamous cell carcinoma, radiograph and CT image ▼

Note the appearance of a large hilar mass (◆). The chest CT reveals the large squamous cell carcinoma involving right upper lobe and extending around the right main bronchus (■), invading into the mediastinum and involving hilar lymph nodes (▲).

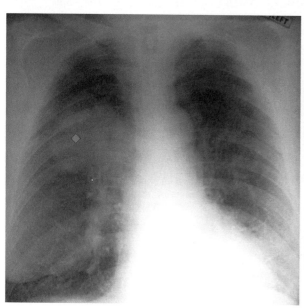

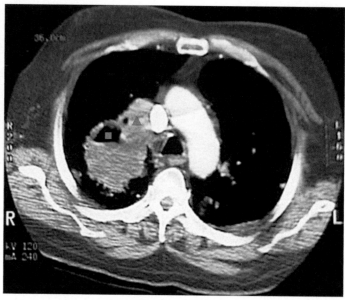

◀ **FIGURE 5–98 Squamous cell carcinoma, microscopic**

The cells with their pink cytoplasm containing keratin along with distinct cell borders and intercellular bridges (▲) are characteristic of squamous cell carcinoma, seen here at high magnification. A mitotic figure (◆) is present. Such features are seen in well-differentiated tumors (those that more closely mimic the cell of origin). Most bronchogenic carcinomas, however, are poorly differentiated. *RB, p53*, and *p16* gene mutations are often present. The most common paraneoplastic syndrome seen with pulmonary squamous cell carcinoma is hypercalcemia from production of parathormone-related peptide.

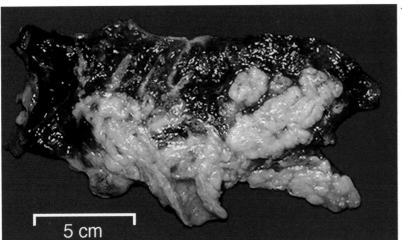

◄ **FIGURE 5–99 Small cell carcinoma, gross**

Arising centrally in this lung and spreading extensively is a small cell anaplastic (oat cell) carcinoma. The cut surface of this tumor has a soft, lobulated, white to tan appearance. The tumor seen here has caused obstruction of the main bronchus to the left lung so that the distal lung is collapsed (atelectatic). Oat cell carcinomas are very aggressive and often metastasize widely before the primary tumor mass in the lung reaches a large size. These neoplasms are more amenable to chemotherapy than radiation therapy or surgery, but the prognosis is still poor. Oat cell carcinomas occur almost exclusively in smokers.

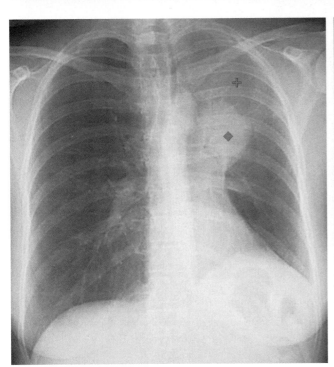

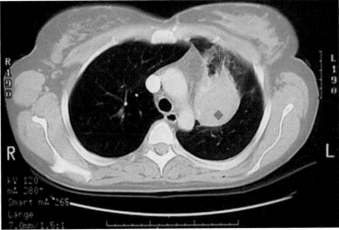

FIGURES 5–100 and 5–101 Bronchogenic carcinoma, radiograph and CT image

There is a carcinoma (◆) at the left hilum in the upper lobe that has caused postobstructive atelectasis (with mediastinal shift to the left) and a lipid pneumonia, marked by haziness (+) and infiltrates distal to the mass. Primary lung neoplasms that arise centrally, such as small cell carcinoma, can produce these complications. The chest CT at the right shows the same hilar mass and distal lipid pneumonia, and the mediastinum is shifted to the left.

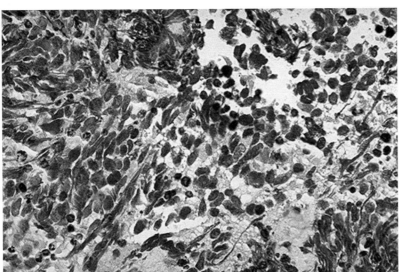

◄ **FIGURE 5–102 Small cell carcinoma, microscopic**

The microscopic pattern of a small cell (oat cell) carcinoma has small dark blue cells with minimal cytoplasm (high nuclear-to-cytoplasmic ratio) packed together in sheets. The cells often show "crush artefact" from handling the specimen. Mutations in *p53* and *RB* tumor suppressor genes, and antiapoptotic *BCL2* gene, are often present. Oat cell carcinomas, which are a highly malignant form of neuroendocrine tumor, are often associated with paraneoplastic syndromes from hormonal effects. Ectopic adrenocorticotropic hormone producing Cushing syndrome and the syndrome of inappropriate antidiuretic hormone leading to hyponatremia are two such syndromes.

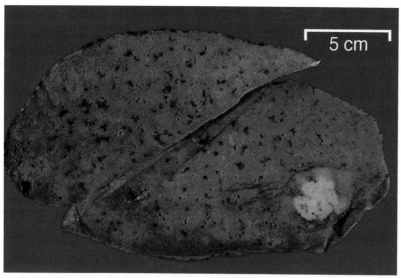

◀ **FIGURE 5–103 Adenocarcinoma, gross**

Note the peripheral location of this mass in the left lung. Adenocarcinomas and large cell anaplastic carcinomas tend to arise peripherally in lung. Adenocarcinoma is the one cell type of primary lung tumor that occurs more often in nonsmokers and in smokers who have quit. If this neoplasm were confined to the lung (a lower stage), then resection would have a greater chance of cure. The solitary appearance of this neoplasm suggests that the tumor is primary rather than metastatic.

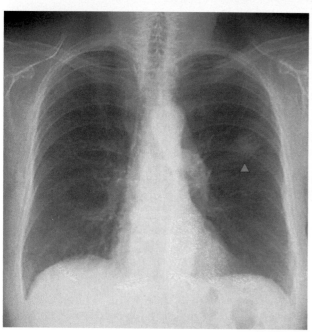

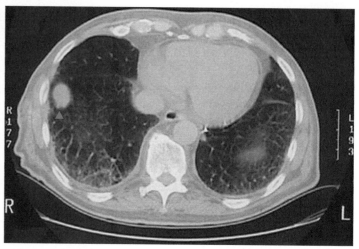

FIGURES 5–104 and 5–105 Adenocarcinoma, radiograph and CT image

A peripheral adenocarcinoma (▲) appears in this chest radiograph of a nonsmoker. Lung cancers in nonsmokers are rare, but if they occur, they are likely to be adenocarcinomas. The chest CT in lung window density demonstrates a peripheral right lung adenocarcinoma that was removed easily with a wedge resection.

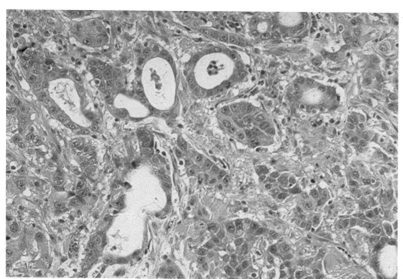

◀ **FIGURE 5–106 Adenocarcinoma, microscopic**

The glandular structures formed by this neoplasm are consistent with a moderately differentiated adenocarcinoma. Droplets of mucin may be found within the tumor cell cytoplasm. Prominent nucleoli are often present. However, many bronchogenic carcinomas, including adenocarcinomas, are poorly differentiated, making diagnosis of the cell type challenging. From a therapeutic standpoint, a designation of non–small cell carcinoma may be sufficient, depending upon the tumor stage. *RB*, *p53*, and *p16* gene mutations are often present. *K-RAS* gene mutations are more likely to be present in smokers.

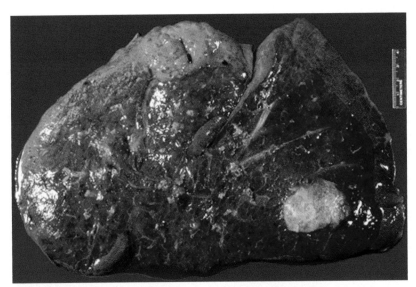

FIGURE 5–107 Large cell carcinoma, gross

The peripheral lung mass seen here in a smoker (note the centriacinar emphysema) proved to be a large cell anaplastic carcinoma. This particular type of bronchogenic carcinoma is poorly differentiated, without light microscopic features of either adenocarcinoma or squamous cell carcinoma. From a treatment standpoint, it is still a non–small cell carcinoma (like adenocarcinoma and squamous cell carcinoma), for which the stage is the most important determinant of therapy and prognosis.

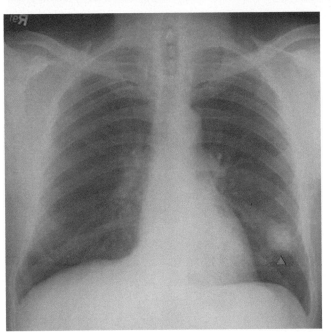

FIGURE 5–108 Large cell carcinoma, radiograph

This chest radiograph demonstrates a mass lesion (▲) in the left lower lobe that proved to be a non–small cell carcinoma, which was best termed *large cell anaplastic carcinoma* on microscopic examination. Large cell carcinomas are seen with increased frequency in smokers.

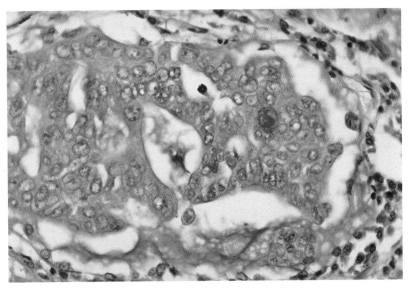

FIGURE 5–109 Poorly differentiated carcinoma, microscopic

The large cell carcinoma is distinguished by its distinct lack of glandular or squamous differentiation. Many of them are probably adenocarcinomas or squamous carcinomas that are so poorly differentiated that it is difficult to determine the cell of origin. Seen here with PAS stain are droplets of intracellular mucin that suggest an adenocarcinoma. Non–small cell pulmonary carcinomas are less frequently associated with paraneoplastic syndromes than small cell carcinomas. Other extrapulmonary manifestations of bronchogenic carcinoma include Lambert-Eaton myasthenic syndrome, acanthosis nigricans, peripheral neuropathy, and hypertrophic pulmonary osteoarthropathy.

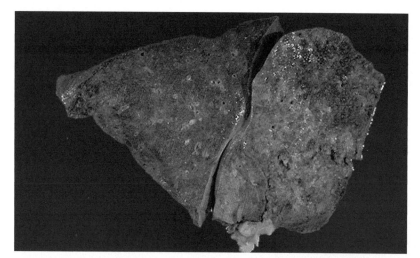

FIGURE 5–110 Bronchioloalveolar carcinoma, gross

This is a less common variant of lung carcinoma that appears grossly (and on chest radiograph) as a less well-defined area resembling pneumonic consolidation. A poorly defined mass involving the lung lobe toward the right here has a pale tan to gray appearance.

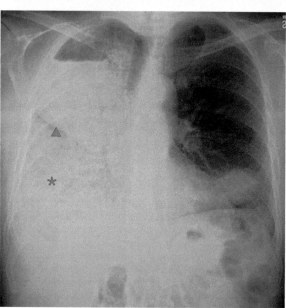

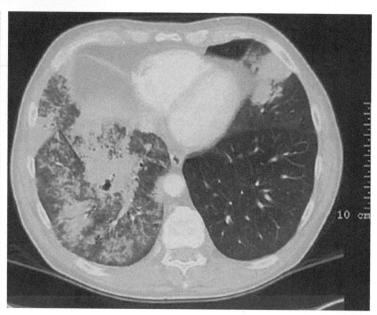

FIGURES 5–111 and 5–112 Bronchioloalveolar carcinoma, radiograph and CT image

The PA chest radiograph at the left and the chest CT at the right show extensive bronchioloalveolar carcinoma involving most of the right lung. The extensive spread of the tumor within the lung leads to an appearance resembling areas of consolidation (*) similar to those seen with pneumonia. There is a loculated pleural effusion (▲) above the neoplasm, as seen at the left.

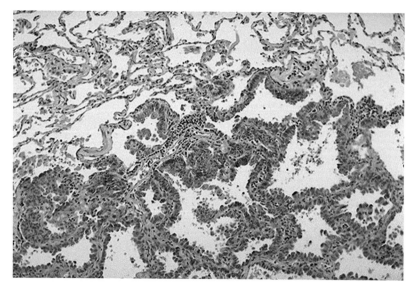

FIGURE 5–113 Bronchioloalveolar carcinoma, microscopic

The bronchioloalveolar carcinoma is composed of columnar cells that proliferate along the framework of alveolar septae. These neoplastic cells are well differentiated. These neoplasms, a form of adenocarcinoma, in general have a better prognosis than most other primary lung cancers, but they may not be detected at a low stage. Nonmucinous variants are usually solitary nodules that are amenable to resection. Mucinous variants tend to spread and form satellite tumors or pneumonia-like consolidation.

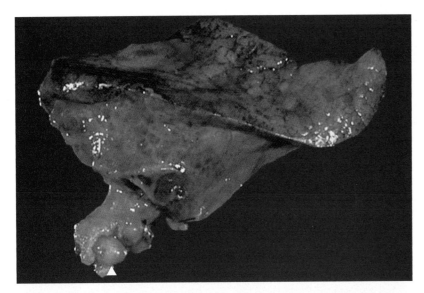

FIGURE 5–114 Bronchial carcinoid, gross

This lung resection was necessitated by the presence of a bronchial carcinoid tumor (▲) that caused hemoptysis and obstruction with distal atelectasis. These endobronchial, discrete, polypoid masses can occur in young to middle-aged adults. Their appearance is not related to smoking. They are not common. They are a form of neuroendocrine tumor that arises from neuroendocrine cells found within the mucosa of the airways.

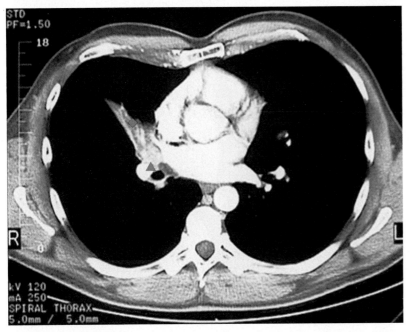

FIGURE 5–115 Bronchial carcinoid, CT image

This chest CT in bone window demonstrates a bronchial carcinoid tumor (▲) that is causing obstruction with atelectasis (◆) of the right middle lobe. Typical clinical findings may include cough and hemoptysis. These highly vascular lesions may bleed profusely when biopsied. There are other bronchial adenomas that are low-grade endobronchial neoplasms that can be locally invasive or even metastasize; these include adenoid cystic and mucoepidermoid tumors.

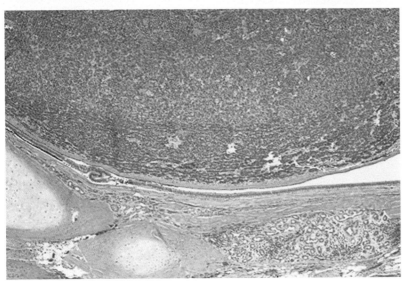

FIGURE 5–116 Bronchial carcinoid, microscopic

Here is a well-circumscribed mass arising from the bronchial wall and composed of uniform small blue cells in sheets and nests. Since these tumors are of neuroendocrine origin, immunohistochemical staining may be positive for compounds such as chromogranin, serotonin, and neuron-specific enolase. This carcinoid tumor is considered the benign counterpart of the small cell carcinoma, at opposite ends of the spectrum of neuroendocrine tumors of the lung. In between are the atypical carcinoids. Bronchial carcinoids usually reach 1 to 2 cm in size before producing symptoms related to obstruction and bleeding. They are unlikely to produce hormonal effects.

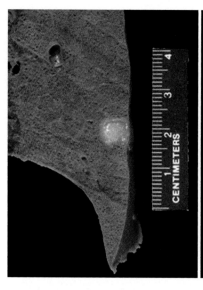
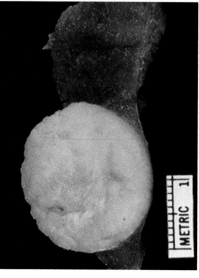

◀ **FIGURE 5–117 Hamartoma, gross**

Here are two examples of a benign lung tumor known as a *pulmonary hamartoma*. These uncommon lesions appear on chest radiograph as a "coin lesion" that has a differential diagnosis of granuloma and localized malignant neoplasm. They are firm and discrete and often have calcifications in them that also appear on radiography. Most are small (<2 cm).

FIGURES 5–118 and 5–119 Hamartoma, radiograph and CT image ▼

The PA chest radiograph at the left shows a discreet coin lesion (▲) that did not greatly increase in size over time. The chest CT in lung window density at the right reveals the presence of a small rounded mass (▲) in the right lung of this rather large individual. The differential diagnosis could include a granuloma, peripheral carcinoma, solitary metastasis, or hamartoma. This mass lesion proved to be a hamartoma, a good diagnosis to have—but not a common one.

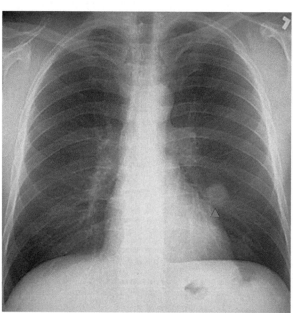
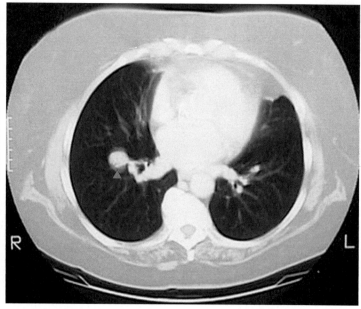

◀ **FIGURE 5–120 Hamartoma, microscopic**

This pulmonary hamartoma microscopically is composed mostly of benign elements: cartilage on the right that is jumbled with a fibrovascular stroma and scattered bronchial glandular structures on the left. The cartilaginous nature of this mass causes it to bounce off a biopsy needle like a ping-pong ball. A hamartoma is a neoplasm in an organ that is composed of tissue elements normally found at that site, but growing in a haphazard mass.

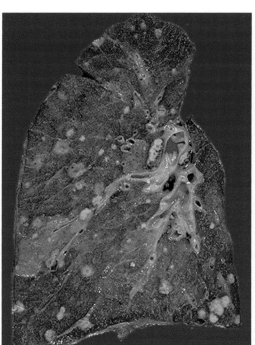
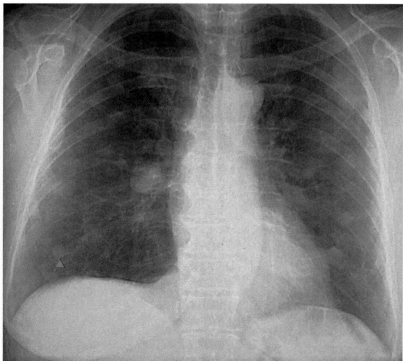

FIGURES 5–121 and 5–122 Metastases, gross and radiograph

Multiple variable-sized masses (▲) are seen in all lung fields in the gross and PA chest radiographic images. These tan-white nodules are characteristic of metastatic carcinoma. Metastases to the lungs are more common even than primary lung neoplasms simply because so many other primary tumors can metastasize to the lungs. The hilar nodes also demonstrate nodules of metastatic carcinoma. Such nodules are often in the periphery and do not cause major airway obstruction.

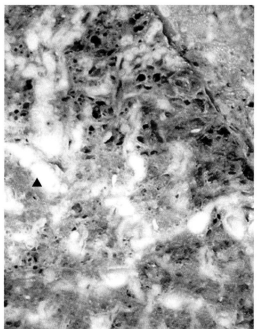
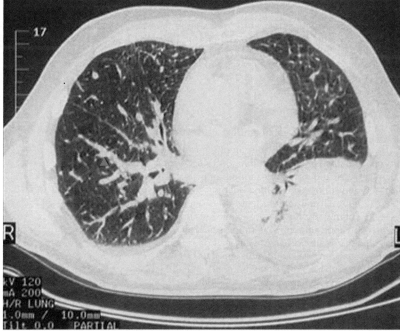

FIGURES 5–123 and 5–124 Metastases, gross and CT image

The cut surface of the lung reveals linear interstitial markings (▲) and nodules in a case of lymphangitic metastatic carcinoma, one of the less common patterns of metastasis. The chest CT shows a diffuse reticular and nodular pattern of involvement by metastatic carcinoma spreading into the lymphatic channels of the lung. There is also a large malignant pleural effusion at the lower left.

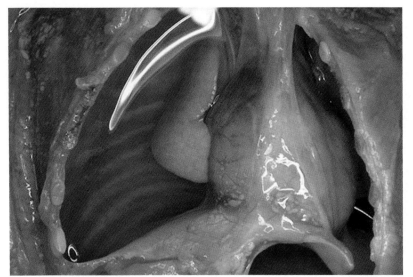

FIGURE 5–125 Serous pleural effusion, gross

Here is an example at autopsy of fluid collection into a body cavity, or an effusion. This is a right pleural effusion (in a baby). Note the clear, pale yellow appearance of the fluid. This is a serous effusion. Extravascular fluid collections can be classified as follows:

Exudate: An extravascular fluid collection that is rich in protein, cells, or both. The fluid appears grossly cloudy.

Transudate: An extravascular fluid collection that is basically an ultrafiltrate of plasma with little protein and few or no cells. The fluid appears grossly clear.

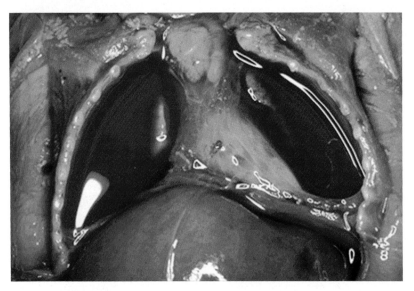

FIGURE 5–126 Serosanguineous pleural effusion, gross

Note that the fluid within the pleural cavities appears reddish because there has been hemorrhage into the effusion. Effusions into body cavities can be further described as follows:

Serous: A transudate with mainly edema fluid and few cells

Serosanguineous: An effusion with RBCs

Fibrinous (serofibrinous): Fibrin strands are derived from a protein-rich exudate

Purulent: Numerous polymorphonuclear leukocytes are present (also called *empyema* in the pleural space)

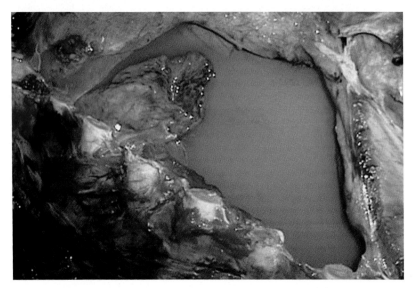

FIGURE 5–127 Chylous pleural effusion, gross

The right pleural cavity is filled with a cloudy yellowish-tan to milky fluid, characteristic of a chylothorax, which is uncommon. The fluid has numerous fat globules and few cells, mainly lymphocytes. Penetrating trauma or obstruction of the thoracic duct, usually by a primary or metastatic neoplasm, may lead to chylothorax formation. In this case, malignant lymphoma involving the lymphatics of the chest and abdomen led to the collection of chylous fluid. The right lung is markedly atelectatic from external compression by the pleural fluid collection.

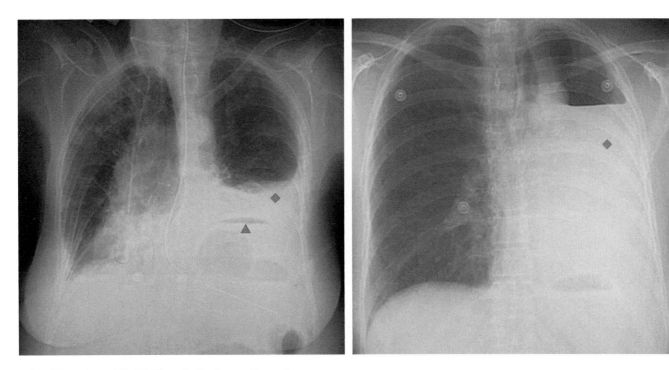

FIGURES 5–128 and 5–129 Pleural effusion, radiographs

The PA chest radiograph at the left demonstrates fluid (◆) in the left pleural cavity in a patient with lung carcinoma causing obstruction and pneumonia. An air-fluid level (▲) is seen in the stomach below the dome of the left diaphragmatic leaf, which is much higher than the right, consistent with atelectasis on the left. The PA chest film at the right shows a large pleural effusion (◆) nearly filling the left chest cavity. This fluid collection occurred postoperatively after a left pneumonectomy.

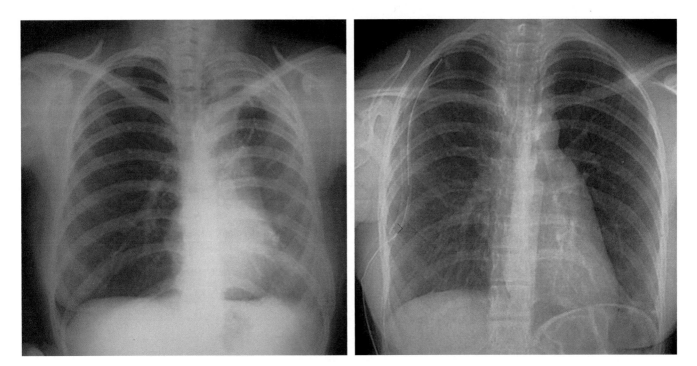

FIGURES 5–130 and 5–131 Pneumothorax, radiographs

These PA chest radiographs reveal a right pneumothorax. Note the displacement of the heart to the left. A pneumothorax occurs with a penetrating chest injury, inflammation with rupture of a bronchus to the pleura, rupture of an emphysematous bulla, or positive pressure ventilation. The escape of air into the pleural space collapses the lung. The examples seen here are of a tension pneumothorax shifting the mediastinum because a ball–valve air leak is increasing the air in the right chest cavity. The radiograph at the right shows a chest tube (◆) inserted to help reexpand the lung.

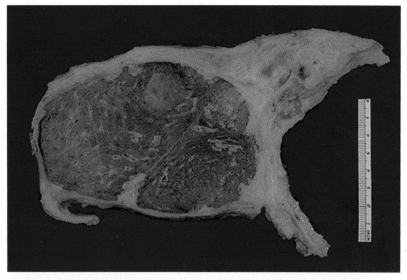

FIGURE 5–132 Malignant mesothelioma, gross

The dense white encircling tumor mass is arising from the visceral pleura and is a malignant mesothelioma. These are big, bulky tumors that can fill the chest cavity. The risk factor for mesothelioma is asbestos exposure. Asbestosis more commonly predisposes to bronchogenic carcinomas, increasing the risk by a factor of five. Smoking increases the risk for lung cancer by a factor of ten. Thus, smokers with a history of asbestos exposure have a 50-fold greater likelihood of developing bronchogenic lung cancer.

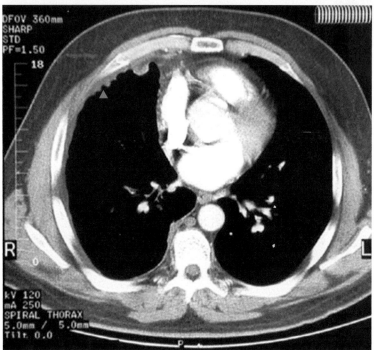

FIGURE 5–133 Malignant mesothelioma, CT image

This chest CT scan in the bone window setting demonstrates a malignant mesothelioma involving the right pleura, with thickening (▲) and nodularity. This may obscure pleural plaques that may have been present. The neoplasm is seen near the base of the lung. The development of mesothelioma may follow the initial asbestos exposure by 25 to 45 years, and the amount and duration of the initial exposure may have been minimal. Adjacent lung, in cases of more significant asbestos exposure, may have interstitial fibrosis. Asbestos (ferruginous) bodies are increased in number within the lung parenchyma.

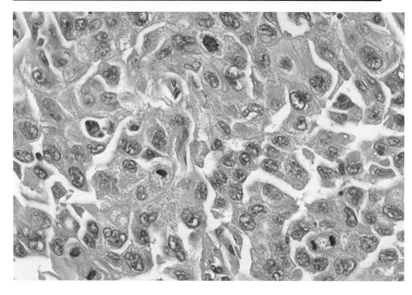

FIGURE 5–134 Malignant mesothelioma, microscopic

Mesotheliomas have either spindle cells or plump, rounded cells forming glandlike configurations. Cytogenetic abnormalities are often present, as are *p53* mutations. They are very difficult to diagnose cytologically. At high magnification as shown here, the rounded, epithelioid cells of a malignant mesothelioma are seen. Mesotheliomas are rare, even in people with asbestos exposure, and are virtually never seen in people without a history of asbestos exposure. In addition to the pleura, other but less common sites of occurrence of this neoplasm are the peritoneum, pericardium, and testicular tunica.

CHAPTER 6

Head and Neck

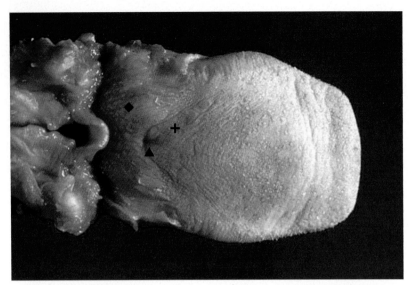

FIGURE 6–1 Normal tongue, gross

The tongue and the epiglottis are seen superiorly. The abundant submucosal lymphoid tissue (lingual tonsil) gives the posterior tongue (◆) a lobulated surface. The small indentation at the posterior tongue represents a vestigial foramen cecum (▲). The tongue surface has papillae. The filiform papillae impart a velvety texture to the dorsal (upper) surface and allow for a scraping function. Circumvallate papillae (+) are arranged in a V pattern toward the back of the tongue and have associated taste buds. Foliate papillae at the posterolateral aspects have associated taste buds. Fungiform papillae have a rounded surface and are nonkeratinized to give the appearance of a red dot pattern on the dorsum of the tongue and have associated taste buds.

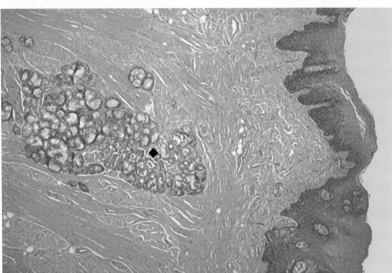

FIGURE 6–2 Normal tongue, microscopic

The tongue is covered with thick stratified squamous epithelium. The bulk of the tongue consists of the genioglossus muscle with the muscle bundles arranged in three planes to provide movement in any direction. The squamous mucosa extends across the floor of the oral cavity to become the gingiva at the base of the teeth. Scattered throughout the tongue, but more prominent toward the back of the tongue, are minor salivary glands (◆).

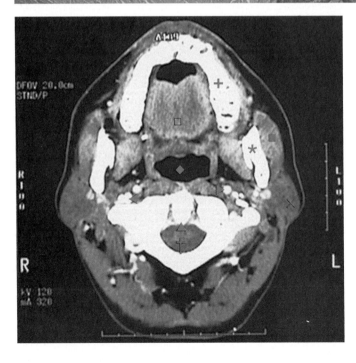

FIGURE 6–3 Normal head, CT image

This normal axial head and neck CT demonstrates the relationships of the maxilla (+) with teeth and nasopharynx (◆), tongue (□), ramus of mandible (*), masseter muscle (■), C2 and dens (▲), spinal canal (†), internal jugular vein (◄), internal carotid artery (►), and parotid gland (×).

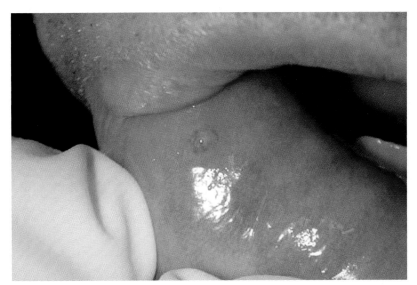

FIGURE 6–4 Cold sore, gross

The small "cold sore" seen here on the buccal mucosa just inside the lower lip is the result of herpes simplex virus type 1 (HSV-1) infection. Most adults have had past HSV-1 infection, but it remains latent, only to produce this small sore during periods of stress, from local trauma, or with environmental changes such as exposure to cold. This vesicle may rupture to produce an ulcer, which can then become secondarily infected. A similar lesion is the aphthous ulcer, or "canker sore," which can appear under conditions of stress, local trauma, or hormonal changes, but does not have an infectious etiology. About 5% to 25% of the population have had aphthous ulcers, particularly during the second decade of life.

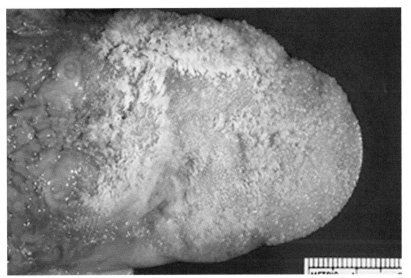

FIGURE 6–5 Oral candidiasis, gross

The tongue is covered with a tan, matted layer of *Candida* organisms enmeshed in a fibrinopurulent exudate, forming the pseudomembranous form of candidiasis. This can be scraped off to reveal an erythematous base. *Candida albicans* is a frequent oral commensal, present in half of the population; it is normally held in check by normal oral flora. The "thrush" as seen here is most likely to occur in immunocompromised people.

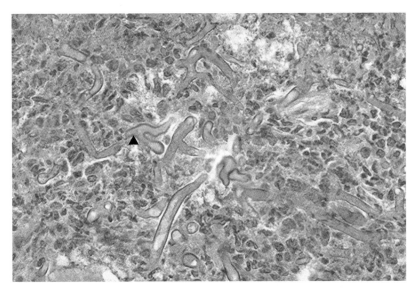

FIGURE 6–6 Mucormycosis (zygomycosis), microscopic

Note here the broad, nonseptate hyphae (▲) (6 to 50 μm wide) with necrotizing inflammation. Infection with *Mucor circinelloides* and related genera *Rhizopus* and *Absidia* of the "true" sexual fungi (Zygomycetes) can produce extensive tissue invasion and necrosis. Inhalation of airborne spores by immunocompromised people, particularly those with diabetes mellitus and ketoacidosis, corticosteroid therapy, and neutropenia, can lead to nasopharyngeal, pulmonary, and gastrointestinal infection. Spread of these organisms into the orbit and intracranial cavity (rhinocerebral mucormycosis) is a feared complication.

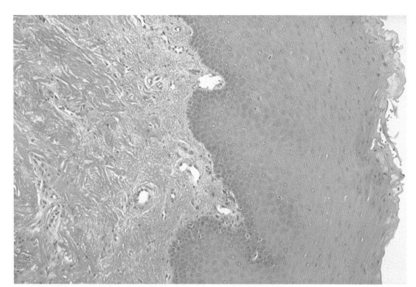

FIGURE 6–7 Leukoplakia, microscopic

In this excised lesion from the buccal mucosa, the overlying squamous epithelium is thickened (acanthotic), producing the gross appearance of a white plaque or leukoplakia on the oral mucosal surface. In addition, the underlying submucosa has increased collagen deposition, leading to the diagnosis of irritation fibroma in this patient with ill-fitting dentures. Although no cellular atypia is seen here, persistent leukoplakia can be a precursor to squamous atypia and carcinoma. Besides mechanical irritation, use of tobacco, alcohol, and betel nut can predispose to leukoplakia. Areas of grossly red and eroded epithelium denote erythroplakia, which carries a higher risk for malignant transformation.

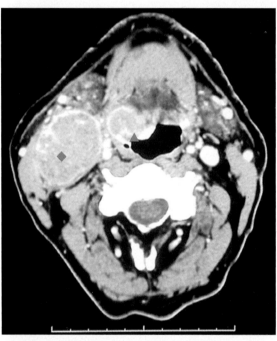

FIGURE 6–8 Squamous cell carcinoma, CT image

Shown is a prominent mass (▲) involving the right posterior base of the tongue in the region of the lingual tonsil. There is a large confluent mass of adjacent lymph nodes (◆) involved with metastatic squamous carcinoma. The oral cavity, floor of the mouth, tongue, and soft palate are the most common locations for squamous carcinoma to arise, but multiple lesions may occur. Distant metastases may involve lungs, liver, and bone marrow. The major risk factors are tobacco use (particularly the "smokeless" tobacco products) and alcohol abuse. In regions where chewing betel nut is popular, the incidence of oral cavity cancers is higher. Half of oropharyngeal cancers are associated with human papillomavirus infection. Chronic mucosal irritation from trauma or infection may promote the neoplastic process. About 95% of head and neck primary carcinomas are squamous cell carcinomas, and these now constitute the sixth most common malignant neoplasm in the world. Mutations of *p16* and *p53* tumor suppressor genes are common. Amplification and overexpression of cyclin D1 often occurs with progression of the tumor.

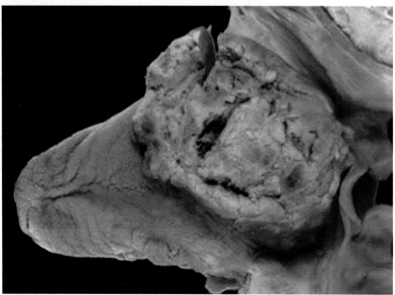

FIGURE 6–9 Squamous cell carcinoma of tongue, gross

The large fungating mass seen here involving the right posterior tongue has extensive surface ulceration. This large mass led to difficulty swallowing and progressive cachexia. Squamous cell carcinomas may progress from *in situ* lesions to invasive lesions over a variable time that can range from months to years. Smaller lesions discovered earlier have a lower stage, are more easily excised, and have a better prognosis, but most of these oropharyngeal cancers are discovered at a higher stage.

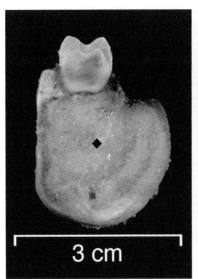
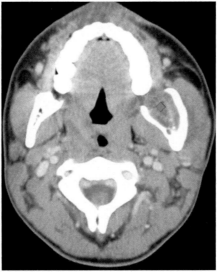

FIGURES 6–10 and 6–11 Ameloblastoma, gross and CT image

At the left, a coronal section through an excised portion of the mandible reveals a mass lesion (◆) that is below a molar tooth. This lesion is slow growing and locally invasive but has a benign course in most cases. The head CT in the "soft tissue window" shows the mass lesion (◆) expanding the left mandibular ramus of a teenage male. The histologic pattern of an ameloblastoma mimics the enamel organ of the tooth. Neoplasms of a related histologic appearance include craniopharyngiomas of the sella turcica and adamantinomas of long bone.

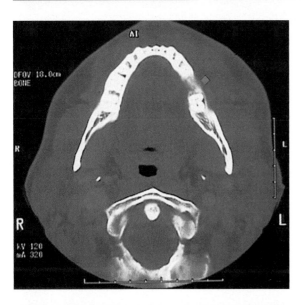

FIGURE 6–12 Odontogenic abscess, CT image

This head CT scan demonstrates an odontogenic abscess (◆) involving the first molar of the left mandible. Lack of dental care can lead to serious complications from dental caries. Once the tooth enamel is breached, infection can reach the inner tooth pulp and extend down the tooth root to the tooth socket and the bone of the mandible or maxilla. One measure of the health of a society is directly proportional to the level of dental care.

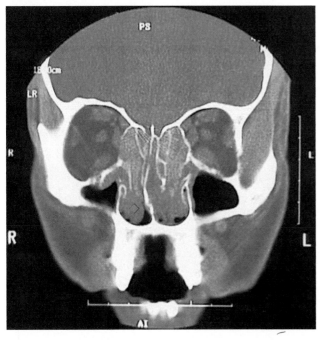

FIGURE 6–13 Nasal polyps, CT image

There are lobulated soft tissue densities (◆) in the nasal cavities extending into paranasal sinuses. These are inflammatory, or allergic, nasal polyps. Although benign, they can obstruct the nasal passages and cause discomfort from difficulty breathing and mass effect. The polyps start as local inflammation with areas of edema and enlargement of the turbinates. Patients with such polyps may have a history of allergic rhinitis, or "hay fever," from increased inflammatory reactivity with type I hypersensitivity to allergens such as plant pollens. The allergens contact and cross-link immunoglobulin E (IgE) bound to mast cells, causing degranulation with immediate release of vasoactive amines such as histamine that cause vasodilation and fluid exudation. There is also mast cell synthesis of arachidonic acid metabolites such as prostaglandins that produce more vasodilation. Mast cell cytokines such as tumor necrosis factor and interleukin-4 attract neutrophils and eosinophils. However, only about 0.5% of atopic people develop nasal polyps. The polyps can reach 3 to 4 cm in length and produce nasal airway obstruction.

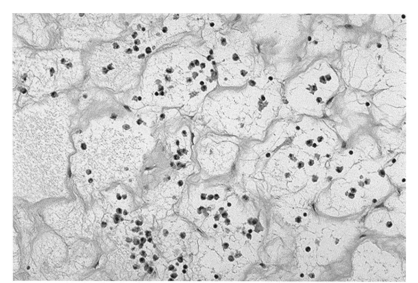

FIGURE 6–14 Allergic nasal polyp, microscopic

Recurrent attacks of rhinitis may lead to the development of nasal polyps, which may be multiple and from a few millimeters to several centimeters in size. There is overlying respiratory mucosa, beneath which seen here is an edematous stroma with inflammatory cells, including the eosinophils, which can be characteristic of allergic inflammatory responses. However, neutrophils, plasma cells, and occasional clusters of lymphocytes can also be seen. Such polyps are rare in children and are most often seen in people older than 30 years of age. Sometimes these polyps can become eroded and secondarily infected. Such polyps can be excised.

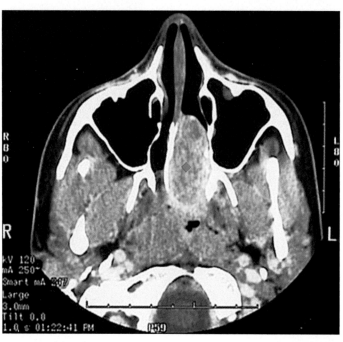

FIGURE 6–15 Nasopharyngeal angiofibroma, CT image

This CT image reveals an angiofibroma (◆) filling and expanding the nasal cavity on the left. The maxillary sinuses are not involved. It can cause nosebleeds and nasal obstruction, and sometimes proptosis or facial deformity. Angiofibromas arise in the posterior or lateral nasopharynx. This lesion, which is not common, is most always seen in adolescent males. Although circumscribed, it can slowly invade into surrounding bone, nasal cavities, paranasal sinuses, and orbits. Larger masses may even extend intracranially.

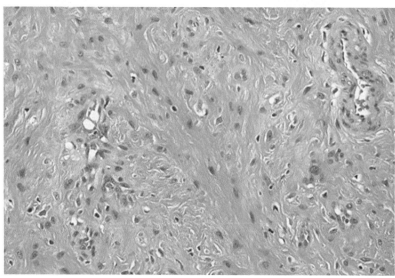

FIGURE 6–16 Nasopharyngeal angiofibroma, microscopic

The nasal angiofibroma is histologically benign but can block the nasal passages, erode adjacent structures, ulcerate, and bleed. The tumor is composed of a fibrous stroma with plump fibroblastic cells along with scattered capillaries.

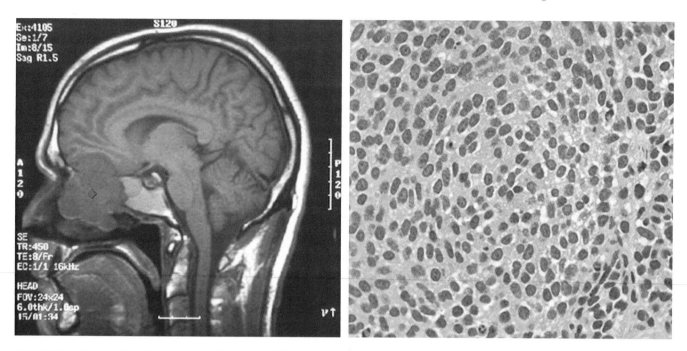

FIGURES 6–17 and 6–18 Olfactory neuroblastoma, MRI and microscopic

The sagittal MRI at the left demonstrates an olfactory neuroblastoma (◆) (also known as a *primitive neuroectodermal tumor*, or PNET) filling the nasopharyngeal region, eroding the orbital plate superiorly, and extending to the inferior frontal lobe. It can cause unilateral nasal obstruction, epistaxis, headaches, and visual disturbances. At the right on microscopic examination, sheets of primitive small blue cells form this neoplasm. These lesions have a propensity to spread locally and metastasize hematogenously.

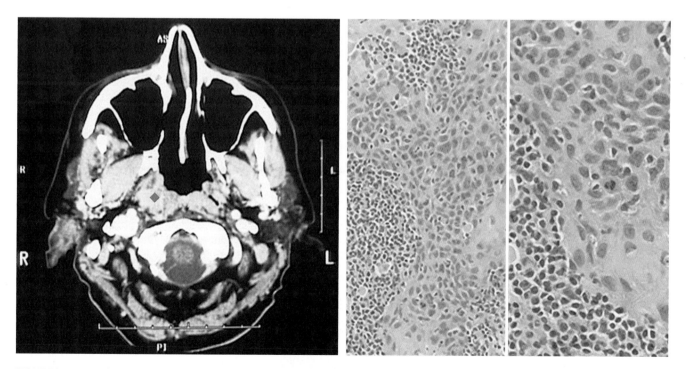

FIGURES 6–19 and 6–20 Nasopharyngeal carcinoma, CT image and microscopic

This head CT with contrast demonstrates a 3-cm mass (◆) on the right between the pterygoid plate anteriorly and the prevertebral and right carotid space posteriorly. These carcinomas have features of squamous cell carcinoma with a prominent lymphoid component. Many are associated with Epstein-Barr virus infection. The tumor often infiltrates locally into orbits and even the cranial cavity. Metastases occur most often to cervical lymph nodes.

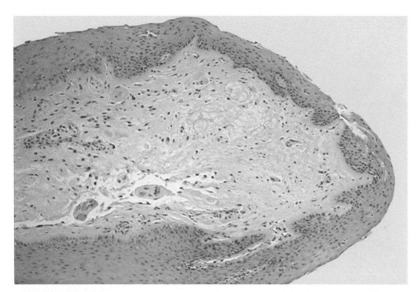

FIGURE 6–21 Laryngeal nodule, microscopic

This laryngeal nodule, also known as a *reactive nodule* or *laryngeal polyp*, occurs most frequently in people who abuse their voice (e.g., a "singer's nodule") or who are smokers. Such polypoid lesions are typically found on the true vocal cord and are covered by nonkeratinizing stratified squamous epithelium surrounding an edematous submucosa. The overlying epithelium may become hyperkeratotic or hyperplastic. The nodule may impart a hoarse quality to the voice, or a change in the character of the voice, but is very unlikely to predispose to malignancy. Larger nodules (up to 1 cm) may ulcerate.

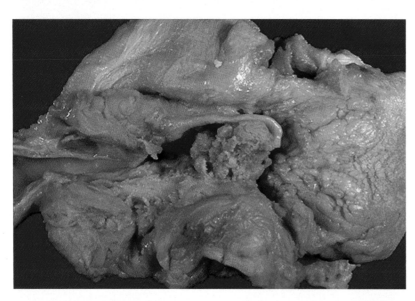

FIGURE 6–22 Laryngeal carcinoma, gross

The region from tongue at the right to upper trachea at the left is shown here. A large fungating squamous cell carcinoma is extending from the larynx to the epiglottis, and a portion of the right epiglottis is eroded. Such large masses can have presenting symptoms including hoarseness, cough, and dysphagia. More advanced lesions may ulcerate and lead to hemoptysis. Metastases to local lymph nodes are often found, producing nontender lymphadenopathy. Most cases are related to tobacco and alcohol use. The precursor lesions begin with focal epithelial hyperplasia that progresses to dysplasia, but these early lesions are often clinically inapparent.

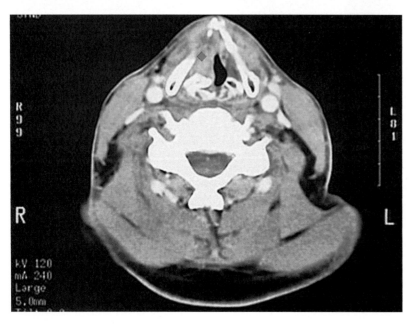

FIGURE 6–23 Laryngeal carcinoma, CT image

This CT scan of the region of the mid-neck demonstrates irregular thickening (◆) of the right vocal fold, representing a squamous cell carcinoma. This carcinoma is invading laterally into the region of the hyoid bone on the right, indicating a worse overall prognosis because it has become extrinsic to the larynx. Intrinsic lesions confined to the larynx would have a better prognosis. Resection can be accompanied by radiation therapy and chemotherapy to eradicate or to control the disease.

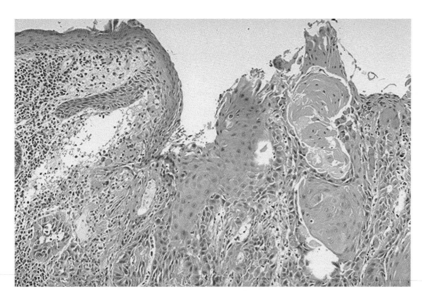

FIGURE 6–24 Laryngeal carcinoma, microscopic

The normal respiratory tract pseudostratified columnar epithelium has been replaced by the metaplastic squamous epithelium seen at the left. Arising at the center and extending to the right is a well-differentiated squamous cell carcinoma with overlying ulceration. This neoplasm infiltrates downward into the submucosa. Many of the cells are arranged in nests and demonstrate keratinization with abundant pink cytoplasm. Ninety-five percent of laryngeal carcinomas have squamous differentiation.

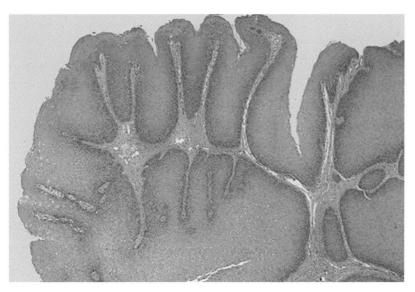

FIGURE 6–25 Laryngeal papilloma, microscopic

A squamous papilloma of the larynx is found on the true vocal fold. Note the long projections of orderly, benign squamous epithelium overlying fibrovascular cores. These uncommon lesions are solitary in adults and may cause some bleeding. Although rare in children, juvenile papillomas of the larynx tend to be multiple and continually recur after resection. With laryngeal papillomatosis, dozens of lesions may be resected over many years. However, some may regress with onset of puberty. Infection with human papillomavirus types 6 and 11 typically drives this process. Such papillomas are unlikely to progress to carcinoma.

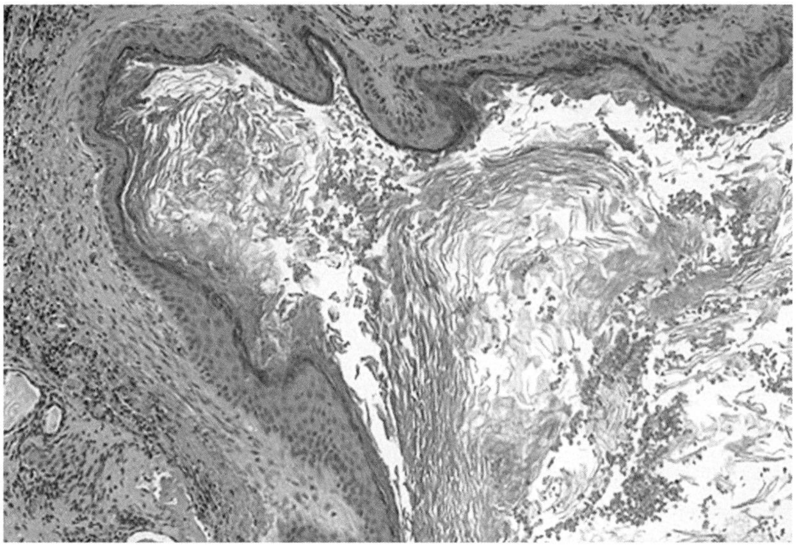

FIGURE 6–26 Cholesteatoma, microscopic

Severe inflammation from otitis media or rupture of the tympanic membrane of the middle ear may result in the trapping of squamous epithelium that starts to grow, expanding as a cystic mass lesion that can rupture and erode surrounding structures such as the mastoid. Shown here is the wall of such an excised non-neoplastic cyst. The center of the cyst is filled with keratinaceous debris. The cholesteatoma can elicit an inflammatory reaction since the keratinaceous debris acts as a foreign body, with foreign body giant cells and mononuclear cells. Hemorrhage and necrosis lead to formation of cholesterol clefts. Cholesteatomas require surgical removal.

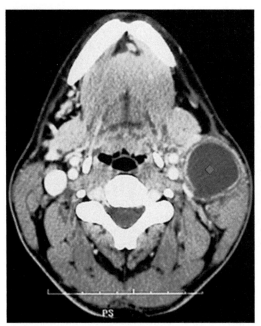
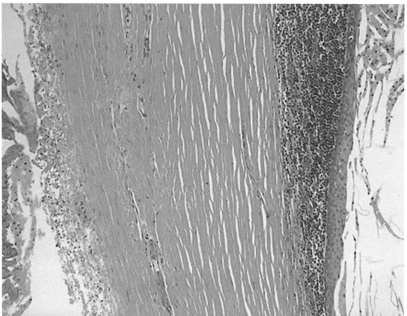

FIGURES 6–27 and 6–28 Branchial cyst, CT image and microscopic

The CT image in the region of the upper neck (with the inferior, anterior portion of the mandible seen here) demonstrates a large but circumscribed branchial cyst (◆) in the neck. Such lesions typically occur in the anterolateral neck region and grossly have a cystic cavity filled with cellular debris formed from desquamation of the epithelial lining. A branchial cyst (lymphoepithelial cyst) enlarges slowly over time. Microscopically, branchial cleft cysts are lined by benign stratified squamous epithelium and are often surrounded by lymphoid tissue, as shown.

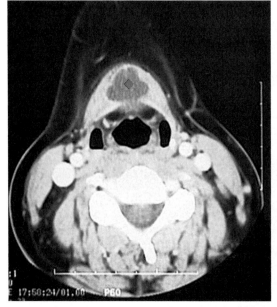
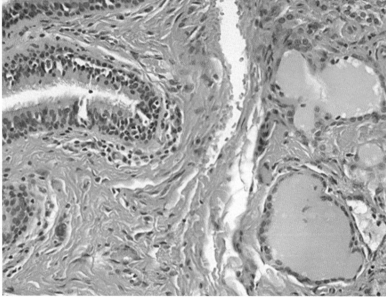

FIGURES 6–29 and 6–30 Thyroglossal duct cyst, CT image and microscopic

This CT image in the region of the mid-neck at the level of the hyoid bone demonstrates a circumscribed midline thyroglossal duct cyst (◆). Such cysts are embryologic remnants of the traverse made by the primordial thyroid tissue from the foramen cecum of the tongue down to the final location of the thyroid anterior to the thyroid cartilage. Microscopically, a thyroglossal duct cyst most typically has a lining of respiratory epithelium as shown here, but there may also be squamous epithelium. Around the cyst, there may be thyroid follicles and lymphoid aggregates.

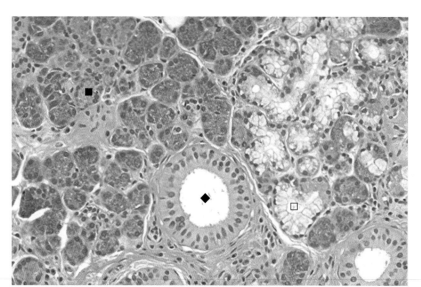

FIGURE 6–31 Normal salivary gland, microscopic

Major and minor salivary glands composed of tubuloalveolar glands produce serous and mucous secretions that aid in chewing and swallowing. Ducts from the major salivary glands drain into the oral cavity. The major salivary glands include the submandibular gland and the parotid gland. Salivary gland amylase provides some initial digestion of carbohydrates. The histologic appearance of normal submandibular gland with both serous (■) and mucinous (□) acini, as well as ducts (◆), is shown here.

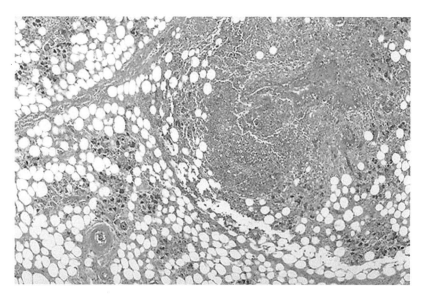

FIGURE 6–32 Sialadenitis, microscopic

Obstruction of salivary gland ducts from lithiasis or inspissated secretions predisposes to stasis and infection. An acute parotitis is seen here, with neutrophils infiltrating the parotid gland and formation of an abscess around a duct at the upper right. Elderly people are more prone to develop this problem. *Staphylococcus aureus* is the most common infectious agent isolated. Bilateral inflammation of salivary glands can also occur acutely with mumps virus infection, but the inflammatory infiltrates are mainly composed of macrophages and lymphocytes. Sialadenitis is often patchy and resolves with minimal scarring.

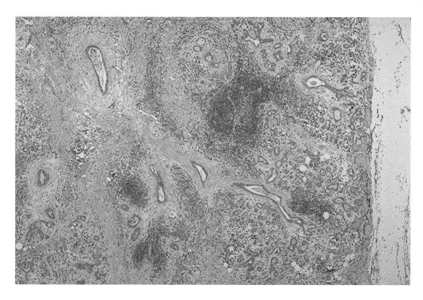

FIGURE 6–33 Sialadenitis, microscopic

Chronic obstruction of a salivary gland duct can lead to chronic inflammatory cell infiltrates along with fibrosis and acinar atrophy. The chronic sialadenitis seen here is due to ductal obstruction. A similar appearance can occur with Sjögren syndrome, an autoimmune disease that involves salivary glands (with xerostomia) and lacrimal glands (with xerophthalmia). There can be extensive lymphoid infiltrates and even formation of lymphoid follicles with reactive germinal centers. Sjögren syndrome is often accompanied by serologic testing that is positive for autoantibodies to the ribonucleoprotein antigens SS-A and SS-B, and there is an increased risk for subsequent development of non-Hodgkin lymphoma.

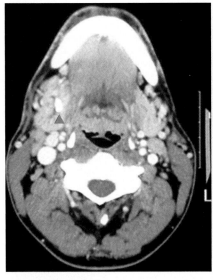
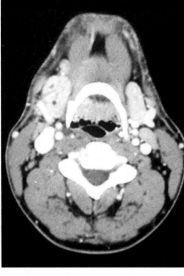

FIGURE 6–34 Sialolithiasis, CT images

This head CT scan reveals a calculus (▲) within the submandibular gland in the panel on the left. Obstruction has resulted in inflammation and duct dilation, producing more brightness in this gland, compared with the normal left submandibular gland. The inflamed gland is enlarged, seen in the panel on the right. Salivary gland duct lithiasis leads to obstruction with localized pain and swelling of the gland with microscopic findings of acute or chronic inflammation.

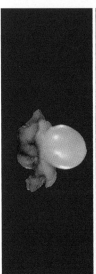
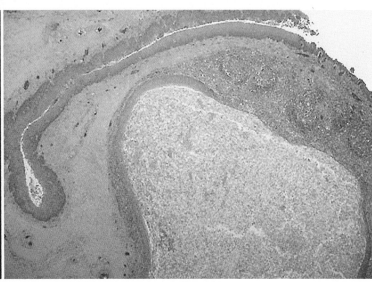

FIGURE 6–35 Mucocele, gross and microscopic

This mucocele (mucous retention cyst) involving a minor salivary gland of the oral cavity was removed surgically. The duct from the small gland became obstructed and led to the expansion of the gland with secretions to form the small, smooth-surfaced mass seen here. Sometimes, the mucocele can rupture and produce a surrounding foreign body granulomatous response with pain and enlargement. At the right, microscopically, the mucocele is filled with pale blue mucinous material.

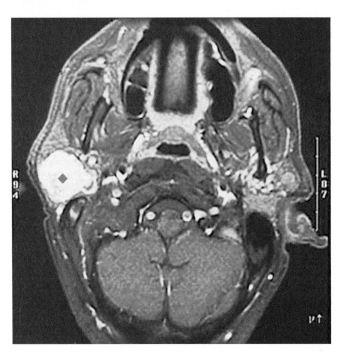

FIGURE 6–36 Pleomorphic adenoma, MRI

This axial MRI of the head demonstrates a mass lesion (◆) involving the superficial aspect of the right parotid gland. This is a pleomorphic adenoma, or mixed tumor, of the salivary gland. Such pleomorphic adenomas are the most common salivary gland tumor (65% of all salivary gland tumors), and the most common location for them is in the parotid gland (usually the superficial lobe). The highest incidence occurs in older adults. These neoplasms usually present as a painless, persistent, movable swelling, which has often been present for a long time. They are solid masses that are circumscribed but not encapsulated. Most act in a benign manner, although they can recur after incomplete resection since they are not strictly encapsulated. If not removed, about 10% will have malignant transformation after 15 years.

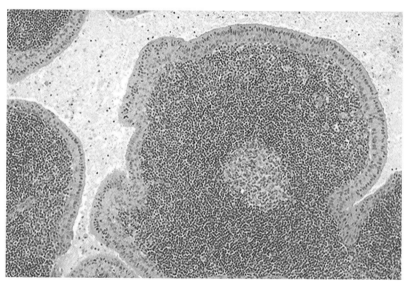

FIGURE 6–37 Pleomorphic adenoma, microscopic

At low magnification, the pleomorphic adenoma (mixed tumor) of salivary gland borders the surrounding normal parotid gland. This neoplasm has a mixed proliferation of both ductal epithelium, myoepithelial cells, and a chondroid, hyaline, or a mesenchyme-like myxomatous stroma (thus, these lesions are also called *mixed tumors*). The facial nerve nearby can be involved, making a nerve graft necessary with a wide tumor excision.

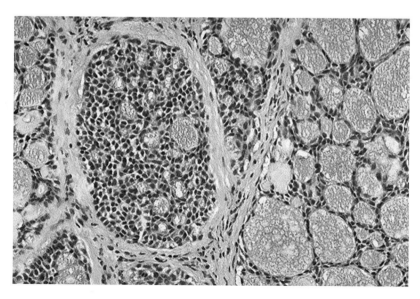

FIGURE 6–38 Warthin tumor microscopic

This neoplasm has papillary fronds projecting into cystic spaces, with cystic to cleftlike spaces filled with pale pink mucinous to serous secretions. The spaces are lined by a double layer of pink (oncocytic) cuboidal to columnar epithelial cells over the papillary fronds. The fronds beneath the epithelium are filled with lymphocytes, sometimes with germinal centers. Oncocytic cells by electron microscopy are filled with mitochondria. This neoplasm, also known as *papillary cystadenoma lymphomatosum*, is the second most common salivary gland tumor. It is almost always found in the parotid gland and is much more common in males and in smokers. About 10% of cases are multifocal, and 10% are bilateral.

FIGURE 6–39 Adenoid cystic carcinoma, microscopic

This type of neoplasm is not common in the parotid gland, but it is the most common neoplasm of minor salivary glands. The microscopic pattern is that of a solid to tubular to cribriform pattern, with the neoplastic cells surrounding mucinous secretions. Although often small and slow growing, these neoplasms are infiltrative and have a tendency to invade perineural spaces and recur locally, as well as spread hematogenously. Thus, distant metastases are more likely to occur than regional lymph node metastases, and half of adenoid cystic carcinomas eventually metastasize to a distant site, even years after the original resection of the mass.

CHAPTER 7

The Gastrointestinal Tract

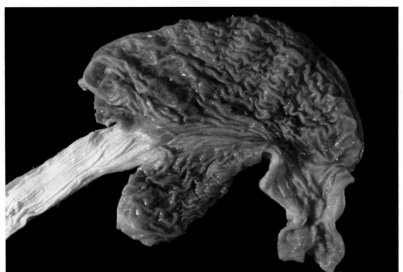

FIGURE 7–1 Normal esophagus and stomach, gross

The normal esophagus at the left has the usual white to tan mucosa. The gastroesophageal junction with the lower esophageal sphincter (LES), whose physiologic function is maintained by muscle tone, is at the center-left, and the normal stomach is at the right, opened along the greater curvature. In the fundus can be seen the lesser curvature. Just beyond the antrum is the pylorus with thick surrounding muscle that empties into the first portion of duodenum at the lower right. The rugal folds of the normal stomach are prominent.

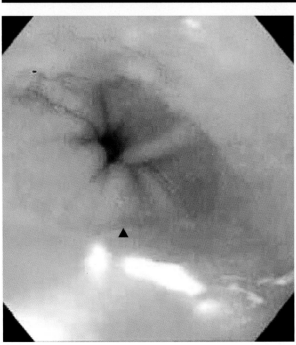

FIGURE 7–2 Normal esophagus, endoscopy

This is the normal upper GI endoscopic view of the transition from the pale pink to tan squamous mucosa of the esophagus to the darker pink columnar mucosa of the stomach at the gastroesophageal junction (▲). The LES is a physiologic sphincter maintained by normal muscle tone. Distention of the lower esophagus by food produces relaxation of the LES and receptive relaxation of the proximal stomach through a vasovagal reflex with release of vasoactive intestinal peptide (VIP) from postganglionic peptidergic vagal nerve fibers. A loss of this tone allows reflux of gastric contents into the lower esophagus. Reflux of acid contents into the lower esophagus often produces a burning retrosternal or substernal chest pain (heartburn). An abnormality of the esophageal sphincter can also produce difficulty in swallowing (dysphagia). Lesions of the esophageal mucosa may cause pain on swallowing (odynophagia). Abnormalities in intrinsic or extrinsic esophageal innervation may lead to failure of LES relaxation, leading to achalasia and progressive dysphagia with esophageal dilation above the LES.

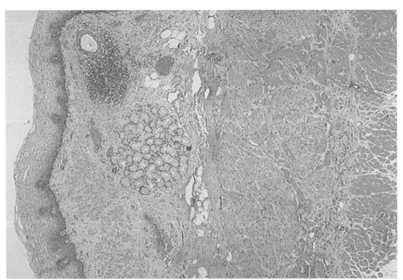

FIGURE 7–3 Normal esophagus, microscopic

The normal squamous mucosa is at the left, with underlying submucosa containing minor mucus glands and a duct surrounded by lymphoid tissue. The muscularis is at the right. Predominantly voluntary striated muscle to initiate swallowing in the upper esophagus merges and changes to involuntary smooth muscle distally in lower esophagus that provides propulsive peristalsis of food and liquid boluses into the stomach. There is a physiologic LES of smooth muscle with muscle tone providing an effective barrier to regurgitation. At the gastroesophageal junction, the squamous epithelium interdigitates with the glandular epithelium of the stomach.

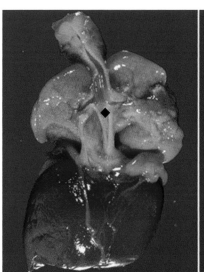
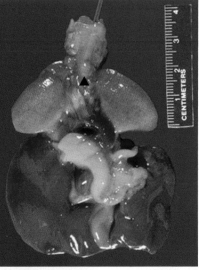

FIGURE 7–4 Tracheoesophageal fistula, gross

Congenital anomalies involving the esophagus include atresia and fistula with the trachea. Embryologically, the lung buds off the esophagus, an endodermal derivative, so both are intimately associated in development. The esophageal atresia (▲) shown here is present in the mid-esophagus in the right panel. The tracheoesophageal fistula (◆) is located below the carina in the left panel. Depending on the location of the atretic portion or the fistula, a baby at birth may exhibit vomiting or aspiration. Additional congenital anomalies are often present. Agenesis (complete absence) of the esophagus is very rare.

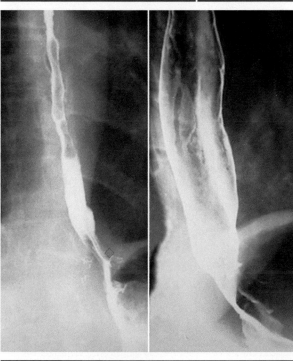
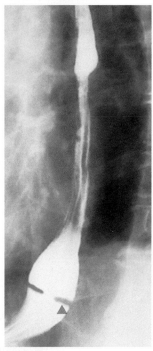

FIGURES 7–5 and 7–6 Esophageal stricture and Schatzki ring, barium swallow radiographs

The two panels at the left demonstrate stricture (◆) (stenosis) of the lower esophagus. This can occur from inflammation with reflux, scleroderma with submucosal fibrosis, radiation injury, or ingestion of caustic chemicals. The lateral view at the right reveals a Schatzki ring (▲) of the lower esophagus. There is an infolding of the muscular wall just above the diaphragm. With these conditions, there is progressive dysphagia, more marked for solid foods than liquids initially.

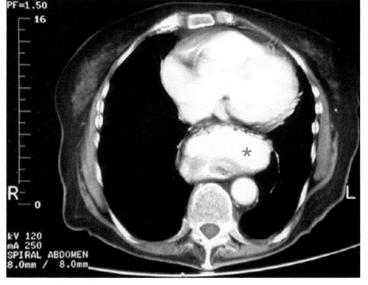

FIGURE 7–7 Hiatal hernia, CT image

This chest CT scan shows a hiatal hernia (✳) with a dilated portion of gastric fundus sliding through a widened esophageal hiatus into the lower chest. About 95% of hiatal hernias are of this sliding type. About 9% of patients with hiatal hernias have associated symptoms of acid reflux with gastroesophageal reflux disease (GERD). Conversely, some cases of GERD are associated with a hiatal hernia. The widened esophageal hiatus interferes with maintenance of the normal LES function. Patients may have symptoms of "heartburn" from reflux of gastric contents into the lower esophagus, with retrosternal burning pain, particularly after eating, and exacerbated by lying down after a meal.

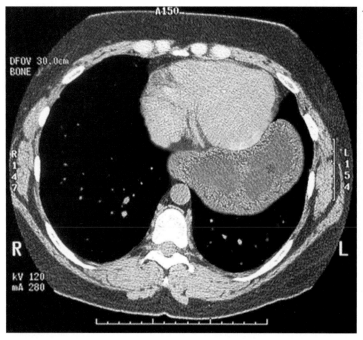

◀ **FIGURE 7–8 Paraesophageal hernia, CT image**

This chest CT without contrast reveals that much of the stomach (∗) is present in the left chest cavity adjacent to the heart. This is a complication of a hiatal rolling hernia known as *paraesophageal hernia*, an uncommon but serious form of hernia. The vascular supply to the stomach becomes compromised when the stomach herniates upward through the small opening, leading to ischemia and infarction.

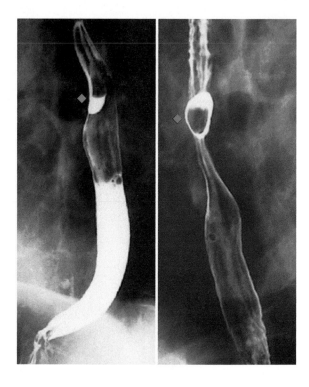

FIGURE 7–9 Esophageal pulsion diverticulum, barium swallow radiographs ▶

These two views from an upper GI series with barium contrast material reveal a pulsion diverticulum (◆) in the upper esophagus. Note the contrast that fills this small outpouching. Such a diverticulum represents enlargement and outpouching of esophagus through a weak point in the muscular wall, typically between the constrictor muscles in the upper esophagus or through the muscularis just above the diaphragm. Such a lesion is also known as a *Zenker diverticulum*. This lesion can produce a mass effect, interfere with swallowing, and collect food that decays and produces marked halitosis.

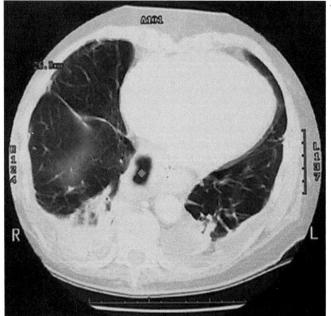

◀ **FIGURE 7–10 Mallory-Weiss syndrome, CT image**

Longitudinal tears in the esophagus leading to hemorrhage may occur from bouts of severe or forceful vomiting. The rare complication of rupture (Boerhaave syndrome) is shown on this chest CT scan with contrast that demonstrates a lucency (◆) representing an air leak from the esophageal rupture into the mediastinum. The point of rupture in the lower esophagus lies just above the gastroesophageal junction. Leakage of esophageal contents into the mediastinum leads to infection with inflammation that can quickly spread to other areas of the chest cavity.

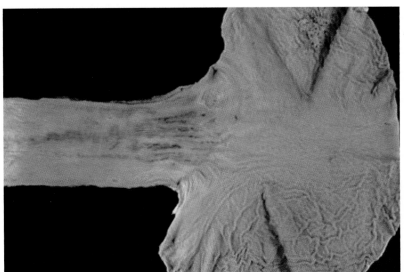

FIGURE 7–11 Esophageal varices, gross

These prominent purplish varices near the gastroesophageal junction are a source of bleeding with hematemesis. Submucosal dilated veins known as *varices* occur in patients with portal hypertension (usually from micronodular cirrhosis from chronic alcoholism) because the submucosal esophageal plexus of veins is a collateral channel for venous drainage. This plexus of veins also drains part of the upper stomach, but it is generically called the *esophageal plexus of veins*; hence, bleeding here is termed *esophageal variceal bleeding*.

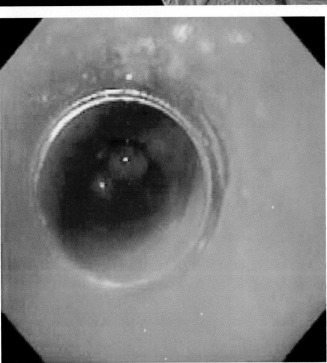

FIGURE 7–12 Esophageal varices, endoscopy

The dilated submucosal veins of the esophageal plexus bulge into the lower esophageal lumen as here on upper GI endoscopy. This venous dilation is most often a complication of portal hypertension with hepatic cirrhosis. Eventually, about two thirds of patients with cirrhosis develop esophageal varices. With erosion and rupture of these delicate submucosal veins, there can be sudden massive life-threatening hematemesis. Banding of the varices, or injection of sclerosing agents (sclerotherapy), and balloon tamponade have been employed as therapeutic measures to halt or prevent blood loss.

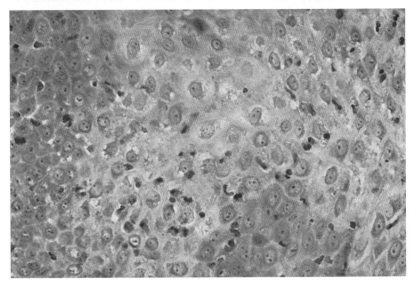

FIGURE 7–13 Esophagitis, microscopic

Reflux of acidic gastric contents into the lower esophagus from incompetence of the LES leads to GERD with reflux esophagitis. Histologic findings in mild reflux esophagitis include epithelial hyperplasia with basal zone hyperplasia and lengthened papillae, and inflammation with neutrophils, eosinophils, and lymphocytes (eosinophils, especially in children, have been reported to be a sensitive and specific indicator of reflux, as seen here with a Giemsa stain). Causes of GERD with esophagitis include hiatal hernia, neurologic disorders, scleroderma, lack of esophageal clearance, and delayed gastric emptying. Severe reflux esophagitis can be complicated by ulceration and subsequent stricture.

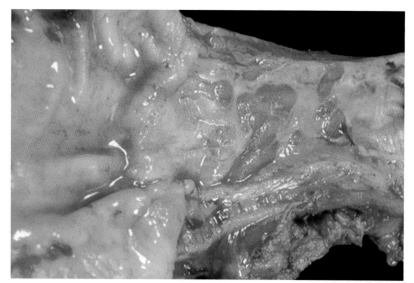

FIGURE 7–14 Barrett esophagus, gross

Chronic GERD with esophageal mucosal injury can lead to metaplasia of the normal esophageal squamous mucosa into gastric-type columnar mucosa, but with intestinal-type goblet cells, known as *Barrett esophagus*. Up to 10% of patients with chronic gastric reflux may develop Barrett esophagus. Seen here are islands of reddish metaplastic mucosa in the lower esophagus, above the gastroesophageal junction, with remaining surrounding white squamous mucosa. Ulceration leads to bleeding and pain; inflammation with stricture may ensue. Endoscopy with biopsy is required for diagnosis.

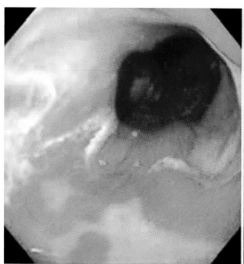
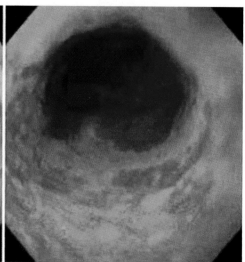

FIGURE 7–15 Barrett esophagus, endoscopy

These endoscopic views of lower esophagus show areas of red metaplastic mucosa typical of Barrett esophagus along with islands of normal pale esophageal squamous mucosa. If the area of Barrett mucosa extends less than 2 cm above the normal squamocolumnar junction, then the condition is called *short-segment Barrett esophagus*.

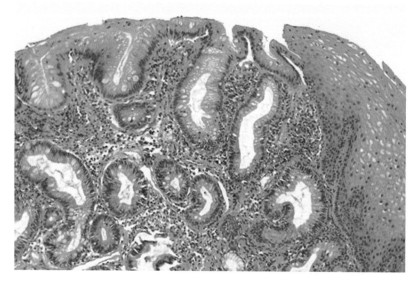

FIGURE 7–16 Barrett esophagus, microscopic

Note the abnormal columnar epithelium in the left image and the normal squamous epithelium at the right. This is "typical" Barrett mucosa at the left because there is intestinal metaplasia as well (note the goblet cells in the columnar mucosa). Chronic reflux of gastric contents into the lower esophagus over many years predisposes to development of this metaplasia. Most people diagnosed with Barrett esophagus are 40 to 60 years of age. There is a long-term risk (more than 30- to 40-fold compared with the general population) for development of esophageal adenocarcinoma when more than 3 cm of Barrett mucosa is present in the esophagus.

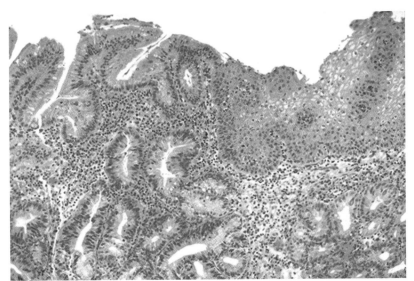

FIGURE 7–17 Barrett esophagus with dysplasia, microscopic

Adjacent to remaining squamous mucosa at the right is an area of high-grade dysplasia of the metaplastic columnar epithelium in the Barrett mucosa. Note the crowded, hyperchromatic nuclei in the columnar cells, and a few remaining goblet cells at the upper surface on the left, as well as the architectural irregularity of these glands. Because the columnar cell nuclei are basally oriented, this is a low-grade dysplasia, but an apical orientation is part of high-grade dysplasia that has a much greater likelihood of going on to adenocarcinoma. Dysplasia may develop after years of untreated Barrett esophagus.

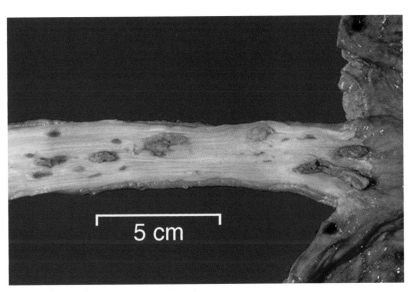

FIGURE 7–18 Herpes esophagitis, gross

The lower esophagus shows sharply demarcated, oblong ulcerations that have a brown-red base, contrasted with the surrounding normal pale white esophageal squamous mucosa. These ulcerations have a "punched-out" appearance suggestive of herpes simplex virus (HSV) infection. Opportunistic infections such as HSV, *Candida*, and cytomegalovirus are most often seen in immunocompromised patients. Odynophagia is a typical symptom. Herpetic esophagitis usually remains localized, rarely causes significant bleeding or obstruction, and is unlikely to become disseminated.

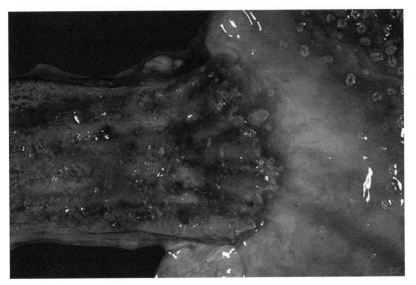

FIGURE 7–19 *Candida* esophagitis, gross

Tan-yellow plaques are seen in the lower esophagus, along with mucosal hyperemia. The same lesions also appear at the upper right in the upper gastric fundus. *Candida* infections involving the oral cavity ("oral thrush") and upper gastrointestinal tract tend to remain superficial, but invasion and dissemination occasionally occur in immunocompromised patients. A few *Candida* organisms can be part of the normal flora of the mouth. These lesions rarely cause significant hemorrhage or obstruction. These lesions may coalesce to form pseudomembranes.

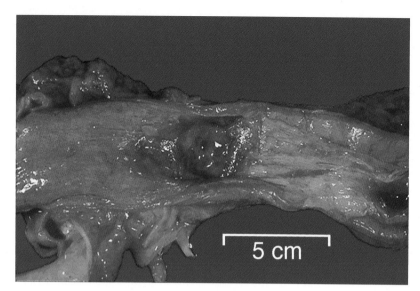

FIGURE 7–20 Squamous cell carcinoma, gross

Note the irregular reddish, ulcerated, exophytic mid-esophageal mass seen here on the esophageal mucosal surface. The distensibility of the esophagus ameliorates the mass effect so that early symptoms are uncommon, and by the time a diagnosis is made, there is often extensive mediastinal invasion that precludes a surgical cure. Thus, the overall prognosis for this tumor is poor. Risk factors for esophageal squamous carcinoma include smoking and alcohol abuse in the United States. In other parts of the world dietary factors such as a high nitrate/nitrosamine content, deficiency of zinc or molybdenum, or human papillomavirus infection, may play a role.

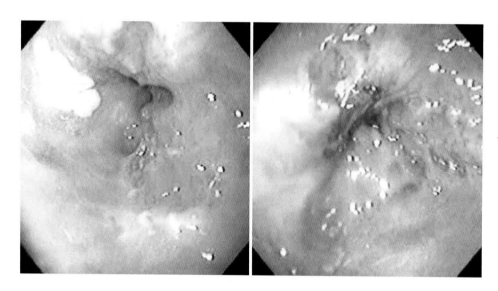

FIGURE 7–21 Squamous cell carcinoma, endoscopy

Endoscopic views of an ulcerated mid-esophageal squamous cell carcinoma causing luminal stenosis are seen here. Pain and dysphagia are typical presenting problems. Interference with swallowing leads to cachexia with weight loss.

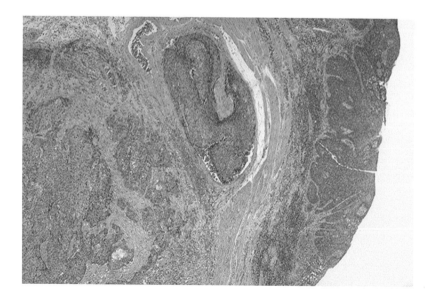

FIGURE 7–22 Squamous cell carcinoma, microscopic

At the lower right is a small remnant of normal squamous esophageal mucosa that merges into abnormal, thick squamous cell carcinoma. Solid nests of neoplastic cells are infiltrating down through the submucosa at the left. Esophageal cancers often spread to surrounding structures, making surgical removal difficult. The cells have abundant pink cytoplasm and distinct cell borders typical of squamous cell carcinoma. Half of these cancers have *p53* tumor suppressor gene mutations. The *p16/CDKN2A* tumor suppressor gene is abnormal in some cases, while *CYCLIN D1* may be amplified in others. These mutations can arise in the setting of chronic inflammation with increased epithelial cell proliferation.

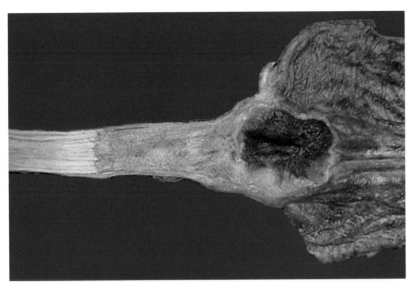

FIGURE 7–23 Adenocarcinoma, gross

Normal tan upper esophageal mucosa is at the far left. The distal esophagus is replaced by Barrett mucosa, producing a darker, slightly erythematous gross appearance. In the distal esophagus arising near the gastroesophageal junction is a large ulcerating adenocarcinoma that extends into the upper stomach. Adenocarcinomas most often arise in Barrett esophagus, with the *p53* tumor suppressor gene often mutated, followed by nuclear translocation of β-catenin and c-*ERB B2* amplification. As with squamous cell carcinoma, there are often no early symptoms, so that the cancer is advanced at the time of diagnosis, with a poor prognosis.

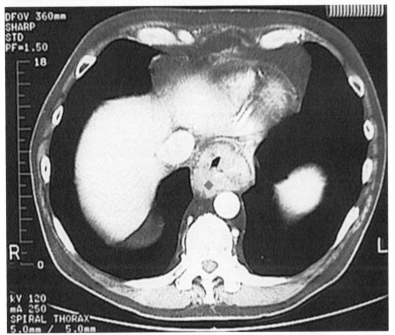

FIGURE 7–24 Adenocarcinoma, CT image

This abdominal CT with contrast demonstrates a mass (◆) surrounding the central esophageal lumen, which is a lower esophageal adenocarcinoma extending to the upper stomach. This tumor arose in a Barrett mucosa that resulted from chronic GERD. Preexisting dysplasia arising in Barrett mucosa increases the risk for development of subsequent adenocarcinoma. By the time an adenocarcinoma arises, untreated GERD has usually been present for years, and the patient is older than 40 years of age. The increased epithelial cell turnover with increased proliferative activity in Barrett mucosa is the background for mutations to arise with subsequent loss of cell cycle control.

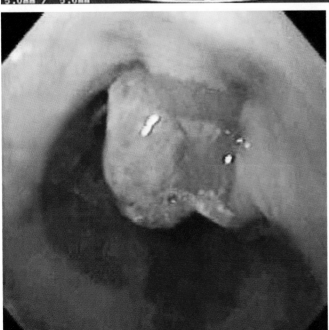

FIGURE 7–25 Adenocarcinoma, endoscopy

In this view of the lower esophagus seen on endoscopy, note the areas of dark red friable mucosa representing Barrett esophagus. Note the polypoid mass extending into the esophageal lumen, which on biopsy proved to be a moderately differentiated adenocarcinoma. This patient had a 30-year history of poorly controlled GERD. Clinical findings with esophageal carcinomas include hematemesis, dysphagia, chest pain, and weight loss.

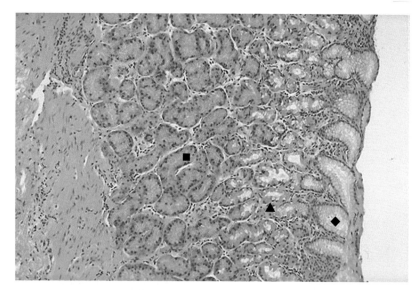

FIGURE 7–26 Normal gastric mucosa, microscopic

The mucosa of the fundus has short gastric pits (◆), beneath which are long glands (■). These fundic glands contain parietal cells (▲) secreting hydrochloric acid and intrinsic factor. Acid is secreted through the H^+-K^+ATPase ("proton pump") in parietal cells under the influence of acetylcholine secreted from the vagus nerve acting on muscarinic receptors, histamine from mast cells acting on H_2 receptors, and gastrin. Fundic glands also have chief cells secreting pepsinogen, a proteolytic enzyme. Cuboidal mucous neck cells in the glands secrete mucus to protect the mucosa against the acid and enzyme secretions.

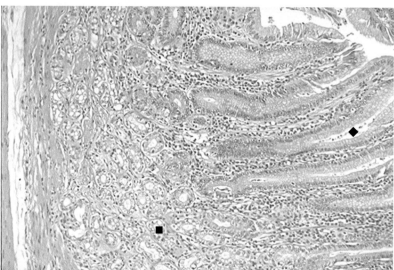

FIGURE 7–27 Normal gastric mucosa, microscopic

The gastric antral epithelium has long pits (◆) with shorter glands (■) than the fundus. In the antrum and pyloric regions distally in the stomach, there are columnar mucous cells in pits and glands. Mucosal cells produce prostaglandins that favor production of mucus and bicarbonate and increase mucosal blood flow to protect the mucosa from the effects of gastric acid. Peristaltic movements in the stomach mix the chyme. The rate of gastric emptying is in part controlled by the amount of H^+ and fat entering the duodenum. Duodenal fat increases the secretion of cholecystokinin (CCK), which slows the rate of gastric emptying.

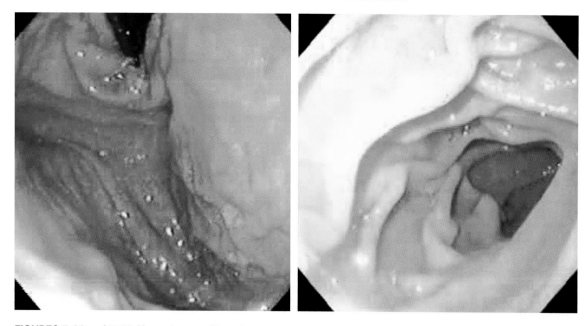

FIGURES 7–28 and 7–29 Normal upper GI, endoscopy

The normal appearance of the gastric fundus is shown below at the left, with the normal duodenal appearance at the right.

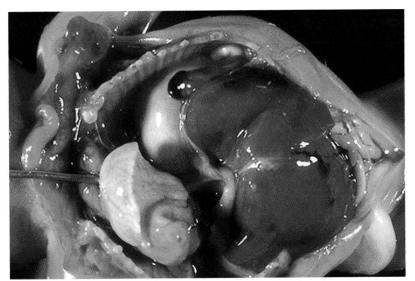

FIGURE 7-30 Congenital diaphragmatic hernia, gross

The left diaphragmatic dome is absent, allowing herniation of abdominal contents into the chest cavity during fetal development. The metal probe is positioned behind the left lung, which has been displaced into the right chest by the herniated stomach. Below the stomach is a dark spleen that overlies the left lobe of liver herniating upward. Incursion of abdominal contents into the chest cavity results in pulmonary hypoplasia. Although diaphragmatic hernia may occur as an isolated congenital anomaly that is potentially reparable, most are associated with multiple anomalies and often with chromosomal abnormalities such as trisomy 18.

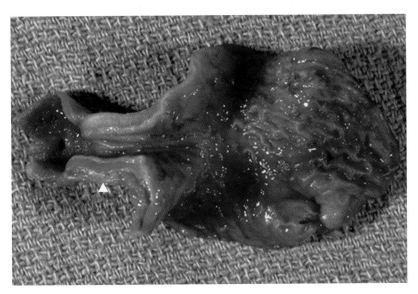

FIGURE 7-31 Pyloric stenosis, gross

Note the hypertrophied muscle (▲) at the gastric outlet. Pyloric stenosis is uncommon but is a cause of "projectile" vomiting in an infant about 3 to 6 weeks of age. The muscle hypertrophy may be so prominent that there is a palpable mass. Pyloric stenosis manifests the genetic phenomenon of "threshold of liability" above which the disease is manifested when more genetic risks are present. The incidence is 1 in 300 to 900 live births, with males affected more often than females because more risks must be present in females for the disease to occur.

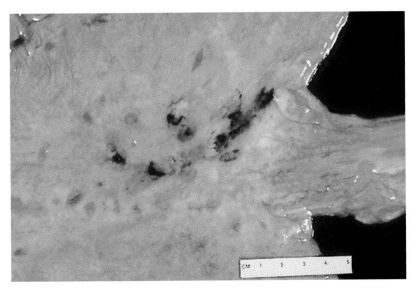

FIGURE 7-32 Gastropathy, gross

Shown are some larger irregular areas of gastric hemorrhage that could best be termed *erosions* because the superficial mucosa is eroded away, but not completely gone. Such erosions are typical of the pathologic process termed *gastropathy*, a clinical term that describes several different patterns of gastric mucosal epithelial or endothelial injury with mucosal damage and hemorrhage but without significant inflammation. Causes of gastropathy are similar to those of acute gastritis and include drugs such as NSAIDs, alcohol, stress, bile reflux, uremia, portal hypertension, radiation, and chemotherapy. The findings here fit with acute erosive gastropathy.

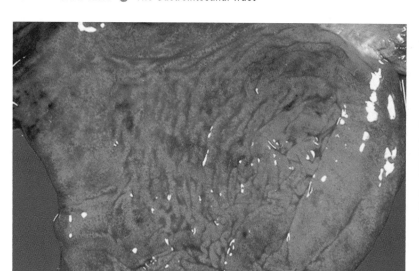

FIGURE 7–33 Acute gastritis, gross

The gastric mucosa of the fundus is diffusely hyperemic, with multiple petechiae, but no erosions or ulcerations are present. Acute gastritis (also called *hemorrhagic gastritis*, or *acute erosive gastritis* if mucosal erosions are present) can be caused by ischemia (shock, burns, or trauma), or toxins such as alcohol, salicylates, or NSAIDs. Damage to the mucosal barrier allows back diffusion of acid. Patients may be asymptomatic or have massive hemorrhage. The lesions can progress to erosions or ulcerations. The stress of burn injuries (Curling ulcer) or CNS trauma (Cushing ulcer) can cause acid hypersecretion.

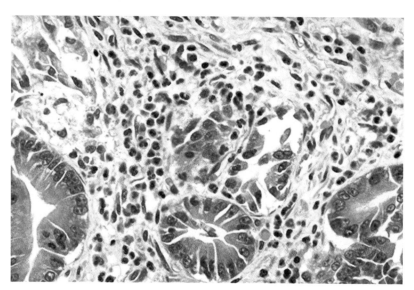

FIGURE 7–34 Acute gastritis, microscopic

Microscopic findings include hemorrhage, edema, and variable degrees of acute inflammation with neutrophilic infiltrates. The gastric mucosa here shows infiltration of glands and lamina propria by neutrophils. Typical clinical findings range from mild to severe epigastric pain, nausea, and vomiting. In severe cases, there can be significant hematemesis, particularly in patients with a history of chronic alcohol abuse, and this can be termed *acute hemorrhagic gastritis*. Although the presence of gastric acid is a necessary antecedent to ulceration, the amount of acid is not typically the determining factor for development of most gastric ulcerations.

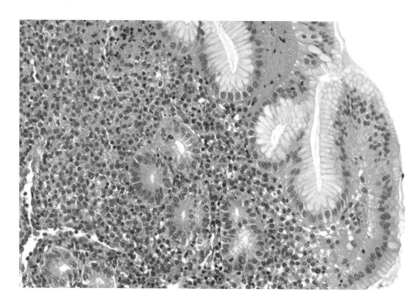

FIGURE 7–35 Chronic gastritis, microscopic

Chronic nonspecific (antral) gastritis is typically the result of *Helicobacter pylori* infection. Other causes include bile reflux and drugs (salicylates and alcohol). The inflammatory cell infiltrates are mainly composed of lymphocytes and plasma cells, and occasionally some neutrophils. Mucosal atrophy and intestinal metaplasia are sequelae that can be the first step toward development of gastric adenocarcinoma. An autoimmune form of gastritis can occur when antiparietal or intrinsic factor antibodies are present, leading to atrophic gastritis and pernicious anemia. Fasting serum gastrin levels are inversely proportional to gastric acid production, and a high serum gastrin suggests atrophic gastritis.

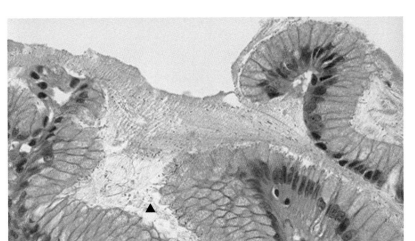

FIGURE 7–36 Helicobacter pylori, microscopic

H. pylori is a small, spiral rod-shaped gram-negative bacterium residing under microaerobic conditions in a neutral microenvironment between the mucus and the superficial columnar mucosal cells. The organisms here are pale pink rods (▲) with H+E staining. *H. pylori* strains that possess the *cag* pathogenicity island induce more severe gastritis and augment the risk for developing peptic ulcer disease and gastric cancer. These organisms do not invade or directly damage the mucosa, but rather change the microenvironment of the stomach to promote mucosal damage. The *H. pylori* organisms contain urease and produce a protective surrounding cloud of ammonia to resist gastric acid. The urea breath test is used to detect the presence of *H. pylori*.

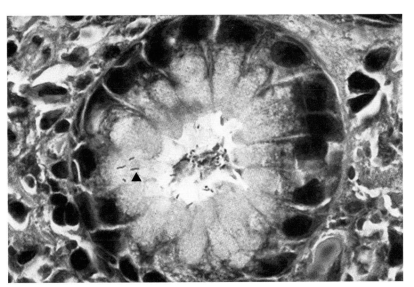

FIGURE 7–37 Helicobacter pylori, microscopic

The *H. pylori* organisms (▲) stimulate cytokine production by epithelial cells that recruit and activate immune and inflammatory cells in the underlying lamina propria. This infection is generally considered to be acquired in childhood, but the inflammatory changes progress throughout life. Only a minority of the many patients (20% of the US population) infected with *H. pylori* develop the complications of chronic gastritis, gastric ulcers, duodenal ulcers, mucosa-associated lymphoid tissue (MALT) lymphoma, or adenocarcinoma. *H. pylori* is found in the surface epithelial mucus of most patients with active gastritis. The organisms are shown here with methylene blue stain.

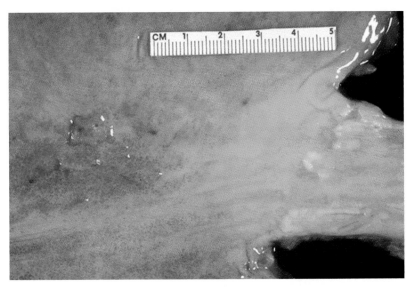

FIGURE 7–38 Acute gastric ulcer, gross

An ulcer is an area of full-thickness loss of the mucosa (an erosion is just a partial-thickness loss). Ulcers can be complicated by hemorrhage, penetration (extension into an adjacent organ), perforation (communication with the peritoneal cavity), and stricture (due to scarring). A 1-cm shallow and sharply demarcated acute gastric ulcer with surrounding hyperemia is shown here in the upper fundus. This ulcer is probably benign. However, all gastric ulcers should undergo biopsy to rule out a malignancy. Isolated gastric ulcers may be seen with chronic atrophic gastritis; they are usually located in the antrum and lesser curve or at the junction of antrum and body. *H. pylori* is the most common cause, followed by NSAIDs. Patients are usually normochlorhydric or hypochlorhydric.

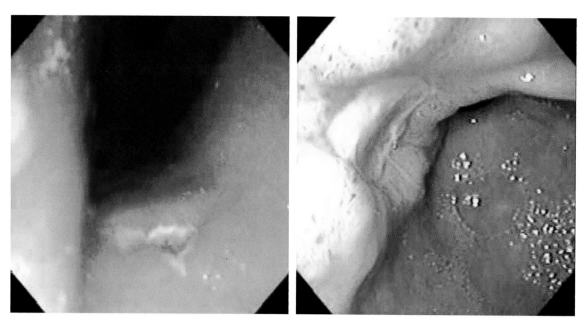

FIGURES 7–39 and 7–40 Acute gastric ulcers, endoscopy

There is a small prepyloric ulcer in the left panel, and a larger antral ulcer in the right panel. All gastric ulcers undergo biopsy because gross inspection alone cannot determine whether a malignancy is present. Smaller, more sharply demarcated gastric ulcerations are more likely to be benign.

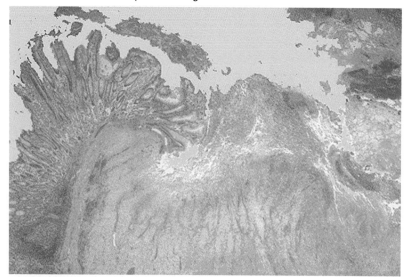

FIGURE 7–41 Acute gastric ulcer, microscopic

Note the loss of the epithelium and extension of the ulcer downward to the muscularis. This ulcer is sharply demarcated, with normal gastric mucosa on the left falling away into a deep ulcer crater whose base contains inflamed, necrotic debris. An arterial branch at the ulcer base is eroded and bleeding. Ulcers will penetrate more deeply over time if they remain active and do not heal. Penetration leads to pain. If the ulcer penetrates through the muscularis and through adventitia, the ulcer is said to "perforate," leading to an acute abdomen with peritonitis, and an abdominal radiograph may demonstrate free air with a perforation.

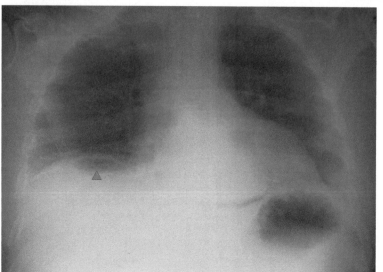

FIGURE 7–42 Perforated gastric ulcer, radiograph

The AP portable upright chest radiograph shown here demonstrates free air (▲) under the right diaphragmatic dome. This patient had a perforation of a duodenal peptic ulcer. The intraluminal air released from a perforated viscus can be detected as free peritoneal air, and a good place to detect it is under a diaphragmatic leaf on an upright abdominal plain film radiograph. Such patients have an "acute abdomen" with pain and sepsis. The pathogenesis of duodenal ulcers is hyperacidity. These ulcers occur in the proximal duodenum and are associated with peptic duodenitis. Almost all duodenal ulcers are associated with *H. pylori* infection in the stomach.

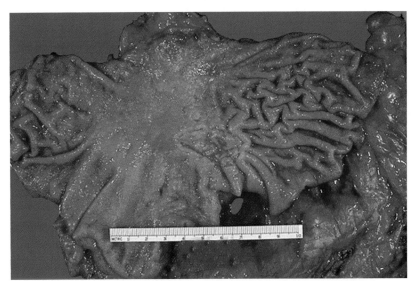

FIGURE 7–43 Adenocarcinoma, gross

Here is a gastric ulcer. It is shallow and is about 2 to 4 cm in size. This ulcer on biopsy proved to be malignant, so that the stomach was resected as shown here. In the United States, most gastric cancers are discovered at a late stage when the neoplasm has invaded or metastasized. *All* gastric ulcers and *all* gastric masses must undergo biopsy because it is not possible to determine malignancy from gross appearance. In contrast, virtually all duodenal peptic ulcers are benign. Worldwide, gastric carcinoma is the second most common cancer, but the incidence has been dropping for decades in the United States.

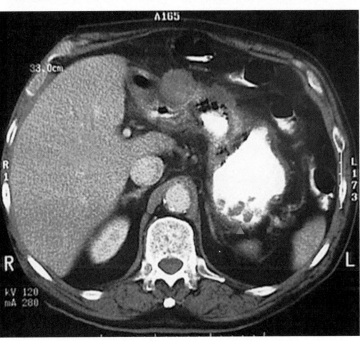

FIGURE 7–44 Adenocarcinoma, CT image

This abdominal CT with contrast reveals an exophytic mass (▲) lesion distorting the gastric antrum. This is an adenocarcinoma. This patient had *H. pylori* infection with chronic gastritis for many years. However, few people with *H. pylori* infection develop gastric cancer. Risks, including dietary factors such as ingestion of pickled or smoked foods, nitrosamines derived from ingested nitrites, and excessive salt intake, predispose to development of the intestinal type of gastric cancer, and changes in dietary patterns have led to a steady decrease in the incidence of this form of cancer. Risk factors for the diffuse form of gastric cancer are less well defined. Clinical manifestations include nausea, vomiting, abdominal pain, hematemesis, weight loss, altered bowel habits, and dysphagia. Early gastric cancers confined to the mucosa are usually asymptomatic and detected by endoscopic screening.

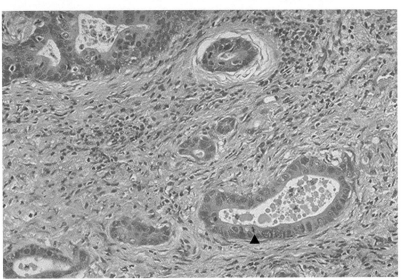

FIGURE 7–45 Adenocarcinoma, microscopic

This intestinal type of gastric adenocarcinoma has neoplastic glands infiltrating into the submucosa. Some of the cells demonstrate mitoses (▲). The cells have an increased nuclear-to-cytoplasmic ratio and nuclear hyperchromatism. There is a desmoplastic stromal reaction to these infiltrating glands. Genetic abnormalities in the intestinal type of gastric cancer include *p53* mutation, abnormal E-cadherin expression, and instability of *TGFβ* and *BAX* genes.

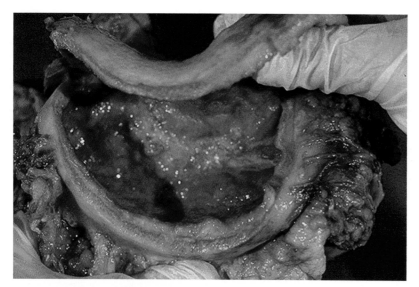

FIGURE 7–46 Adenocarcinoma, gross

This is an example of linitis plastica, a diffuse infiltrative gastric adenocarcinoma that gives the stomach a shrunken "leather bottle" appearance with extensive mucosal erosion, ulceration, and a markedly thickened gastric wall. This type of gastric carcinoma has a very poor prognosis. More localized gastric cancers are most likely to arise on the lesser curvature and demonstrate ulceration. The intestinal type of gastric cancer is more likely to arise from precursor lesions and be related to *H. pylori* infection. The declining incidence of intestinal-type gastric cancers in the United States is probably related to diminishing prevalence of *H. pylori* infection. The incidence of the diffuse type of gastric cancer shown here has remained constant over time.

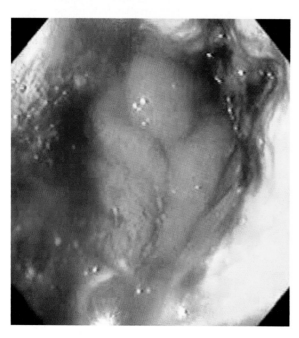

FIGURE 7–47 Adenocarcinoma, endoscopy

The endoscopic view of the linitis plastica appearance of the diffuse type of gastric adenocarcinoma reveals extensive mucosal erosion.

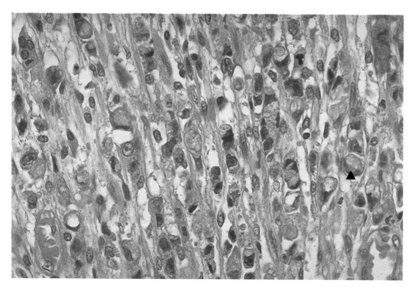

FIGURE 7–48 Adenocarcinoma, microscopic

This diffuse type of gastric adenocarcinoma is so poorly differentiated that glands are not visible. Instead, rows of infiltrating neoplastic cells with marked pleomorphism are seen. Many of the neoplastic cells have their cytoplasm filled with clear vacuoles of mucin (▲), displacing the cell nucleus to the periphery. This is the "signet ring" cell pattern that is typical of the diffuse type of gastric adenocarcinoma, which tends to be highly infiltrative and thus has a poor prognosis.

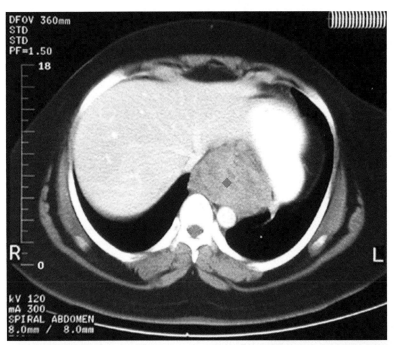

Figure 7–49 Gastrointestinal stromal tumor, abdominal CT scan

There is a large mass (◆), a gastrointestinal stromal tumor (GIST), involving the lower esophagus and extending to the upper gastric fundus. The mass has decreased attenuation and some variability in attenuation from necrosis and cystic change. The margins are discrete. These lesions used to be classified as smooth muscle tumors but are now thought to arise from the interstitial cell of Cajal, a cell that forms part of the myenteric plexus that controls gastrointestinal peristalsis.

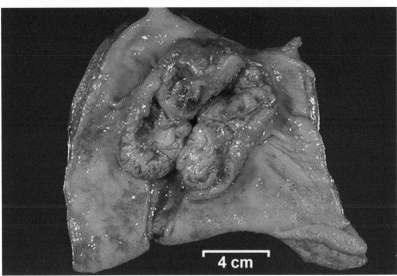

Figure 7–50 Gastrointestinal stromal tumor, gross

The GIST shown is a prominent mass that arose in the muscular wall of the stomach and grew exophytically toward the lumen, retaining a covering of mucosa except in the central ulcerated area. GISTs can be solitary or multiple.

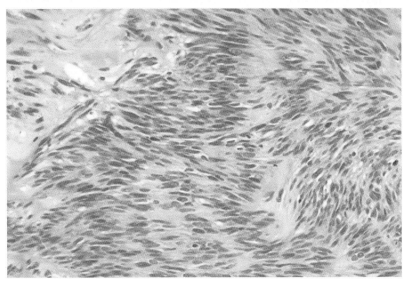

Figure 7–51 Gastrointestinal stromal tumor, microscopic

GISTs can be subclassified into spindle, epithelioid, or mixed types. Here are bundles of spindle cells, which are typical of a GIST. Immunohistochemical staining for c-*KIT* (CD117) is positive in 95% of GISTs, and staining for CD34 is positive in 70% of GISTs. In addition to c-*KIT* mutations, platelet-derived growth factor receptor, A chain (*PDGFA*) mutations are found in 35% of GISTs. The biologic potential of these tumors is difficult to evaluate. The most important features are mitotic count, size, and cellularity. A newly designed tyrosine kinase inhibitor (STI571) has been shown to be effective in treating this tumor.

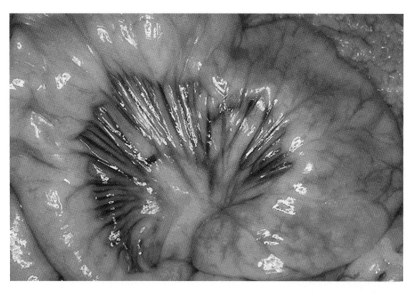

FIGURE 7–52 Normal small intestine and mesentery, gross

Seen here is a loop of bowel attached through the mesentery. Note the extensive venous drainage, which will flow into the portal venous system draining into the liver. Arcades of arteries supplying blood to the bowel run in the same mesenteric location. The bowel is supplied by branches and collaterals from the celiac axis, superior mesenteric artery, and inferior mesenteric artery, providing an extensive anastomosing arterial blood supply to the bowel, making it more difficult to infarct. Note the smooth, glistening peritoneal surfaces of the small intestine.

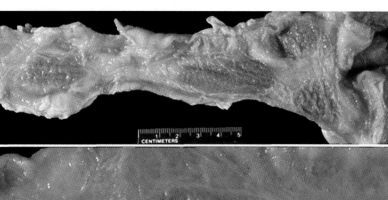
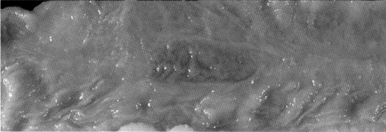

FIGURE 7–53 Normal small intestine, gross

This is the normal appearance of terminal ileum. In the upper frame, note the ileocecal valve, and several darker oval Peyer patches are present on the mucosa. In the lower frame, note the prominent oval Peyer patch, which is a concentration of submucosal lymphoid tissue. In the duodenum, the lamina propria and the submucosa have proportionately more lymphoid tissue than the rest of the GI tract. The ileum has more prominent submucosal lymphoid tissue, which appears as small nodules or as the elongated ovoid Peyer patches. However, gut-associated lymphoid tissue (GALT) is present from the back of the tongue all the way to the rectum and is collectively the largest lymphoid organ of the body.

FIGURE 7–54 Normal small intestine, microscopic

The small intestinal mucosa has surface villi lined by columnar cells (♦) and scattered goblet cells (▲). The villi terminate in the lamina propria as glandular lumina known as *crypts of Lieberkühn* (■). The villi greatly increase the surface absorptive area. The jejunum has more prominent folds (plicae) of the mucosa to increase absorptive area. Each intestinal villus contains a blind-ended lymphatic channel known as a *lacteal*. The major immunoglobulin secreted by plasma cells of the gastrointestinal tract (and respiratory tract) is immunoglobulin A (IgA), so-called secretory IgA. This is bound to protein on the glycocalyx overlying the microvilli of the brush border to neutralize harmful agents such as infectious organisms.

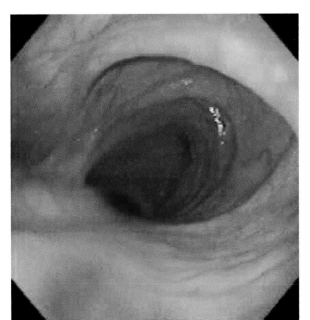

FIGURE 7–55 Normal transverse colon, endoscopy

Note the mucosal haustral folds typical of the colon. The function of the colon is primarily to absorb most of the remaining water and electrolytes passed from the small intestine in order to concentrate the volume of stool, so that only about 100 mL of water is lost per day in the stool. There are about 7 to 10 liters of gas traversing the colon each day, primarily as a result of growth of normal bacterial flora, although only about half a liter is passed as flatus. The gaseous components include swallowed air (nitrogen and oxygen) along with methane and hydrogen from digestive processes and bacterial growth. Irritable bowel disease (IBD) has no gross or microscopic findings, but results from an abnormally exaggerated sensory responses to physiologic stimuli from gas in the bowel, worsened by stress, and anticholinergic drugs may provide temporary relief.

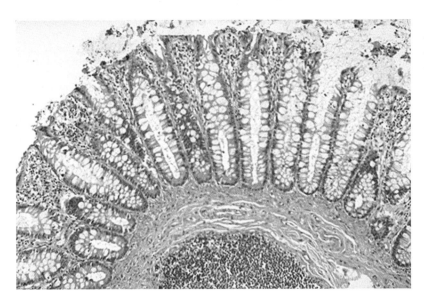

FIGURE 7–56 Normal colon, microscopic

The colon has a mucosal architecture of long tubular glands (crypts of Lieberkühn) lined by columnar mucous cells. Goblet cells are numerous and provide lubrication for transit of stool. Lymphoid nodules are in the lamina propria and submucosa. The outer longitudinal layer of muscle is coalesced into long bands known as *taenia coli*. At the anorectal junction, there is a mucosal transition from columnar cells lining crypts to stratified squamous mucosa. Both above and below this junction are prominent submucosal veins (internal and external hemorrhoidal veins), which when dilated form hemorrhoids with itching and bleeding. A layer of skeletal muscle at the anus provides a sphincter under voluntary control.

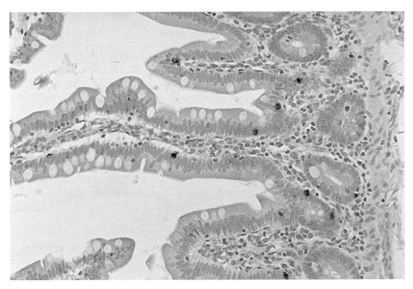

FIGURE 7–57 Normal intestinal endocrine cells, microscopic

The areas of black, stippled staining identify the scattered enteroendocrine (neuroendocrine) cells in the mucosal crypts of the small intestine (Kulchitsky cells). These cells are scattered within the glands and become more numerous distally in small intestine. There are a variety of enteroendocrine cells in the mucosa of the gut. When food passes into the small intestine, some of them release cholecystokinin (CCK), which delays gastric emptying while promoting digestion by causing the gallbladder to contract and release bile that aids in digestion of lipids. CCK also causes release of a variety of enzymes from pancreatic acinar cells.

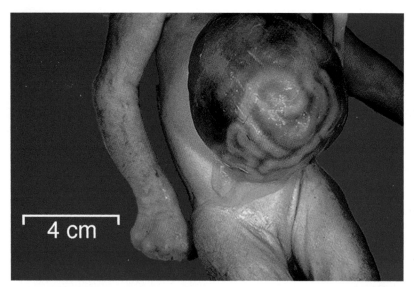

FIGURE 7–58 Omphalocele, gross

Here is a ventral midline abdominal wall defect in a newborn infant girl. This defect involves the region of the umbilical cord, so this is called an *omphalocele*. Note that there is a thin membrane covering the herniated abdominal contents (including loops of bowel as well as liver). Since this bowel has mainly developed outside of the abdominal cavity during fetal life, it is malrotated, and the abdominal cavity is not properly formed (too small). Thus, such a defect would have to be repaired in several stages. An omphalocele may occur sporadically, but most are associated with other congenital malformations and may be the result of a genetic abnormality such as trisomy 18.

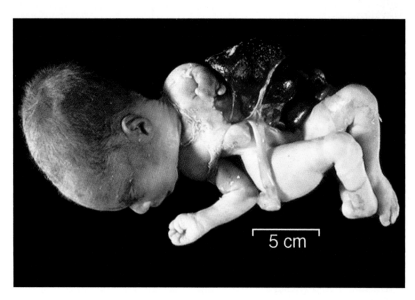

FIGURE 7–59 Gastroschisis, gross

This is a large lateral abdominal wall defect, which does not involve the cord and is not covered by a membrane. Much of the bowel, stomach, and liver have developed outside the abdominal cavity. This gastroschisis is associated with limb–body wall (LBW) complex, sometimes called *amnionic band syndrome*, but such fibrous bands may only be present in half of cases of LBW complex. It results from early amnion disruption, which occurs sporadically in embryonic development and is not part of a defined genetic abnormality. Seen here in association with LBW complex are reductions of the extremities, particularly the left upper extremity, and scoliosis. Not seen here are craniofacial clefts and defects that can also occur with LBW complex.

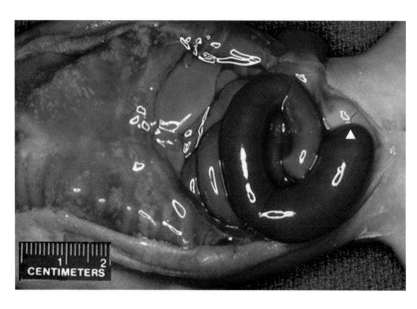

FIGURE 7–60 Intestinal atresia, gross

The meconium-filled intestine shown here ends in a blind pouch (▲). This is complete obstruction, or atresia. Partial or incomplete obstruction is called *stenosis*. Such a defect, like many anomalies, often occurs in conjunction with other anomalies. Bowel atresias *in utero* are accompanied by polyhydramnios since the swallowing and absorption of amniotic fluid by the fetus is impaired. Atresia is uncommon, but one place it can be seen is the duodenum, and half of all duodenal atresias occur with Down syndrome, although conversely, few cases of Down syndrome have duodenal atresia. By ultrasound, there is a "double-bubble" sign from duodenal enlargement proximal to the atresia accompanying the normal stomach bubble.

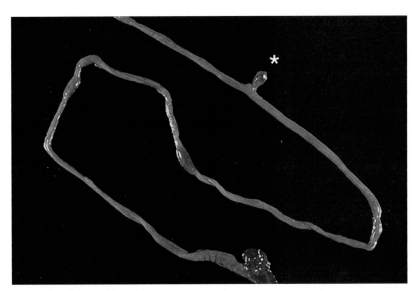

FIGURE 7–61 Meckel diverticulum, gross

Congenital anomalies of bowel consist mainly of diverticula or atresias, which often occur in association with other congenital anomalies. Seen here is the most common congenital anomaly of the GI tract—a Meckel diverticulum (∗). Remember the number 2: about 2% of people have them; they are usually located 2 feet from the ileocecal valve. This "true" diverticulum with all three bowel wall layers is an incidental finding from an adult unless it must be excised because of blood loss from ulceration because this diverticulum may contain ectopic gastric mucosa (which can ulcerate surrounding mucosa with consequent pain and possible iron deficiency anemia) or ectopic pancreas (which is of little consequence unless it forms a mass large enough predisposing to intussusception).

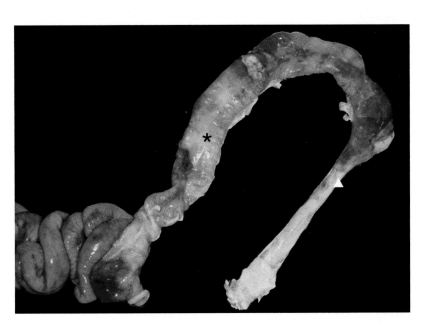

FIGURE 7–62 Hirschsprung disease, gross

Shown here is dilation of bowel (megacolon) caused by failure of migration of neuroblasts that form the myenteric plexus in the lower bowel wall. This dilation (∗) is proximal to the affected aganglionic region (▲) at the lower left center in the sigmoid colon. The result is intestinal obstruction, marked by delayed passage of meconium following birth, from lack of normal peristalsis in affected neonates. The incidence is 1 per 5000 live births, mostly males. A variety of genetic defects can cause Hirschsprung disease, but about half of familial cases and one sixth of sporadic cases result from *RET* gene mutations. Mucosal damage and secondary infection may follow.

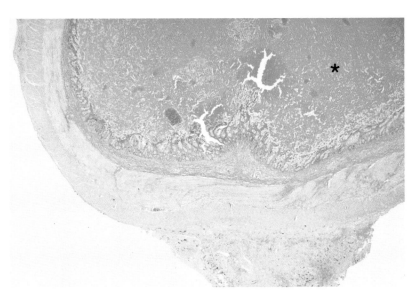

FIGURE 7–63 Meconium ileus, microscopic

This form of bowel obstruction most often occurs in neonates with cystic fibrosis, but can rarely occur in normal infants. In cystic fibrosis, the abnormal pancreatic secretions lead to inspissated meconium with intestinal obstruction. The dilated ileum is shown filled with meconium (∗) (the gross appearance is dark green, and meconium may also be tarry or gritty). Little or none of this highly viscid meconium is passed per rectum following birth. A potential complication is meconium peritonitis with bowel rupture. Calcifications in the spilled meconium may be seen radiographically. Another complication of meconium ileus is volvulus.

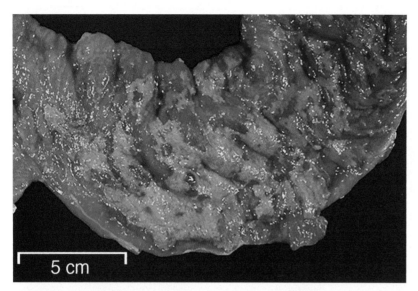

FIGURE 7–64 Pseudomembranous colitis, gross

The mucosal surface of the colon seen here is partially covered by a yellow-green exudate. The mucosa itself is erythematous and superficially denuded but not eroded. It may cause an acute or chronic diarrheal illness. Broad-spectrum antibiotic usage (such as clindamycin) or immunosuppression allows overgrowth of normally suppressed intestinal bacterial flora such as *Clostridium difficile* or *Staphylococcus aureus* or fungi such as *Candida* to cause this antibiotic-associated colitis. Exotoxins elaborated by the bacteria damage the mucosa by inducing cytokine production to cause cellular apoptosis.

5 cm

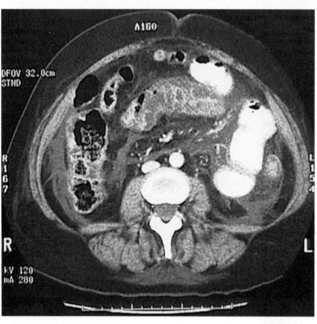

FIGURE 7–65 Pseudomembranous colitis, CT image

This abdominal CT scan reveals a narrowed lumen with thickened, edematous transverse colon (▲) and colonic splenic flexure as a consequence of antibiotic-associated (pseudomembranous) colitis. This appearance can also be present with ischemic colitis and neutropenic colitis (typhlitis). Typhlitis typically involves the cecum, where blood flow is most likely to be diminished, in an immunocompromised patient with neutropenia.

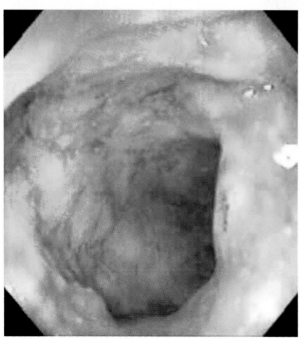

FIGURE 7–66 Pseudomembranous colitis, endoscopy

On colonoscopy, there is a tan to green exudate overlying the surface of the colonic mucosa. This appearance may also be seen with ischemia and with severe acute infectious colitis. Patients with this disorder may have abdominal pain and develop a severe diarrhea. With progression of disease there can be sepsis and shock. The affected bowel may need to be resected.

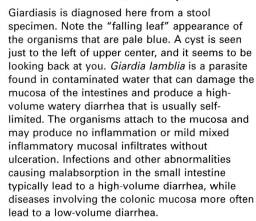

FIGURE 7–67 Giardiasis, microscopic

Giardiasis is diagnosed here from a stool specimen. Note the "falling leaf" appearance of the organisms that are pale blue. A cyst is seen just to the left of upper center, and it seems to be looking back at you. *Giardia lamblia* is a parasite found in contaminated water that can damage the mucosa of the intestines and produce a high-volume watery diarrhea that is usually self-limited. The organisms attach to the mucosa and may produce no inflammation or mild mixed inflammatory mucosal infiltrates without ulceration. Infections and other abnormalities causing malabsorption in the small intestine typically lead to a high-volume diarrhea, while diseases involving the colonic mucosa more often lead to a low-volume diarrhea.

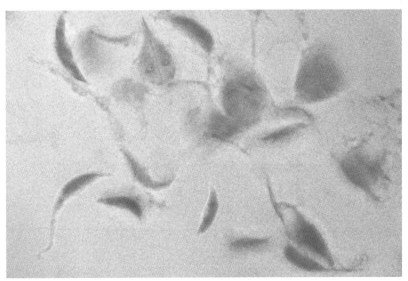

FIGURE 7–68 Amebiasis, microscopic

Entamoeba histolytica organisms (▲) are seen in the region of colonic mucosal ulceration with this H+E stain. Amebiasis, a disease acquired through ingestion of contaminated food or water, can lead to an acute inflammatory bowel disease with diarrhea, which may be bloody. It is most often diagnosed by examination of a stool specimen. Since the organisms can invade the mucosa, there can be ulceration and hemorrhage along with abdominal pain. If these protozoa gain access to the small mucosal or submucosal vessels, they can disseminate through the portal system to the liver, or rarely other sites. In the liver, they may produce an amebic abscess.

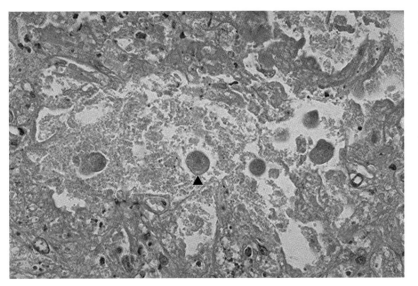

FIGURE 7–69 Cryptosporidiosis, microscopic

The small round blue objects (▲) at the luminal border or within a vacuole in peripheral enterocyte cytoplasm are *Cryptosporidium parvum* organisms. The organisms rarely invade or disseminate. There is no inflammation, necrosis, or hemorrhage. This infectious agent most frequently affects immunocompromised patients, particularly those with AIDS. Immunocompetent patients may just develop a mild watery diarrhea, but with diminished cell-mediated immunity, cryptosporidiosis produces a copious watery diarrhea. Diagnosis is typically made by examination of a stool specimen, and the organisms can be highlighted with an acid-fast stain.

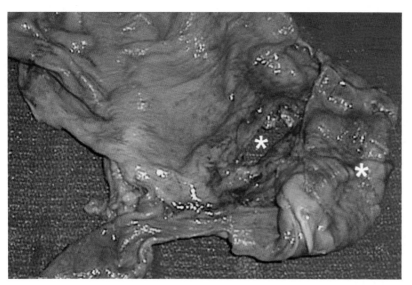

FIGURE 7–70 Neutropenic colitis, gross

This is typhlitis, inflammation of the cecum, with perforation seen at the left asterisk. The serosal surface seen at the right (∗) demonstrates a green-brown exudate with peritonitis from rupture and release of feculent material. Typhlitis is uncommon but can occur in immunocompromised patients, including those with neutropenia and leukemia. The term *neutropenic enterocolitis* is used when there is more extensive bowel involvement. The combination of impaired mucosal immunity and compromised blood supply promote this inflammatory process.

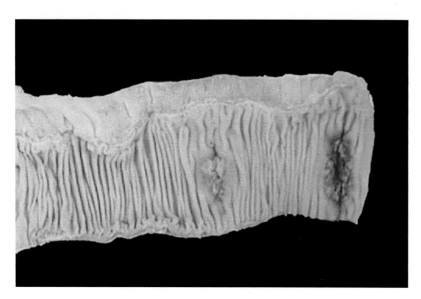

FIGURE 7–71 Tuberculous enteritis, gross

Shown here are circumferential ulcerations, one larger as well as a smaller ulcer, that are characteristic of infection by *Mycobacterium bovis* (rare now because of pasteurization of milk). Swallowed pulmonary secretions with *M. tuberculosis* may rarely produce this finding. The circumferential ulcerations may heal with stricture, producing bowel obstruction.

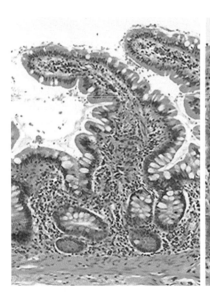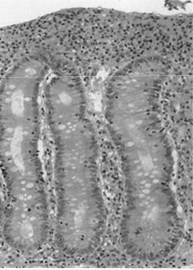

FIGURE 7–72 Celiac sprue, microscopic

Normal small intestinal mucosa is seen in the left panel, and mucosa involved by celiac sprue in the right panel with blunting and flattening of villi (in severe cases, a loss of villi with flattening of the mucosa, as seen here), loss of crypts, increased mitotic activity, loss of brush the border, and infiltration with CD4 cells and plasma cells sensitized to gliadin. Celiac sprue has a prevalence of about 1 in 2000 in the white population, but is rarely seen in other races. More than 95% of affected patients have the HLA DQ2 or DQ8 antigen, which suggests a genetic basis. There is sensitivity to gluten, which contains the protein gliadin, found in wheat, oats, barley, and rye. Removing these grains from the diet results in the enteropathy subsiding.

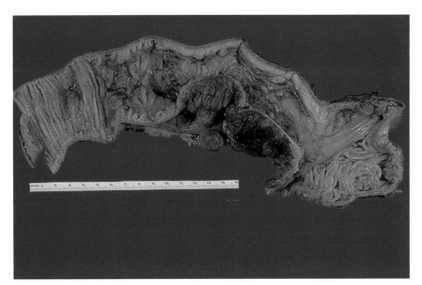

FIGURE 7–73 Crohn disease, gross

The middle portion of bowel seen here has a thickened wall, and the mucosa has lost the regular folds and contains deep fissures. The serosal surface demonstrates reddish indurated adipose tissue that creeps over the surface. The areas of inflammation tend to be discontinuous throughout the bowel ("skip" lesions). Although any portion of the GI tract may be involved with Crohn disease, the small intestine—and the terminal ileum in particular—is most likely to be affected. This disease is more common in the United States and Western Europe; women are affected more often than men. There is a genetic susceptibility that may be related to the presence of certain HLA types and to *NOD2* gene mutations that may be related to the microbe receptor triggering NF-κB transcription factor production that promotes cytokine release driving inflammation.

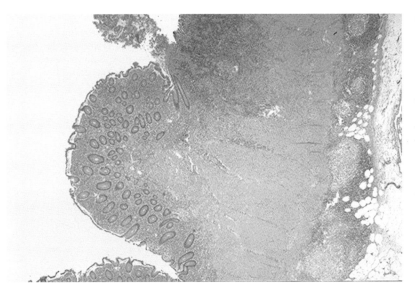

FIGURE 7–74 Crohn disease, microscopic

Note the transmural inflammation with inflammatory cells (the bluish infiltrates) extending from the ulcerated mucosa through submucosa and muscularis and to the serosa, appearing as nodular granulomatous infiltrates on the serosal surface. This transmural inflammation predisposes to formation of adhesions and fistulae with adjacent intra-abdominal structures from serosal involvement. Enteroenteric fistulae between loops of bowel, and perirectal fistulae, are common complications. Mucosal injury predisposes to malabsorption, particularly of vitamin B_{12}, and steatorrhea from loss of bile salt recirculation, because of terminal ileal involvement.

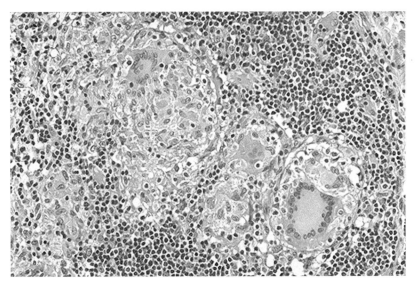

FIGURE 7–75 Crohn disease, microscopic

The granulomatous nature of the inflammation of Crohn disease is shown here with epithelioid cells, giant cells, and many lymphocytes. Special stains for organisms are negative. Most patients have a relapsing course over decades, while some have quiescent disease for many years and others have continuously active disease after onset. Anti–*Saccharomyces cerevisiae* antibodies (ASCAs) are highly specific and sensitive for Crohn disease and are unlikely to be present with ulcerative colitis (UC). Antineutrophil cytoplasmic autoantibodies with perinuclear staining (pANCA) can be found in 75% of patients with Crohn disease but in only 11% with UC.

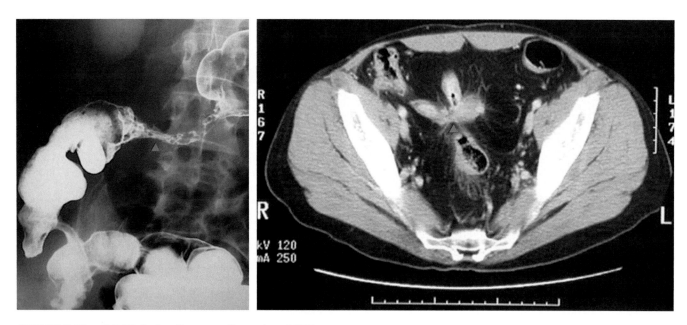

FIGURES 7–76 and 7–77 Crohn disease, radiograph and CT image

The upper GI series at the left with bright barium contrast media filling the bowel lumen reveals a long area of narrowing (▲) involving nearly the entire terminal ileum, a favorite site of involvement of Crohn disease, but the remaining small bowel, as well as the colon, may also be involved. The stomach is rarely involved. The abdominal CT without contrast at the right demonstrates enteroenteric fistula formation. Loops of small bowel converge (▲) because of the adhesions resulting from the transmural inflammation.

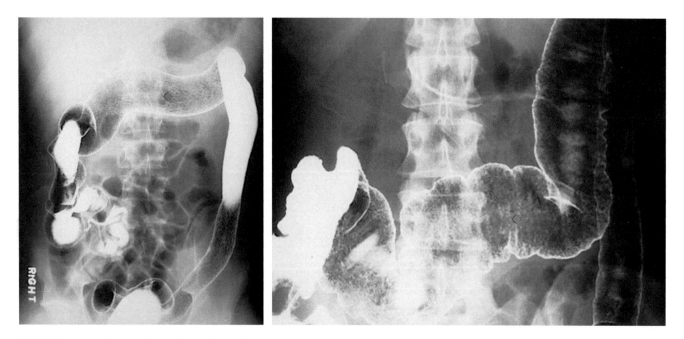

FIGURES 7–78 and 7–79 Ulcerative colitis, radiographs

The barium enema at the left has fine granularity (◆) of the mucosa from the rectum to the transverse colon, typical of earlier involvement of the mucosa with UC. UC, along with Crohn disease, is a form of idiopathic inflammatory bowel disease. The barium enema at the right demonstrates a closer view of an area of coarse granularity (◆) of the mucosa from the rectum to the transverse colon, typical of a more severe involvement of the mucosa with UC. UC typically involves the colonic mucosa in a continuous pattern, starting from the rectum and extending a variable distance proximally.

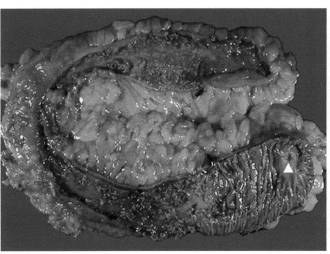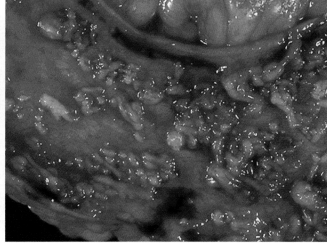

FIGURES 7–80 and 7–81 Ulcerative colitis, gross

At the left is a colectomy specimen with extensive UC beginning in the rectum and extending all the way to the ileocecal valve (▲). There is diffuse mucosal inflammation with focal ulceration, erythema, and granularity. As the disease progresses, the mucosal erosions coalesce to linear ulcers that undermine remaining mucosa, leaving islands of residual mucosa called *pseudopolyps.* At the right, these pseudopolyps are seen in a case of severe UC. The remaining mucosa has been ulcerated away, leaving only hyperemic submucosa and muscularis.

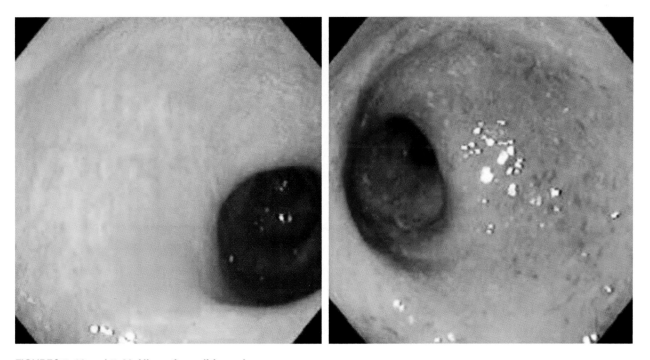

FIGURES 7–82 and 7–83 Ulcerative colitis, endoscopy

A colonoscopic view of less severe UC is seen at the left, with friable, erythematous mucosa and reduction in haustral folds. A view of active UC, but not so eroded as to produce pseudopolyps, is seen at the right. UC is idiopathic and occurs more frequently in the United States and Europe than in other areas of the world. UC is a chronic disease with a relapsing course in most patients, although a few patients have only one or two bouts, and some unfortunate patients may have continuous active disease. The onset of active UC is marked by low volume but bloody, mucoid diarrhea along with abdominal cramping pain, tenesmus, and fever. Extraintestinal manifestations often develop over the course of an inflammatory bowel disease and include sclerosing cholangitis, migratory polyarthritis, sacroiliitis, uveitis, and acanthosis nigricans. There is a long-term risk for development of colonic adenocarcinoma. Extraintestinal manifestations occur with Crohn disease as well, although the risk for adenocarcinoma is not as great for Crohn disease as for UC.

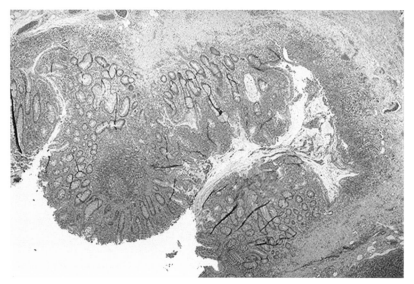

FIGURE 7–84 Ulcerative colitis, microscopic

The inflammation of UC is confined primarily to the mucosa, which is shown here as an inflammatory process that undermines the surrounding mucosa to produce a flask-shaped ulceration. An exudate is present over the surface. Both acute and chronic inflammatory cells can be present. The stools are typically of low volume, but may contain blood and mucus. A relapsing but mild course is most common, seen in 60% of patients, although some patients may have a single episode, while others have almost continuous attacks. One third of patients may undergo colectomy within 3 years of onset because of uncontrolled colitis. Toxic megacolon with marked dilation and thinning of the bowel is a feared complication because of risk for rupture.

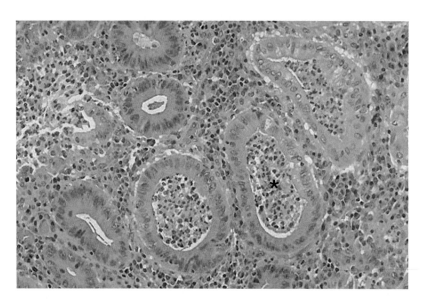

FIGURE 7–85 Ulcerative colitis, microscopic

The colonic mucosa of active UC shows "crypt abscesses" in which a neutrophilic exudate (∗) is found within the glandular lumens of the crypts of Lieberkühn. The submucosa shows intense inflammation. These inflamed glands with architectural distortion demonstrate loss of goblet cells and hyperchromatic nuclei with inflammatory atypia. Crypt abscesses are a histologic finding more typical with UC than Crohn disease, but there is overlap between these two forms of idiopathic inflammatory bowel disease, and not all cases can be classified completely in all patients.

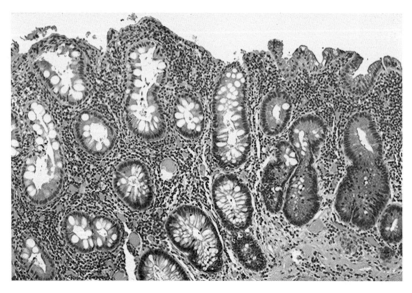

FIGURE 7–86 Ulcerative colitis, microscopic

Here, more normal colonic glands with goblet cells are seen at the left, but the glands at the right demonstrate crypt distortion with dysplasia, the first indication that there is a move toward development of neoplasia from chronic UC. There is DNA damage with microsatellite instability. Over time, after 10 to 20 years of pancolitis, there is such a significant risk for adenocarcinoma that total colectomy may be performed. Patients with UC may undergo screening colonoscopies to detect development of dysplasia.

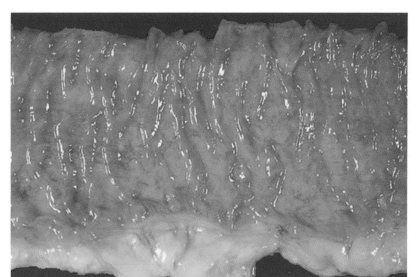

FIGURE 7–87 Ischemic bowel disease, gross

This small intestinal mucosa demonstrates marked hyperemia of the tips of the villi as a result of early ischemic enteritis. Such ischemia most often results from hypotension (shock) from cardiac failure, from marked blood loss, or from loss of blood supply from mechanical obstruction (as with the bowel incarcerated in a hernia or with volvulus or intussusception). Less frequently, thrombosis or embolization with occlusion of one or more mesenteric arterial branches can produce acute intestinal ischemia. Venous thrombosis from hypercoagulable states is less frequent. If the blood supply is not quickly restored, the bowel will become infarcted.

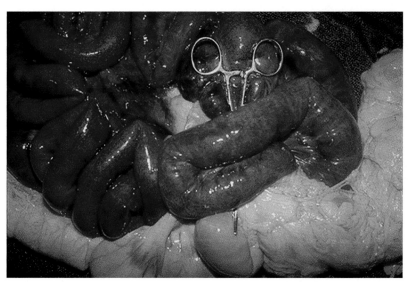

FIGURE 7–88 Ischemic enteritis, gross

The small intestine is infarcted. The dark red to gray infarcted bowel contrasts with the pale pink normal bowel at the bottom. Some organs, such as bowel with anastomosing blood supplies or liver with a dual blood supply, are harder to infarct. This bowel was caught in a hernia created by internal adhesions from prior surgery. A similar finding could result from incarceration of bowel in an inguinal hernia sac. The mesenteric blood supply was constricted here by the small opening to the hernia, located here by the Kelly clamp. Bowel ischemia often produces acute abdominal pain with distention. Lack of peristalsis, marked by absence of bowel sounds, is known as ileus.

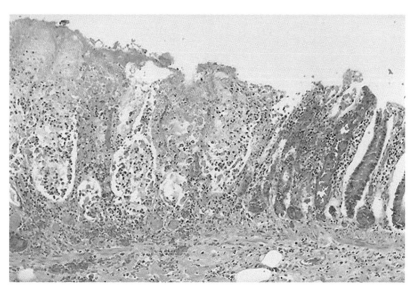

FIGURE 7–89 Ischemic enteritis, microscopic

The mucosal surface of the bowel seen here shows necrosis with hyperemia extending all the way from mucosa to submucosal and muscular wall vessels. The submucosa and muscularis, however, are still intact. With more advanced ischemia and necrosis, the small intestinal mucosa can show hemorrhage with acute inflammation. Progression of ischemia will produce transmural necrosis extending into submucosa and muscularis. Patients can have abdominal pain, vomiting, and bloody or melanotic stools. With ischemic necrosis, intestinal bacterial organisms can gain access to blood, producing septicemia, or to peritoneal cavity, producing peritonitis and leading to shock.

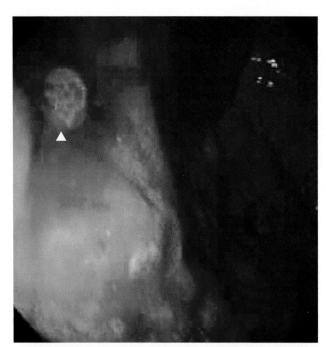

FIGURE 7–90 Angiodysplasia, endoscopy

On upper GI endoscopy is seen an area of angiodysplasia (▲), a condition more common in older people and a cause for GI tract bleeding. This bleeding is often intermittent and rarely severe. One or more foci of irregular, tortuous, thin-walled, dilated venous or capillary channels are present in the mucosa or submucosa, typically of the colon, but occasionally elsewhere. The lesions are often quite small, less than 0.5 cm, making them hard to find. Colonoscopy and mesenteric angiography can be performed for diagnosis, and affected areas can be resected. Some cases are associated with the uncommon systemic disorder known as *hereditary hemorrhagic telangiectasia* (Osler-Weber-Rendu syndrome). A similar "Dieulafoy lesion" is a focal submucosal arterial or arteriovenous malformation of the gut submucosa with overlying mucosal disruption, most often found in the stomach, that can produce bleeding.

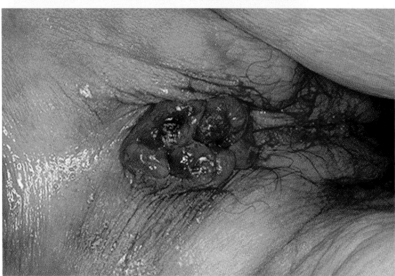

FIGURE 7–91 Hemorrhoids, gross

Seen here is the anus and perianal region with prominent prolapsed true (internal) hemorrhoids, which consist of dilated submucosal veins predisposed to thrombose and rupture with hematoma formation. External hemorrhoids form beyond the intersphincteric groove to produce an "acute pile" at the anal verge. Chronically increased venous pressure leads to venous dilation. Hemorrhoids can itch and bleed (usually bright red blood, during defecation). Rectal prolapse is another complication. Hemorrhoids may become ulcerated. Healing of a thrombosed hemorrhoid results in a fibrous polyp, or anal tag.

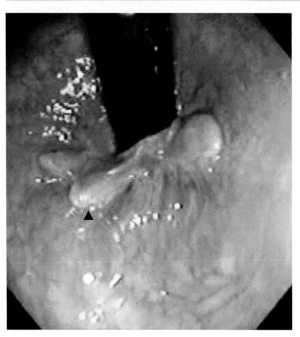

FIGURE 7–92 Hemorrhoids, endoscopy

These polypoid lesions (▲) are hemorrhoids at the anorectal junction. The vessels forming them have undergone at least partial thrombosis and have become shrunken, with a whitened appearance. Chronic constipation, low-fiber diet, chronic diarrhea, pregnancy, and portal hypertension enhance hemorrhoid formation. They are rarely present before the age of 30.

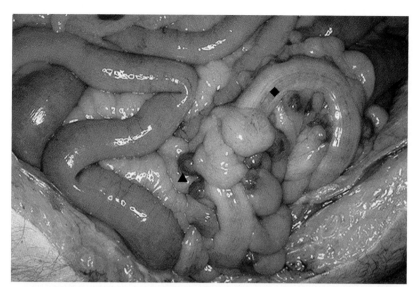

FIGURE 7–93 Diverticular disease, gross

The sigmoid colon at the right has a band of taenia coli (◆) muscle running longitudinally and appears lighter in color than the adjacent small intestine. Protruding from the sigmoid colon are multiple rounded bluish-gray outpouchings (▲) known as diverticula. Diverticula average 0.5 to 1 cm in diameter, are much more common in the colon than in small intestine, and are more common in the left colon. Diverticula are more common in people living in developed nations and may be related to the usual diet, which has less fiber, leading to diminished motility and increased intraluminal pressure. The number of diverticula increases with age.

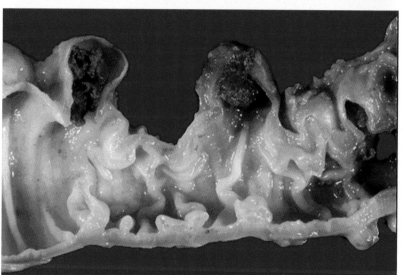

FIGURE 7–94 Diverticular disease, gross

Sectioning the colon longitudinally reveals that the diverticula have an opening to the colonic lumen through a narrow neck. Colonic diverticula are rarely larger than 1 cm in diameter. These are not true diverticula because only the submucosa and mucosa are herniated through an acquired focal weakness in the muscularis. Peristalsis does not empty them, so they become filled with stool. Focal weaknesses in the bowel wall and increased luminal pressure contribute to the formation of multiple diverticula, collectively termed *diverticulosis*. They rarely occur in people younger than the age of 30.

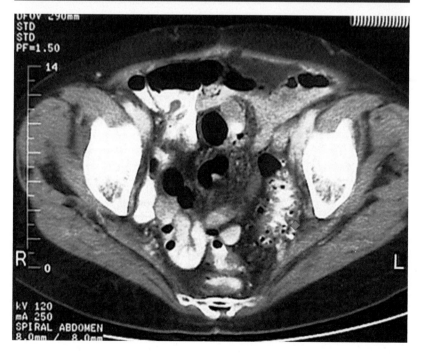

FIGURE 7–95 Diverticular disease, CT image

This abdominal CT with contrast in the pelvic region demonstrates diverticulosis (◆) most pronounced in the sigmoid colon in the pelvis. Note that the small, rounded outpouchings are dark because they are filled with stool and air, not contrast. Most diverticula are asymptomatic. Complications can develop in about 20% of patients with diverticulosis, including abdominal pain, constipation, intermittent bleeding, and inflammation (diverticulitis), with possible perforation and peritonitis.

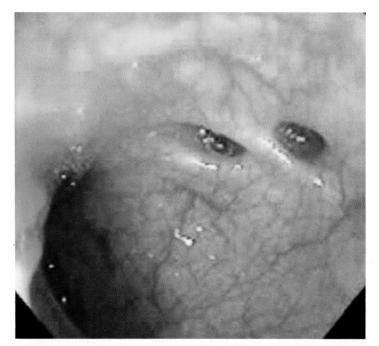

FIGURE 7–96 Diverticular disease, endoscopy

This colonoscopic view of sigmoid colon shows two diverticula, which proved to be incidental findings. The presence of multiple diverticula, or diverticulosis, may become complicated by inflammation, typically initiated at the narrow neck of a diverticulum, with mucosal erosion and irritation. The inflammation causes diverticulitis. Lower abdominal cramping pain, constipation (or less commonly, diarrhea), and occasional intermittent bleeding are possible problems. Diverticulosis and diverticulitis can be causes for iron deficiency anemia. Rarely, there can be more extensive inflammation extending through the diverticular wall, leading to rupture of a diverticulum with peritonitis.

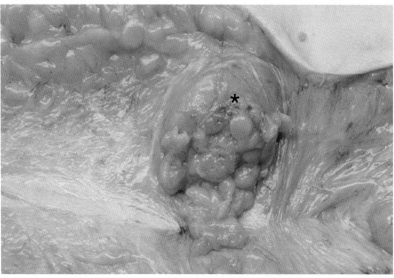

FIGURE 7–97 Hernia, gross

External hernias represent an outpouching of peritoneum through a defect or weakness in the abdominal wall. This most often occurs in the inguinal region, but it can also occur in the umbilical region, as seen here. An "internal" herniation of bowel can result from an abnormal opening formed by adhesions. The defect may be large enough to admit a portion of omentum or bowel. In this abdominal incision can be seen a small hernia sac (∗) that contains adipose tissue from omentum. A reducible hernia contains bowel that can slip in and out of the opening; bowel can become trapped, or incarcerated within the hernia, which predisposes to strangulation of the bowel, with ischemia from a compromised blood supply.

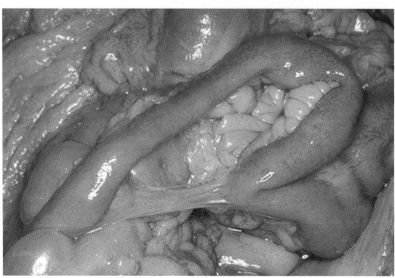

FIGURE 7–98 Adhesion, gross

Note the bandlike adhesion between loops of small intestine. Such adhesions are most likely to form after abdominal surgery. More diffuse adhesions may also form after peritonitis. Adhesions may therefore predispose to bowel obstruction when loops of bowel become trapped in the abnormal opening created by adhesions. In populations where prior abdominal surgery for a variety of conditions, such as acute appendicitis, has been performed, adhesions are often the most common cause of bowel obstruction. The presence of abdominal scars on physical examination of a patient presenting with acute abdominal pain, distention, and ileus is a clue to this diagnosis.

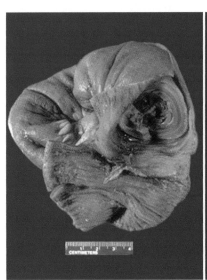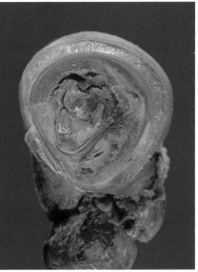

FIGURE 7–99 Intussusception, gross

One rare form of bowel obstruction occurs when a segment of bowel telescopes on itself, a process called intussusception. The blood supply to that segment becomes compromised, predisposing to infarction. In the left panel, the dark red resected portion of infarcted bowel is opened to reveal the telescoped segment within. The cross-section in the right panel shows the "bowel within a bowel" appearance. When this condition occurs in children, it is typically idiopathic. In adults, a polyp or diverticulum driven by peristalsis may lead to intussusception.

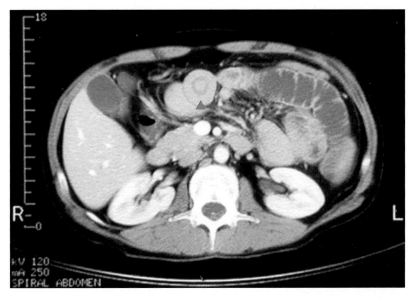

FIGURE 7–100 Intussusception, CT image

This abdominal CT scan demonstrates a thickened portion of small intestine that contains a target appearance (▲) from the presence of an intussuscepted portion of bowel, a "bowel within a bowel" characteristic of intussusception. An abdominal plain film radiograph will typically demonstrate loops of small bowel dilated with air, or air-fluid levels from ileus, as a consequence of bowel obstruction. Patients can present with abdominal pain, abdominal distention, obstipation, and diminished or abnormal bowel sounds on physical examination.

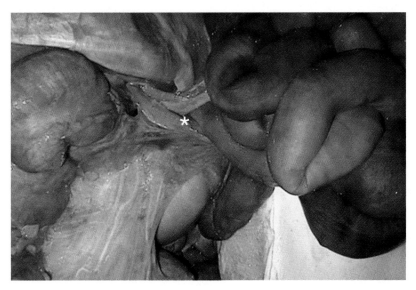

FIGURE 7–101 Volvulus, gross

Volvulus is twisting of the bowel so that the blood supply becomes obstructed, as well as the bowel itself, leading to ischemia with infarction. Obstruction of venous outflow can produce marked congestion. If caught early, the bowel can be untwisted to restore blood supply, but this is often not the case. Seen here is twisting (∗) of the mesentery so that the entire small intestine from jejunum through ileum has become ischemic and is dark red from infarction. Volvulus is rare, but most often seen in adults, where it occurs with equal frequency in small intestine (around a twisted mesentery) and colon (in either sigmoid or cecum, which are more mobile). In very young children, volvulus almost always involves the small intestine.

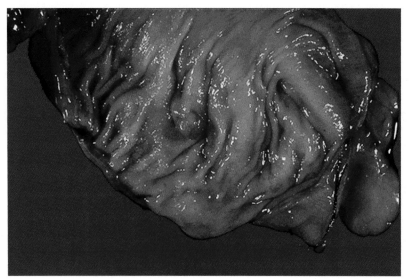

FIGURE 7–102 Adenoma, gross

A small "adenomatous polyp" is seen here in the left colon. A polyp is a structure that protrudes above the surrounding mucosa. It may be pedunculated or sessile. This lesion is called a *tubular adenoma* because of the rounded nature of the neoplastic glands that form it. It has smooth surfaces and is circumscribed. Such lesions are common in adults. An adenoma is the benign precursor to adenocarcinomas Small ones are virtually always benign. Those larger than 2 cm carry a much greater risk for development of a carcinoma. These adenomas can collect mutations in *APC, SMAD4, K-RAS, p53*, and DNA mismatch repair genes over the years.

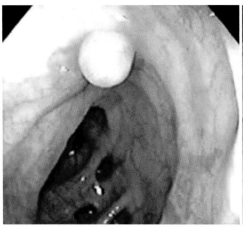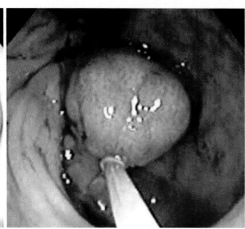

FIGURE 7–103 Adenoma, endoscopy

The colonoscopic appearance of rectal polyps that proved to be tubular adenomas is seen here. Note the smooth, rounded appearance and slight pedunculating of the polyp in the left panel. The adenoma in the right panel is larger and has prominent vasculature, explaining the common appearance of occult blood in the stool in association with polyps.

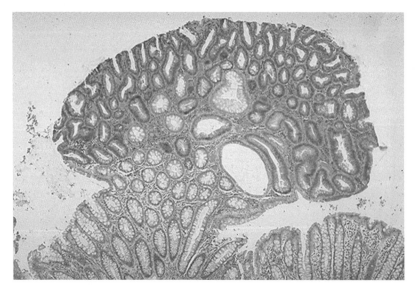

FIGURE 7–104 Adenoma, microscopic

A colonic adenoma is a benign neoplasm with formation of new glands or villi having dysplastic epithelium. This small pedunculated adenomatous polyp on a small stalk is seen to have more crowded, disorganized but rounded glands (a tubular pattern) than the normal underlying colonic mucosa. Goblet cells are less numerous in the polyp, and the crowded cells lining the glands of the polyp have hyperchromatic nuclei. However, this small benign neoplasm is still well-differentiated and circumscribed, without invasion of the stalk. Accumulation of additional mutations over time and with continued growth of the polyp could give rise to malignant transformation.

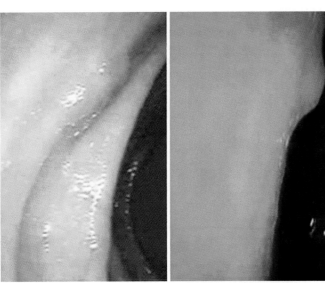

FIGURE 7–105 Hyperplastic polyp, microscopic

In each of these panels, a small flat mucosal polyp is present, no more than about 0.5 cm in diameter. These are excrescences that represent mucosal crypt enlargement. They are most frequent in the rectum. They increase in number with age, and overall half of all people have at least one of them. They are non-neoplastic, carry no risk for development of cancer within them, and are unlikely to be a cause of an occult blood–positive stool. However, they occur more frequently in patients with tubular adenomas and may gradually enlarge. Hyperplastic polyps are typically incidental findings observed on colonoscopy.

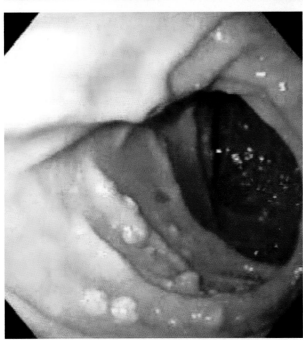

FIGURE 7–106 Peutz-Jeghers polyps, endoscopy

Peutz-Jeghers syndrome is characterized by mucocutaneous pigmentation with gastrointestinal hamartomatous polyps. Polyps can occur in all parts of the GI tract, but mostly in small intestine. Shown on upper endoscopy are multiple small polyps in the duodenum that proved to be hamartomatous polyps on biopsy. This rare autosomal dominant condition can be associated with polyps anywhere in the GI tract. Patients with this syndrome are at increased risk for developing malignant neoplasms in various organs, such as breast, ovary, testis, or pancreas, but malignancies do not directly arise within the polyps. Mucocutaneous freckle-like pigmentation is often seen on buccal mucosa, genital region, hands, and feet. These polyps can be large enough to cause obstruction or intussusception.

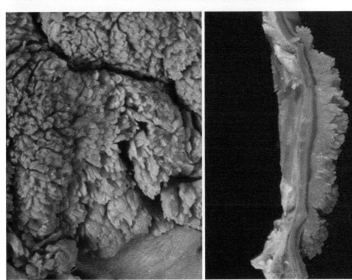

FIGURE 7–107 Villous adenoma, gross

The cauliflower-like gross appearance of a villous adenoma is shown from above the surface in the left panel and in cross-section through the bowel wall in the right panel. Note that this type of adenoma is broad based and sessile, rather than pedunculated, and much larger than the typical tubular adenoma (adenomatous polyp). A villous adenoma averages several centimeters in diameter, and may be as large as 10 cm. The risk for adenocarcinoma arising in the larger villous adenoma is high. Polyps with both tubular and villous features may be termed *tubulovillous adenomas*.

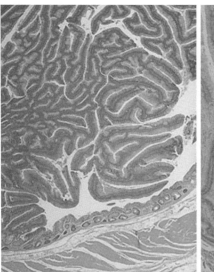 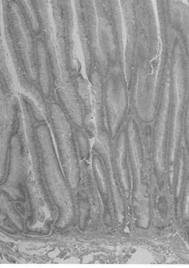

FIGURE 7–108 Villous adenoma, microscopic

A villous adenoma is shown at its edge in the left panel and projecting above the basement membrane in the right panel. The cauliflower-like appearance is due to the elongated glandular structures covered by dysplastic epithelium. Although villous adenomas are less common than adenomatous polyps, they are much more likely to harbor invasive carcinoma in them (about 40% of villous adenomas).

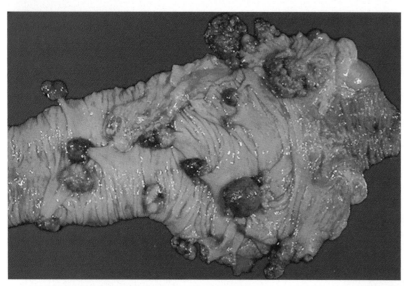

FIGURE 7–109 Hereditary nonpolyposis colon carcinoma, gross

Hereditary non-polyposis colon carcinoma (HNPCC or Lynch syndrome when a genetic basis is defined) leads to right-sided colon cancer in young individuals. HNPCC is associated with extraintestinal malignancies (endometrium, urinary tract) due to germ line mutations in mismatch repair genes with abnormal expression levels of hMLH1 and hMSH2 proteins. Tumors associated with HNPCC exhibit microsatellite instability (10% to 15% of sporadic cancers also show microsatellite instability). There are far fewer polyps than in familial adenomatous polyposis with *APC* mutations, but the polyps are aggressive. Here are multiple adenomatous polyps of the cecum (there is a terminal ileum at the right).

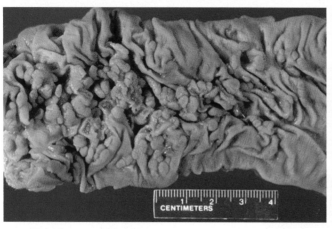 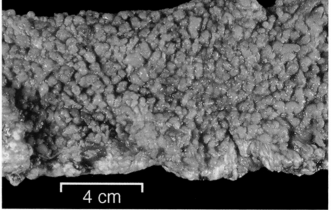

FIGURES 7–110 and FIGURE 7–111 Familial adenomatous polyposis, gross

Faulty *APC* genes in familial adenomatous polyposis (FAP) lead to accumulation of β-catenin translocating to the nucleus and activating transcription of genes such as *MYC* and *cyclin D1*. This autosomal dominant condition leads to development by adolescence of more than 100 colonic adenomas that carpet the mucosa (right panel). If untreated by total colectomy, nearly all individuals develop adenocarcinoma. An "attenuated" form of *APC* (left panel) has fewer, more variable numbers of polyps, with older age of onset of colon cancer. Gardner syndrome, also with mutated *APC* gene, has in addition osteomas, periampullary adenocarcinoma, thyroid cancer, fibromatosis, dental abnormalities, and epidermal inclusion cysts.

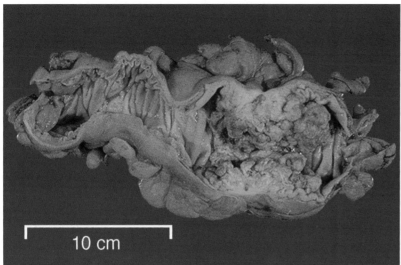

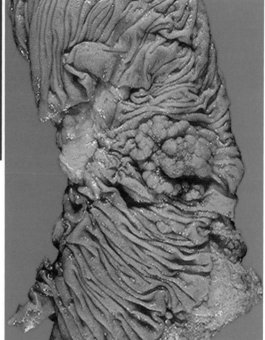

◄ FIGURE 7–112 Adenocarcinoma, gross

The exophytic growth pattern can obstruct the colonic lumen. Thus, one of the complications of a carcinoma is obstruction (usually partial). A change in stool or bowel habits can be created by the mass effect.

FIGURE 7–113 Adenocarcinoma, gross ►

At the right is an adenocarcinoma arising in a villous adenoma. The surface of the neoplasm is polypoid and reddish pink. Hemorrhage from the surface of the tumor creates a guaiac-positive stool. This neoplasm was located in the sigmoid colon, just out of reach of digital examination, but easily visualized with sigmoidoscopy. A variety of genetic abnormalities precede development of colonic carcinogenesis, including the *APC/β-catenin* pathway, *K-RAS* mutations, loss of *SMADs*, loss of *p53*, activation of telomerase, and the microsatellite instability pathway.

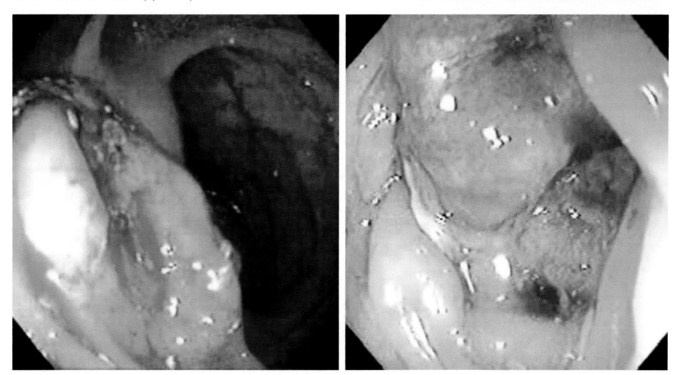

FIGURES 7–114 and 7–115 Adenocarcinoma, endoscopy ▲

Here are colonoscopic views of colonic adenocarcinoma. The mass in the left panel has a central ulcerated crater with hemorrhage, explaining why testing for occult blood in the stool provides a good screening tool for detection of this lesion. In the right panel is another bulky mass that produces partial intraluminal obstruction.

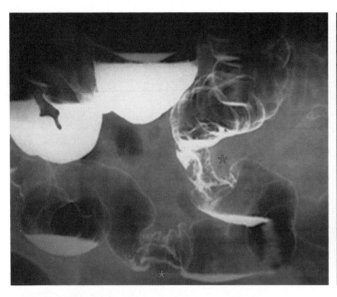
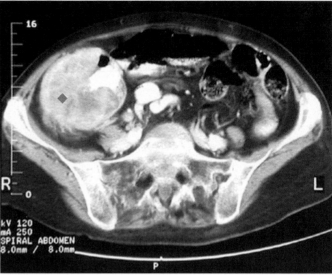

FIGURES 7–116 and 7–117 Adenocarcinoma, barium enema and CT image

The barium enema technique instills the radiopaque barium sulfate into the colon, producing a contrast with the wall of the colon that highlights any masses present. In the left panel, the procedure was performed with the patient in a lateral position (head toward the right of the image) and shows two encircling masses (*), one in the transverse colon and one in the descending colon, representing an adenocarcinoma that constricts the lumen. The large mass lesion (◆) seen in the abdominal CT with contrast in the right panel is a large adenocarcinoma distending the cecum. Cecal carcinomas often become bulky masses and may first be manifested by iron deficiency anemia from blood loss.

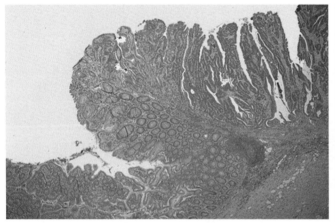
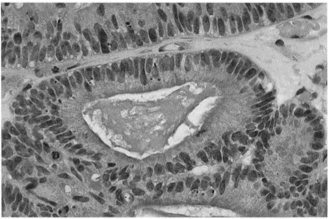

FIGURES 7–118 and 7–119 Adenocarcinoma, microscopic

In the left panel can be seen the edge of an adenocarcinoma. The neoplastic glands are long and frondlike, similar to those seen in a villous adenoma, but more disorganized. The growth is primarily exophytic (outward into the lumen), and invasion is not seen at this point. Grading and staging of the tumor are done by the surgical pathologist, who will examine multiple histologic sections of the tumor. In the right panel at high magnification, the neoplastic glands of adenocarcinoma have crowded nuclei with hyperchromatism and pleomorphism. No normal goblet cells are seen. A series of genetic mutations may precede development of colon cancer. The *APC* gene may be mutated, followed by mutation of *K-RAS*, *SMAD4*, and *p53*. Epidermal growth factor receptor (EGFR) is a surface membrane receptor that has been shown to occur in a variety of solid malignancies, including colonic adenocarcinoma. The monoclonal antibody cetuximab directed against EGFR can be used for treatment for colonic adenocarcinomas expressing EGFR.

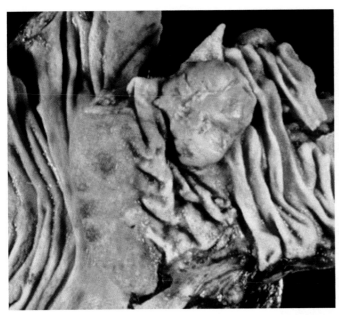
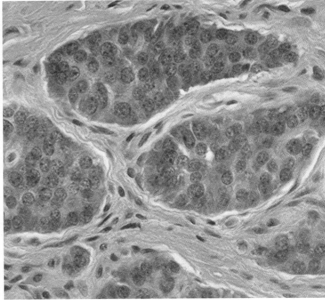

FIGURES 7–120 and 7–121 Carcinoid tumor, gross and microscopic

Neoplasms of the small intestine are uncommon. Benign tumors can include leiomyomas, fibromas, neurofibromas, and lipomas. Seen in the left panel at the ileocecal valve is another tumor that has a faint yellowish color. This is a carcinoid tumor. Most benign tumors are incidental submucosal lesions, although rarely they can be large enough to obstruct the lumen. At high magnification, the nests of carcinoid tumor in the right panel have a typical endocrine appearance, with small round cells having small round nuclei and pink to pale blue cytoplasm. Rarely, a malignant carcinoid tumor can occur as a large bulky mass. Metastatic carcinoid tumor to the liver can rarely result in the carcinoid syndrome.

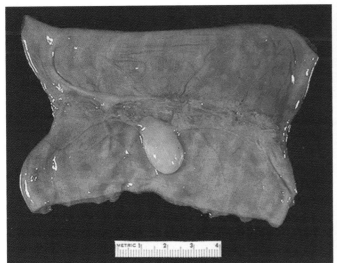
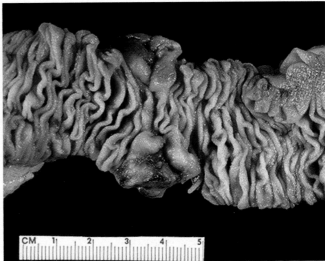

FIGURES 7–122 and 7–123 Lipoma and Non-Hodgkin Lymphoma, gross

The small discrete yellow subserosal mass at the left is a lipoma of the small intestine found incidentally at autopsy; it is composed of cells essentially resembling mature adipose tissue. Benign neoplasms closely resemble the cell of origin, are circumscribed, and slow-growing. The multifocal irregular tan-to-brown masses seen at the right on the mucosal surface of the small intestine are non-Hodgkin lymphoma arising in the bowel in a patient with AIDS. Lymphomas in AIDS are high-grade. In contrast, the mucosa-associated lymphoid tissue (MALT) lesion is sporadic, and in the stomach may result from chronic *Helicobacter pylori* infection. Over 95% of gastrointestinal lymphomas are of B-cell origin. They may produce thickening of the bowel wall with loss of motility, or larger masses that may ulcerate or obstruct the lumen.

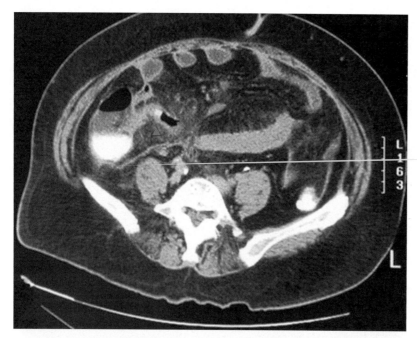

FIGURE 7–124 Acute appendicitis, CT image

Shown is an enlarged appendix (▲) with a fecalith that appears bright because it is partly calcified. The cecum to the left is partially filled with bright contrast. Distal to the fecalith, the appendiceal lumen is dark because it is full of air. There is stranding of brighter areas of attenuation from inflammation extending to surrounding adipose tissue. Patients with acute appendicitis typically present with sudden onset of abdominal pain that localizes to the right lower quadrant, and on physical examination, there is often rebound tenderness. Leukocytosis is often present. This patient presents an increased operative risk because of obesity (note the large amount of dark adipose tissue beneath the skin).

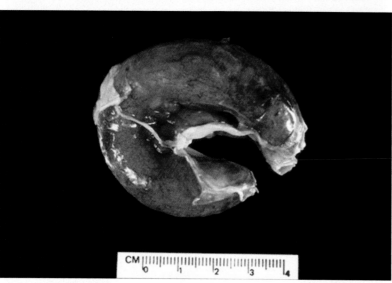

FIGURE 7–125 Acute appendicitis, gross

Here is the resected appendix from abdominal laparoscopic surgery. Note that there is a serosal tan-yellow exudate, but the main features of this early acute appendicitis are edema and hyperemia. This patient had a fever and an elevated total white blood cell count with a left shift (increased band neutrophils) noted on the peripheral blood smear. However, this patient had minimal abdominal pain, but had flank pain because the appendix had a retrocecal orientation.

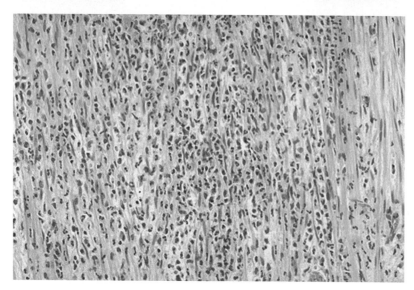

FIGURE 7–126 Acute appendicitis, microscopic

Acute appendicitis is marked by mucosal inflammation and necrosis. As shown here, numerous neutrophils extend into and through the wall of the appendix. A peripheral neutrophilia with bandemia is often present as well. This condition is treated surgically by removal of the inflamed appendix before potential complications of rupture or sepsis occur. If the inflammation is limited to the serosa (periappendicitis), it is likely that the instigating process is somewhere else in the abdomen and that the appendix is just an "innocent bystander."

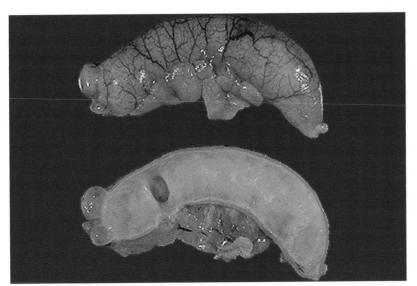

FIGURE 7–127 Mucocele, gross

The lumen of the appendix shown here is markedly dilated. It was filled with a clear, viscous mucoid material. Mucoceles that persist probably represent true neoplasms, most often a mucinous cystadenoma, rather than just an obstructed appendix. Rupture of a mucocele can fill and distend the peritoneal cavity with mucin. Mucinous cystadenocarcinomas of appendix, colon, and ovary can also spread throughout the abdominal cavity and produce much the same pattern, except malignant cells are present, and the condition is known as *pseudomyxoma peritonei.*

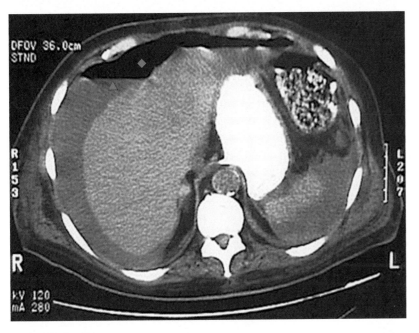

FIGURE 7–128 Perforation with free air, CT image

This abdominal CT reveals free air (◆) from perforation of a viscus. Inflammation or ulceration of the bowel, stomach, or gallbladder can be complicated by perforation. The presence of free air is a good indication that some viscus has ruptured or perforated within the peritoneal cavity. Also seen here is ascitic fluid adjacent to the liver on the right and forming an air-fluid level (▲). Peritonitis may occur in the absence of perforation, a condition known as *spontaneous bacterial peritonitis,* which usually occurs when there is ascites, most often in children with nephrotic syndrome or adults with chronic liver disease.

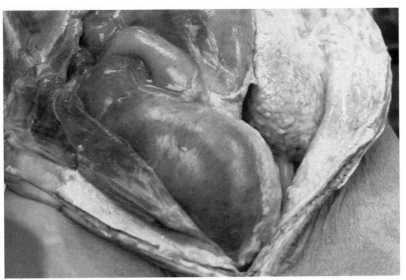

FIGURE 7–129 Peritonitis, gross

Perforation of GI tract within the peritoneal cavity (anywhere from the lower esophagus to colon) can result in peritonitis, as seen here at autopsy. A thick yellow purulent exudate covers peritoneal surfaces. A variety of bacterial organisms can contaminate the peritoneal cavity, including Enterobacteriaceae, streptococci, and *Clostridium* species. An ovarian carcinoma caused sigmoid colonic obstruction (the sigmoid is the markedly dilated gray-black bowel in the pelvis seen here) with perforation. Peritonitis can cause functional bowel obstruction from paralytic ileus, seen with abdominal plain-film radiographs as dilated loops of bowel with air-fluid levels.

CHAPTER 8

Liver and Biliary Tract

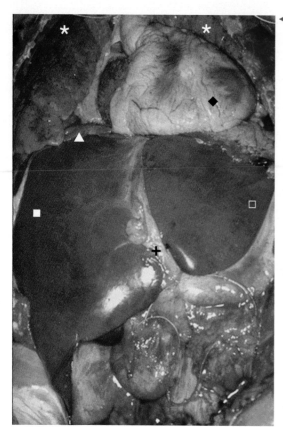

◄ **FIGURE 8–1 Normal liver in situ, gross**

Here is the normal liver in situ in the upper abdomen, as seen at autopsy. The liver lies below the diaphragm (▲), and the chest cavity is above with heart (◆) and lungs (*). As can be seen, the liver is the largest parenchymal organ. The right lobe (■) (here at the left) is larger than the left lobe (□). The falciform ligament (+) is the rough dividing line between the two lobes. Embryologically, the liver is derived from an endodermal bud of foregut.

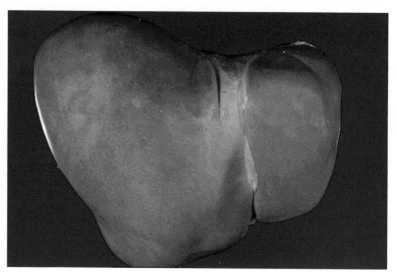

FIGURE 8–2 Normal liver, gross ►

This is the external surface of a normal liver. The color is brown, and the surface is smooth. The normal liver in adults weighs between 1400 and 1600 gm. There is a dual blood supply, with one third of the blood flow but most of the oxygenated blood supplied by the hepatic artery, and two thirds of the blood flow coming through the portal venous system draining from the intestines. Bile formed in the liver drains from the canaliculi of hepatic lobules through increasing diameters of branching ducts to coalesce into right and left hepatic ducts that join at the hilum just outside the inferior hepatic surface to form the common bile duct.

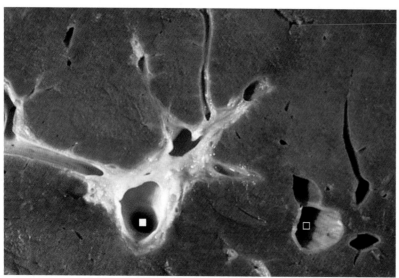

◄ **FIGURE 8–3 Normal liver, gross**

The cut surface of a normal liver has a uniform brown color. Near the hilum here, note the portal vein (■) carrying blood to the liver, which branches at center left, with accompanying hepatic artery and bile ducts. At the lower right is a branch of hepatic vein (□) draining blood from the liver to the inferior vena cava. The liver performs numerous metabolic functions, including the processing of dietary amino acids, carbohydrates, and lipids. It detoxifies and excretes waste products through the bile and synthesizes many plasma proteins.

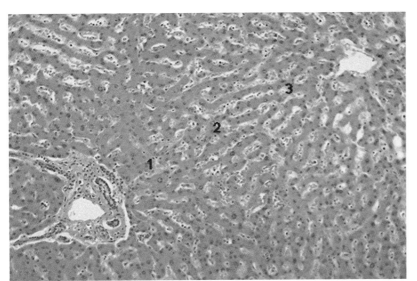

FIGURE 8–4 Normal liver zones, microscopic

The liver is functionally divided into lobules with a central vein and peripheral triads. Hepatic cords radiate from the central vein as single plates of one hepatocyte thickness sandwiching a bile canaliculus flowing toward the triad. Hepatocytes adjacent to the triad form a "limiting plate." The lobule has three zones defined by their relationship to the portal triad at the lower left and the central vein at the upper right. Zone 1 is periportal and receives blood with the highest oxygen concentration. Zone 2 encompasses the central portion of a liver lobule (mid-zonal). Zone 3 is centrilobular. Within the triad are branches of bile ducts, hepatic artery, and portal vein.

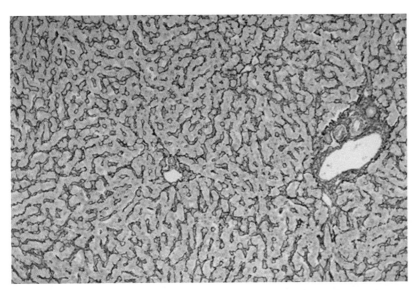

FIGURE 8–5 Normal liver, microscopic

The normal liver is seen at low power with a reticulin stain to outline the connective tissue support by the dark reticulin fibers. The hepatic cord architecture, with plates of hepatocytes staining pink, and sinusoids between, is outlined. A portal triad appears at the right, and a central vein in the center. Hepatocytes are in the resting phase of the cell cycle and in response to injury can reenter the cycle and proliferate to regenerate hepatic parenchyma. Perisinusoidal stellate cells in the space of Disse can be transformed into myofibroblasts in response to hepatic inflammation.

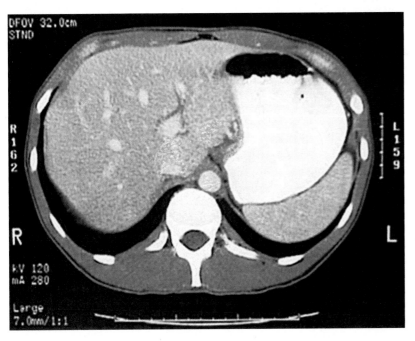

FIGURE 8–6 Normal liver, CT image

An abdominal CT scan with contrast demonstrates the appearance of the normal liver. The attenuation (brightness) of the liver and spleen is similar. Bright orally administered contrast fills the stomach seen here between the liver and spleen. Intravenous contrast material in the hepatic veins is brighter than the surrounding hepatic parenchyma. The right lobe of the liver is much larger than the left lobe, which extends across the midline. Since the liver is the largest abdominal organ, it may be injured with blunt abdominal trauma, producing surface lacerations through the thin Glisson's capsule, leading to hemoperitoneum.

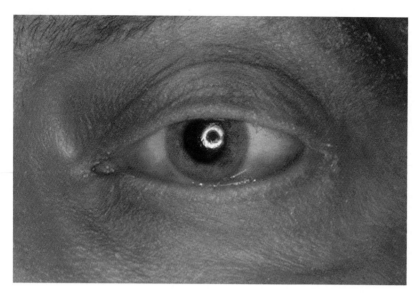

FIGURE 8–7 Jaundice, gross

The end product of heme degradation is bilirubin, which is an extrahepatic metabolic process. The hepatocytes take up unconjugated bilirubin and conjugate it with glucuronic acid and excrete it into bile. Increased bilirubin production, decreased hepatic conjugation and excretion, or biliary tract obstruction leads to increasing bilirubin levels in the blood. This is observed as the physical exam finding of jaundice, or icterus. The normally white sclera of the eye is yellow here because the patient has jaundice; this is a good place on physical examination to look for icterus. Transient neonatal jaundice results from β-glucuronidases in maternal milk that deconjugate bilirubin diglucuronides in the gut that are reabsorbed.

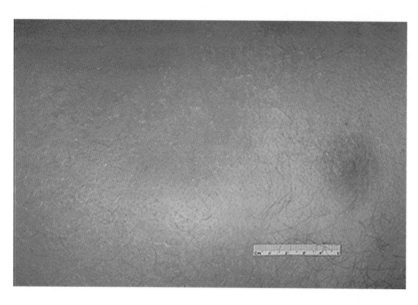

FIGURE 8–8 Jaundice, gross

Increased amounts of circulating bilirubin in the blood can lead to the physical examination finding of "icterus," or jaundice, as seen here from the yellowish hue of the skin. With hemolysis of erythrocytes, there is an increase in unconjugated (indirect) bilirubin to produce icterus. An increase in the conjugated (direct) fraction of bilirubin suggests intrahepatic disease, such as hepatitis, or biliary tract obstruction. Both direct and indirect bilirubin concentrations in serum add to the total serum bilirubin. An elevation in the serum alkaline phosphatase suggests biliary tract obstruction because an isoenzyme of alkaline phosphatase is produced in bile ductular epithelium and in hepatocyte canalicular membranes.

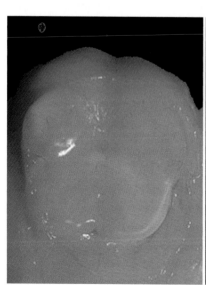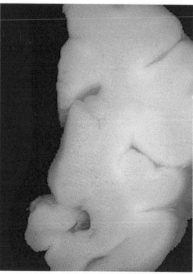

FIGURE 8–9 Kernicterus, gross

Unconjugated bilirubin is tightly bound to circulating albumin and is not excreted in urine; thus, in premature newborns without the mature hepatic capacity to clear bilirubin, blood levels will rise and accumulate in the brain to cause neurologic damage. The yellow staining in the brain of a neonate is known as *kernicterus*. Shown is a coronal section of medulla in the left panel and cerebral hemisphere in the right panel demonstrating kernicterus in deep gray matter. Increased unconjugated bilirubin, which accounts for the kernicterus, is toxic to the brain tissue. Kernicterus is more likely to occur with prematurity, low birth weight, and increased bilirubin levels.

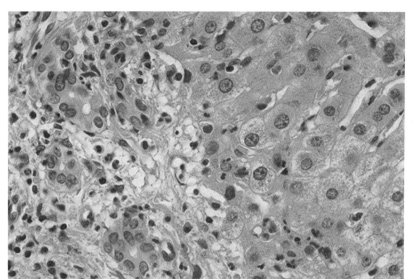

FIGURE 8–10 Cholestasis, microscopic

The yellowish pigmentation seen here in the hepatocyte cytoplasm at the right is due to the accumulation of bile pigments. Intrahepatic cholestasis can be a consequence of hepatocyte dysfunction or of biliary tract obstruction. In addition to intrahepatic bile stasis, there is also intracanalicular bile stasis seen here. The biliary tract obstruction in this case also led to bile duct proliferation, seen here at the left. The catabolism of heme derived from developing, damaged, and senescent erythrocytes produces bilirubin loosely bound to albumin in the blood. Bilirubin is taken up into hepatocytes, bound to cytosolic glutathione S-transferases, conjugated with glucuronic acid by uridine diphosphate-glucuronyl transferase, and excreted into the bile canaliculus.

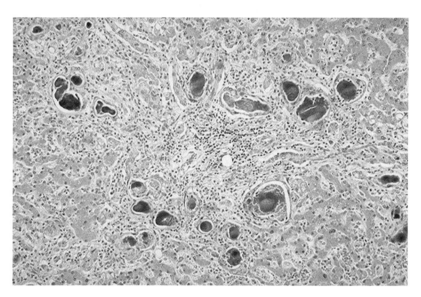

FIGURE 8–11 Cholestasis, microscopic

The yellowish green accumulations of pigment seen here in liver are bile pigments. Obstruction of the biliary tree leads to intrahepatic bile stasis and formation of bile lakes. Proliferation of bile ducts may occur in response to chronic obstruction. If prolonged, there can be portal fibrosis with "biliary" cirrhosis. Bile acts as an emulsifier and is an important component of lipid digestion in the small intestine. Lack of bile secretion into the duodenum leads to acholic (clay-colored) stools and possible steatorrhea with increased stool fat. Malabsorption of the fat-soluble vitamins A, D, E, and K can then occur. Some vitamin D and K can be made endogenously.

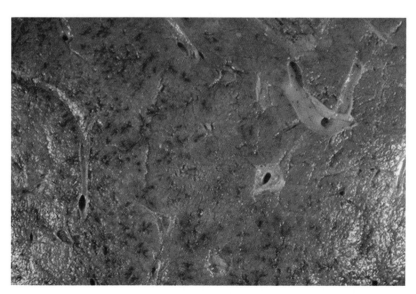

FIGURE 8–12 Hepatic necrosis, gross

Necrosis and hepatic lobular collapse are seen here as areas of hemorrhage and irregular furrows and granularity on the cut surface. Extensive necrosis can follow hepatocyte injury from toxins, infections (such as fulminant viral hepatitis), and ischemia. Alanine aminotransferase (ALT) and aspartate aminotransferase (AST) enzymes are released into the blood (the former more specific for liver injury). Extensive loss of hepatocyte function can lead to decreased protein synthetic function, with hypoalbuminemia and decreased production of clotting factors II, VII, IX, and X (initially manifested by an elevated prothrombin time, and decreased metabolic function, as in the urea cycle, with hyperammonemia.

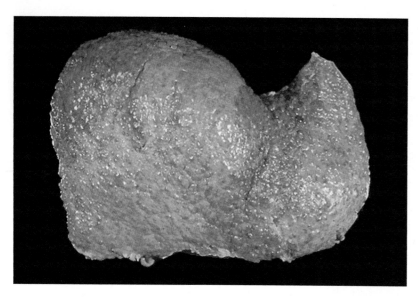

FIGURE 8–13 Cirrhosis, gross

Cirrhosis occurs when diffuse chronic hepatic injury leads to formation of fibrous septae that extend between portal tracts, disrupting the normal hepatic architecture with formation of regenerative nodules of parenchyma. The normal vascular inflow and outflow patterns are disrupted, with development of portal hypertension. The external appearance of micronodular cirrhosis, with a markedly bumpy appearance to the liver capsule, is shown here. Fibrous septae surround regenerative hepatocyte nodules. Cirrhosis requires at least a decade to develop from chronic liver injury. Once established, cirrhosis regresses so slowly that it is essentially irreversible. The cirrhotic liver tends to shrink in size with time.

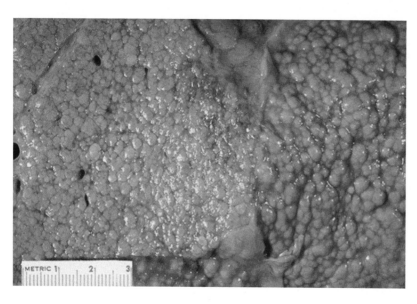

FIGURE 8–14 Cirrhosis, gross

In micronodular cirrhosis, the regenerative nodules average 3 mm or less in size. The yellow-brown appearance of these nodules is due to concomitant hepatic steatosis. The most common cause of micronodular cirrhosis and steatosis is chronic alcohol abuse. A fine reticulin network of type IV collagen is normally present in the liver, but with cirrhosis, there is extensive deposition of type I and III collagen generated from activated perisinusoidal stellate cells. Cirrhosis may remain clinically silent for many years until complications of portal hypertension, such as esophageal varices or ascites, develop, or there is significant loss of liver parenchyma with diminished metabolic function.

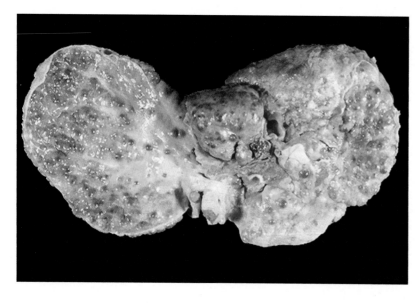

FIGURE 8–15 Cirrhosis, gross

Macronodular cirrhosis is seen here from the inferior hepatic surface, with nodules larger than 3 mm in size. There is extensive deposition of tan-appearing collagen surrounding these regenerative nodules. This is end-stage cirrhosis with hepatic failure marked by increasing hyperbilirubinemia, as evidenced by the green-tinged appearance of the nodules after formalin fixation (with oxidation of bilirubin to biliverdin). The most common cause of macronodular cirrhosis is viral hepatitis. Most causes of cirrhosis can produce both patterns, as well as a mixed micronodular and macronodular cirrhosis; hence, the pattern of nodules provides no reliable clue to the underlying etiology.

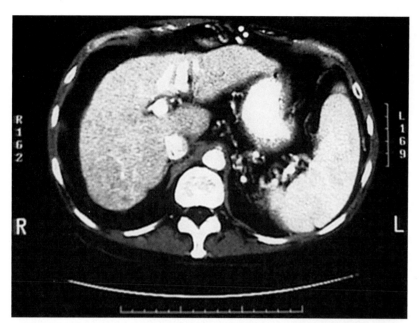

FIGURE 8–16 Cirrhosis, CT image

This abdominal CT scan shows a small, nodular cirrhotic liver with more parenchymal heterogeneity (light and dark areas) than a normal liver. The abnormal blood flow in the cirrhotic liver leads to an elevation in portal venous pressure. Portal hypertension leads to splenomegaly, as shown here. Increased collateral venous blood flow may also lead to formation of esophageal varices, dilated superficial abdominal veins, and hemorrhoids. In addition to chronic alcohol abuse, nonalcoholic fatty liver, viral hepatitis B and C, biliary tract disease, hereditary hemochromatosis, Wilson disease, and α_1-antitrypsin deficiency can lead to cirrhosis. When no identifiable cause is found, the term *cryptogenic cirrhosis* is employed.

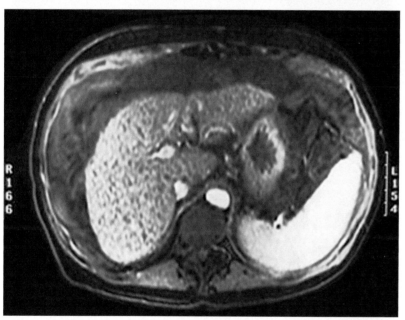

FIGURE 8–17 Cirrhosis, MRI

This abdominal T2-weighted MRI in axial view demonstrates a small, shrunken cirrhotic liver. The spleen is larger than normal due to portal hypertension and can reach up to 1 kg in size. Transudation from the intravascular compartment producing an ascites often accompanies cirrhosis. This ascites results from multiple mechanisms, including hepatic sinusoidal hypertension, hypoalbuminemia, increased lymph drainage into the peritoneal cavity, leakage from intestinal capillaries, and secondary hyperaldosteronism with renal sodium and water retention. In addition, "hepatorenal syndrome" occurs with decreased renal function caused by diminished renal perfusion coupled with renal afferent arteriolar vasoconstriction.

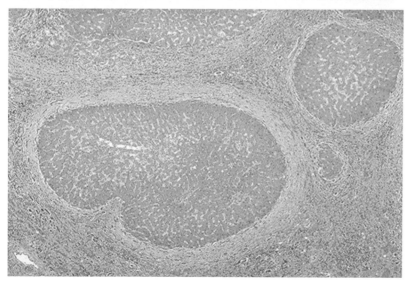

FIGURE 8–18 Cirrhosis, microscopic

This is micronodular hepatic cirrhosis at low power, with regenerative nodules of hepatocytes ringed by thick bands of collagenous fibrosis. Within the fibrous bands are lymphocytic infiltrates and a proliferation of bile ductules. The increased proliferation of hepatocytes from the nodular regeneration increases the risk for hepatocellular and (to a lesser extent) cholangiolar carcinoma. Liver injury leads to Kupffer cell activation with release of cytokines such as platelet-derived growth factor and tumor necrosis factor that stimulate stellate cells in the space of Disse to proliferate into myofibroblastic cells that contribute to the fibrogenesis.

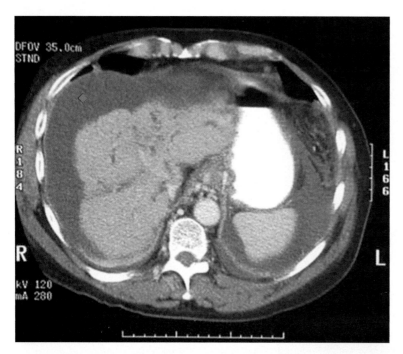

FIGURE 8–19 Cirrhosis and ascites, CT image

A complication of cirrhosis of the liver with portal hypertension seen in this abdominal CT scan is ascites with extensive fluid collections (◆) in the peritoneal cavity. The cirrhotic liver has diminished protein synthetic function, leading to hypoalbuminemia and diminished intravascular oncotic pressure. This is combined with increased sodium and water retention by the kidneys along with increased hydrostatic pressure in veins and capillaries to promote this extravascular fluid collection. The patient may note increasing abdominal girth, and a fluid wave may be observed on physical examination.

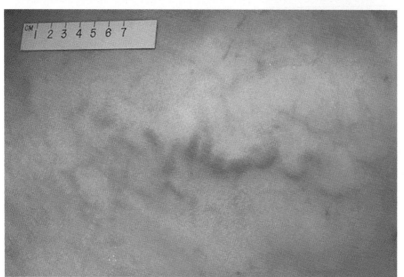

FIGURE 8–20 Portal hypertension, gross

Portal hypertension results from the abnormal blood flow pattern in liver created by cirrhosis. The increased pressure is transmitted to collateral venous channels. These venous collaterals may become dilated. Seen here is "caput medusae," which consists of dilated veins radiating from the umbilicus toward the rib margins, as seen here on the abdomen of a patient with cirrhosis of the liver. Other venous collateral affected by portal hypertension include the esophageal plexus and the hemorrhoidal veins. In addition to cirrhosis, portal hypertension may result from infiltrative granulomatous diseases, schistosomiasis, and marked steatosis.

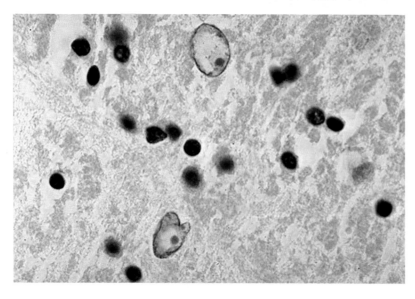

FIGURE 8–21 Hepatic encephalopathy, microscopic

On microscopic examination of the brain in hepatic encephalopathy, Alzheimer type 2 cells are found in the lower layers of the cortex and in the basal ganglia. These are enlarged protoplasmic astrocytes that are responding to the toxins (primarily ammonia) that are not cleared by the urea cycle in the failing liver. These cells have an enlarged watery nucleus with no visible cytoplasm and prominent nucleoli. Patients may exhibit muscular rigidity, hyperreflexia, and asterixis before onset of confusion progressing to stupor and coma.

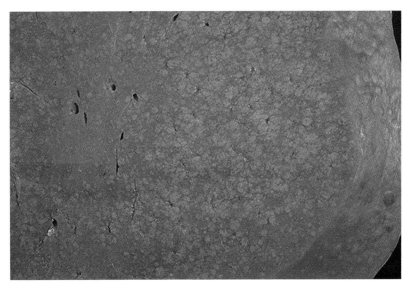

FIGURE 8–22 Viral hepatitis, gross

This liver involved with acute viral hepatitis demonstrates areas of necrosis with collapse of the liver lobules. The necrosis is seen here as ill-defined pale yellow areas between more viable areas of light brown hepatic parenchyma. Note the irregularity of the capsular surface at the right from lobular collapse. If a significant portion of the parenchyma becomes necrotic, the liver becomes pale and shrunken—diffuse massive necrosis—a rare complication most likely to occur with the ordinarily subclinical hepatitis A infection or in some cases of hepatitis B infection. Patients with acute viral hepatitis may present with nausea, anorexia, malaise, and fever, then icterus and progress to hepatic encephalopathy.

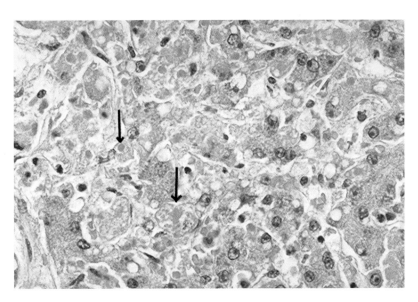

FIGURE 8–23 Viral hepatitis, microscopic

There is ballooning degeneration of many hepatocytes (*arrows*) in this case of a more acute fulminant hepatitis. This ballooning is a manifestation of apoptosis (single cell necrosis). Hepatitis A, a picornavirus with single-stranded RNA in a capsid, may be directly cytotoxic. In contrast, hepatocyte necrosis with hepatitis B, an enveloped virus with double-stranded DNA, or hepatitis C, an enveloped virus with a single-stranded RNA genome, may be induced by cytotoxic CD8 lymphocytes attacking the virally infected hepatocytes. Drugs and toxins that produce hepatic necrosis, such as halothane or isoniazid, may be directly cytotoxic to hepatocytes.

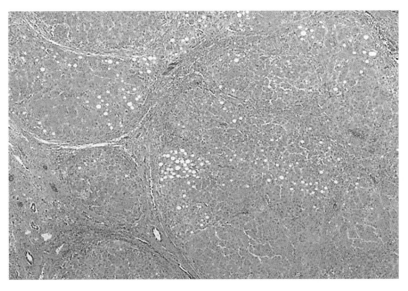

FIGURE 8–24 Viral hepatitis, microscopic

With chronic hepatitis, there is lobular irregularity, with fibrosis and inflammation seen between the lobules. In this case of hepatitis C viral infection, there is a minimal degree of steatosis as well. This case is at a high stage, with extensive fibrosis and beginning progression to macronodular cirrhosis, as evidenced by the large regenerative nodule at the center right. Serologic testing for diagnosis of this form of viral hepatitis includes the hepatitis C virus (HCV) antibody test. Polymerase chain reaction testing for HCV RNA can identify HCV subtypes. Hepatitis C accounts for most (but not all) cases formerly called *non-A, non-B hepatitis*. About 85% of HCV cases proceed to chronic hepatitis, which remains stable in 80% but leads to cirrhosis in 20%.

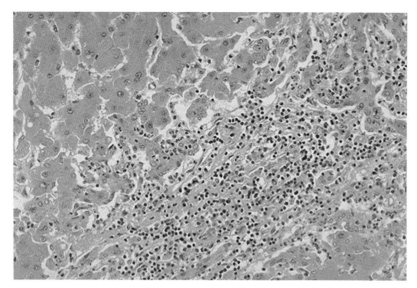

FIGURE 8–25 Viral hepatitis, microscopic

At medium-power magnification, this portal triad is expanded by mainly mononuclear inflammatory cell infiltrates, and the limiting plate of hepatocytes around the triad has been breached, with extension of the inflammation into adjacent hepatic parenchyma, along with focal (piecemeal) necrosis of the hepatocytes. This is typical of a chronic active form of hepatitis. The AST and ALT enzymes would be expected to remain elevated in the patient's serum. In this case, the hepatitis B surface antigen (HBsAg) and hepatitis B core antibody (HBcAb) were positive. A similar appearance can also be seen with chronic hepatitis C viral infection.

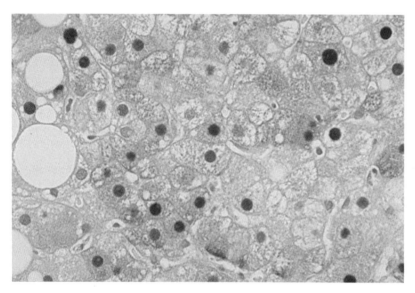

FIGURE 8–26 Viral hepatitis, microscopic

An immunohistochemical stain with antibody to hepatitis B virus (HBV) reveals nuclear staining in the hepatocytes. HBV, a hepadnavirus, has a partially double-stranded circular DNA genome, along with a nucleocapsid "core" protein (detected serologically as antibody to the protein: HBcAb). The surrounding envelope glycoprotein is detected serologically as the surface antigen (HBsAg), and an antibody response that indicates prior hepatitis B viral infection or vaccination yields the antibody designated HBsAb. Vaccination provides immunity to HBV, important to health care workers who have increased risk from exposure to blood and body fluids of patients. HBV and HCV can be transmitted sexually and through needles shared by injection drug users.

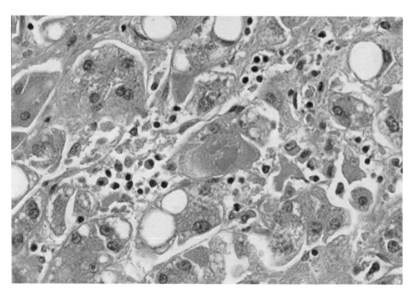

FIGURE 8–27 Viral hepatitis, microscopic

This is a case of HCV that has progressed to chronic hepatitis. The extent of chronic hepatitis can be graded by the degree of activity (necrosis and inflammation) and staged by the degree of fibrosis. In this case, necrosis and inflammation are prominent, and there is some steatosis as well. Regardless of the grade or stage, the etiology of the hepatitis must be sought because the treatment may depend on knowing the cause, and chronic liver diseases of different etiologies may appear microscopically and grossly similar. α-Interferon therapy can be useful in treating HCV infection.

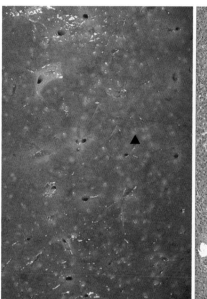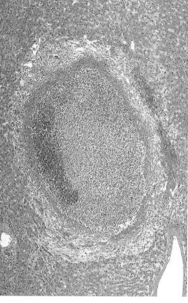

FIGURE 8–28 Hepatic abscesses, gross and microscopic

Pyogenic abscesses in liver are often bacterial and result from spread of infection to hepatic parenchyma with septicemia through the arterial supply, or abdominal infection through portal vein, through an ascending biliary tract infection (cholangitis), with direct spread from an adjacent intra-abdominal infection, or by direct introduction of organisms with penetrating trauma. In the left panel are multiple microabscesses (▲) in a patient with septicemia. The right panel shows a microabscess containing numerous neutrophils producing focal liquefactive necrosis. The beginning of an organizing abscess wall with some pink fibrin is also seen. Patients with abscesses can have fever, right upper quadrant pain, and hepatomegaly. Parasitic and helminthic infections may also cause hepatic abscesses.

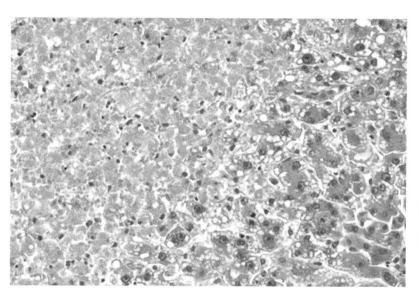

FIGURE 8–29 Acetaminophen toxicity, microscopic

The rate of serum AST and ALT rise indicate the extent of hepatic necrosis. Acetaminophen toxicity may be more severe with accidental overdose in many cases because of an additional risk factor of chronic alcohol abuse. Therapeutic drug levels are metabolized by hepatic conjugation with glucuronidation and sulfation, but acute ingestion of more than 140 mg/kg overwhelms normal metabolic pathways, so that more acetaminophen is metabolized to the toxin N-acetyl-p-benzoquinoneimine (NAPQI) by cytochrome P450. NAPQI is normally detoxified by glutathione, but chronic alcoholism and malnutrition can deplete glutathione and induce P450, increasing the toxicity.

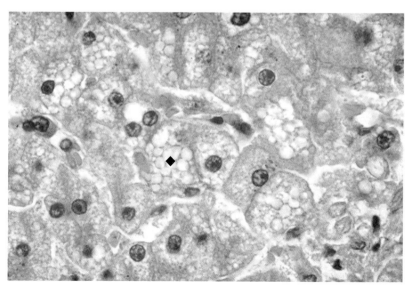

FIGURE 8–30 Reye syndrome, microscopic

There are many small lipid droplets (◆) within these hepatocytes (microvesicular steatosis). Reye syndrome is a rare disease that may result from mitochondrial dysfunction associated with drug ingestion, particularly aspirin given to children for a febrile illness. Laboratory findings can include hypoglycemia, elevated transaminases, hypoprothrombinemia, and hyperammonemia. The serum bilirubin is usually not elevated. A similar appearance can occur with acute fatty liver of pregnancy, a rare complication associated with preeclampsia and a defect in intramitochondrial fatty acid oxidation.

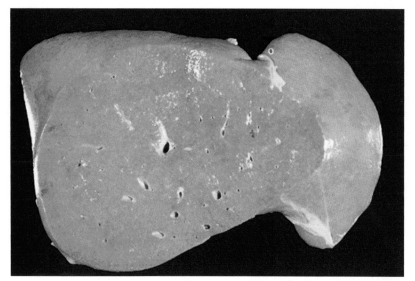

FIGURE 8–31 Hepatic steatosis, gross

This fatty liver is pale yellow-brown because of the increased lipid content within hepatocytes. The capsule is smooth, and the cut surface has a uniform texture. Hepatomegaly is present, 2 to 3 times normal liver size. Hepatic steatosis is a consequence of increased lipid biosynthesis from generation of more NADH, deranged lipoprotein synthesis and secretion, and increased peripheral fat catabolism. The most common cause is excessive alcohol consumption. Toxic injury from methotrexate or corticosteroids may also produce steatosis. Steatosis can result in diminished hepatocytic function detected by hypoalbuminemia and hypoprothrombinemia.

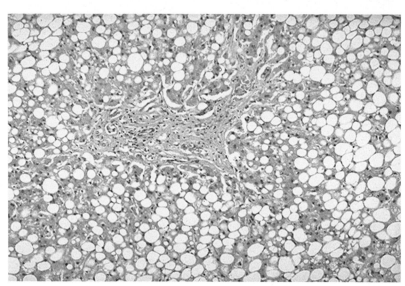

FIGURE 8–32 Hepatic steatosis, microscopic

Many hepatocytes have their cytoplasm filled with large, clear lipid droplets. This is severe macrovesicular steatosis. This process is potentially reversible in a matter of weeks to months with cessation of alcohol abuse or discontinuation of a toxic drug. Chronic injury may be accompanied by varying degrees of portal fibrosis. Some degree of steatosis accompanies all cases of chronic alcohol abuse, but only about 10% to 15% of these patients go on to develop cirrhosis.

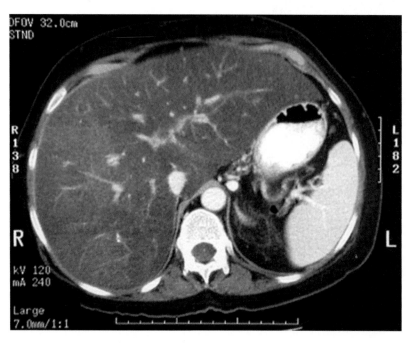

FIGURE 8–33 Hepatic steatosis, CT image

This abdominal CT scan illustrates a fatty liver with hepatomegaly and decreased attenuation (brightness) from the increased lipid content (compare the brightness of the normal spleen with that of the fatty liver). A form of steatosis similar to that seen with alcohol-induced injury is known as *nonalcoholic fatty liver* (NAFL) disease, which most often accompanies diabetes mellitus type II and obesity. More extensive injury may lead to *nonalcoholic steatohepatitis* (NASH). There may be progression to cirrhosis. Life style modification with cessation of alcohol abuse or weight reduction can lead to reversal of hepatic steatosis.

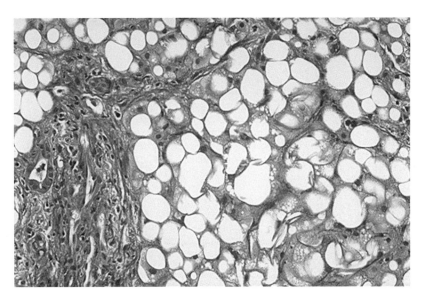

FIGURE 8–34 Nonalcoholic steatohepatitis, microscopic

This is NASH with trichrome stain demonstrating blue-staining collagenous fibrosis within the liver parenchyma. This patient had a body mass index (BMI) of 30, in the obese range, a risk factor for NAFL. A BMI of more than 25 indicates an overweight condition. Note that virtually every hepatocyte is filled with a clear lipid droplet (macrovesicular steatosis). Patients may be asymptomatic for many years, with only mild elevations of serum ALT and AST.

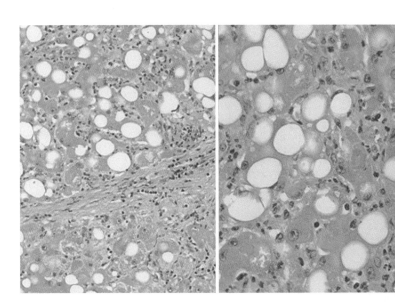

FIGURE 8–35 Alcoholic hepatitis, microscopic

A complication superimposed on alcoholic liver disease in patients with a history of alcohol abuse is acute alcoholic hepatitis. Mallory hyaline is seen here, but there are also neutrophils, necrosis of hepatocytes, collagen deposition, and fatty change (steatosis). Such inflammation can occur in a person with a history of alcohol abuse who goes on a drinking binge and consumes large quantities of alcohol over a short time. In this case, note a band of fibrosis in the left panel, with inflammatory cell infiltrates identified as neutrophilic in the right panel. The serum AST and ALT are markedly increased in these cases.

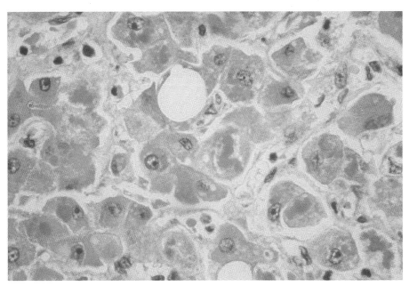

FIGURE 8–36 Alcoholic hepatitis, microscopic

This case of acute alcoholic hepatitis has prominent intracellular deposits of red globular alcoholic hyalin (Mallory bodies). This hyalin represents an intracellular accumulation of cytoskeletal elements, including cytokeratins, with the toxic hepatocellular injury. Mallory hyaline is also known as *alcoholic hyaline* because it is most often seen in conjunction with liver injury from chronic alcohol abuse. It may also be seen in cases of Wilson disease, primary biliary cirrhosis, and chronic cholestasis, and within hepatocellular neoplasms.

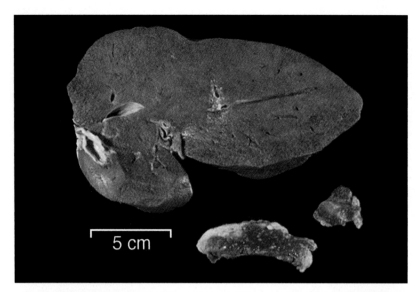

FIGURE 8–37 Hemochromatosis, gross

The dark brown color of this liver, as well as the pancreas and lymph nodes on cross-sectioning, is due to extensive iron deposition with hereditary hemochromatosis (HH). HH results from a mutation involving the hemochromatosis gene (HFE) that leads to increased iron absorption from the gut. The prevalence is between 1 in 200 and 1 in 500 people in the United States. About 1 in 10 people of northern European ancestry carries an abnormal recessive *HFE* gene, and most of these are due to a single missense C282Y mutation, although some are the H63D or S65C mutations associated with a milder phenotype. Excessive iron deposition in tissues generates free radicals producing lipid peroxidation, fibrosis, and DNA damage.

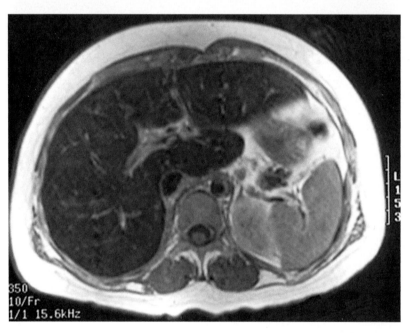

FIGURE 8–38 Hemochromatosis, MRI

There is markedly decreased signal intensity in this T1-weighted axial MRI of the abdomen within the liver due to marked iron deposition in a patient with hereditary hemochromatosis. Compare the attenuation (brightness) of the liver with that of the normally equivalent spleen. Total body iron stores normally average 3 to 6 gm, but in HH, these stores can exceed 20 gm by age 40 in men or age 60 in women, with onset of organ dysfunction from excessive iron stores. The normal HFE protein forms a complex with β_2-microglobulin and transferrin, and a mutation eliminates this interaction so that the mutant HFE protein remains trapped intracellularly, reducing transferrin receptor-mediated iron uptake by the intestinal crypt cell. This may up-regulate divalent metal transporter (DMT-1) on the intestinal brush border, leading to inappropriate iron absorption.

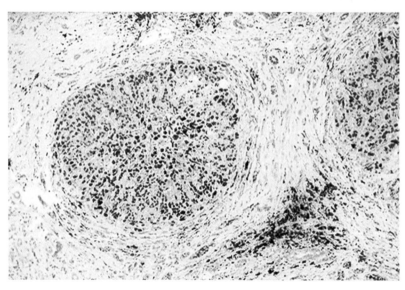

FIGURE 8–39 Hemochromatosis, microscopic

This Prussian blue iron stain reveals extensive hepatic hemosiderin deposition microscopically in this case of HH. Note that there is also cirrhosis. Excessive iron deposition in patients with HH is toxic to tissues in many organs, but heart (congestive failure), pancreas (diabetes mellitus), liver (cirrhosis and hepatic failure), joints (pseudogout with polyarthropathy), skin (dark pigmentation), and pituitary and gonads (loss of libido, impotence, amenorrhea, testicular atrophy, gynecomastia) are the most severely affected. Treatment consists of periodic phlebotomy to remove 250 mg of iron with each unit of blood. Screening for *HFE* gene mutations in family members of affected patients should be done.

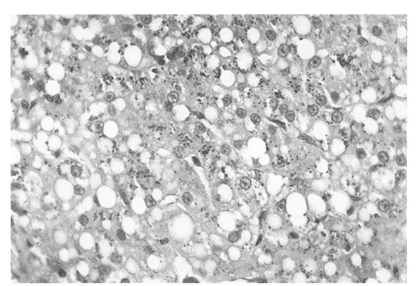

FIGURE 8–40 Wilson disease, microscopic

The red-brown granular material seen here with a copper stain is excessive lysosomal copper due to the rare autosomal recessive disorder Wilson disease from mutation of the *WD* gene encoding a copper-transporting ATPase. Decreased hepatic excretion of copper into bile leads to excessive copper accumulation in brain, eye, and liver. There is neuronal degeneration of basal ganglia, especially putamen. Kayser-Fleischer rings are seen on slit-lamp examination of the cornea. Hepatic copper accumulation results in fatty change, cholestasis, acute or chronic hepatitis, and eventual cirrhosis. Urinary copper excretion is increased, and serum ceruloplasmin is decreased. Chelation therapy is employed to remove the excess copper.

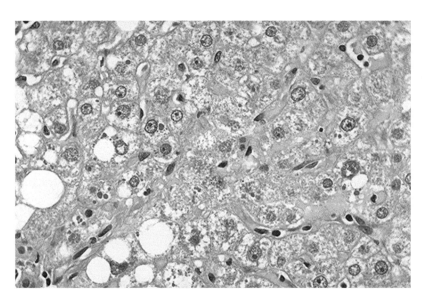

FIGURE 8–41 α_1-Antitrypsin deficiency, microscopic

The periportal red hyaline globules seen here with PAS stain are characteristic of α_1-antitrypsin (α_1-AT) deficiency. The serum α_1-AT is low. The normal allele is PiM, and a single gene mutation leads to PiZ or PiS. One in ten persons of European ancestry may have an abnormal phenotype (PiMM is normal). Homozygotes PiSS and PiZZ, and the heterozygote PiSZ, are more likely to develop panlobular emphysema and/or chronic liver disease than heterozygotes PiMS and PiMZ. The globules are collections of abnormally folded and polymerized α_1-AT not excreted from hepatocytes, resulting in chronic hepatitis, cirrhosis, and hepatocellular carcinoma. α_1-AT deficiency sometimes leads to neonatal hepatitis that may progress to cirrhosis.

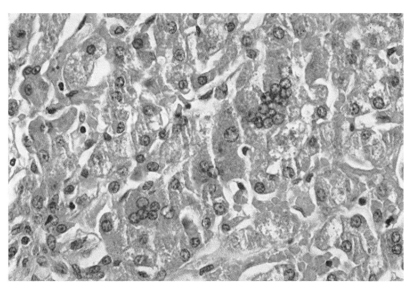

FIGURE 8–42 Neonatal cholestasis with hepatitis, microscopic

Seen here is lobular disarray with focal hepatocyte necrosis, along with giant cell transformation, lymphocytic infiltration, Kupffer cell hyperplasia, and cholestasis. Neonatal cholestasis with hepatitis may be idiopathic or the result of viral infection, or inborn errors of metabolism. Many neonates with idiopathic or viral etiologies of this disease recover within several months. The major differential diagnoses of neonatal hepatitis include biliary atresia and α_1-AT deficiency. All these conditions are rare and can present with icterus and liver failure.

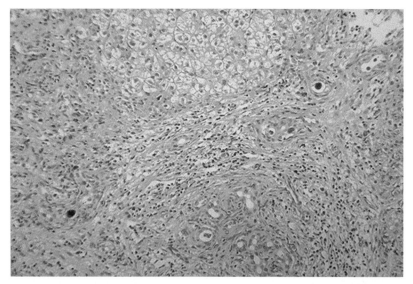

FIGURE 8–43 Extrahepatic biliary atresia, microscopic

Secondary biliary cirrhosis from prolonged extrahepatic biliary tract obstruction leads to the appearance of numerous brown-green bile plugs, bile ductular proliferation (at the lower center), and extensive fibrosis. Unlike neonatal hepatitis, multinucleated cells are infrequent here. If a large enough bile duct can be found to anastomose and provide bile drainage, then surgery can be curative. A complication of the obstruction can be ascending cholangitis. Without bile drainage, secondary biliary cirrhosis will develop.

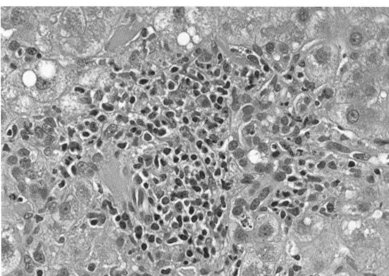

FIGURE 8–44 Primary biliary cirrhosis, microscopic

This rare autoimmune disease, seen mostly in middle-aged women, causes intense pruritus along with hepatomegaly and xanthomas. Destruction of bile ductules within hepatic triads is seen with intense mononuclear infiltrates and occasional granulomatous inflammation. Serum antimitochondrial antibody is often detectable. Additional findings include marked elevations in serum alkaline phosphatase, cholesterol, and serum globulins. Micronodular cirrhosis ensues. Jaundice is a late finding that suggests incipient liver failure. Patients sometimes have other autoimmune phenomena.

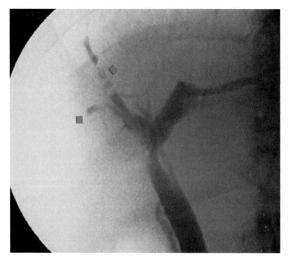
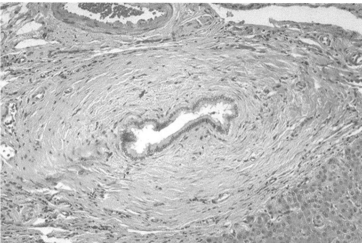

FIGURES 8–45 and 8–46 Primary sclerosing cholangitis, radiograph and microscopic

The cholangiogram shows a beaded pattern with bile ductular narrowing (◆) and pruning (■) from irregular segmental strictures. This leads to fibrous obliteration of extrahepatic and intrahepatic bile ducts. Microscopic examination shows a bile duct surrounded by marked collagenous connective tissue deposition with epithelial atrophy and luminal narrowing. Patients can have marked alkaline phosphatase elevation along with icterus and pruritus. Idiopathic cases most often affect men 20 to 50 years of age. About 70% of cases occur with idiopathic inflammatory bowel disease, particularly ulcerative colitis.

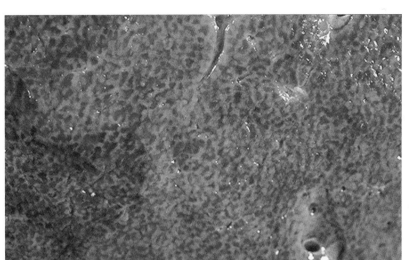

FIGURE 8–47 Centrilobular congestion, gross

This is a "nutmeg" liver with chronic passive congestion. Note the dark red congested regions that represent accumulation of red blood cells within centrilobular regions. The nutmeg pattern results from congestion around the central veins, usually from right-sided heart failure. If the passive congestion is pronounced and heart failure leads to ischemia, there can be centrilobular necrosis because the oxygenation in zone 3 of the hepatic lobule is diminished, and the AST and ALT will be elevated. Rarely, chronic passive congestion leads to fibrosis extending between central veins—a "cardiac cirrhosis." Extensive hepatic congestion can accompany disseminated intravascular coagulation and hemoglobinopathies such as sickle cell disease.

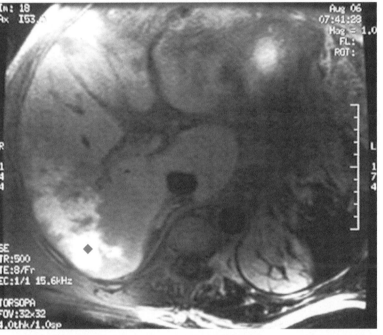

FIGURE 8–48 Hepatic infarction, MRI

This axial T1-weighted abdominal MRI shows a bright area (◆) of liver infarction caused by portal vein thrombosis. Infarcts are uncommon because the liver has two blood supplies: portal venous system and hepatic arterial system. Hepatic infarcts typically have irregular geographic borders with surrounding hyperemia. About half of liver infarcts occur with arteritis involving the hepatic artery and its branches, such as classic polyarteritis nodosa, and the remaining half have a variety of causes.

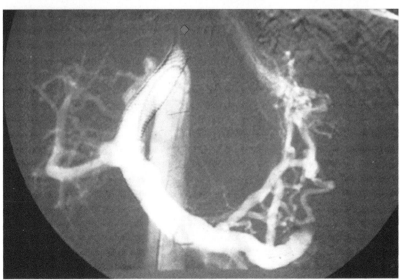

FIGURE 8–49 Budd-Chiari syndrome, angiogram

Injection of contrast material into the portal vein demonstrates lack of flow (◆) from portal vein through a transjugular intrahepatic portosystemic shunt to the hepatic venous drainage, which is blocked by thrombosis. This patient had recurrent thrombosis of the inferior vena cava and hepatic venous system, leading to an enlarged liver, reduced hepatic function, and complications of portal hypertension. Causes of Budd-Chiari syndrome, which is rare, include polycythemia, pregnancy, coagulopathies, and paroxysmal nocturnal hemoglobinuria. It is also a complication of hepatocellular carcinoma, which can invade into the intrahepatic vasculature.

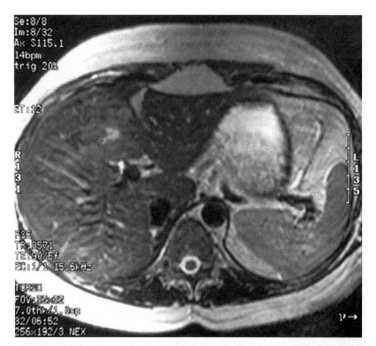

FIGURE 8–50 Focal nodular hyperplasia, MRI

This abdominal T1-weighted MRI in axial view shows an area of abnormal signal (+) in the medial aspect of the right lobe of liver with a central bright scar. This is focal nodular hyperplasia, a slow-growing, hamartomatous process that is uncommon. It occurs more often in women than in men.

In contrast, nodular hyperplasia, or nodular regenerative hyperplasia, is a diffuse process distinguished from cirrhosis by the lack of portal bridging fibrosis. It may occur in up to 5% of elderly patients. It is associated with myeloproliferative disorders (primarily polycythemia vera), rheumatoid arthritis, classic polyarteritis nodosa, primary biliary cirrhosis, HCV infection, and liver, kidney, and marrow allogeneic transplantation. It is also associated with thioguanine therapy. The pathogenesis is thought to be related to impaired blood flow ischemia with reactive hepatocyte proliferation. Although myeloproliferative disorders do contribute to splenomegaly, they do not cause portal hypertension.

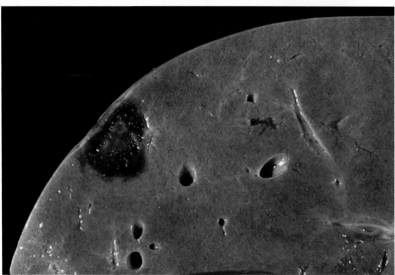

FIGURE 8–51 Hemangioma, gross

This discrete, dark red, benign hemangioma lies just beneath Glisson's capsule, surrounded by normal, uniform brown hepatic parenchyma. About 1 person in 50 has such a neoplasm, which is typically just an incidental finding on abdominal CT scan or at autopsy, since most are 2 cm or smaller, unless one is unlucky enough to put a percutaneous biopsy needle into it. They can sometimes be multiple. Hemangiomas can be subcapsular, as seen here, or periportal. Most have a cavernous pattern of vascular spaces on microscopic examination.

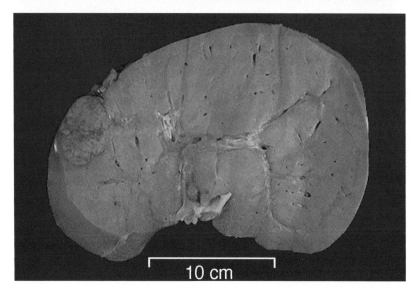

FIGURE 8–52 Hepatic adenoma, gross

A benign circumscribed neoplasm arising from a proliferation of cells resembling hepatocytes is known as a *liver cell adenoma*. There is an association with oral contraceptive use in women and anabolic steroid use in men. A subcapsular adenoma such as the one seen here may rupture, producing a hemoperitoneum. The cells of this neoplasm can produce bile, leading to the green appearance with formalin fixation seen here. Microscopically, these neoplasms are composed of cells resembling normal hepatocytes, but without a lobular pattern, so that normal triads and central veins are not recognized. Such adenomas must be distinguished from metastatic or primary malignant neoplasms.

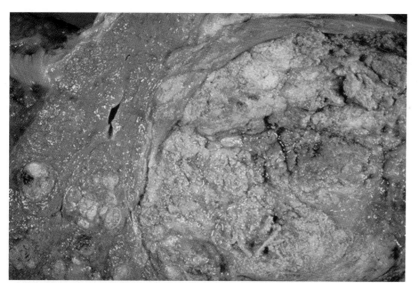

FIGURE 8–53 Hepatocellular carcinoma, gross

Primary liver cancers typically arise in the setting of chronic hepatitis and cirrhosis from increased hepatocellular proliferative activity. Worldwide, viral hepatitis B and C are the most common causes, but in the United States, chronic alcohol abuse is a common cause. Other causes include aflatoxin exposure, hemochromatosis, α_1-AT deficiency, and tyrosinemia. These large, bulky tumors have a greenish cast because bile is present. In addition to the main mass are smaller satellite nodules that represent either intrahepatic spread or multicentric origin of the tumor. There may be an elevated serum α-fetoprotein (AFP). Such masses can focally obstruct the biliary tract to increase the serum alkaline phosphatase.

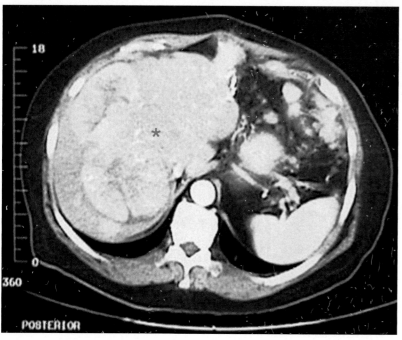

FIGURE 8–54 Hepatocellular carcinoma, CT image

This large irregular mass (∗) in the hepatic right lobe is a hepatocellular carcinoma (HCC), which most often arises in liver involved with chronic hepatitis or cirrhosis. These cancers can appear as one large mass, or there may be small surrounding satellite nodules, or multifocal masses. HCCs are very prone to undergo necrosis and hemorrhage. In fact, hemorrhage from such an HCC at the liver capsule may lead to a hemoperitoneum. Intrahepatic mass lesions are unlikely to completely obstruct the biliary tract, so that hyperbilirubinemia is infrequent. The highest incidence of HCC occurs in areas of the world with high rates of chronic hepatitis B infection. Clinical findings include malaise, fatigue, weight loss, abdominal pain, and abdominal enlargement.

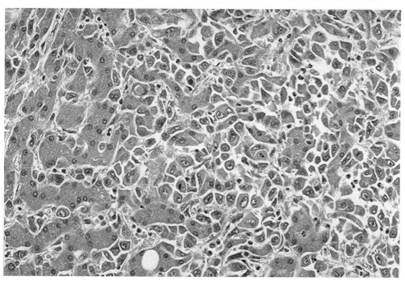

FIGURE 8–55 Hepatocellular carcinoma, microscopic

The malignant cells of this HCC, here seen mostly on the right, are well differentiated and interdigitate with normal, larger hepatocytes, seen mostly at the left. An HCC can form cords that are much wider than the normal liver plate, and there is no discernable normal lobular architecture, so that triads and central veins are absent. Irregular vascular structures are present. Larger neoplasms may have areas of necrosis. Invasion of vascular channels, particularly portal vein branches, is frequent. Most patients with this neoplasm survive less than a year because it is unlikely to be discovered at an early stage.

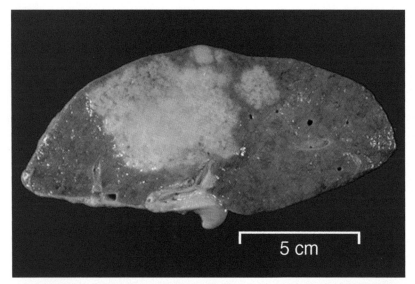

FIGURE 8–56 Cholangiocarcinoma, gross

This white mass with a few satellite nodules, but lack of bile staining, is a cholangiocarcinoma, which is less common than hepatocellular carcinoma, although identifiable risk factors can be similar. Viral hepatitis B and C infections are more strongly associated with hepatocellular carcinoma. Chronic alcoholism has been reported as a risk in both. The most common risk factor for cholangiocarcinoma in the United States is primary sclerosing cholangitis, although it is more common in parts of the world in which people can be infected with trematodes (liver flukes) such as *Clonorchis sinensis*. Most cholangiocarcinomas are diagnosed at a high stage and have a poor prognosis.

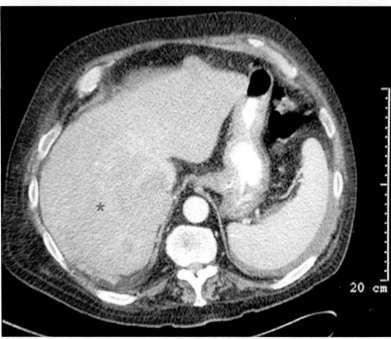

FIGURE 8–57 Cholangiocarcinoma, CT image

The ill-defined, subtle mass (∗) with heterogenous density and irregular margins in the superior aspect of the right hepatic lobe seen in this abdominal CT scan is a cholangiocarcinoma, a primary liver cancer that occurs less frequently than HCC, and many of the same risk factors apply. In fact, primary liver cancers with elements of both HCC and cholangiocarcinoma can occur. Clinically, the presentation and course of cholangiocarcinomas resembles that of HCCs. Note the presence of a small amount of ascitic fluid in this scan.

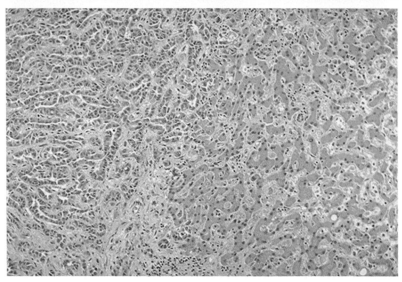

FIGURE 8–58 Cholangiocarcinoma, microscopic

The carcinoma seen at the left has a glandular appearance consistent with a cholangiocarcinoma, although HCCs can occasionally have such areas within them. A primary liver cancer may have both hepatocellular and cholangiolar differentiation. Cholangiocarcinomas do not make bile, but the cells do make mucin, and they can be almost impossible to distinguish from metastatic adenocarcinoma. Immunohistochemical staining in cholangiocarcinoma is positive for CK-7 and negative for CK-20 and AFP. Metastases are more likely to be CK-20 positive. HCCs are often AFP positive.

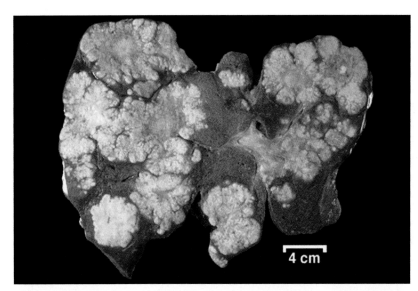

FIGURE 8–59 Hepatic metastases, gross

Note the numerous mass lesions of variable size. Some of the larger masses demonstrate central necrosis, producing a grossly umbilicated appearance when seen beneath the hepatic capsule. These masses are metastases to the liver. The obstruction from such masses generally elevates the serum alkaline phosphatase, but not all bile ducts are obstructed, so that hyperbilirubinemia is typically not present. Also, the transaminases are usually not greatly elevated. Of all neoplasms involving the liver, metastases are the most common because the liver is a good place for circulating neoplastic cells to settle down and grow. Metastases are usually multiple throughout the liver.

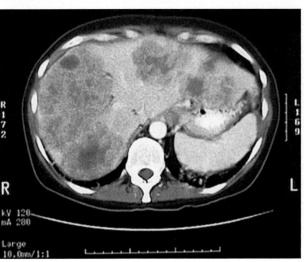
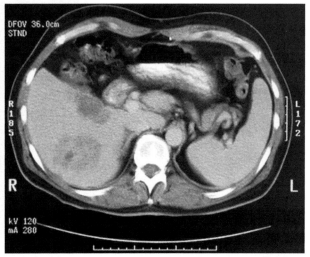

FIGURES 8–60 and 8–61 Hepatic metastases, CT images

These abdominal CT images without intravenous contrast show multiple mass lesions (◆) with focal darker areas of necrosis, resulting in a markedly enlarged liver in the left panel that extends from the right side to nearly the left side of the upper abdomen. These are metastases from a primary colonic adenocarcinoma. A normal-sized spleen is seen at the lower left in both panels.

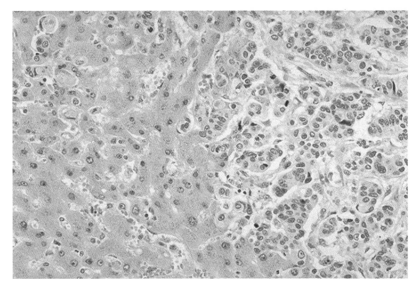

FIGURE 8–62 Hepatic metastases, microscopic

Metastatic infiltrating ductal carcinoma from a breast primary is seen on the right, with normal liver parenchyma on the left. As the metastases enlarge, they outgrow their blood supply, leading to central necrosis.

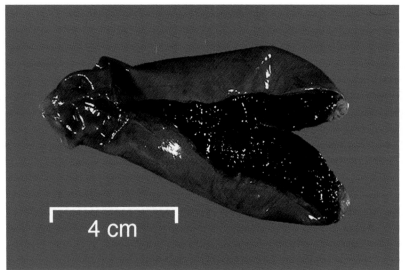

FIGURE 8–63 Normal gallbladder, gross

A normal gallbladder has a velvety dark green mucosa and a thin wall. One minor variation is the small yellowish bulbous projection at the right known as a *Phrygian cap* resulting from a folded fundus. The gallbladder serves as a storage organ for bile secreted by the liver. The muscularis of the gallbladder contracts under the influence of cholecystokinin secreted by enteroendocrine cells of the small intestine with passage of food from the stomach into the duodenum, particularly fatty food. Thus, modern gallbladders are working harder than ancient gallbladders, due to increasing dietary fat from such sources as "fast food" and ice cream.

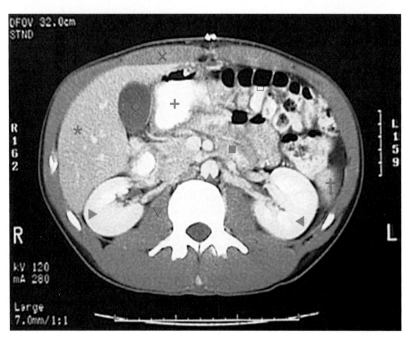

FIGURE 8–64 Normal gallbladder, CT image

This abdominal CT scan with contrast at the L2-L3 level demonstrates normal structures including the liver (∗), gallbladder (♦), gastric antrum (+), jejunum (■), colon (+), right kidney (▶), left kidney (◀), spleen (†), aorta (▲), psoas muscle (▼), and rectus abdominis muscle (×). The gallbladder normally stores about 50 mL of concentrated bile. The location of the gallbladder on the inferior surface of the hepatic right lobe varies somewhat among 5% to 10% of the population, but congenital gallbladder anomalies such as agenesis are rare. Hypoplasia of all or part of the biliary tract may lead to biliary atresia.

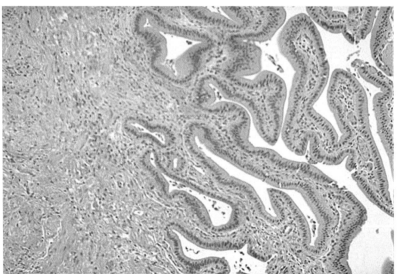

FIGURE 8–65 Normal gallbladder, microscopic

The columnar mucosa is arranged in folds over the lamina propria, allowing expansion as bile fills the gallbladder. Beneath the lamina propria is a muscularis, and not seen here surrounding the gallbladder are a connective tissue layer and serosa. The gallbladder mucosa transports sodium out of the bile, passively followed by chloride and water, leading to bile concentration. Thus, bile excreted by the liver and stored in the gallbladder becomes more concentrated. The bile includes bile salts such as cholic and chenodeoxycholic acid, lecithin, calcium bilirubinate, and cholesterol. An imbalance in the relative concentrations of these bile components predisposes to precipitation and stone formation.

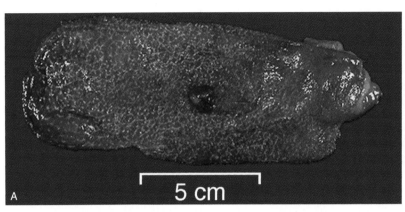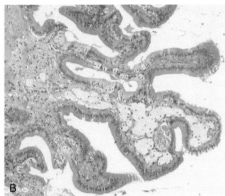

FIGURE 8–66*A* and *B* Cholesterolosis, gross and microscopic

The mucosa contains many foamy macrophages in the lamina propria, shown in the right panel (*B*), which produce the grossly visible strawberry-like appearance shown in the left panel (*A*), along with a solitary gallstone.

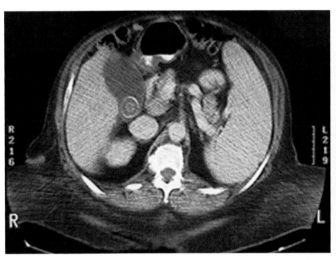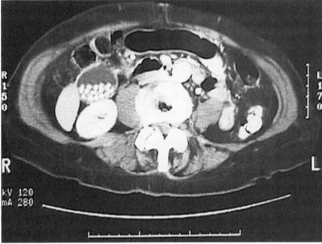

FIGURES 8–67 and 8–68 Cholelithiasis, CT images

In the left panel is a solitary gallstone within a dilated gallbladder. Gallstones may contain varying portions of cholesterol, calcium, and bilirubin. They are often built through apposition of layers, leading to the laminated appearance seen here. In the right panel are multiple small gallstones within the gallbladder. A small stone or a portion of a stone broken off may pass into the neck of the gallbladder and become impacted, or may pass down the cystic duct and impact at the ampulla.

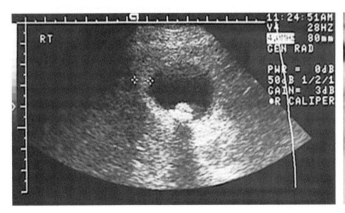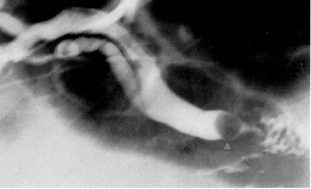

FIGURES 8–69 and 8–70 Cholelithiasis, ultrasound, and choledocholithiasis, radiograph

Note the gallstones (▲) in the gallbladder lumen on abdominal ultrasound in the left panel. The cursors mark the thickened wall of the gallbladder, a finding consistent with chronic cholecystitis. The cholangiogram in the right panel reveals the outline of a gallstone (▲) occluding the distal dilated common bile duct near the ampulla.

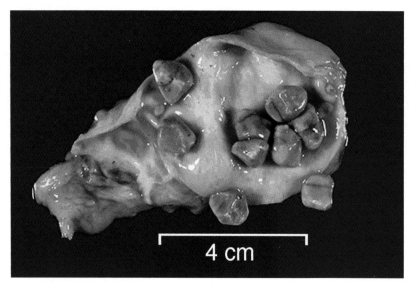

FIGURE 8–71 Cholelithiasis, gross

Yellow-tan faceted gallstones are present in this gallbladder that shows evidence of chronic cholecystitis because the mucosa is tan and the wall and surface are pale, suggesting collagenization as a result of scarring from chronic inflammation. Repeated bouts of acute cholecystitis can lead to chronic cholecystitis. About 10% to 20% of adults have gallstones, and most of them are asymptomatic. Most gallstones have a preponderance of cholesterol, giving them a yellow gross appearance. However, some calcium bilirubinate is often present, and these are termed *mixed* stones. Stones mainly composed of calcium bilirubinate are dark green to black and are known as *pigment* stones.

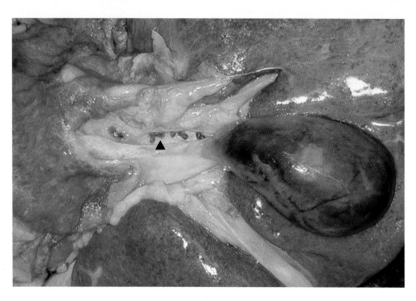

FIGURE 8–72 Choledocholithiasis, gross

The common bile duct emptying into the duodenum at the left is opened here to reveal several small calculi (▲) within the lumen. Note that the gallbladder to the right is dilated from obstruction by calculi at the gallbladder neck. Stones from the gallbladder, if small enough, can pass through (or impact within) the neck of the gallbladder and gain access to the common bile duct, a condition known as *choledocholithiasis*. Biliary tract obstruction can produce colicky right upper quadrant pain. In about two thirds of the population, the common bile duct joins the main pancreatic duct before emptying through the ampulla of Vater, and this allows a stone to obstruct the pancreatic duct, causing pancreatitis.

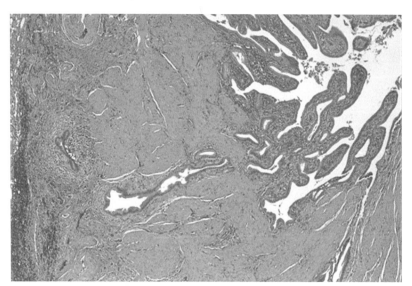

FIGURE 8–73 Chronic cholecystitis, microscopic

Chronic cholecystitis is almost always seen in association with gallstones, although precipitation of bile alone may be sufficient to produce inflammation. The term *acalculous cholecystitis* applies when inflammation is present but cholelithiasis is absent. There may not be a history of bouts of acute cholecystitis. Seen here is a thickened gallbladder wall beneath the mucosa with chronic inflammatory infiltrates and containing outpouchings of the mucosa termed *Rokitansky-Aschoff sinuses*. In contrast, acute cholecystitis has neutrophilic infiltrates. Bacterial infection is typically absent from cases of acute and chronic cholecystitis.

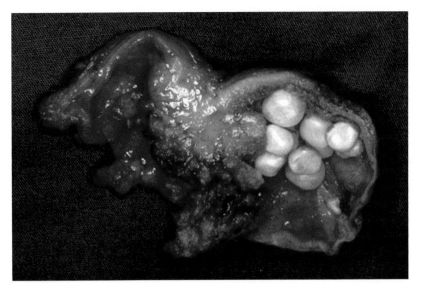

FIGURE 8–74 Adenocarcinoma, gross

This gallbladder has been opened, and to the left of the pale porcelain gallstones (averaging 1 cm in size) is a fungating mass that extends into the gallbladder lumen and into the gallbladder wall. This is a primary adenocarcinoma of gallbladder. Gallstones accompany such carcinomas in up to 60% to 90% of cases. Adenocarcinomas of the biliary tract are not common and typically occur in elderly people. Larger tumors, or tumors arising in the extrahepatic bile ducts, may lead to biliary tract obstruction, with laboratory findings including direct hyperbilirubinemia and elevated serum alkaline phosphatase.

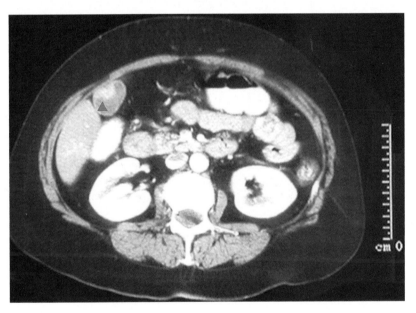

FIGURE 8–75 Adenocarcinoma, CT image

In this abdominal CT scan, there is an irregular bright mass (▲) within the lower portion of the gallbladder, with the inferior tip of the right lobe of liver adjacent to it. This mass proved to be an adenocarcinoma of the gallbladder. There often are no early signs or symptoms; therefore, most adenocarcinomas of the gallbladder are nonresectable at diagnosis, and the prognosis is poor. There may be clinical signs and symptoms similar to cholelithiasis with cholecystitis.

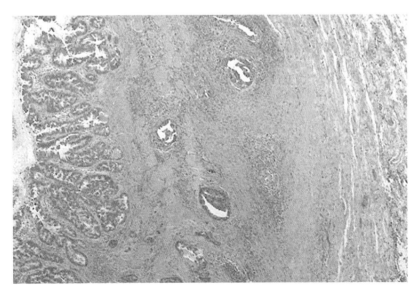

FIGURE 8–76 Adenocarcinoma, microscopic

The dysplastic epithelium can be seen at the left, and neoplastic glandular structures are invading into the muscular wall. Adenocarcinoma of the gallbladder is more common in elderly people and more frequently seen in women. Carcinomas can arise in the rest of the biliary tree, but these are associated with gallstones in only one third of cases and are slightly more common in men.

CHAPTER 9

The Pancreas

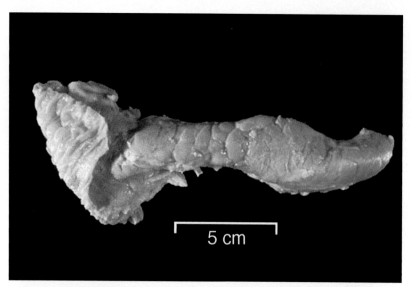

FIGURE 9-1 Normal pancreas, gross

The normal adult pancreas weighs 85 to 90 gm and has indistinct regions, including a head adjacent to the duodenum (a small portion of duodenum appears here at the left), a body, and a tail (at the right) with a tan, lobular architecture. Adjacent adipose tissue and lymph nodes are closely apposed. Ninety-nine percent of the pancreatic mass is acinar parenchyma producing digestive enzymes and bicarbonate, with the remainder islets of Langerhans. The pancreas forms embryologically from a larger dorsal and smaller ventral endodermal bud from the duodenum; the buds fuse along with their respective developing ducts of Wirsung and Santorini. The pancreatic duct runs the length of the pancreas to empty into the duodenum at the ampulla of Vater.

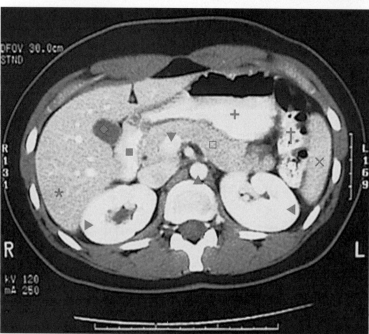

FIGURE 9-2 Normal pancreas, CT image

This is a normal abdominal CT scan with contrast at the L1 level demonstrating the upper abdomen with the liver (*), gallbladder (◆), stomach (+) and duodenum (■), pancreas (□), colon (†), spleen (✕), portal vein, inferior vena cava (▼), right kidney (▶), left kidney (◀), and aorta (▲). The pancreas forms embryologically from dorsal and ventral buds that form from gut outpouchings; these fuse to form the pancreas. Failure of fusion may produce pancreas divisum, with exocrine pancreatic tissue draining into the duodenum through both a larger duct of Santorini and a smaller duct of Wirsung that normally forms the papilla of Vater. Much rarer is abnormal fusion of dorsal and ventral buds to form an annular pancreas that encircles the duodenum and can produce bowel obstruction. Pancreatic ectopia in gastrointestinal tract mucosa is common (2% of the population) but incidental since the mass of tissue is typically less than 1 cm in diameter.

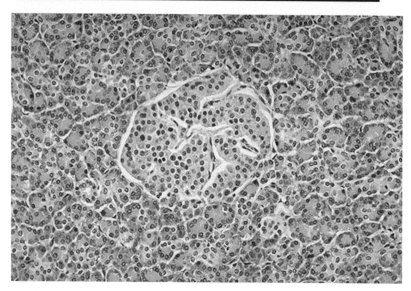

FIGURE 9-3 Normal pancreas, microscopic

Normal exocrine pancreas is composed of acini that secrete enzymes including the proenzymes phospholipases A and B, trypsin, chymotrypsin, and elastase under the influence of cholecystokinin. These proenzymes require activation in the gut. Amylase and lipase are secreted as active enzymes. Secretin triggers release of bicarbonate and water from ductal cells. The pancreas produces about 2 L/day of fluid that flows into the duodenum. Interspersed within the exocrine acini are the islets of Langerhans with endocrine function, one of which is seen here in the center. Small capillaries within the islet receive the secretions of islet α cells (glucagon), β cells (insulin), and δ cells (somatostatin).

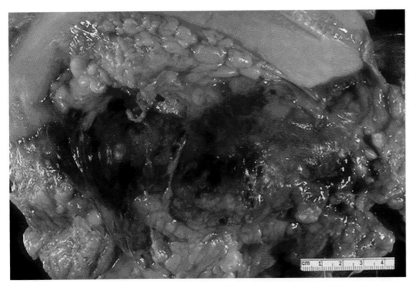

FIGURE 9–4 Acute pancreatitis, gross

At autopsy, the stomach is reflected superiorly and the spleen can be seen at the far upper right. The pancreas is swollen and does not show the typical tan, lobulated architecture. Instead, it shows hemorrhagic necrosis that appears as blotchy black to red areas. Both serum amylase and lipase are typically elevated. Several mechanisms are implicated in triggering activation of pancreatic enzymes causing the inflammation, including pancreatic duct obstruction (the most common cause, typically from gallstone impaction), acinar cell injury (typical of viral infections), and defective intracellular transport of acinar cell proenzymes (typical of alcohol-induced pancreatitis).

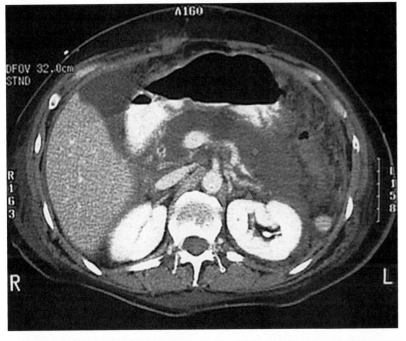

FIGURE 9–5 Acute pancreatitis, CT image

This abdominal CT image with contrast reveals acute pancreatitis with decreased enhancement of a swollen pancreas (◆) from edema, hemorrhage, and fat necrosis. In this case, as a consequence of the inflammation, can be seen splenic vein thrombosis (▲). Pancreatitis is a medical emergency that can lead to "acute abdomen." Patients have severe abdominal pain and paralytic ileus. The clinical course can quickly be complicated by disseminated intravascular coagulation, shock, and secondary bacterial infection with sepsis. Chalky deposits of fat necrosis can involve the pancreas and even adipose tissue within the abdomen. There can be intraperitoneal fluid collection (ascites).

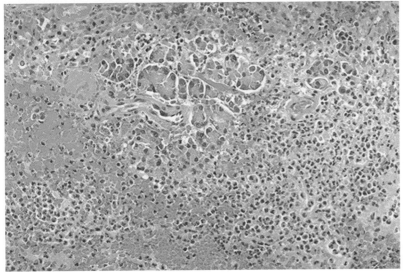

FIGURE 9–6 Acute pancreatitis, microscopic

Acute inflammation with necrosis and hemorrhage is seen here along with residual pancreatic acini. The damage involves primarily the acinar cells, but the vasculature is also affected, and if severe and extensive, even the islets of Langerhans may be destroyed. Less common causes of pancreatitis include hypertriglyceridemia (typically more than 1 gm/dL), hypercalcemia, and drugs such as azathioprine, didanosine, pentamidine, and thiazides. In 10% to 20% of cases, an underlying cause cannot be identified.

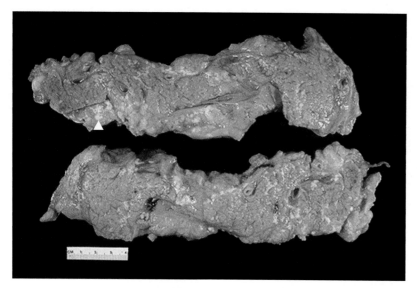

FIGURE 9–7 Fat necrosis, gross

Yellow-tan foci of fat necrosis (▲) are visible throughout the pancreas, seen here sectioned in half. There is some edema, but no hemorrhage, in this case of mild acute pancreatitis. Enzymatic release from the exocrine pancreas leads to autodestruction. Trypsin activation triggers a cascade of additional proenzyme activation, including proelastase and prophospholipase, which disintegrate adipocytes and pancreatic parenchyma. Trypsin release also activates prekallikrein to bring the kinin system into play, with vascular thrombosis and damage.

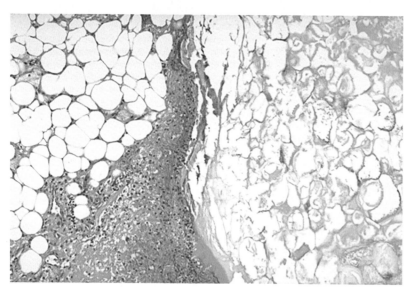

FIGURE 9–8 Fat necrosis, microscopic

Fat necrosis consists of steatocytes that have lost their nuclei and whose cytoplasm has a granular pink appearance, most pronounced here at the right. The rare autosomal dominant condition of hereditary pancreatitis results from germ line mutations in the *PRSS1* gene that lead to abnormally activated trypsin. Another rare inherited autosomal recessive *SPINK1* gene mutation reduces inhibition of trypsin activity and leads to pancreatitis. These inherited forms of pancreatitis often have a chronic, relapsing course.

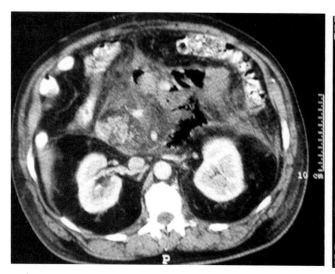
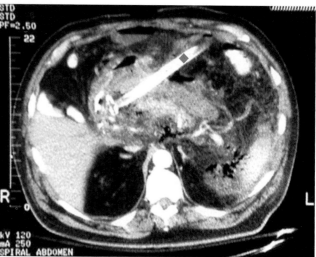

FIGURES 9–9 and 9–10 Pancreatic phlegmon, CT images

In these abdominal CT images without contrast, there is a phlegmon that represents a swollen, inflamed mass (◆) in the region of the pancreas. This complication may occur if acute pancreatitis persists. Infection of a phlegmon results in a pancreatic abscess. In the right panel, a drain (◆) is in place after laparotomy with débridement of the abscess.

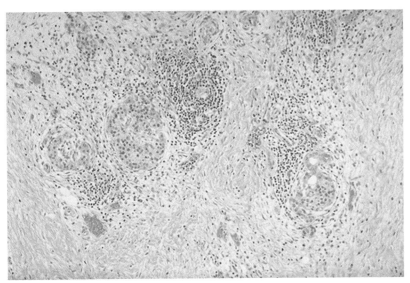

FIGURE 9–11 Chronic pancreatitis, microscopic

There are scattered chronic inflammatory cells in a collagenous stroma with absence of acini but a few remaining islets of Langerhans in a case of chronic pancreatitis. Chronic alcohol abuse is a common cause of this condition, which typically occurs after repeated bouts of mild to moderate acute pancreatitis. However, about 40% of the time, no specific etiology is identified. Depending on the amount of remaining functional parenchyma, there can be pancreatic insufficiency with malabsorption and steatorrhea, and even diabetes mellitus from loss of islets of Langerhans, although most of the islets are typically spared. Compound heterozygotes with variant *CFTR* gene mutations may develop chronic pancreatitis.

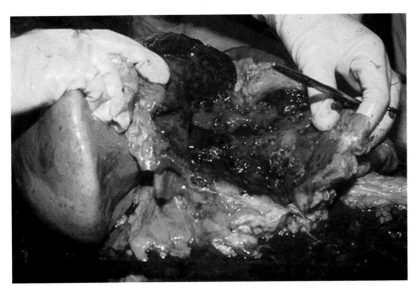

FIGURE 9–12 Pancreatic pseudocyst, gross

This structure at autopsy is hardly recognizable as pancreas because a large pancreatic pseudocyst has formed. Seen here is an opened pseudocyst involving most of the pancreas. The yellowish liver with blunted edge is consistent with steatosis from alcohol abuse. This pseudocyst has an irregular red to brown to black inner surface. A pseudocyst is a localized area of liquefactive necrosis bounded by granulation tissue. It appears grossly and radiographically as a cystic structure, and like a pancreatic phlegmon (which appears as a mass), it can become secondarily infected to form a pancreatic abscess.

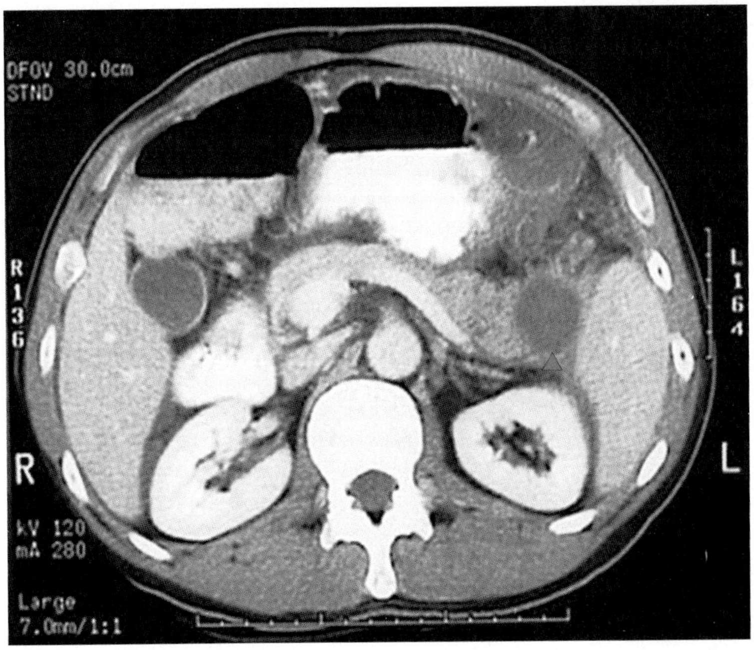

FIGURE 9–13 Pancreatic pseudocyst, CT image

This pancreatic pseudocyst (▲) demonstrates low attenuation in its liquefied center. This lesion is located in the tail of the pancreas next to the spleen. Most pseudocysts involve the lesser sac. This one is small, but some may reach 30 cm in diameter. Inflammation with fluid collection extends to the adjacent omentum near the stomach, in the region of the lesser omental sac. A pancreatic pseudocyst is a serious complication of pancreatitis because hemorrhage, peritonitis, and sepsis may occur. Pseudocysts may be treated by drainage.

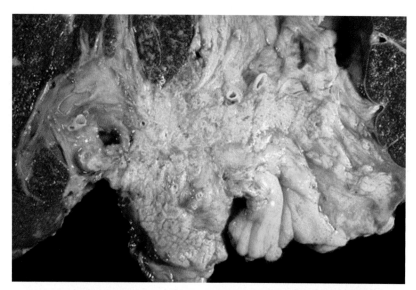

FIGURE 9–14 Adenocarcinoma, gross

This pancreatic adenocarcinoma is very extensive, sparing only the uncinate process at the lower left center. Chronic biliary tract obstruction from this mass produced icterus, marked by the green color of the liver after formalin fixation. Tumor invades into the hilum of liver, and small parenchymal metastases to liver are also present. Pancreatic cancer is the fourth most frequent cause of death from cancer in the United States. Few cases are diagnosed early, so the prognosis overall is poor, with a 5-year survival rate of less than 5%. Pain is typically the initial presenting complaint. About 60% of cases involve the head of the pancreas, causing biliary tract obstruction with jaundice and direct hyperbilirubinemia.

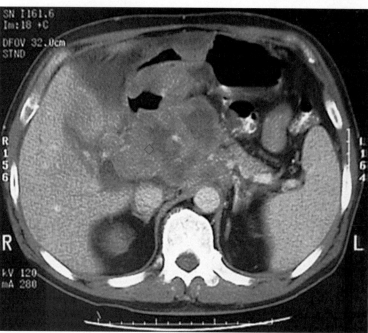

FIGURE 9–15 Adenocarcinoma, CT image

This large adenocarcinoma (◆) involves the head and body of the pancreas, and it infiltrates into the hilum of the liver. Most pancreatic adenocarcinomas have infiltrated surrounding structures or have metastasized at the time of diagnosis. The *K-RAS* oncogene and the *p53*, *SMAD*4, and *p16* tumor suppressor genes are frequently found to have mutations in this condition. More than 80% of cases occur in people older than 60 years. Cigarette smoking is a risk for pancreatic carcinoma, as are chronic pancreatitis and diabetes mellitus. Rare risk factors include Peutz-Jeghers syndrome and hereditary pancreatitis. Regardless of the etiology, clinical findings may include abdominal pain, anorexia, and weight loss. Trousseau syndrome, a hypercoagulable state with arterial or venous thromboses, occurs in 10% of cases.

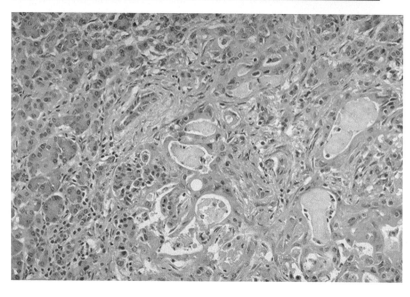

FIGURE 9–16 Adenocarcinoma, microscopic

This pancreatic adenocarcinoma is moderately differentiated, showing some irregular gland formation with both intracytoplasmic mucin production and gland luminal mucin accumulation. These neoplasms often have significant desmoplasia (elaboration of a collagenous connective tissue stroma). Some residual normal pancreas is seen at the upper left. These neoplasms infiltrate locally and are difficult to resect because they are invariably diagnosed at a high stage. Perineural invasion is common and accounts for the constant pain typical of cancer. A serum marker, not specific for pancreatic cancer, is the CA19-9 antigen.

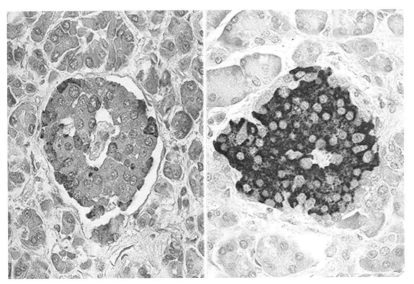

FIGURE 9–17 Normal islet of Langerhans, microscopic

The endocrine function of the pancreas resides in the islets of Langerhans scattered within the parenchyma, but concentrated more in the tail. With the immunohistochemical staining seen here, an islet contains β cells that secrete insulin (at the left), α cells secreting glucagon (at the right), and unstained δ cells producing somatostatin. The hormones are secreted directly into the bloodstream. Since there are multiple hormones that oppose insulin, loss of glucagon or somatostatin production from islets has minimal clinical consequence.

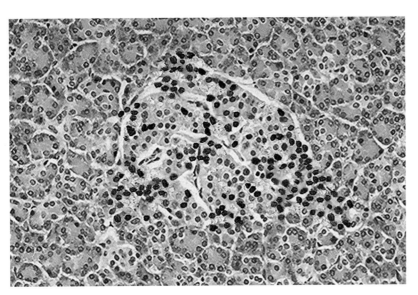

FIGURE 9–18 Insulitis, microscopic

The rarely seen hallmark of type 1 diabetes mellitus is inflammation of the islets, which occurs before the onset of clinical findings. A genetic susceptibility, coupled with viral or toxic agents that damage the islet cells, culminates in an autoimmune reaction with islet destruction that underlies type 1 diabetes The autoimmune nature of type 1 diabetes is shown by insulin autoantibody, glutamic acid decarboxylase (GAD65), and islet cell antigen (IA-2). Islets are nearly absent by the onset of overt diabetes with hyperglycemia, polyuria, polydipsia, and polyphagia, and there is an absolute lack of circulating insulin. Insulin lack leads to catabolism of adipose tissue and muscle, leading to metabolic acidosis (ketoacidosis) and muscle wasting.

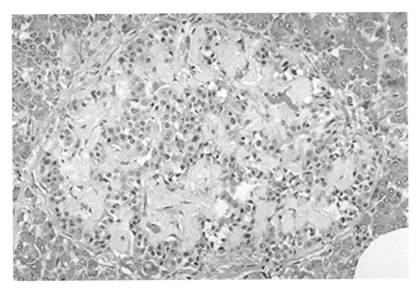

FIGURE 9–19 Islet amyloid deposition, microscopic

This islet of Langerhans demonstrates pink hyaline material (with deposition of amyloid) around many of the islet cells. The amyloid is derived from amylin, a protein secreted along with insulin. This finding is typical in patients with type 2 diabetes mellitus, who have a relative lack of insulin, but in whom islets are still present. There may be deranged secretion of insulin by β cells or peripheral insulin resistance. Islet β-cell dysfunction leads to decreased insulin and islet amyloid polypeptide (amylin) secretion. Most patients with type 2 diabetes are obese. Not all type 2 diabetic patients have amyloid in islets; thus, its role in the pathogenesis of the disease is not clear.

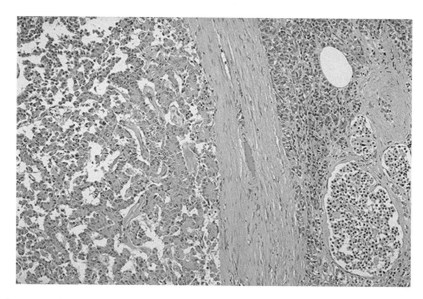

FIGURE 9–20 Islet cell adenoma, microscopic

The islet cell adenoma at the left contrasts with the normal pancreas with islets at the right, separated by a capsule of collagenous connective tissue. Some of these adenomas function hormonally. Like carcinoid tumors seen in the gastrointestinal tract, they are endocrine neoplasms that can potentially secrete a variety of hormonal products. β-Cell (insulin-producing) neoplasms are the most common islet cell tumors. The excess circulating insulin causes hypoglycemia with resulting mental confusion, weakness, or even convulsions. G-cell (gastrin-producing) tumors are the second most common islet cell tumor and may give rise to the Zollinger-Ellison syndrome (gastric hypersecretion leading to gastric, duodenal, and even jejunal peptic ulcers). The serum gastrin levels in such patients will generally be at least 5 times normal. α-Cell (glucagon-producing) tumors are uncommon and present with a clinical syndrome of mild diabetes mellitus and a peculiar widespread dermatitis known as *necrolytic migratory erythema*. Most of the cases have distant metastases, particularly to the liver. δ-Cell (somatostatin-producing) tumors are very rare and produce diabetes mellitus, steatorrhea, and diarrhea. Most are malignant. Less commonly, islet cell tumors may produce adrenocorticotropic hormone, causing Cushing syndrome, or serotonin, producing the carcinoid syndrome. Vasoactive intestinal polypeptide may also be produced and probably gives rise to the Verner-Morrison syndrome of watery diarrhea, hypokalemia, and achlorhydria.

Islet cell tumors may be part of an autosomal dominant disorder known as *multiple endocrine neoplasia syndrome, type I*. In addition to the islet cell tumors, these patients may have hyperplasia or adenomas of the pituitary and parathyroid glands and may thus present with a variety of problems depending on the hyperfunctioning tissue. The islet cell tumors usually produce either insulin or gastrin.

CHAPTER 10

The Kidney

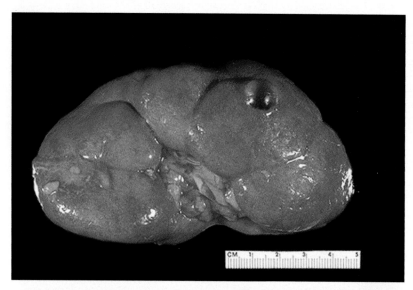

FIGURE 10–1 Normal kidney, gross

This normal adult kidney with the capsule removed has a pattern of fetal lobulations that still persists, as it sometimes does in adults. The hilum at the center contains some adipose tissue. An adult kidney can range from 11 to 15 cm in length and weigh 125 to 200 gm, depending on the size of the person. There is ordinarily enough renal reserve function that it is possible to survive with just half of one normal kidney. At the right is a smooth-surfaced, small, clear fluid-filled simple renal cyst. Such cysts occur either singly or scattered around the renal parenchyma and are not uncommon in adults. The amount of renal reserve capacity is remarkable, and it is possible to survive with only half of one kidney.

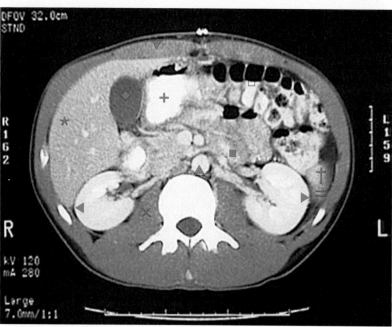

FIGURE 10–2 Normal kidneys, CT image

This normal abdominal CT scan with contrast at the L2-L3 level demonstrates the right (▶) and left (◀) kidneys, liver (*), gallbladder (◆), gastric antrum (+), jejunum (■), colon (□), spleen (†), aorta (▲), psoas muscle (×), and rectus abdominis muscle (▼). The kidneys are located in the retroperitoneum and are well protected by surrounding connective tissues with fat and skeletal muscle. Normal renal blood flow, which is about 25% of the cardiac output, is indicated here by the bright attenuation of the kidneys from the inflow of the injected intravenous contrast material. Branches of renal artery within each kidney have no anastomoses; thus, branch arterial occlusion leads to focal infarction. Also, since renal tubular capillary beds derive from efferent arterioles, glomerular disease leads to parenchymal ischemia, and glomerular loss with aging results in diminution of renal size.

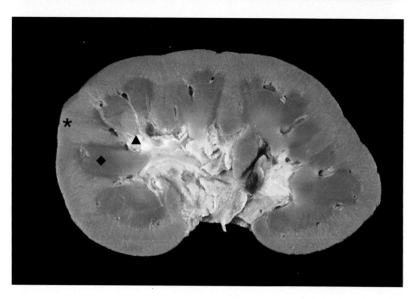

FIGURE 10–3 Normal kidney, gross

In cross-section, this normal adult kidney demonstrates the lighter outer renal cortex (*), normally 5 to 10 mm in thickness, and darker inner medulla (◆) with central pelvis containing adipose tissue. Note the renal papillae (▲) projecting into the calyces, through which collecting ducts drain the excreted urine into the renal pelvis. The amount of renal reserve capacity is remarkable, and it is possible to survive with only half of one kidney. This explains why renal failure is not associated with aging. In addition to excretion of waste products, the kidney contributes to acid-base balance, salt and water volume with regulation of blood pressure, and maintenance of red blood cell mass through elaboration of erythropoietin.

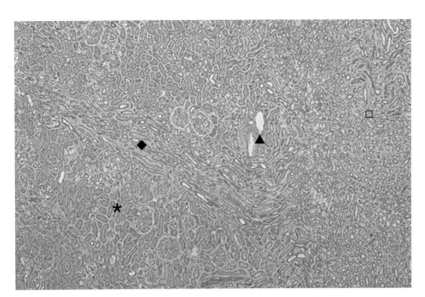

FIGURE 10–4 Normal kidney, microscopic

The corticomedullary junction of the kidney is seen here. The cortex contains a medullary ray (renal column (◆)) extending to the medulla (□). Within the cortex (*) are glomeruli and tubules. Arcuate arteries (▲) arising from interlobar arteries course along the corticomedullary junction, giving rise to interlobular arteries from which the afferent arterioles originate to supply blood to individual glomeruli.

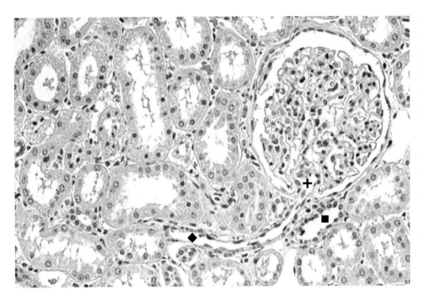

FIGURE 10–5 Normal kidney, microscopic

Here the afferent arteriole (◆) enters the glomerulus at the vascular pole (+). The juxtaglomerular apparatus is a region of specialized smooth muscle cells called *JG cells* located in the afferent arteriole, which, along with a set of columnar cells called the *macula densa* in the adjacent segment of distal convoluted tubule (■), sense changes in blood pressure and sodium concentration. The JG cells secrete renin, which catalyzes conversion of angiotensinogen to angiotensin I (AI). AI is biologically inactive and converted to angiotensin II (AII) by angiotensin-converting enzyme (ACE). AII is a potent vasoconstrictor and regulator of aldosterone secretion, which promotes sodium reabsorption and potassium excretion by the kidneys.

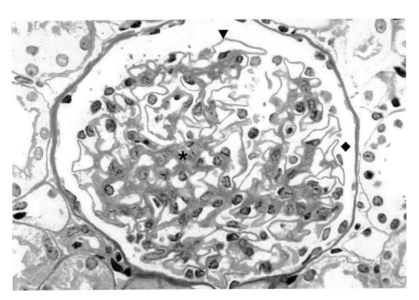

FIGURE 10–6 Normal kidney, microscopic

The normal glomerulus of the kidney at high power with PAS stain has thin, delicate capillary loops around the mesangial regions (*), which are not prominent, containing two to four mesangial cells. Most glomerular filtration occurs through the capillary loops into Bowman space (◆). The mesangium accounts for about 16% of filtration and serves a macrophage-like function as well as a reparative function. The visceral epithelial cells (podocytes) that surround the capillary loops (▼) are not easily recognized by light microscopy; parietal epithelial cells line the external surface of Bowman space.

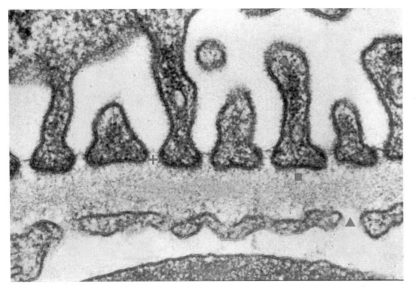

FIGURE 10–7 Normal kidney, electron microscopy

A glomerular capillary loop at high magnification has a visceral epithelial cell (podocyte) with interdigitating foot processes (♦) embedded in and adherent to the lamina rara externa (■) of the basement membrane. Adjacent foot processes (pedicels) are separated by 20- to 30-nm wide filtration slits (+). The basement membrane of uniform thickness (composed mainly of type IV collagen) has thin endothelial cell cytoplasm with fenestrations (▲) on the opposite surface. The exclusion of molecules such as albumin from the glomerular filtrate is a function of anionic charges from polyanionic proteoglycans as well as the anatomic size of the slit pores.

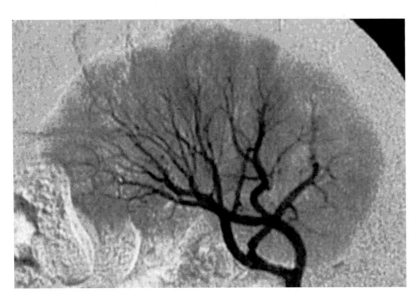

FIGURE 10–8 Normal kidney, angiogram

Seen here is the normal distribution of blood flow in the kidney, extending distally from the main renal artery and branches to arcuate branches at the corticomedullary junction. The kidneys receive about 25% of the cardiac output, and the renal cortex receives 90% of this renal blood flow. Decreasing renal blood flow triggers release of renin, which triggers generation of angiotensin I converted to angiotensin II, elevating blood pressure both through vasoconstriction to increase peripheral vascular resistance and from stimulation of aldosterone secretion from adrenal cortical glomerulosa cells that promotes distal tubular sodium reabsorption to increase blood volume.

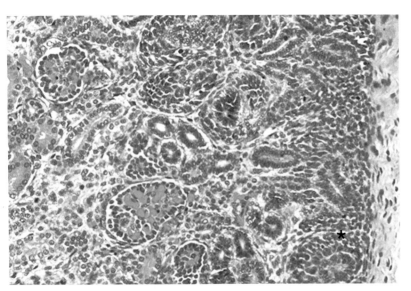

FIGURE 10–9 Normal fetal kidney, microscopic

Beneath the capsule of the developing fetal kidney is a nephrogenic zone (*) composed of primitive dark blue cells in which development of glomeruli and tubules is taking place and from which the new cortex will form. At the time of birth, most of this formative process has occurred, with just a small remnant of the nephrogenic zone persisting for up to 3 months. At birth, the infant's urine is quite dilute since the solute concentration of the medulla has not yet increased to the point that the countercurrent mechanism is fully operational.

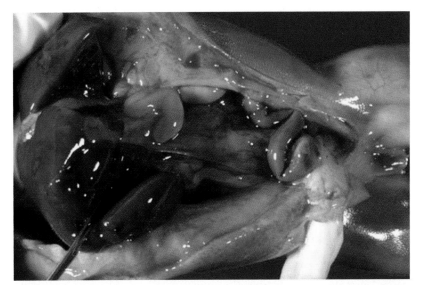

FIGURE 10–10 Renal agenesis, gross

Agenesis refers to absence of formation of a body part during embryogenesis. Here the kidneys are absent from the retroperitoneum, and this will result in oligohydramnios in utero because amniotic fluid is mainly derived from fetal urine. Bilateral renal agenesis is rare, present in about 1 in 4500 births. Unilateral renal agenesis is still rare but survivable, and the opposite kidney will develop to about twice the size of a normal kidney from compensatory hyperplasia. Bilateral renal agenesis is incompatible with life. At birth, there will be severe pulmonary hypoplasia from the oligohydramnios sequence.

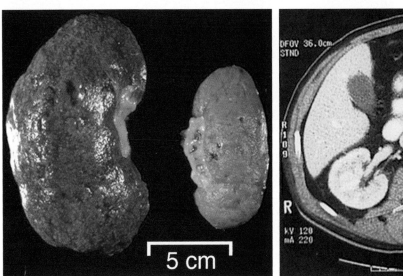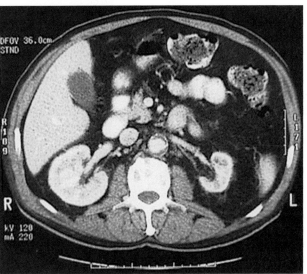

FIGURES 10–11 and 10–12 Renal acquired hypoplasia, gross and CT image ▲

There is one relatively normal-sized right kidney with a granular surface and a few scattered, shallow cortical scars as a result of left renal arterial occlusion from severe atherosclerosis. (The renal veins in the CT image are highlighted by contrast.) The increased renin secretion from the left kidney led to hypertension (Goldblatt kidney), which eventually damaged the opposite kidney. The atherosclerosis is marked by prominent aortic mural thrombus in the CT image. True congenital hypoplasia is quite rare, without scars, and there is a reduced number and size of renal lobes and pyramids.

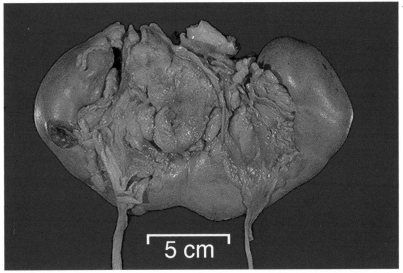

◄ FIGURE 10–13 Horseshoe kidney, gross

This congenital anomaly most often occurs in association with other anomalies or syndromes or with specific genetic defects such as trisomy 18. However, horseshoe kidney occurs as an isolated anomaly in about 1 in 500 people. Because the ureters take an abnormal course across the "bridge" of renal tissue, there is a potential for partial ureteral obstruction with resultant hydronephrosis. However, in many cases, this is just an incidental finding since renal filtration function is not affected and the total mass of renal tissue is normal. Abnormal fusion usually occurs at the lower renal poles.

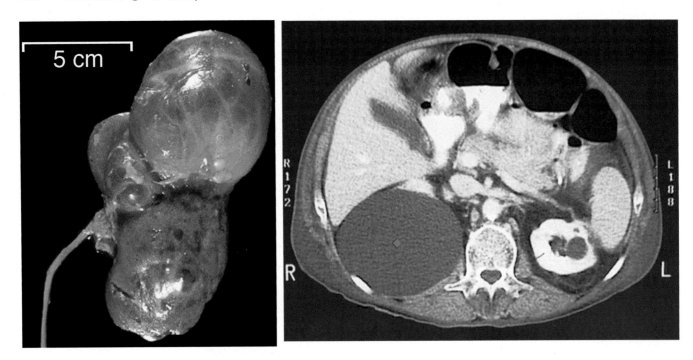

FIGURES 10–14 and 10–15 Simple renal cyst, gross and CT image

This is a large simple cyst of the right upper pole. Other smaller cysts are also scattered within the renal cortex in the left panel. Simple renal cysts are a common incidental finding in adults. A large renal cyst (♦) can be seen in this CT image, but it can be distinguished from a neoplasm by its fluid density and thin wall. In the CT image, a smaller simple cyst on the left has the characteristic features of low fluid attenuation and discrete borders. There is sufficient remaining functional renal cortex to provide adequate renal function in nearly all people with simple renal cysts.

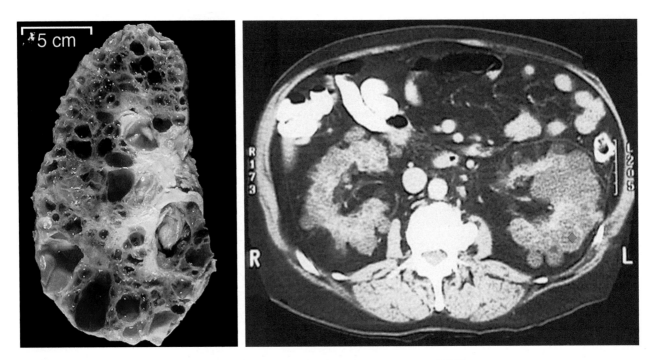

FIGURES 10–16 and 10–17 Autosomal dominant polycystic kidney disease, gross and CT image

The right kidney shown here grossly weighed 3 kg, as did the left kidney. Autosomal dominant polycystic kidney disease (ADPKD) is a bilateral process. The cysts (♦) are not typically present at birth, but develop slowly over time, so that onset of renal failure occurs in middle age to later adult life. An initial laboratory finding is often hematuria, followed by proteinuria (rarely more than 2 gm/day). Patients often have polyuria and hypertension. Cysts may appear in other organs such as liver, pancreas, and spleen. About 4% to 10% of patients with ADPKD have an intracranial berry aneurysm.

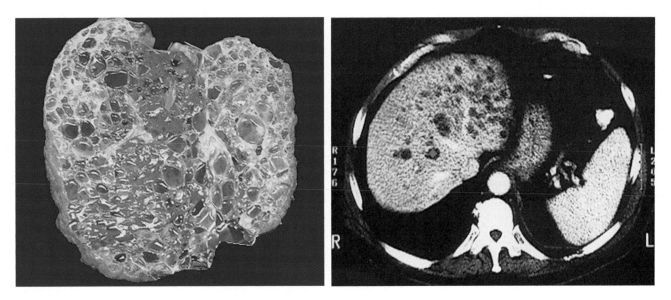

FIGURES 10–18 and 10–19 Autosomal dominant polycystic kidney disease, gross and CT image

Cysts appear within the liver in about 40% of patients with ADPKD. The hepatic cysts (♦), as well as the renal cysts, develop over the course of many years. Polycystic liver change, if extensive, may lead to hepatic failure, but liver function is normal in most cases. Cysts may rupture, bleed, or become sites for infection. Less commonly, the pancreas is involved. Mitral valve prolapse and other congenital cardiac defects are seen in up to 25% of ADPKD patients. The underlying genetic defect involves the *PKD1* gene in 80% of cases and the *PKD2* gene in about 10%. The polycystin gene product is a membrane-associated protein involved in cell–cell interactions during tubular epithelial cell growth and differentiation.

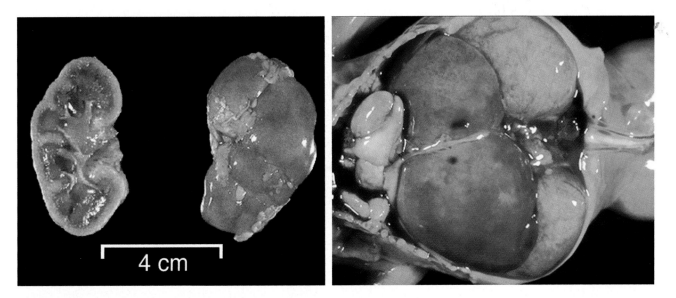

FIGURES 10–20 and 10–21 Normal fetal kidney and autosomal recessive polycystic kidney disease, gross

The normal term infant kidneys in the left panel reveal typical fetal lobulations and smooth cortical surfaces with some attached adipose tissue. Note the well-defined corticomedullary junctions on cut section. In the right panel, note the bilaterally massively enlarged kidneys that nearly fill the abdomen below the liver, consistent with autosomal recessive polycystic kidney disease (ARPKD) in this baby at 23 weeks' gestation who died from pulmonary hypoplasia as a consequence of oligohydramnios. There are perinatal, neonatal, infantile, and juvenile subcategories depending on the nature of the *PKHD1* gene (which encodes a large novel protein, *fibrocystin*) mutation, the time of presentation, and presence of associated hepatic lesions. The first two are the most common; serious manifestations are usually present at birth, typically with renal failure from birth. The latter two are compatible with longer survival, but patients often develop congenital hepatic fibrosis leading to complications from portal hypertension. There are many *PKHD1* mutations, and cases of ARPKD are compound heterozygotes.

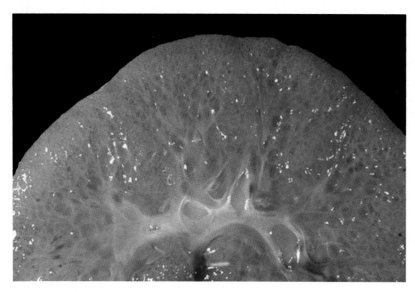

FIGURE 10–22 Autosomal recessive polycystic kidney disease, gross

One of the bilaterally and symmetrically enlarged kidneys with ARPKD is shown here on cut surface. Note that the numerous cysts are small, about 1 to 2 mm in diameter, but uniformly distributed throughout the parenchyma to produce a spongy appearance, and there is no distinguishable cortex or medulla. This condition is most often present from birth (hence the synonym "infantile" polycystic kidney disease). In utero, this condition results in reduced production of fetal urine, which forms amniotic fluid. Thus, fetal ultrasound will show oligohydramnios, or anhydamnios if severe.

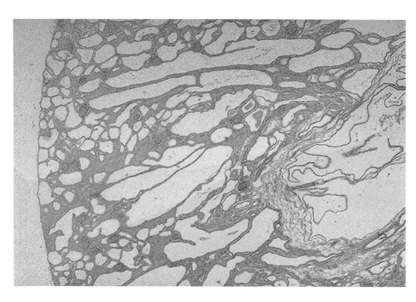

FIGURE 10–23 Autosomal recessive polycystic kidney disease, microscopic

The microscopic appearance of ARPKD is characterized by many cysts involving the collecting ducts, often elongated and radially arranged, or saccular. Within the residual renal cortex are a few scattered glomeruli. The cysts have a uniform lining of cuboidal cells. Consequent oligohydramnios leads to a deformation sequence from constriction of the fetus in utero. In addition to pulmonary hypoplasia, there can be varus deformities of the lower extremities, glovelike redundant skin on hands, and flattened (Potter) facies.

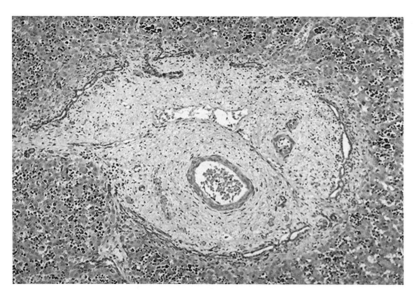

FIGURE 10–24 Autosomal recessive polycystic kidney disease, microscopic

Characteristic of ARPKD is the appearance of congenital hepatic fibrosis, seen as expanded portal regions with collagenous fibrosis and a proliferation of radially arranged portal bile ducts, as shown here. The surrounding normal hepatic parenchyma contains islands of extramedullary hematopoiesis, typical for second- and third-trimester fetal liver. In cases in which the patient survives, this may result in portal hypertension with splenomegaly in childhood.

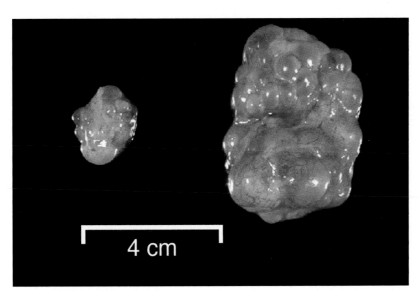

4 cm

FIGURE 10–25 Multicystic renal dysplasia, gross

Multicystic renal dysplasia (or multicystic dysplastic kidney, or cystic renal dysplasia) must be distinguished from ARPKD because it can occur sporadically without a defined inheritance pattern, and it is more common than ARPKD. It may be part of a syndrome, such as Meckel-Gruber syndrome. Many cases are associated with additional urinary tract anomalies such as ureteropelvic obstruction, ureteral agenesis, or atresia. The cysts are larger than those of ARPKD and are variably sized. Often, multicystic dysplastic kidney is unilateral. If bilateral, it is often asymmetric, as seen here. If bilateral, oligohydramnios and its complications can ensue, just as with ARPKD.

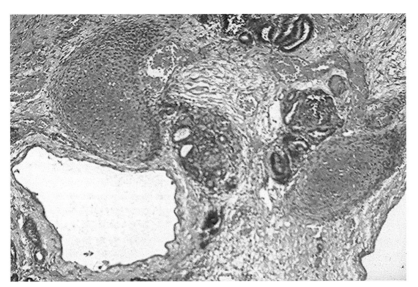

FIGURE 10–26 Multicystic renal dysplasia, microscopic

Dysplasia in pediatric terms implies disordered organ development, not an epithelial precursor of neoplasia. This is evident here in the renal parenchyma composed of irregular vascular channels, islands of cartilage, undifferentiated mesenchyme, and scattered immature collecting ductules in a fibrous stroma with cysts. There is also abnormal lobar organization. If the process is unilateral, or involves just a part of a kidney, there is enough renal reserve capacity with compensatory hyperplasia of the remaining renal tissue for adequate renal function to live a normal life. In fact, a person could survive with just half of one normal kidney.

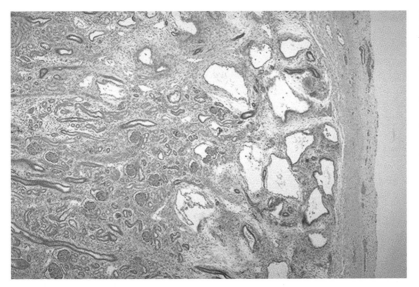

FIGURE 10–27 Congenital urinary tract obstruction with cystic change, microscopic

Urinary tract obstruction in utero can lead to renal cystic change in addition to hydronephrosis. The cysts appear near the nephrogenic zone because the developing glomeruli are most sensitive to the increased pressure. Thus, cortical microcysts develop as shown here. Causes of congenital urinary tract obstruction can include posterior urethral valves (in males) or urethral atresia (in both sexes). Obstruction below the bladder is detected by bladder enlargement on ultrasound scans, and diminished (or absent) fetal urine production leads to oligohydramnios (or anhydramnios) with a diminished amniotic fluid index.

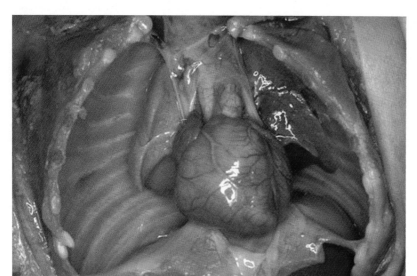

FIGURE 10–28 Pulmonary hypoplasia, gross

Congenital renal diseases or urinary tract outflow anomalies lead to the oligohydramnios sequence, which constricts lung development in utero, causing pulmonary hypoplasia. An ultrasound scan will show marked oligohydramnios because fetal urine forms the bulk of the amniotic fluid volume. The chest cavity opened here at autopsy reveals a normal-sized heart but very small lungs, which become the rate-limiting step for survival after birth. Additional features of oligohydramnios sequence include Potter facies with flattened nose and prominent infraorbital creases. Deformations of the extremities are common, with talipes equinovarus and joint contractures.

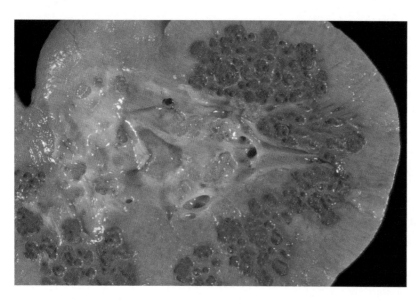

FIGURE 10–29 Medullary sponge kidney, gross

Note the 1- to 7-mm cysts involving the medulla of this kidney that resulted from nonprogressive dilation of the distal portion of the collecting ducts and tubules in the renal papillae. Most cases are bilateral and are discovered incidentally with imaging studies, and renal function is usually normal because the cortex is not involved. However, up to 20% of cases of medullary sponge kidney may be complicated by formation of renal calculi which predispose to infection (pyelonephritis) and hematuria in middle-aged people. Some cases appear in conjunction with Marfan syndrome, Ehlers-Danlos syndrome, and Caroli disease.

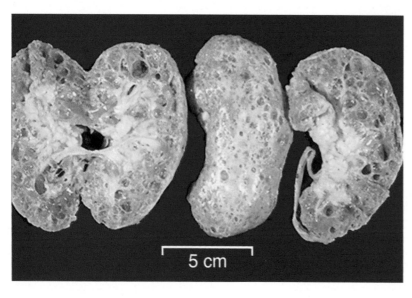

FIGURE 10–30 Acquired renal cystic disease, gross

Patients with chronic renal failure (CRF) who undergo hemodialysis for many years may develop multiple cysts in their renal cortices. This is probably the result of obstruction with progressive interstitial fibrosis in end-stage renal disease. When such cysts develop, they are more numerous than the common simple renal cysts, but usually less numerous than the cysts with ADPKD, and the size of the kidneys with dialysis-induced cystic disease is usually not markedly increased, as it is with ADPKD, since it is superimposed on chronic renal disease. There may be hemorrhage into the cysts. There is an increased risk for development of renal cell carcinoma.

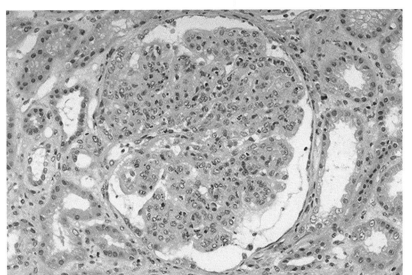

FIGURE 10–31 Post-infectious glomerulonephritis, microscopic

This glomerulus is hypercellular with increased inflammatory cells, and capillary loops are poorly defined. This type of acute proliferative glomerulonephritis (GN) is known as *postinfectious* GN, but is better known as *poststreptococcal* GN because historically most cases followed streptococcal pharyngitis (a different bacterial strain than that producing acute rheumatic fever). Other infections may include staphylococcal endocarditis, pneumococcal pneumonia, hepatitis B or C, HIV, or malaria. The infectious agent induces an immune response with antibodies that cross-react with glomerular antigens or lead to antigen–antibody complex formation with glomerular deposition.

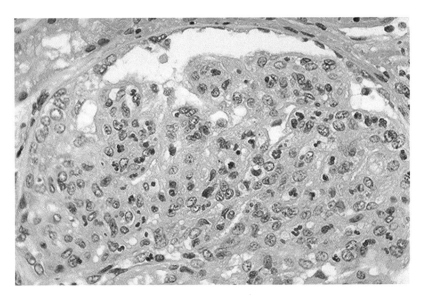

FIGURE 10–32 Postinfectious glomerulonephritis, microscopic

At higher magnification, the hypercellularity of postinfectious glomerulonephritis is due to increased numbers of epithelial, endothelial, and mesangial cells as well as neutrophils infiltrating in and around the capillary loops. This disease may occur 1 to 4 weeks after recovery from infection with certain (nephritogenic) strains of group A β-hemolytic streptococci that involve the pharynx ("strep throat") or skin (impetigo). These patients typically have elevated anti–streptolysin O (ASO), anti–DNase B, or antihyaluronidase titers. Patients may have microscopic hematuria, mild proteinuria, and mild to moderate hypertension.

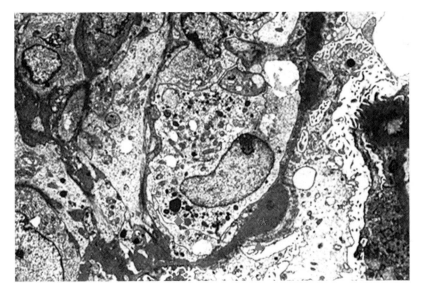

FIGURE 10–33 Postinfectious glomerulonephritis, electron microscopy

The immune deposits that appear in a bumpy granular pattern consist mainly of immunoglobulin G (IgG), IgM, and C3, as shown by immunofluorescence, and seen here by electron microscopy to be predominantly subepithelial. There are electron-dense subepithelial "humps" (٭) above the basement membrane and below the epithelial cell (podocyte) foot processes (▲). The capillary lumen is filled with a leukocyte having multiple cytoplasmic granules (◆). More than 95% of children with this disease recover, but a minority may evolve to rapidly progressive glomerulonephritis (RPGN). About 40% of adults with this condition go on to develop chronic renal disease.

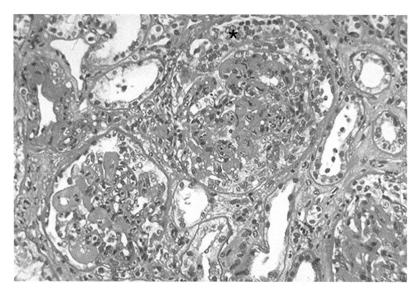

FIGURE 10–34 Rapidly progressive glomerulonephritis, microscopic

Seen here within three glomeruli are crescents (∗) composed of proliferating epithelial cells. Crescentic glomerulonephritis is known as *rapidly progressive glomerulonephritis* (RPGN) because this disease has a fulminant course. RPGN may be idiopathic or may result from anti–glomerular basement membrane (anti-GBM) antibody disease such as Goodpasture syndrome (type 1), from immune complex deposition with diseases such as systemic lupus erythematosus (SLE) or postinfectious GN (type 2), and from various types of vasculitis (type 3), often "pauci-immune" forms. Note in the lower left glomerulus that the capillary loops are markedly thickened (the so-called wire-loop lesion of lupus nephritis).

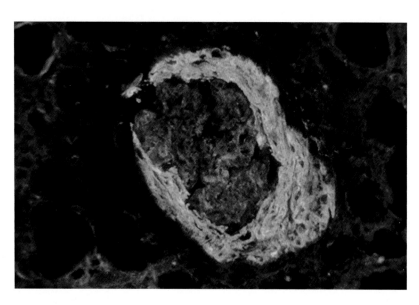

FIGURE 10–35 Rapidly progressive glomerulonephritis, immunofluorescence

This glomerulus demonstrates bright green immunofluorescence with antibody to fibrinogen. With RPGN, the glomerular damage is so severe that fibrinogen leaks into the Bowman space, leading to proliferation of the epithelial cells and formation of a crescent. Patients typically develop RPGN over a few days. Clinical manifestations include hematuria, moderate to severe proteinuria with edema, and hypertension. Hemoptysis characterizes those patients with Goodpasture syndrome, who also have detectable circulating anti-GBM antibody. Patients with systemic vasculitis, such as microscopic polyangiitis, may have circulating antineutrophil cytoplasmic antibody.

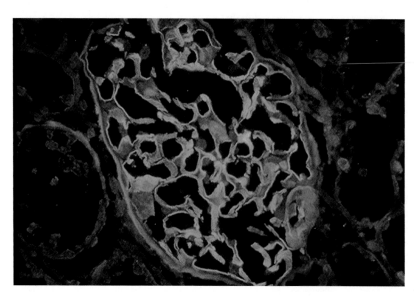

FIGURE 10–36 Rapidly progressive glomerulonephritis, immunofluorescence

There is bright green positivity with antibody to IgG with a smooth, diffuse, linear pattern that is characteristic of RPGN caused by circulating GBM antibody with Goodpasture syndrome. The antibody is directed at the noncollagenous domain of the α_3 chain of type IV collagen. This leads to a form of type II hypersensitivity reaction. Patients with RPGN have rapidly increasing serum urea nitrogen and creatinine, decreasing urine output, and urinary sediment that may contain red blood cells (RBCs) and RBC casts. The presence of the urinary dysmorphic RBCs and RBC casts along with oliguria and hypertension characterizes a nephritic syndrome.

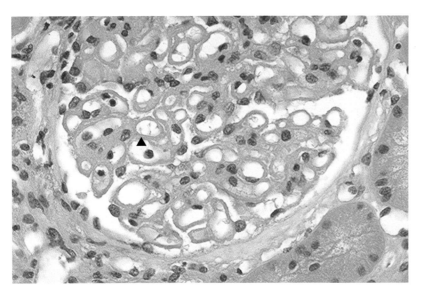

FIGURE 10–37 Membranous glomerulonephritis, microscopic

These capillary loops (▲) are diffusely thickened and prominent, but the overall glomerular cellularity is not increased. Membranous GN is the most common cause of nephrotic syndrome in adults. Nephrotic syndrome is defined as more than 3.5 gm of urine protein (mainly albumin) per day per 1.62 m^2 body surface area. RBCs are typically absent in the urine with pure nephrotic syndrome. Some cases of membranous GN are secondary to an underlying condition, such as a chronic infection like hepatitis B or C, a carcinoma, drugs such as NSAIDs, or SLE. However, many cases of membranous GN are idiopathic. This pattern is similar to experimental Heymann nephritis.

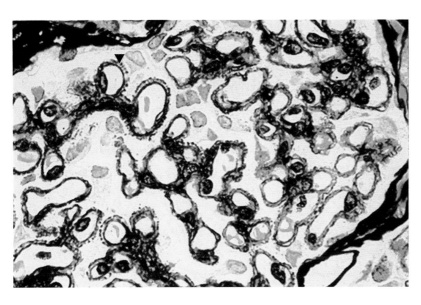

FIGURE 10–38 Membranous glomerulonephritis, microscopic

A Jones silver stain of this glomerulus highlights the proteinaceous basement membranes of capillary loops in black. There are characteristic "spikes" (▼) involving the capillary loops with membranous GN, seen here with black basement membrane material appearing as small projections distributed within the capillary loops. The immune complexes, not highlighted by the Jones stain, lie between the black spikes. Loss of anticoagulant proteins in nephrosis predisposes to thrombosis, including renal vein thrombosis. Urinalysis with nephrotic syndrome may show lipiduria and proteinuria, whereas blood lipids (cholesterol and triglyceride) are increased.

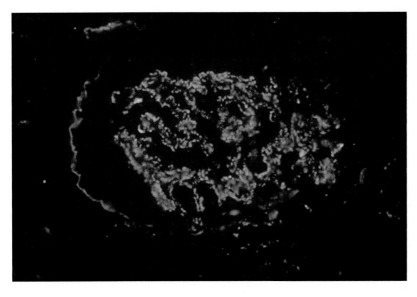

FIGURE 10–39 Membranous glomerulonephritis, electron microscopy

The immunofluorescence pattern here has a "bumpy" or granular staining pattern as a result of irregular deposition of immune complexes within the basement membrane of the glomerular capillary loops. A variety of fluorescein-labeled antibodies can be employed, such as those directed against immunoglobulins or complement components, which commonly compose the immune complexes. The onset of membranous GN is often gradual, with nephrotic syndrome a likely presenting finding. Some patients may have hypertension; hematuria is less common. About 10% of patients go on to develop CRF within 10 years.

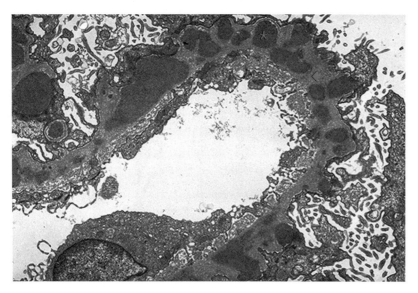

FIGURE 10–40 Membranous glomerulonephritis, electron microscopy

By electron microscopy in membranous GN, the darker electron-dense immune deposits (∗) appear scattered within the thickened capillary basement membrane. The "spikes" seen with the silver stain are the lighter areas (♦) representing the intervening increased matrix of basement membrane between the darker immune deposits. The loss of basement membrane function leads to proteinuria, which is often "selective" because mostly lower-molecular-weight proteins such as albumin are lost.

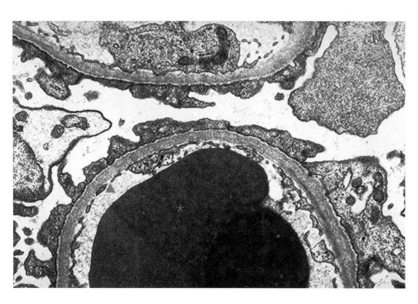

FIGURE 10–41 Minimal change disease, electron microscopy

By light microscopy, the glomerulus is normal with minimal change disease (MCD), the most common cause of nephrotic syndrome in children. In this electron micrograph, the lower capillary loop contains two electron-dense RBCs (∗) in close apposition. Normal fenestrated endothelium (▲) is present, and the basement membranes (♦) are normal in thickness with no immune deposits. However, overlying epithelial cell (podocyte) foot processes are effaced (giving the appearance of fusion) and run together (+), which leads to loss of the normal charge barrier such that albumin selectively leaks out, and proteinuria ensues, often with nephrotic syndrome. Most patients recover completely after a course of corticosteroid therapy.

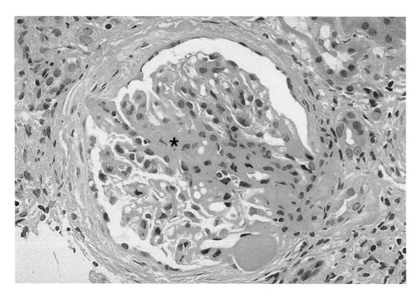

FIGURE 10–42 Focal segmental glomerulonephritis, microscopic

An area of collagenous sclerosis (∗) runs across the middle segment of this glomerulus, and the biopsy showed that the process was focal, with only 3 of 10 glomeruli involved. In contrast to MCD, patients with focal segmental glomerulosclerosis (FSGS) are more likely to have a poor response to corticosteroid therapy with nonselective proteinuria (more proteins than albumin), hematuria, and progression to CRF. FSGS may represent the opposite end of the spectrum of MCD since more than half of FSGS patients progress to CRF within 10 years.

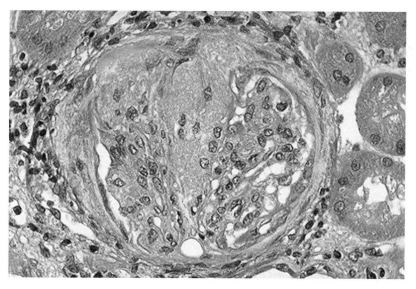

FIGURE 10–43 Focal segmental glomerulosclerosis, microscopic

This trichrome stain of a glomerulus in a patient with FSGS shows blue collagen deposition. FSGS accounts for about one sixth of cases of nephrotic syndrome in adults and children. This disease is focal, involving some glomeruli, and segmental, involving part of the glomerulus. Patients may present with either nephrotic or nephritic syndrome. In some cases, a mutated *NPHS1* gene produces an abnormal nephrin protein, and in others, abnormal podocin is produced by an abnormal *NPHS2* gene. Both proteins are components of the slit diaphragm between podocyte foot processes. Recurrence of FSGS after transplantation is frequent.

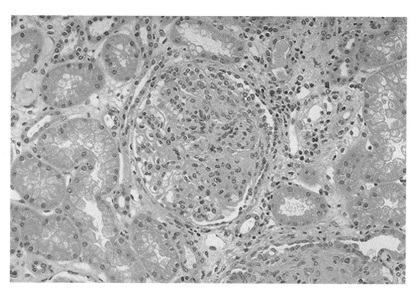

FIGURE 10–44 Membranoproliferative glomerulonephritis, microscopic

This glomerulus has increased overall cellularity, mainly mesangial. Membranoproliferative glomerulonephritis (MPGN), like membranous GN, may be termed *secondary* and follow infections such as hepatitis B or C, malignancies, or immune complex diseases such as SLE. However, most cases of MPGN are idiopathic. MPGN is divided into types I and II by pathologic findings. By light microscopy, the two types are similar, with mesangial proliferation, increased mesangial matrix, accentuation of the lobular architecture, and increased leukocytes. Recurrence of MPGN after renal transplantation is frequent.

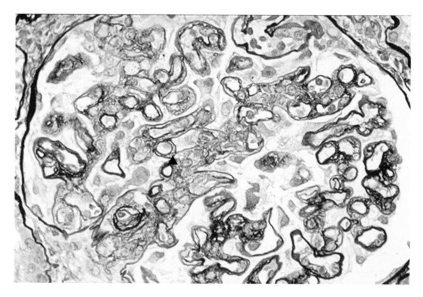

FIGURE 10–45 Membranoproliferative glomerulonephritis type I, microscopic

This Jones silver stain shows a double contour (▲) to many basement membranes, or the "tram-tracking" that is characteristic of MPGN type I that results from basement membrane reduplication. (A *tram* is a streetcar on rails.) The disease results from subendothelial immune complex deposition after both classic and alternate pathway complement activation, but antigens that trigger this process are often unknown; hepatitis B or C infections may account for some cases. Type 1 constitutes two thirds of MPGN cases. Most patients present with nephrotic syndrome, but there can be a nephritic pattern or even RPGN. About half of patients develop CRF within 10 years.

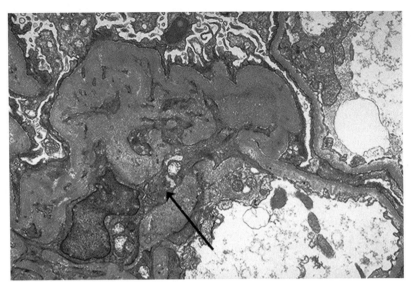

FIGURE 10–46 Membranoproliferative glomerulonephritis type I, electron microscopy

A mesangial cell at the lower left is interposing its cytoplasm at the arrow into the basement membrane, leading to splitting and reduplication of basement membrane that is piled up above the mesangial cytoplasm. These characteristic electron microscopic changes occur when the mesangial cell (which has a macrophage-like function) tries to phagocytose subendothelial immune deposits, but makes a mess of the GBM in the process. Secondary MPGN type I can complicate SLE, hepatitis B or C infections with cryoglobulinemia, infective endocarditis, HIV infection, non-Hodgkin lymphoma/leukemia, hereditary complement deficiencies, and α_1-antitrypsin deficiency.

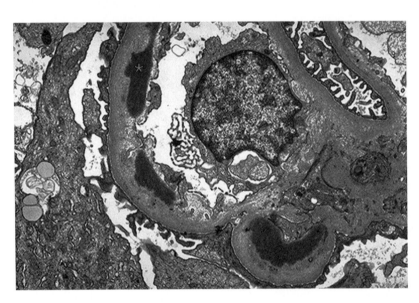

FIGURE 10–47 Membranoproliferative glomerulonephritis type II, electron microscopy

These dense deposits (*) in the basement membrane are typical of MPGN type II ("dense deposit" disease). The dense deposits within the basement membrane often coalesce to form a ribbon-like mass of deposits. The deposits result from activation of the alternative complement pathway, evidenced by a reduced serum C3 with normal C1 and C4. Patients with MPGN type II often have circulating C3 nephritogenic factor (C3NeF).

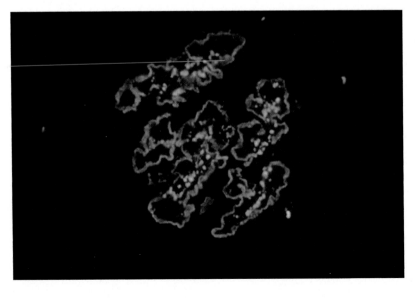

FIGURE 10–48 Membranoproliferative glomerulonephritis type II, immunofluorescence

There are irregular granular to linear foci of bright intramembranous deposits scattered along both the capillary walls and in the mesangium by immunofluorescence microscopy with antibody to C3. Such deposits are typical of MPGN type II. These patients often present with a nephritic syndrome. The rare condition called *partial lipodystrophy with C3NeF activity* may be accompanied by MPGN type II.

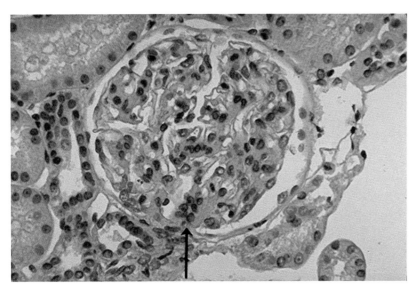

FIGURE 10–49 IgA nephropathy, microscopic

The IgA is deposited mainly in mesangium, which then increases mesangial cellularity, as shown at the arrow. Patients with IgA nephropathy (Berger disease) are usually young men with hematuria after a respiratory, gastrointestinal, or urinary tract infection. Proteinuria is often present, sometimes severe enough to qualify as nephrotic syndrome. Immune dysregulation with either increased production or decreased clearance of IgA is implicated in the pathogenesis, and there is a familial tendency with some HLA types. Some cases occur in patients with celiac disease and some with chronic liver disease from decreased IgA clearance. IgA nephropathy has now become the most common form of glomerulonephritis.

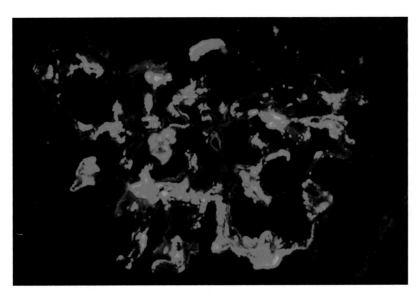

FIGURE 10–50 IgA nephropathy, immunofluorescence

Note the pattern here of mesangial staining with antibody to IgA (of the IgA1 subclass), and there is often accompanying C3 deposition. This disease most often tends to be mild, but recurrent, and continues with normal renal function for years. One fourth to one half of patients develop CRF within 20 years. Patients with IgA nephropathy who are older tend to have hypertension, or more severe proteinuria, and are more likely to have a worse prognosis, with earlier progression to CRF. There is rare presentation as RPGN. Some cases in children are a manifestation of the systemic illness Henoch-Schönlein purpura.

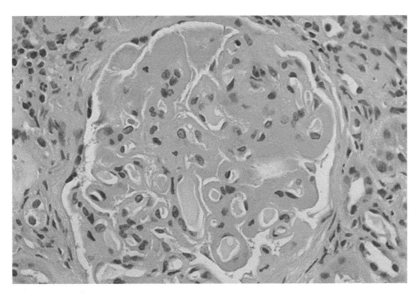

FIGURE 10–51 Focal proliferative glomerulonephritis, microscopic

Proliferative glomerulonephritis may involve just a portion of only some glomeruli. This may be idiopathic or due to an underlying vasculitis, SLE, Goodpasture syndrome, IgA nephropathy, or infection. Glomerular disease with SLE is common, and such a lupus nephritis can have many morphologic manifestations on renal biopsy. In general, the more immune complex deposition and the more cellular proliferation, the worse the disease. In this case, there is extensive immune complex deposition in the thickened glomerular capillary loops, giving a wire-loop appearance. However, a portion of the glomerulus is still intact.

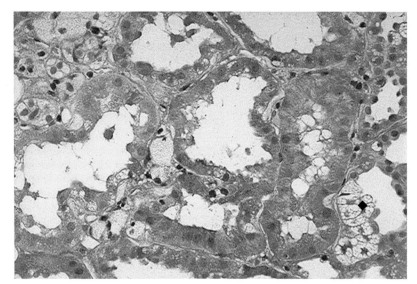

FIGURE 10–52 Alport syndrome, microscopic

This disease is a form of hereditary nephritis accompanied by nerve deafness and eye problems such as lens dislocation, cataracts, and corneal dystrophy. Males are more often and more severely affected since some cases have an X-linked dominant inheritance pattern resulting from mutations in the α_2 chain of type IV collagen (*COLA45*). Although onset of hematuria or proteinuria occurs in childhood, renal failure is more likely to occur in adults. The renal tubular cells appear foamy (◆) because of the accumulation of neutral fats and mucopolysaccharides, seen here imparting a pale red appearance with a fat stain. There is thickening and thinning with splitting of the GBM, resulting from defective GBM production in the X-linked form.

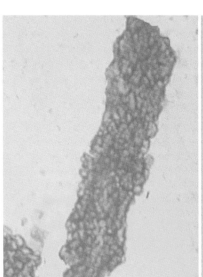
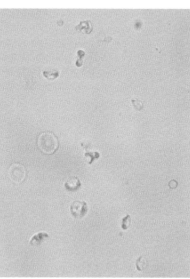

FIGURE 10–53 Hematuria, urine microscopic

"Nephritic" renal diseases with appearance of RBCs in the urine may have casts on examination of the urine. In contrast, renal diseases that are "nephrotic" are characterized by the presence of protein spilled into the urine. Some renal diseases are both nephritic and nephrotic. Shown at the left is a red blood cell cast that formed either in distal convoluted tubules or collecting ducts. At the right at high magnification are seen "dysmorphic" RBCs that are misshapen. The presence of dysmorphic RBCs in urine suggests a glomerular disease such as a glomerulonephritis. Dysmorphic RBCs have odd shapes as a consequence of being distorted by their passage through the abnormal glomerular structure.

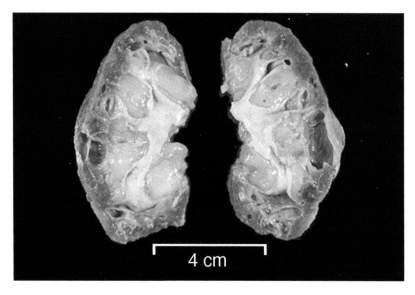

FIGURE 10–54 Chronic glomerulonephritis, gross

Here is the answer to the question regarding the cause of many cases of CRF. If all else fails, call it "chronic glomerulonephritis." Seen here are atrophic kidneys with thin cortices from a patient at autopsy with CRF. About one third to one half of patients with CRF slowly reach end-stage renal disease without significant signs or symptoms along the way, and at the end stage, there are no diagnostic features and, therefore, no point in performing a renal biopsy. Steadily rising serum creatinine and urea nitrogen are clues to this progression. Most patients also have hypertension. (Some incidental simple cysts are also seen here.)

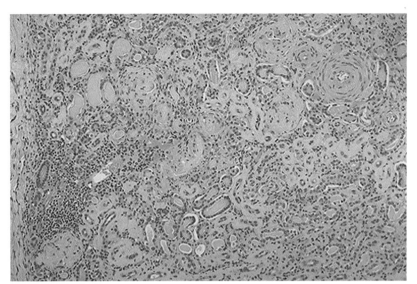

FIGURE 10–55 End-stage renal disease, microscopic

The microscopic appearance of the "end-stage kidney" is similar regardless of cause, which is why a biopsy in a patient with CRF may yield little useful information. The cortex is fibrotic, the glomeruli are sclerotic from hyaline obliteration, there are scattered interstitial chronic inflammatory cell infiltrates, and the arteries are thickened. Tubules are often dilated and filled with pink casts and give an appearance of "thyroidization." Patients placed on hemodialysis may have extensive deposition of calcium oxalate crystals in tubules and interstitium. Diminished renal clearance of phosphate predisposes to secondary hyperparathyroidism.

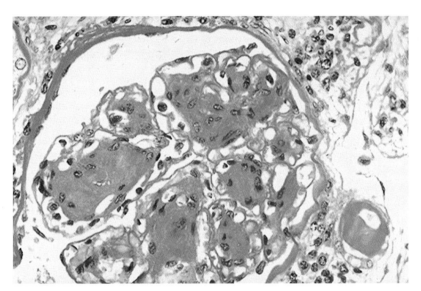

FIGURE 10–56 Nodular glomerulosclerosis, microscopic

Nodular glomerulosclerosis (Kimmelstiel-Wilson disease) of diabetes mellitus (either type 1 or 2) is characterized by nodules of pink hyaline material that form in mesangial regions between glomerular capillary loops, made more prominent here with a PAS stain. This is due to metabolic alterations with hyperglycemia, with a marked increase in mesangial matrix from cellular damage from nonenzymatic glycosylation of proteins. Also note the markedly thickened arteriole at the lower right, which is typical of hyaline arteriolosclerosis seen in diabetic kidneys. In early stages of this disease, microalbuminuria is present, but it progresses to overt proteinuria that presages renal failure. Hypertension is common.

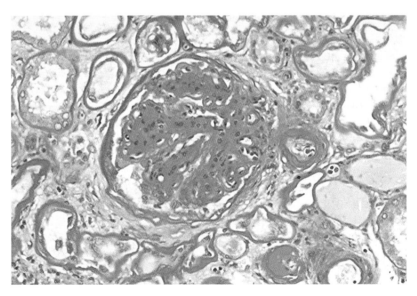

FIGURE 10–57 Diffuse glomerulosclerosis, microscopic

A PAS stain highlights diffuse glomerulosclerosis associated with long-standing type 1 or 2 diabetes mellitus. There is an increase in mesangial matrix, a slight increase in mesangial cellularity, and capillary basement membrane thickening. These changes gradually advance until the entire glomerulus is sclerotic. Changes of glomerulosclerosis with diabetes mellitus take a decade or longer to develop and gradually worsen. Patients with diabetes mellitus, whether type 1 or 2, are at risk for many renal diseases, including nephrosclerosis, pyelonephritis, and papillary necrosis, in addition to glomerulosclerosis. Thus, a major complication of diabetes mellitus is CRF.

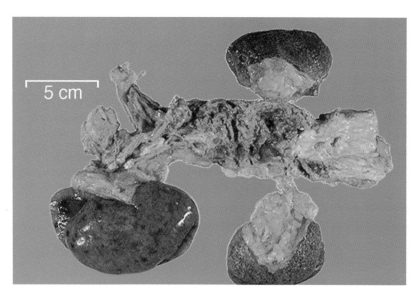

FIGURE 10–58 Atherosclerosis, gross

Accelerated and advanced atherosclerosis in a patient with diabetes mellitus leads to severe atherosclerosis involving the aorta and its branches, including renal arterial stenosis as well as nephrosclerosis. The end-stage renal disease seen here with small native kidneys and granular surfaces was treated with renal transplantation. The transplant kidney is placed in the pelvis because this is technically easier and there is usually no point in trying to remove the native kidneys, which may still produce erythropoietin. In this case, the patient developed chronic rejection, which is why the transplant kidney is slightly swollen with focal hemorrhages.

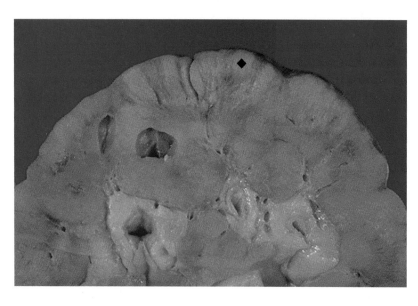

FIGURE 10–59 Amyloidosis, gross

This form of chronic renal disease may actually increase the size of the kidneys. Pale deposits (◆) of amyloid are present in this renal cortex, most prominently at the upper center, which obscure the corticomedullary junction. The most common types of amyloidosis that involve the kidneys are those associated with multiple myeloma and excessive light chain production (AL amyloid) and serum amyloid associated (AA amyloid) conditions, including chronic inflammation or infection. The nephrotic syndrome is common with renal amyloidosis.

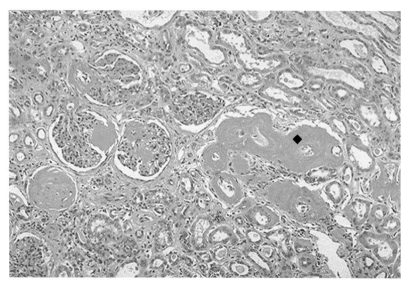

FIGURE 10–60 Amyloidosis, microscopic

Here in the renal cortex, pale pink deposits of amyloid (◆) are seen within glomeruli as well as small renal arterial branches that have become thickened. The amorphous pink deposits of amyloid may be found in and around arteries, in interstitium, or in glomeruli. A Congo red stain will demonstrate the pink material to be amyloid. Such collections of amyloid diminish renal function, resulting in uremia marked by a rising serum creatinine and urea nitrogen. Uremia from CRF of any etiology leads to malaise, nausea, diminished mental function, and development of fibrinous pericarditis.

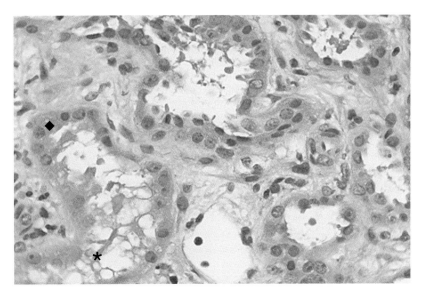

FIGURE 10–61 Acute tubular necrosis, microscopic

The epithelium of these tubules is ragged (∗) from undergoing necrosis with acute tubular necrosis (ATN) from ischemia. In this case, heart failure with hypotension precipitated the ATN. The distribution of the areas of necrosis and apoptosis is more segmental with ischemic injuries, as seen here, with some tubules still having intact epithelium (◆) while others show considerable damage. Lesser degrees of injury with loss of the brush border and cell swelling are common. This is the most common form of acute tubular damage because hypotension from heart failure, sepsis, or disseminated intravascular coagulation is common. ATN is potentially reversible.

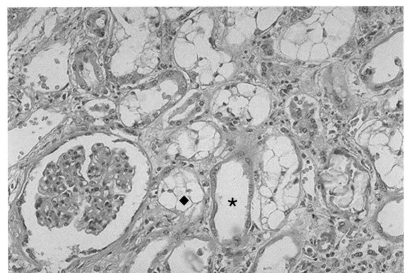

FIGURE 10–62 Acute tubular necrosis, microscopic

ATN from nephrotoxins is more likely to result in diffuse proximal tubular injury. The tubular vacuolization (◆) and dilation (∗) shown here are the result of ethylene glycol poisoning, representative of toxic ATN. The clinical course of ATN is marked by an initiating injury over 1 to 2 days, followed by decreased urine output. The patient can be maintained on dialysis until the recovery phase occurs with polyuria. A nonoliguric form of ATN can be seen in about half of cases of ATN associated with nephrotoxins.

FIGURE 10–63 Vesicoureteral reflux, x-ray

This intravenous urogram shows dilation of the left ureter, beginning at the left ureteral orifice (◆) and extending to the left renal pelvis (■), which is also dilated along with the calyces. Incompetence of the vesicoureteral valve can predispose to reflux with retrograde flow of urine. In children, this is most often due to congenital shortening of the intravesical portion of the ureter. Decreased bladder contraction from autonomic neuropathy or spinal cord injury can lead to reflux in adults. In either case, there is an increased risk for urinary tract infection, and the inflammation from infection further exacerbates the reflux.

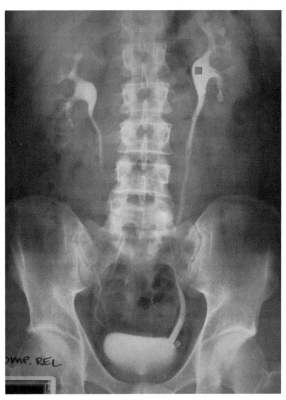

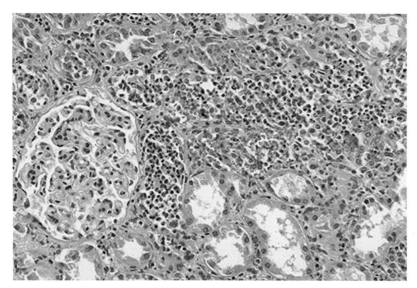

FIGURE 10–64 Acute pyelonephritis, microscopic

There are various forms of tubulointerstitial nephritis. Shown here are numerous inflammatory cells, mainly neutrophils, filling renal tubules and extending into the interstitium. This case of acute pyelonephritis resulted from an ascending urinary tract infection that started in the bladder. Nearly all such cases are due to bacterial organisms, including the Enterobacteriaceae (*Escherichia*, *Klebsiella*, *Proteus*, *Providencia*, *Edwardsiella*, *Enterobacter*) and streptococcal and staphylococcal organisms. Urinary stasis from congenital anomalies, obstructive uropathy, or decreased emptying may predispose to ascending urinary tract infection.

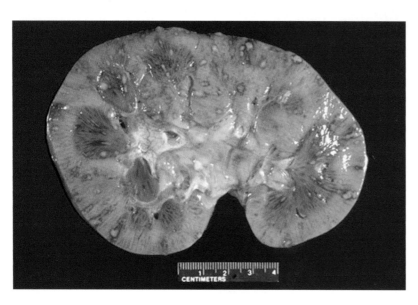

FIGURE 10–65 Acute pyelonephritis, gross

The cut surface of this swollen kidney reveals many small yellowish microabscesses involving both cortex and medulla. This pattern of acute pyelonephritis is most typical of hematogenous dissemination of infection to the kidney in patients with septicemia. Ascending urinary tract infection leading to acute pyelonephritis is more common than the hematogenous route. Clinical findings of acute pyelonephritis include fever, malaise, and flank pain. Costovertebral angle tenderness may be observed on physical examination. A rare complication not seen here is papillary necrosis, which is more likely to occur in patients with diabetes mellitus or urinary tract obstruction.

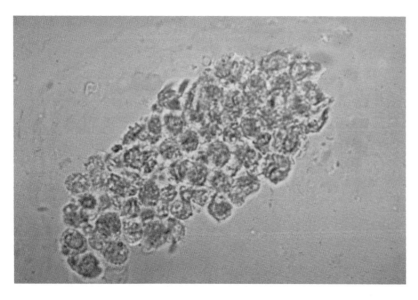

FIGURE 10–66 Acute pyelonephritis, urine microscopic

A characteristic feature of acute pyelonephritis on microscopic urinalysis is the presence of white blood cell (WBC) casts. Findings on dipstick urinalysis can include a positive leukocyte esterase (positive even if the WBCs are lysed and no longer intact) and a positive nitrite test. Urinary casts must come from distal renal tubules, whereas individual neutrophils may originate with acute inflammation from anywhere within the urinary tract. The "cement" holding elements of a cast together includes the Tamm-Horsfall protein normally secreted in small quantities from tubular cells. Urine culture with antibiotic sensitivity testing helps to determine appropriate antibiotic therapy.

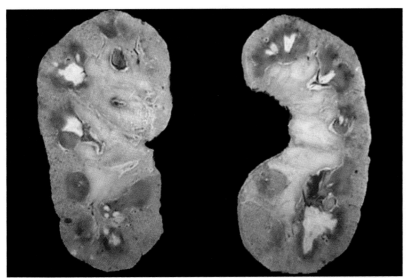

FIGURE 10–67 Papillary necrosis, gross

These pale white areas involving some renal papillae of both kidneys are areas of papillary necrosis, a form of focal coagulative necrosis. This is an uncommon but severe complication of acute pyelonephritis, particularly in patients with diabetes mellitus or urinary tract obstruction. Papillary necrosis may also occur with analgesic nephropathy or sickle cell disease. A necrotic, sloughed renal papilla may be recovered from the urine. Acute renal failure may occur.

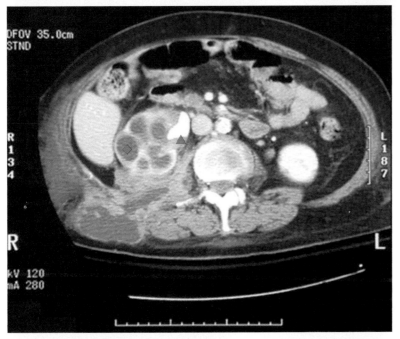

FIGURE 10–68 Perinephric abscess, CT image

This abdominal CT image with contrast demonstrates a staghorn calculus (▲) filling a dilated calyx in this enlarged right kidney, along with marked hydronephrosis (◆) of remaining calyces, as a consequence of chronic urinary tract obstruction. An extensive acute pyelonephritis complicated this process, and the infection became complicated by a perinephric abscess that extended to the right flank region, seen here as irregular areas of decreased attenuation within the skeletal muscle of the posterior flank and back on the right.

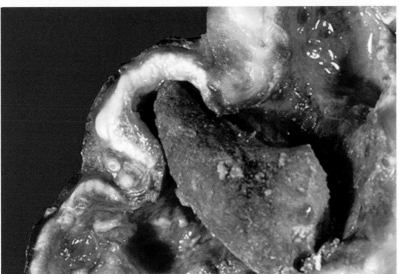

FIGURE 10–69 Pyonephrosis, gross

Sometimes a very large calculus nearly fills the calyceal system, with extensions into calyces that give the appearance of a stag's (deer) horns. Hence, the name "staghorn calculus." Seen here is a hornlike stone extending into a dilated calyx, with nearly unrecognizable pale yellow to tan overlying renal cortex from severe inflammation and atrophy from both hydronephrosis and pyelonephritis. There can be nearly complete or total obstruction with extensive inflammation that destroys renal parenchyma. Note the thin residual cortex and medulla. Nephrectomy may be performed in cases of pyonephrosis because the kidney becomes nonfunctional and serves only as a source of continuing infection.

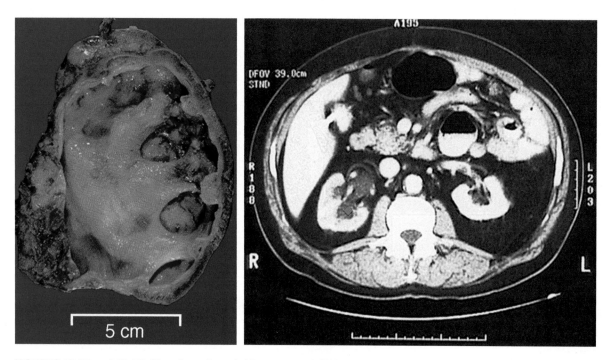

FIGURES 10–70 and 10–71 Chronic pyelonephritis, gross and CT image

This right kidney has advanced chronic pyelonephritis from reflux and consequent hydronephrosis (◆). There is only a thin rim of remaining renal cortex. If this process is unilateral, then the problem originates from a disease involving a location from the ureteral orifice up to the renal pelvis. In this case, an obstructing urinary tract calculus was present for many years. Vesicoureteral reflux, most often presenting in childhood, could produce a similar finding. If the obstructive process were bilateral, then the underlying disease would originate in the bladder trigone or urethra (or the prostate around the urethra of males) or some process (such as a large neoplasm) that could impinge on both ureters or much of the bladder or urethral outlet. Bilateral chronic pyelonephritis is a common cause of end-stage renal disease.

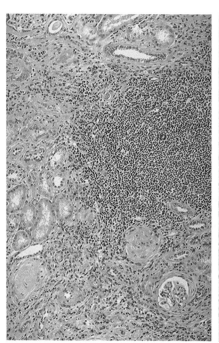 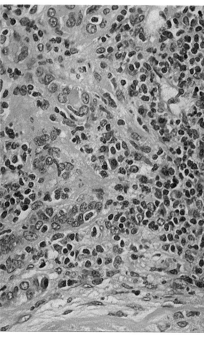

FIGURES 10–72 and 10–73 Chronic pyelonephritis, microscopic

In the left panel at low magnification is a large collection of chronic inflammatory cells in a patient with a long history of multiple recurrent urinary tract infections. Both lymphocytes and plasma cells characteristic of chronic pyelonephritis are seen at high magnification in the right panel. It is not uncommon to see interstitial lymphocytes accompany just about any form of chronic renal disease: glomerulonephritis, nephrosclerosis, or pyelonephritis. However, plasma cells are most characteristic of chronic pyelonephritis. Over time, there is increasing tubular atrophy with prominent proteinaceous casts (so-called thyroidization) and interstitial fibrosis, which eventually affects renal vascular flow, and there is progressive sclerosis of glomeruli leading to CRF.

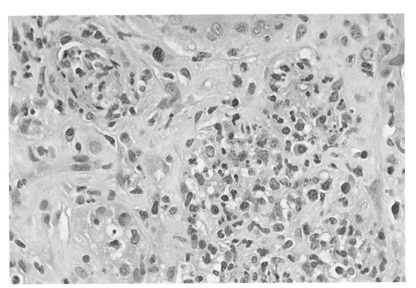

FIGURE 10–74 Interstitial nephritis, microscopic

Cases of tubulointerstitial nephritis may result from drug-induced renal injury. Shown here are scattered eosinophils, along with neutrophils and mononuclear cells in an inflamed interstitium. The patient may have a fever, peripheral blood eosinophilia, and a skin rash, as well as oliguria, hematuria, and proteinuria. Half of cases lead to acute renal failure with increasing serum urea nitrogen and creatinine. A type I hypersensitivity reaction is implicated. In more chronic cases, type IV hypersensitivity with granulomas may occur. Antibiotics (methicillin), NSAIDs, and other drugs such as cimetidine can cause this condition. In one third of cases, the offending agent is unknown.

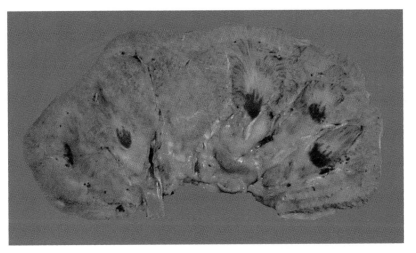

FIGURE 10–75 Analgesic nephropathy, microscopic

The excessive use of analgesics containing phenacetin and aspirin over many years can result in papillary necrosis, shown here, followed by tubulointerstitial nephritis. The aspirin inhibits formation of prostaglandin (a vasodilator) to potentiate ischemic injury. Phenacetin is metabolized to acetaminophen, which is nephrotoxic. A urinary tract infection is present in half of cases. Some patients develop transitional cell carcinoma of the renal pelvis. NSAIDs, particularly the cyclooxygenase-2 inhibitors, can also produce renal injury from reduced prostaglandin synthesis, leading to acute or CRF.

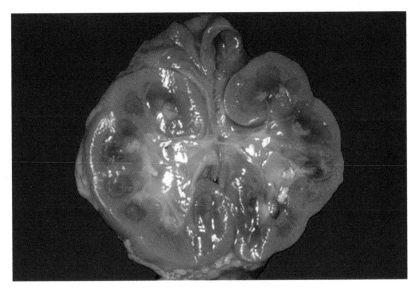

FIGURE 10–76 Urate nephropathy, gross

Chronic urate nephropathy leads to pale yellowish tan tophaceous deposits in the renal medulla. This is most often seen in patients with chronic gout. There is also an acute urate nephropathy that can occur with a "lysis" syndrome resulting from massive cellular necrosis of leukemia or lymphoma cells with chemotherapy. The metabolic breakdown of the many cell nuclei yields large amounts of urate that, when excreted, plug renal tubules. Precipitation of uric acid is enhanced by an acidic urinary pH. An additional complication of hyperuricemia is nephrolithiasis with uric acid calculi.

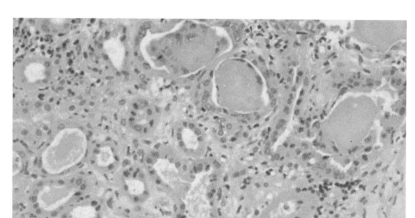

FIGURE 10–77 Multiple myeloma, microscopic

If there is Bence-Jones proteinuria with multiple myeloma, then immunoglobulin light chains may precipitate in renal tubules, forming light-chain casts as shown here that produce a cast nephropathy with renal failure. The pale pink casts may act as a foreign body and have multinucleated giant cells surrounding them. Additional renal problems with multiple myeloma include amyloidosis, light-chain glomerulopathy, hypercalcemia with nephrocalcinosis, hyperuricemia with urate nephropathy, and urinary tract infection with pyelonephritis.

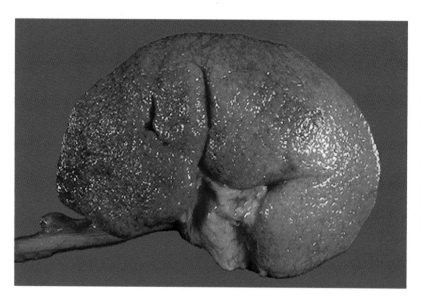

FIGURE 10–78 Benign nephrosclerosis, gross

Intrinsic renal vascular disease with sclerosis and progressive vascular narrowing leads to patchy ischemic atrophy with focal loss of parenchyma that gives the surface of the kidney a characteristic granular appearance. These kidneys are usually slightly smaller than normal. The process is termed *benign* because most patients who have it are aging but continue to have normal renal function, as determined by serum creatinine and urea nitrogen levels in the normal range. There may be a mild reduction in the glomerular filtration rate and mild proteinuria. Patients who have nephrosclerosis associated with hypertension and diabetes mellitus are at increased risk for renal failure.

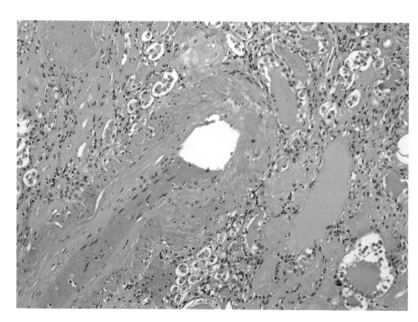

FIGURE 10–79 Benign nephrosclerosis, microscopic

These smaller arteries and arterioles in the kidney have become thickened and narrowed. The medial thickening of small arteries as shown leads to progressive luminal narrowing. Nephrosclerosis leads to interstitial fibrosis. Tubular atrophy and cast formation are common. Glomeruli first undergo collagen deposition within the Bowman space, as well as periglomerular fibrosis, with eventual total glomerular sclerosis. Hyaline arteriolosclerosis with hypertension or diabetes mellitus is also usually present.

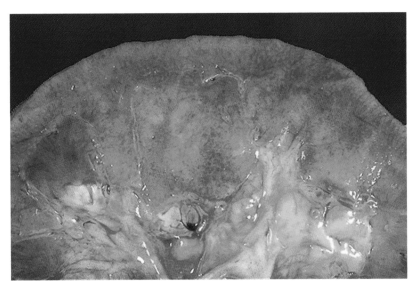

FIGURE 10–80 Malignant nephrosclerosis, gross

This kidney shows focal small hemorrhages in cortex and medulla, and the corticomedullary junction is obscured. This is due to an accelerated phase of hypertension in which blood pressures become very elevated, with diastolic pressures above 130 mm Hg (such as 300/150 mm Hg). This condition typically complicates long-standing essential benign hypertension, but it may occur *de novo*. Systemic sclerosis (scleroderma) may be present in some cases. In any case, it is rare. Patients present with headache, nausea, vomiting, and visual disturbances. Papilledema may be present. Proteinuria and hematuria are common findings.

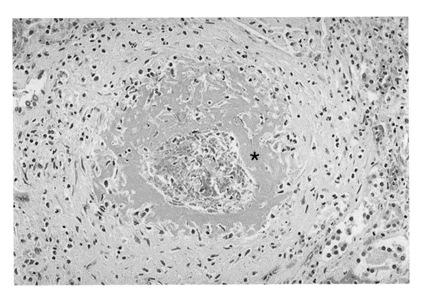

FIGURE 10–81 Malignant nephrosclerosis, microscopic

Malignant hypertension results from endothelial injury and increased permeability to plasma proteins along with platelet activation, leading to fibrinoid necrosis (∗) of small arteries as shown. The damage to this artery is characterized by formation of pink fibrin—hence the term *fibrinoid*. The renin–angiotensin mechanism is stimulated, and very high renin levels develop to produce hypertension. The generation of aldosterone promotes salt retention, which further promotes hypertension. The generation of more angiotensin II leads to further vasoconstriction with ischemic injury.

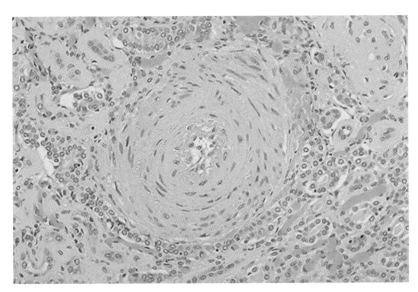

FIGURE 10–82 Malignant nephrosclerosis, microscopic

Thickening of the arterial wall with malignant hypertension also produces a hyperplastic arteriolitis. The arteriole has an onion skin appearance from concentric layering of proliferating smooth muscle with collagen deposition. This arteriolar lumen is nearly obliterated, promoting ischemic injury. Malignant hypertension is a medical emergency. Patients can develop acute renal failure, heart failure, retinopathy, stroke, and encephalopathy. Untreated, half of patients die within 3 months.

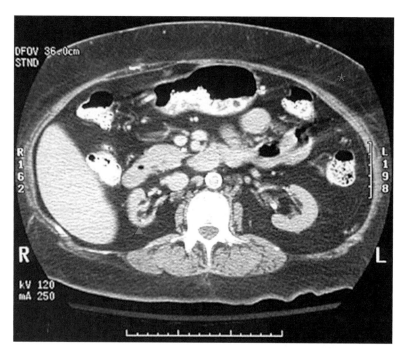

FIGURE 10–83 Nephrosclerosis, CT image

This patient with a body mass index of 34 (note the amount of subcutaneous adipose (∗) tissue seen here) and a long history of poorly controlled diabetes mellitus had decreasing renal function with rising blood urea nitrogen and creatinine. This CT image shows decreased size of both kidneys, although the right kidney (▲) is the smallest. Nephrosclerosis accounted for most of the changes. Patients with vascular disease, whether from arterial or arteriolar nephrosclerosis, can have a similar fate—continuing loss of renal parenchyma. Most causes of chronic renal disease lead to decreased renal size; the exceptions include polycystic kidney disease, amyloidosis, and glomerulosclerosis.

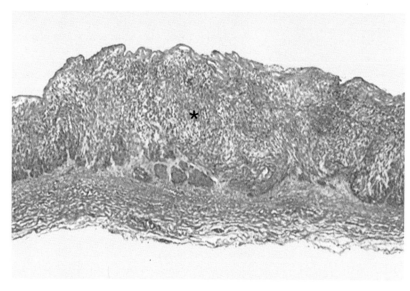

FIGURE 10–84 Fibromuscular dysplasia, microscopic

An uncommon form of vascular obstruction involving medium-sized muscular arteries is produced by fibromuscular dysplasia. In this condition, there are irregular areas of fibrous thickening (∗), mostly involving the media, with an irregular arterial wall and focal luminal narrowing. This process is seen here with trichrome stain at low magnification in a section through carotid artery. However, the renal arteries are most often affected, making this disease one of the surgically correctible causes of hypertension.

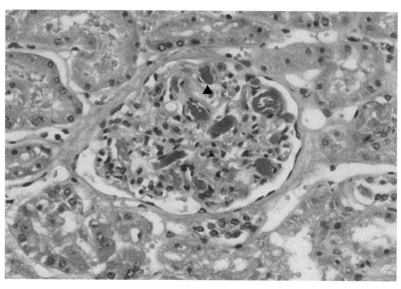

FIGURE 10–85 Thrombotic microangiopathy, microscopic

Platelet-fibrin thrombi (▲) in glomerular capillaries, seen here with trichrome stain, can occur with thrombotic thrombocytopenic purpura (TTP), which mainly affects kidneys, heart, and brain with small arteriolar thrombi. Acute renal failure can occur. Difficult to differentiate from TTP is hemolytic-uremic syndrome (HUS). HUS is a leading cause of acute renal failure in children. Ingestion of foods, such as poorly cooked ground beef, introduces a verotoxin-producing *Escherichia coli* infection into the GI tract. Such strains are often identified by serotyping, typically type O157:H7. A bloody diarrhea is followed in a few days by renal failure caused by endothelial injury from the toxin, leading to the characteristic fibrin thrombi in glomerular and interstitial capillaries. Most patients recover in a few weeks with supportive dialysis.

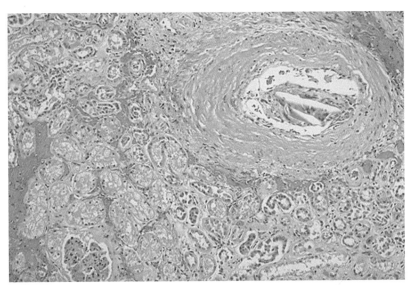

FIGURE 10–86 Atheroembolic renal disease, microscopic

Despite the frequency of aortic atherosclerosis, complications from cholesterol emboli are rare, or at least many such emboli are small and insignificant most of the time. Seen here in a renal artery branch are cholesterol clefts characteristic of such an embolus filling the lumen. This patient had severe ulcerative, friable aortic atheromatous plaques and had undergone angiography, which increases the risk for such emboli. Large numbers of these emboli can compromise renal function. The emboli can produce focal ischemia. Multiple atheroemboli are most likely to be a cause of renal failure in patients with preexisting renal disease.

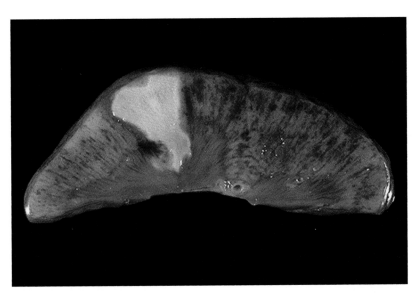

FIGURE 10–87 Renal infarct, gross

Note the wedge shape of this acute infarct, with the pale zone of coagulative necrosis resulting from loss of blood supply with resultant tissue ischemia that progresses to infarction. The small amount of blood from the capsular arteries supplies the immediate subcortical zone, which is spared. The remaining cortex is congested, as is the medulla. Renal infarcts most often occur with emboli that originate from cardiac diseases, such as endocarditis, rheumatic mitral stenosis with left atrial dilation and mural thrombosis, or ischemic heart disease with ventriculomegaly and mural thrombosis. Patients may be asymptomatic, or have costovertebral angle tenderness and hematuria.

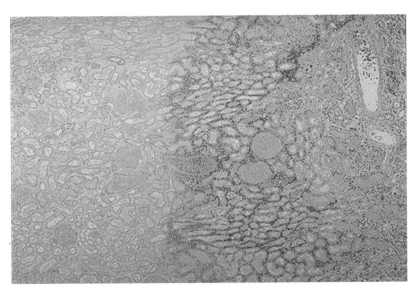

FIGURE 10–88 Renal infarct, microscopic

At the right is normal kidney, then to the left of that hyperemic parenchyma that is becoming necrotic, then to the far left pale pink infarcted kidney in which both tubules and glomeruli have undergone coagulative necrosis, leaving just the cellular outlines of tubules and glomeruli. Renal infarction is most likely a consequence of embolization, although arterial or arteriolar vasculitis may also lead to focal smaller areas of infarction. The renal parenchyma is at increased risk for ischemic injury because there is no collateral blood flow.

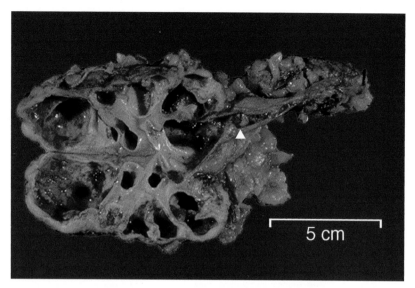

FIGURE 10–89 Obstructive uropathy, gross

Obstruction to the flow of urine in the urinary tract can occur anywhere from the urethral meatus to the kidney calyces. Shown here is a kidney with hydronephrosis, and the cause is a calculus (▲) at the ureteropelvic junction. This kidney demonstrates a marked degree of hydronephrosis with nearly complete loss of cortex. There are many causes of obstruction, including congenital anomalies such as urethral atresia, neoplasms such as transitional cell carcinoma, nodular prostatic hyperplasia, urinary tract calculi, external compression (pregnant uterus), or neurogenic problems such as diabetic neuropathy or spinal cord injury.

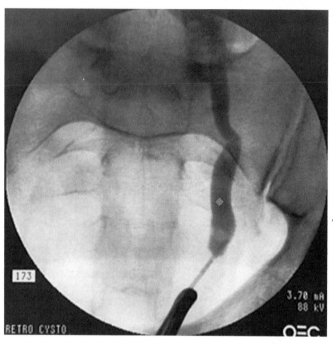

◀ FIGURE 10–90 Obstructive uropathy, radiograph

Injection of contrast into the ureter reveals marked ureteral dilation (◆) consistent with hydroureter from obstruction at the vesicoureteral junction. Most cases of hydronephrosis are clinically silent, although acute obstruction may elicit pain poorly localized to the affected portion of the urinary tract. Initially, urine concentrating ability is lost, followed by reduction in glomerular filtration rate and renal failure.

▼ FIGURES 10–91 and 10–92 Chronic reflux nephropathy, radiograph

The right kidney in the right panel below is decreased in size and demonstrates cortical thinning (◆) with blunted calyces (■) indicative of chronic reflux nephropathy that has led to dilation of the collecting system (*) and overall atrophy. Note that there is compensatory hyperplasia of the unaffected left kidney (×) as seen in this intravenous pyelogram. In the left panel, the right kidney has a less pronounced degree of hydronephrosis.

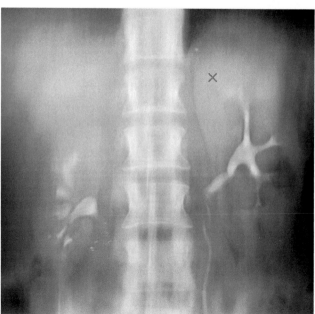

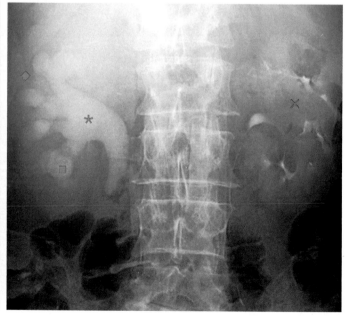

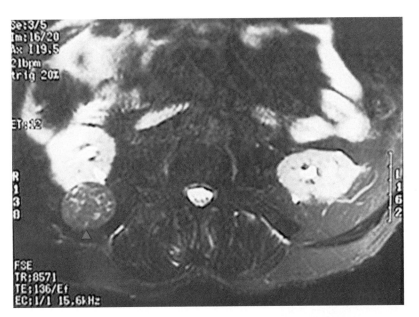

FIGURE 10–93 Renal angiomyolipoma, MRI

This abdominal MRI in axial view demonstrates a rounded, discrete angiomyolipoma (▲) eccentrically positioned in the lower pole of the right kidney, which has bright enhancement. The darker areas of the mass represent the "lipoma" component, while the brighter areas in this neoplasm correspond to vascular tissue (the "angio" component) similar in attenuation to the adjacent normal renal parenchyma with the contrast enhancement. Angiomyolipomas can be multiple and bilateral.

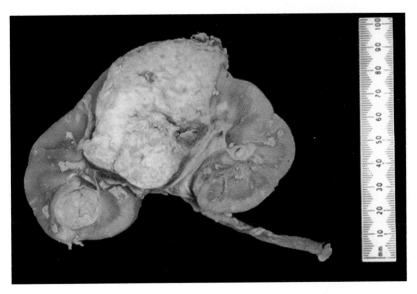

FIGURE 10–94 Angiomyolipoma, gross

This is a rare neoplasm of the kidney. Note that it is solid and has a tan to yellowish tan cut surface. It is also multifocal (a smaller nodule appears in the upper pole. Most of these tumors are incidental findings, but about one fourth to one half of patients with a rare condition known as *tuberous sclerosis* have these tumors. Tuberous sclerosis is an autosomal dominant condition in which mutations of either the *TSC2* or *TSC1* gene lead to formation of hamartomas in brain and other tissues. Other neoplasms include cutaneous angiofibromas and cardiac rhabdomyomas. Otherwise, angiomyolipoma is an uncommon sporadic renal neoplasm.

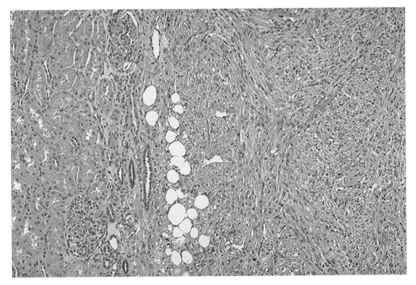

FIGURE 10–95 Renal angiomyolipoma, microscopic

There is normal renal cortical parenchyma with tubules at the left. The tumor has a strip of adipocytes (the "lipoma" part) that blends with interlacing bundles of smooth muscle (the "myo" component) in which are scattered vascular spaces (the "angio" component). These tumor components mimic their non-neoplastic cell counterparts, typical of a benign neoplastic process.

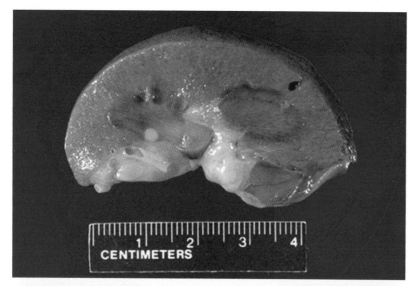

FIGURE 10–96 Renal fibroma, gross

This small round white nodule in the renal medulla is an incidental autopsy finding known as a *medullary fibroma*, also called a *renomedullary interstitial cell tumor*, a designation larger in size than its importance. These lesions generally occur sporadically as a solitary mass 0.5 cm or smaller. They are composed of fibroblast-like cells enmeshed in a collagenous stroma. There are no clinical manifestations.

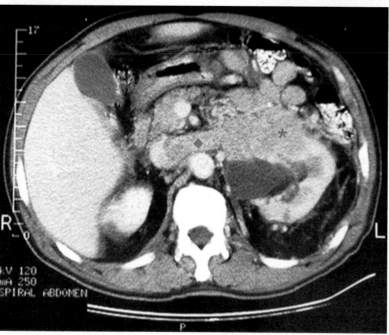

FIGURE 10–97 Renal cell carcinoma, CT image

A renal cell carcinoma (∗) is shown to be invading the left renal vein (◆), distending the vein, and extending into the inferior vena cava (▲). About 85% of primary cancers involving kidneys in adults are renal cell carcinomas. Early signs and symptoms may not be present because the neoplasm has room to grow in the retroperitoneum, but flank pain, a palpable mass, and hematuria are the most common clinical findings. The most important risk factor is tobacco use. Other risks include obesity, unopposed estrogen therapy, and hypertension. However, many cases occur sporadically without an identifiable risk factor. About 4% of cases are familial, occurring with such conditions as von Hippel Lindau (VHL) disease. However, nearly all sporadic renal clear cell carcinomas have a deletion of the *VHL* tumor suppressor gene.

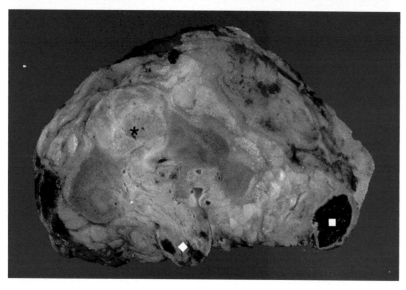

FIGURE 10–98 Renal cell carcinoma, gross

Renal cell carcinomas have a tendency to invade into the renal vein (◆), as shown in a resected kidney surrounded by adipose tissue bounded by Gerota fascia. They may even crawl up the vena cava and into the right heart, but even these can be removed surgically! Here, the tumor (∗) extended up the vena cava and occluded the adrenal vein, leading to hemorrhagic adrenal infarction (■). Renal cell carcinomas may also invade through the renal capsule. Renal cell carcinomas may metastasize to odd locations, they may produce solitary metastases that can successfully be resected without further recurrence, and about one fourth of them first present as metastatic lesions.

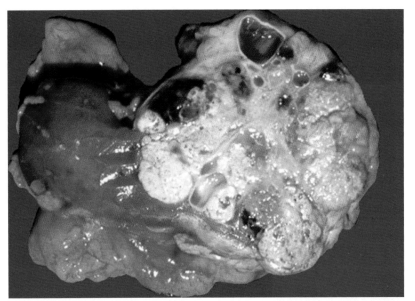

FIGURE 10–99 Renal cell carcinoma, gross

This renal cell carcinoma is arising in the lower pole of the kidney. It is large but still fairly circumscribed, typical for the localized growth pattern for years while the neoplasm remains clinically silent. This cut surface has a variegated appearance with white, yellowish, brown, and hemorrhagic red and cystic areas. Typical presenting signs and symptoms include flank pain and hematuria. Some patients have ongoing constitutional symptoms such as fever. They are uncommon in patients younger than 40 years.

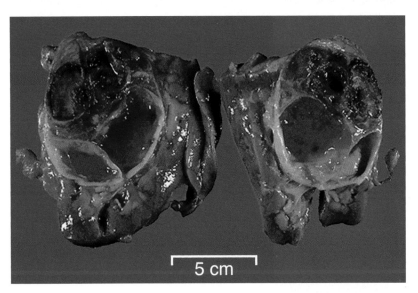

FIGURE 10–100 Renal cell carcinoma, gross

This renal cell carcinoma on sectioning is mainly cystic with extensive hemorrhage. Large simple renal cysts may develop extensive organizing hemorrhage and mimic this appearance. Renal cell carcinomas may also develop in acquired cystic disease with hemodialysis. Renal cell carcinomas can often be associated with various paraneoplastic syndromes, including polycythemia from elaboration of erythropoietin, hypercalcemia with tumor production of parathormone-related peptide, and steroid hormones with Cushing syndrome, feminization, or masculinization.

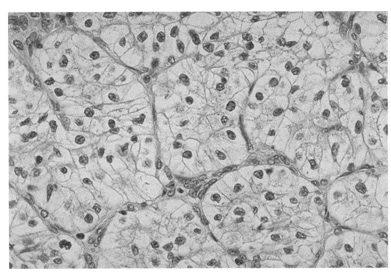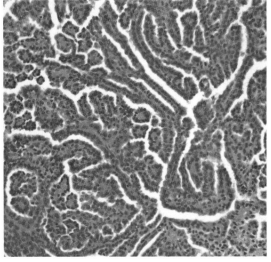

FIGURES 10–101 and 10–102 Renal cell carcinoma, microscopic

In the left panel, the neoplastic cells have abundant clear cytoplasm and are arranged in nests with intervening vessels. About three fourths of renal cell carcinomas have this clear cell pattern. Some will have a papillary pattern as shown at the right, with *MET* proto-oncogene mutations. A rare chromophobe variant has cells with abundant pink cytoplasm resembling the benign renal neoplasm known as oncocytoma.

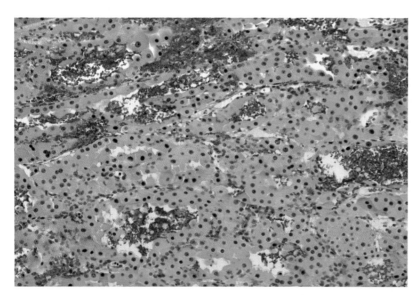

FIGURE 10–103 Oncocytoma, microscopic

An oncocytoma grossly resembles a renal cell carcinoma but tends to have a more uniform tan to brown color. It is thought to arise from intercalated cells of the collecting duct. As shown here, the neoplastic cells are quite uniform in size, with prominent pink cytoplasm. Like other neoplasms with oncocytic differentiation, the cell cytoplasm is seen on electron microscopy to be packed with mitochondria (doing who knows what). This tumor accounts for 5% to 15% of renal parenchymal neoplasms but has a good prognosis because it typically acts in a benign fashion. It is not associated with paraneoplastic syndromes.

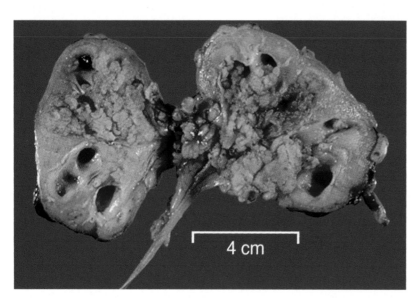

FIGURE 10–104 Urothelial carcinoma, gross

This sagittally sectioned kidney has a multifocal neoplasm arising in the urothelium of the calyceal system and invading into the renal parenchyma. This neoplasm of urothelial origin accounts for about 5% to 10% of renal cancers in adults. Other neoplastic foci may be present in other sites with urothelium, such as ureters and bladder. Hematuria is a frequent presenting symptom, and the onset of hematuria occurs earlier in the course of this tumor than with renal cell carcinoma. However, most urothelial carcinomas are still discovered at a high stage. Like renal cell carcinoma, the major risk factor is smoking.

4 cm

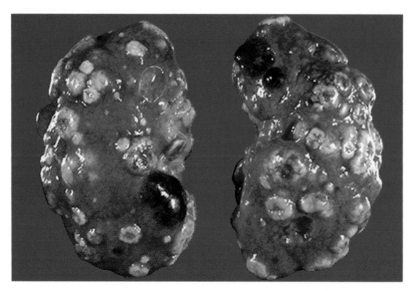

FIGURE 10–105 Renal metastases, gross

These multiple irregular bilateral masses (many of which show central indentations, or "umbilications" from central necrosis) represent metastases of a carcinoma to the kidneys. Some of these metastases have become dark from hemorrhage. The kidneys are not a usual site for metastases, but they can be involved when there are widespread metastases from a primary neoplasm, typically a carcinoma, such as a lung, gastrointestinal tract, or breast primary. The focal nature of the metastases means that there is sufficient residual renal parenchyma to prevent renal failure. Clinical findings of hematuria and flank pain may occur with larger masses.

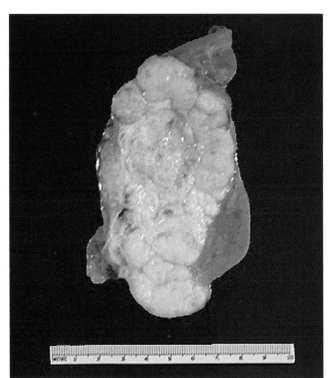

FIGURE 10–106 Wilms tumor, gross

This large circumscribed mass with a lobulated cut surface arose in the kidney of a child. The median age at diagnosis is 3 years. Hypertension due to increased renin activity occurs in 25% of cases. Sixty percent of bilateral and 4% of unilateral Wilms tumors are associated with congenital malformations, including WAGR syndrome (*W*ilms tumor, *a*niridia, *g*enital anomalies, *r*etardation), Beckwith-Wiedemann syndrome (macroglossia, organomegaly, hemihypertrophy, neonatal hypoglycemia, embryonal tumors), and Denys-Drash syndrome (intersexual disorders, nephropathy). This neoplasm is very treatable with an excellent prognosis and higher than 80% cure rate overall.

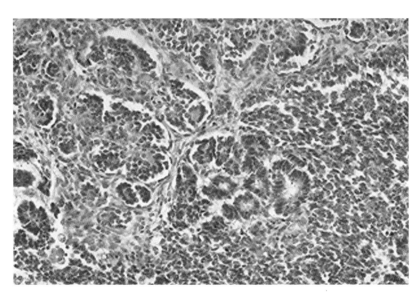

FIGURE 10–107 Wilms tumor, microscopic

Wilms tumor microscopically resembles the primitive nephrogenic zone of the developing fetal kidney, with primitive glomeruloid structures and a cellular stroma. Wilms tumor is associated with tumor suppressor genes: *WT1* is located at chromosome 11p13 and encodes a transcription factor critical to development of normal kidneys and gonads; *WT2* at chromosome 11p15 is linked to Beckwith-Wiedemann syndrome.

CHAPTER 11

The Lower Urinary Tract

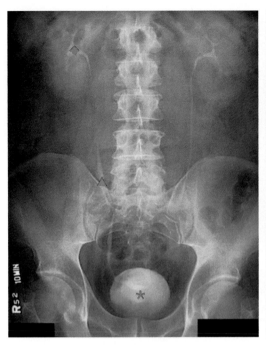

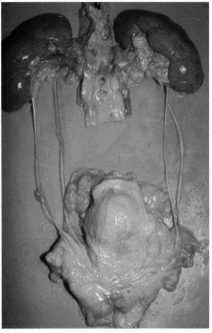

FIGURE 11–1 Urinary tract, x-ray

This intravenous pyelogram shows normal urinary tract, with contrast material that is filling the renal pelves (◆), then the ureters (▲), and finally the bladder (*).

FIGURE 11–2 Double ureters, gross

Two ureters exit from each kidney and extend to a bladder, opened anteriorly. A segment of aorta lies between the normal kidneys. A partial or complete duplication of one or both ureters occurs in 1 in 150 people. There is a potential for urinary obstruction due to abnormal flow of urine and the entrance of two ureters into the bladder in close proximity, but most of the time, this condition is an incidental finding.

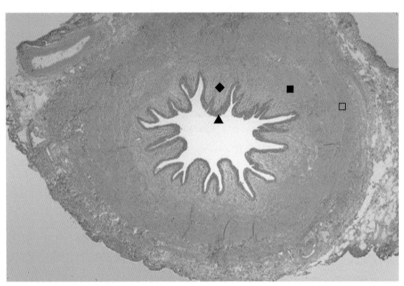

FIGURE 11–3 Normal ureter, microscopic

This normal ureter in cross-section is shown at low magnification, with an inner longitudinal layer (■) and an outer circular layer (□) of smooth muscle (the opposite of the bowel) to supply peristaltic movement of urine down to the bladder from the renal pelvis. There is a urothelium (▲) and underlying lamina propria (◆). Ordinarily, the lumen remains nearly closed since ureters do not store urine. In fact, prolonged stasis of fluids predisposes to infection in the urinary tract.

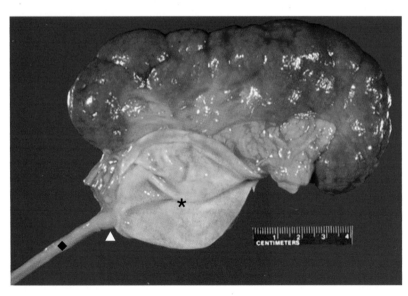

FIGURE 11–4 Ureteropelvic junction stenosis, gross

There is irregular scarring over the cortical surface of this kidney as a consequence of chronic obstruction and development of acute and chronic pyelonephritis. The renal pelvis (*) is markedly dilated, but the ureter (◆) is not, indicating that the point of obstruction is at the ureteropelvic junction (▲). This condition usually presents in childhood and most often affects boys. This is the most common cause of hydronephrosis in infants and children.

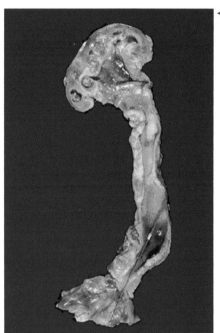

◄ FIGURE 11–5 Hydroureter, gross

A long-standing obstruction (congenital) at the ureteral orifice through which the metal probe passes led to the marked hydroureter and hydronephrosis seen here. This patient had recurrent urinary tract infections complicated by pyelonephritis.

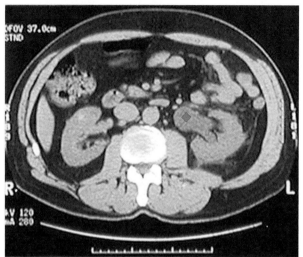

◄ FIGURE 11–6 Hydroureter, CT image

The left ureter (♦) seen near the left renal pelvis in this abdominal CT scan exhibits hydroureter as a consequence of obstruction from the presence of urinary tract calculi.

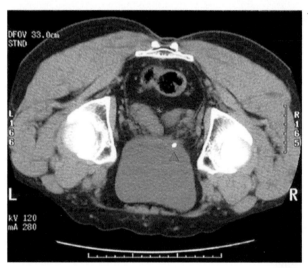

◄ FIGURE 11–7 Ureteral calculus, CT image

The CT scan view seen here is taken in the prone position (the reverse of the usual CT imaging position with the patient supine) and reveals a bright ureteral calculus (▲) at the vesicoureteral junction. Since most urinary tract calculi contain calcium (calcium oxalate or calcium phosphate), they will appear bright with radiographic imaging. Radiolucent stones are likely to be composed of uric acid, and cystine stones are rare.

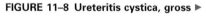

FIGURE 11–8 Ureteritis cystica, gross ►

The small, smooth, glistening bumps seen here over the ureteral mucosa are termed *ureteritis cystica* and represent cystic areas of glandular metaplasia resulting from inflammation, producing cystic nodules from 1 to 5 mm in size. They are more commonly seen in the bladder, where they are called *cystitis cystica*.

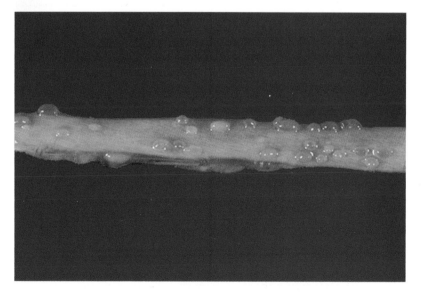

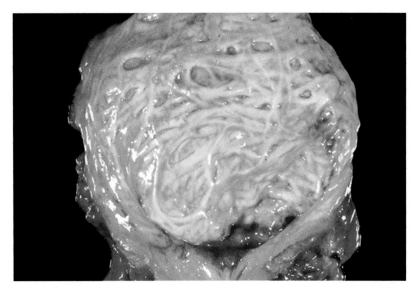

FIGURE 11–9 Urinary bladder, gross

This urinary bladder is opened anteriorly at autopsy and has a normal shape and size, but there is prominent trabeculation seen over the mucosal surface. This is the consequence of bladder muscular hypertrophy from bladder outlet obstruction with nodular prostatic hyperplasia. The outpouchings of mucosa between the muscular trabeculations are "pseudodiverticula," which do not have a complete muscular layer. The stasis from obstruction also predisposes to urinary tract infections because there is incomplete emptying of the bladder with residual urine. The urethral obstruction can also eventually lead to bilateral hydroureter and hydronephrosis.

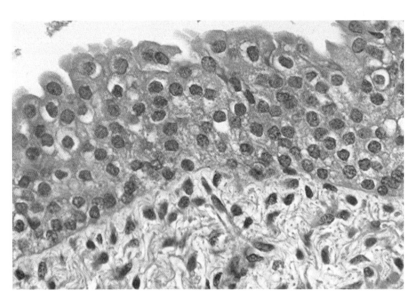

FIGURE 11–10 Normal urinary bladder, microscopic

The appearance at high magnification of normal transitional urothelium with an underlying basement membrane is seen here lining the urinary bladder. The most superficial layer of cells (the "umbrella cell" layer) is quite distensible and provides for bladder filling. The bladder urothelium produces a mucoid secretion with natural antibacterial properties. This feature, along with normal complete emptying of the bladder, helps to prevent urinary tract infections.

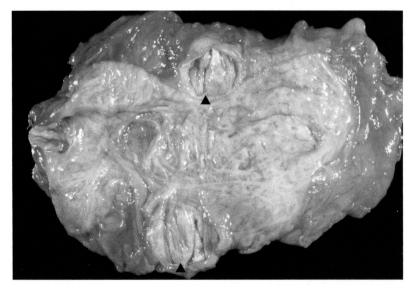

FIGURE 11–11 Urinary bladder diverticulum, gross

There are two diverticula (▲) seen in this urinary bladder, opened anteriorly at autopsy. The urethral outlet is at the left and the dome of the bladder at the right. A diverticulum is a saccular outpouching. Such a lesion of the bladder may be congenital and a "true" diverticulum with a complete muscular layer, as seen here, or it may be acquired with obstruction. A diverticulum represents a region prone to stasis and incomplete emptying that increases the risk for urinary tract infections.

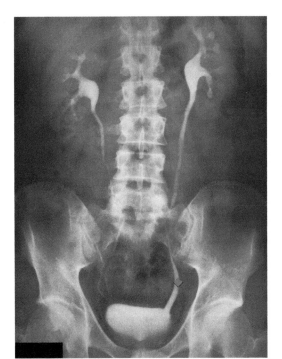

FIGURE 11–12 Vesicoureteral reflux, x-ray

Incompetence of the vesicoureteral valve allows urine to reflux into the ureter, and this predisposes to urinary tract infection, particularly pyelonephritis, from incomplete voiding with residual urine. This intravenous urogram shows dilation of the right ureter (◆), compared with the normal left ureter, in a patient with long-standing vesicoureteral reflux. This condition may be congenital from absence or shortening of the intravesical portion of the ureter, and seen in children, or it may be acquired in adults from loss of bladder innervation after spinal cord injury.

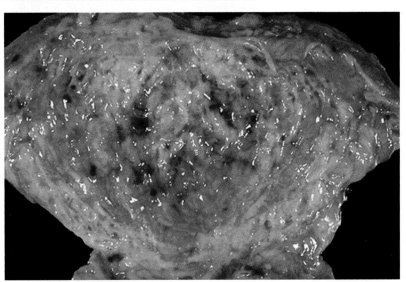

FIGURE 11–13 Cystitis, gross

This bladder has been opened anteriorly at autopsy to reveal mucosal hyperemia with an acute cystitis. This is most likely to result from bacterial infection. The most likely organism is *Escherichia coli*, but *Proteus* and *Klebsiella* species, *Staphylococcus saprophyticus*, enterococci, and group B streptococci may also be implicated. With complicated urinary tract infections (those that are nosocomial or are present with underlying abnormalities such as obstructions, urinary stones, or indwelling catheters), the range of likely causative agents is wider and includes *Pseudomonas aeruginosa*, *Klebsiella* species (including *K. pneumoniae*), *Serratia* species, *E. coli*, and other members of the Enterobacteriaceae family.

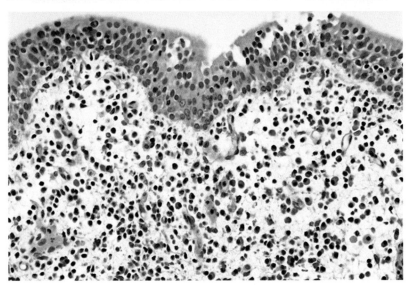

FIGURE 11–14 Cystitis, microscopic

Shown here are increased numbers of inflammatory cells within the submucosa. Urinary tract infections tend to be recurrent, and so episodes of acute cystitis become chronic cystitis with both acute and chronic inflammatory components along with fibrous thickening of the muscularis. The typical clinical findings include increased urinary frequency, suprapubic pain, and dysuria marked by burning or pain on urination. More extensive cases may be marked by fever and malaise. Urinary tract infections are common, particularly in women, in whom the urethra is shorter than in men. Urinary tract obstruction increases the risk for infection.

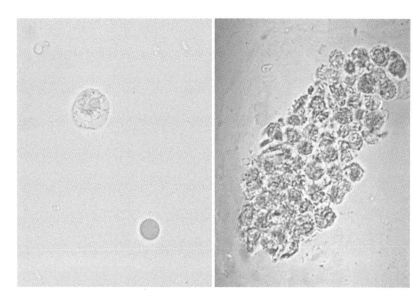

FIGURE 11–15 White blood cells in urine, microscopic

Inflammation of the urinary tract is often accompanied by the presence of leukocytes, typically neutrophils, and usually from urinary tract infection. Most urinary tract infections are caused by bacterial organisms. In addition to infection, calculi, neoplasms, glomerulonephritis, and trauma may also produce inflammation. In the left panel is a white blood cell, along with a red blood cell for comparison of size and morphology. The white blood cell cast seen at the right must form in the distal convoluted tubules or collecting ducts and, therefore, must be due to renal diseases such as glomerulonephritis or interstitial nephritis. Urine dipstick analysis with positive leukocyte esterase suggests that white blood cells are present even if not intact and recognized on microscopic examination.

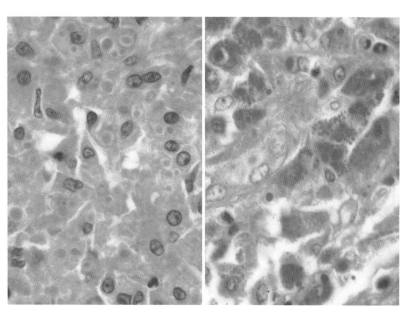

FIGURE 11–16 Malacoplakia, microscopic

Note the rounded Michaelis-Gutmann bodies, which are calcium-containing concretions, within macrophages, seen with H+E in the left panel and with PAS stain in the right panel. Malacoplakia produces grossly visible mucosal plaques on cystoscopy that must be distinguished from carcinoma on biopsy. Malacoplakia is a peculiar inflammatory response to chronic infection, usually with *E. coli* or *Proteus* species. The increased numbers of macrophages suggest phagocytic defects with accumulation of bacterial products.

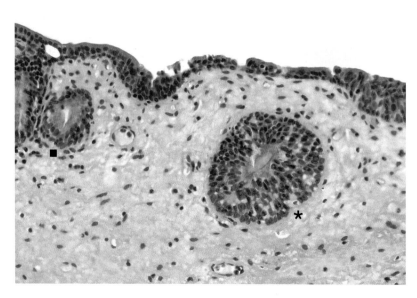

FIGURE 11–17 Cystitis cystica et glandularis, microscopic

Rounded collections of transitional epithelium (Brunn nests) are seen in the lamina propria. The appearance of cystic spaces containing serous fluid within these nests is termed *cystitis cystica*, (∗) and metaplasia in these nests to cuboidal or columnar epithelium is termed *cystitis glandularis* (■). Since both often coexist, the term *cystitis cystica et glandularis* applies. This is a common incidental finding in adults, and since the cysts can range from 0.1 to 1 cm in size, they form a nodule that is resected for biopsy during cystoscopy when carcinoma is suspected; however, they do not carry a risk for malignancy.

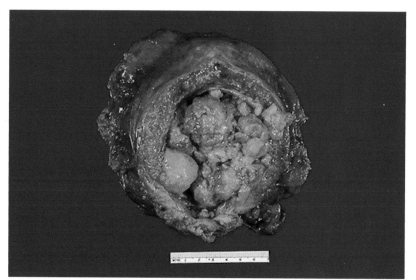

FIGURE 11–18 Urothelial carcinoma, gross

This bladder was removed surgically from a man who had a history of cigarette smoking. He had hematuria. This opened bladder reveals numerous masses of a urothelial carcinoma, which can arise anywhere in the urothelium but is most common in the urinary bladder. Urothelial carcinoma is often multifocal and has a tendency to recur. In addition to smoking, risk factors include exposure to arylamine compounds (such as 2-naphthylamine), chronic infection with *Schistosoma haematobium*, analgesic abuse, extensive exposure to cyclophosphamide, and prior radiation therapy.

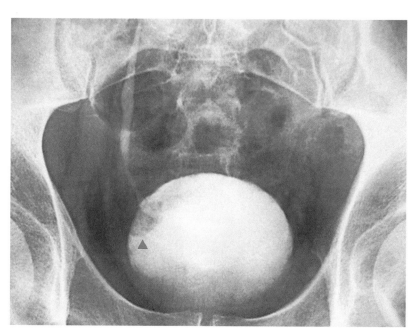

FIGURE 11–19 Urothelial carcinoma, radiograph

This intravenous pyelogram shows a neoplasm (▲) near the right ureteral orifice that produces a filling defect in the urinary bladder. Urothelial carcinoma occurs when there are genetic alterations of tumor suppressor genes, typically 9p deletions (9p21) involving the tumor suppressor gene *p16INK4a,* which encodes an inhibitor of a cyclin-dependent kinase, that are seen in papillary tumors. Other mutations involve the *p53* gene, most often with carcinoma *in situ* (CIS), and *RB* gene, particularly when invasive lesions are present. Once a urothelial carcinoma has been treated, the patient must be followed with periodic cytologic examination of urine for atypical cells and subsequent cystoscopic examination, because of the risk for subsequent multifocal development of additional urothelial carcinomas.

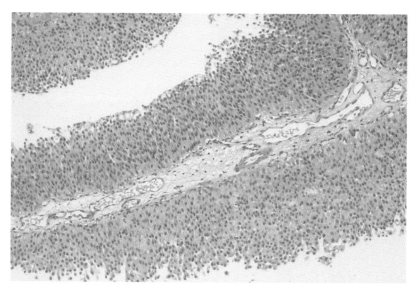

FIGURE 11–20 Urothelial carcinoma, microscopic

Note the finger-like projection of this papillary frond with a fibrovascular core covered by a very thick, disorganized layer of neoplastic transitional cells having marked atypia. Urothelial carcinomas arising from papillary lesions tend to be exophytic and noninvasive. However, CIS gives rise to a "flat" urothelial carcinoma more prone to invasion. The grade and stage determine prognosis. Invasion into the muscularis means that control of the tumor is unlikely to be achieved with local excision alone, and a cystectomy is performed.

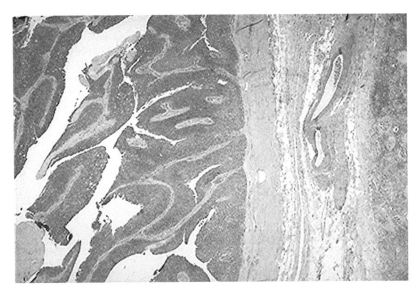

FIGURE 11–21 Urothelial carcinoma, microscopic

The urothelial carcinoma of the urinary bladder shown here at low magnification reveals the frondlike papillary projections of the tumor above the surface extending to the left. It is differentiated enough to resemble urothelium, but is still irregular, with hyperchromatic cells, and is best described as grade 2 (on a scale of 1 to 3). No invasion to the right is seen at this point.

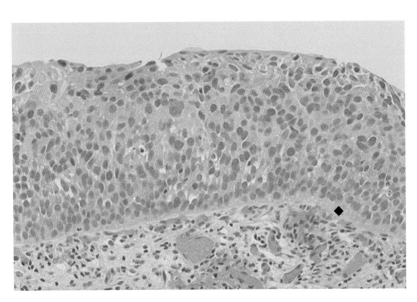

FIGURE 11–22 Urothelial carcinoma, microscopic

This is a urothelial CIS. Note that the atypical cells form a disorganized epithelial layer that occupies the full thickness of the urothelium but does not invade through the basement membrane (◆). However, for the urothelium, *any* malignant cells above the basement membrane qualify as CIS. CIS is often asymptomatic. On cystoscopic examination, it may appear only as a flat area of erythema or granularity. It is often multifocal.

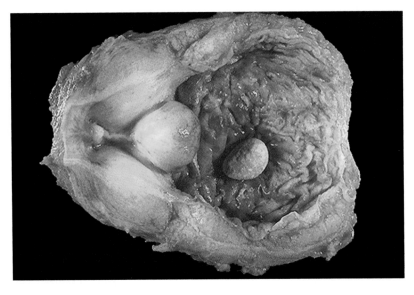

FIGURE 11–23 Bladder outlet obstruction, gross

The markedly enlarged prostate seen here at the left has not only large lateral lobes but also a very large median lobe that obstructed the prostatic urethra and led to chronic urinary tract obstruction. As a result, the bladder became both enlarged and hypertrophied because it had to work against the obstruction with every episode of urination. That is why the surface of the bladder appears trabeculated. Note also the present of another cause for obstruction—a yellowish brown calculus. Obstruction increases the risk for urinary tract infection. Hydroureter and hydronephrosis may occur as well.

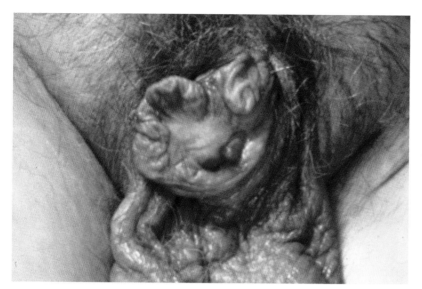

FIGURE 11–24 Urethral caruncle, gross

Note the small rounded red nodule at the urethral orifice. These inflammatory lesions can reach 1 to 2 cm in size. Since they are on the lower abdominal surface, they are easily traumatized, producing pain and bleeding. Caruncles are rare but occur more commonly in adults than children. Note that in the case shown, there is severe hypospadias of the penis, which probably potentiated the inflammation leading to caruncle formation.

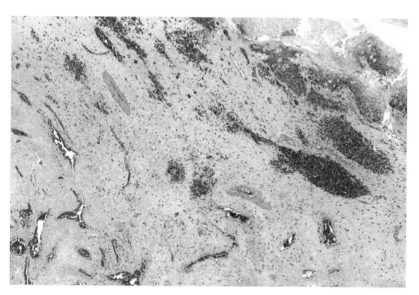

FIGURE 11–25 Urethral caruncle, microscopic

The caruncle is composed of tissue resembling granulation tissue, with multiple vascular channels in a collagenous stroma. In this case, the overlying epithelium is squamous, but it can also be transitional. Scattered inflammatory cells are present. Caruncles are treated by surgical excision.

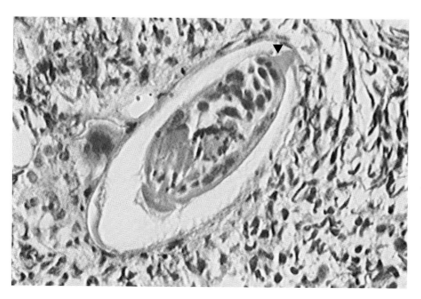

FIGURE 11–26 Schistosomiasis, microscopic

Here in the urinary bladder wall is a *Schistosoma haematobium* egg with a terminal spine (▼) at high magnification. Schistosomes are spread by host snail species through water, with infectious cercariae penetrating human skin. The adult worms of *S. haematobium* reside in pelvic veins, releasing eggs that cut into the bladder and produce chronic to granulomatous inflammation, leading to fibrosis with obstructive uropathy and risk for squamous cell carcinoma. The *Schistosoma mansoni* and *japonicum* species adults inhabit the portal venous system, releasing eggs that travel to liver and induce fibrosing granulomatous inflammation, resulting in portal hypertension.

CHAPTER 12

The Male Genital Tract

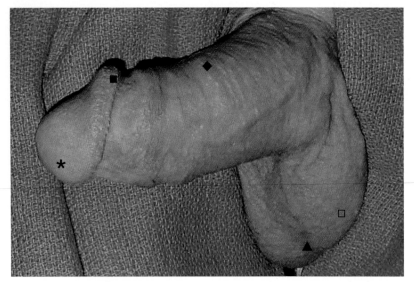

FIGURE 12–1 Normal external genitalia, gross

The normal appearance of the external male genitalia is shown here. Note the glans (∗) and prepuce (■) (mucosal surfaces) but no foreskin in this circumcised penis. The shaft (◆) of the penis is covered by stratified squamous epithelium, as is the scrotum (□), with median (▲) raphe.

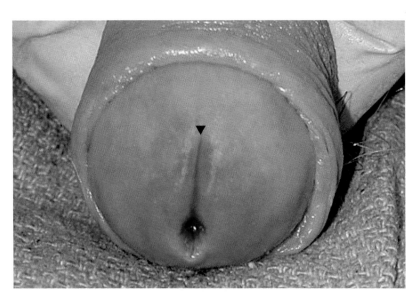

FIGURE 12–2 Epispadias, gross

This groove (▼) on the dorsal aspect of the penis extending for a short distance upward from the urethral meatus is an abnormality termed *epispadias*. This is an uncommon anomaly of varying degrees of severity. This one is not severe. However, when severe and extensive along the dorsum of the penis, it can lead to problems with urination and ejaculation. The opening may be partially constricted, predisposing to urinary tract infections. The foreskin of this uncircumcised penis is retracted here. This anomaly may be associated with other urinary tract anomalies and may also be present along with cryptorchidism.

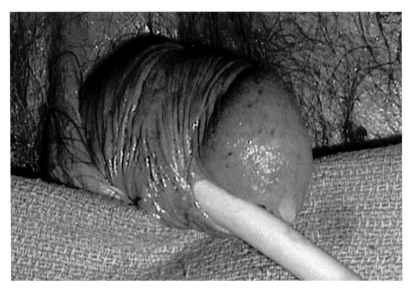

FIGURE 12–3 Hypospadias, gross

The urinary catheter seen here lies in a groove on the undersurface below the tip of the penis and enters the urethra. This abnormal opening is known as a *hypospadias*. Such an anomaly is present in about 1 in 300 male live births, but it can lead to problems with urination and ejaculation. Constriction of the opening may be present, increasing the risk for urinary tract infections.

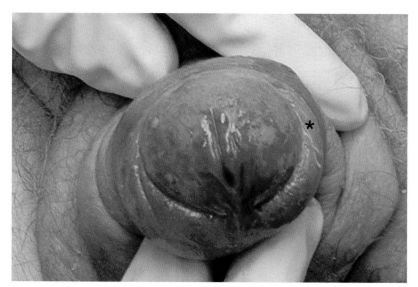

FIGURE 12–4 Balanoposthitis, gross

This glans penis surrounding the penile urethral meatus demonstrates erythema and focal tan exudate, typical of a balanitis. The retracted foreskin (*) is also acutely inflamed, a condition called *posthitis*. Together, this inflammatory condition is known as *balanoposthitis*. Infectious agents driving this process include *Candida albicans*, *Gardnerella* species, and pyogenic bacteria such as *Staphylococcus aureus*. Accumulated smegma (consisting of desquamated squamous epithelial cells and debris) beneath the foreskin predisposes to infection. Persistence of this inflammatory process predisposes to phimosis, a condition in which the prepuce cannot be retracted.

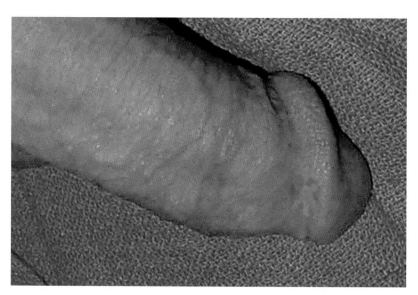

FIGURE 12–5 Bowen disease, gross

Carcinoma in situ (CIS) of the external male genitalia is termed *Bowen disease* when there is a plaquelike lesion. This process is initially painless, but larger lesions may have erythema, ulceration, or crusting. The term *erythroplasia of Queyrat* is reserved for CIS of mucosal surfaces (glans or prepuce). Bowenoid papulosis appears in younger patients as multiple reddish brown papular lesions. Microscopically, all these lesions have dysplastic squamous cells involving the full epithelial thickness without invasion through the basement membrane. Eventually, invasive squamous cell carcinoma occurs in about 10% of cases.

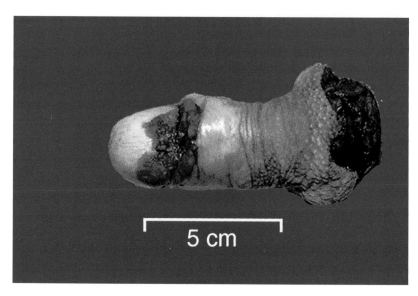

FIGURE 12–6 Squamous cell carcinoma, gross

In this penectomy specimen is a large invasive carcinoma that arose in the region of the head of an uncircumcised penis. The neoplasm is reddish tan and nodular, with an ulcerated surface. Such lesions are strongly associated with human papillomavirus (HPV) infection, particularly types 16 and 18. Other factors, such as a history of smoking and lack of circumcision, are also implicated. Most patients with this disease are older than 40 years. When metastases occur, local inguinal and iliac lymph nodes are most often involved. Denial and fear on the part of the patient may delay treatment.

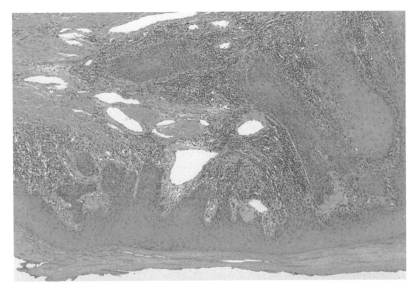

FIGURE 12–7 Squamous cell carcinoma, microscopic

There are tongues of well-differentiated invasive carcinoma extending into the penile corpora cavernosum, with inflammatory cell infiltrates. Like cervical cancer in women, penile carcinoma is most often correlated with HPV infection, and the same types (16 and 18) are the most aggressive. Phimosis with increased accumulation of smegma is another risk factor, and the incidence of penile cancer is rare in circumcised males. Initial metastases occur most often to iliac and inguinal lymph nodes.

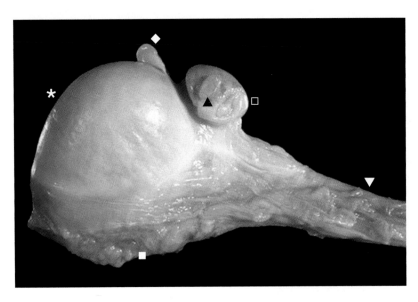

FIGURE 12–8 Normal testis, gross

Here is a normal testis and adjacent structures, including the body of the testis (*), epididymis (□), and spermatic cord (▼). Note the presence of two vestigial structures, the appendix testis (◆) and the appendix epididymis (▲). The pampiniform plexus of veins (■) lies posterior to the body of the testis. The normal testis descends down into the lower abdomen under the influence of müllerian-inhibiting substance. Final descent into the scrotum in the third trimester of fetal development is under the influence of increasing androgens. Failure to normally descend results in cryptorchidism. The Leydig cells of a cryptorchid testis function normally, but the increased body temperature diminishes spermatogenesis.

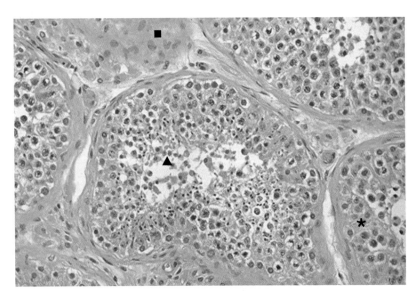

FIGURE 12–9 Normal testis, microscopic

These seminiferous tubules contain numerous germ cells (*). Sertoli (or "nurse") cells are inconspicuous because their attenuated cytoplasm interdigitates with the germ cells. Small dark oblong spermatozoa are seen in the center of the tubules because there is active spermatogenesis. The normal sperm count is 80 to 150 million/mL of ejaculate. Small nodular collections of pink Leydig cells (■) are seen in the interstitium between the tubules, secreting testosterone under the influence of luteinizing hormone. Note the pale golden brown pigment in the interstitium that gives the testicular parenchyma its grossly pale brown color. Sertoli cells secrete inhibin that feeds back on the adenohypophysis to inhibit release of follicle-stimulating hormone, which drives spermatogenesis.

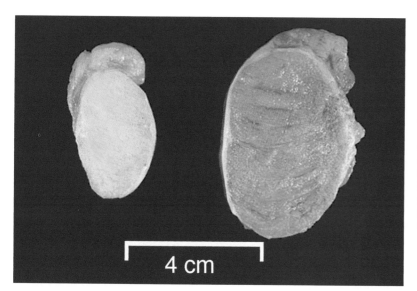

FIGURE 12-10 Cryptorchidism, gross

The testis seen on the left is atrophic, appearing small and pale white, while the opposite testis appears normal. This left testis did not descend into the scrotum during fetal development, but remained in the abdomen, a condition known as *cryptorchidism*, which is unilateral in 75% of cases. There may also be an inguinal hernia. Leydig cell function remains normal. Such a cryptorchid testis fails to develop normal spermatogenesis unless placed in the scrotum by the age of 5 because deterioration begins by age 2. If unilateral, spermatogenesis in the remaining normal testis may prevent infertility. However, cryptorchidism carries an increased risk for testicular carcinoma in either testis.

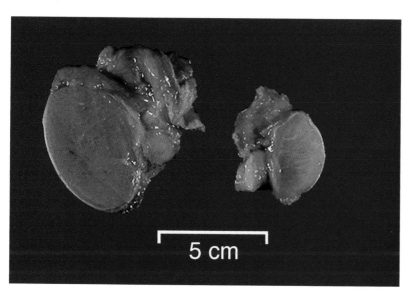

FIGURE 12-11 Testis, atrophy, gross

Seen on the left is a normal testis, but the contralateral testis has undergone atrophy. Bilateral atrophy may occur with a variety of conditions, including chronic alcoholism, hypopituitarism, atherosclerosis, chemotherapy or radiation therapy, and severe prolonged illness. A cryptorchid testis will also become atrophic. Inflammation with orchitis may lead to atrophy. Mumps, the most common infectious cause of orchitis, usually has a patchy and bilateral pattern of involvement that decreases the sperm count but does not usually lead to sterility. Bilateral testicular atrophy may accompany Klinefelter syndrome (47, XXY karyotype). Testicular enlargement may occur with fragile X syndrome.

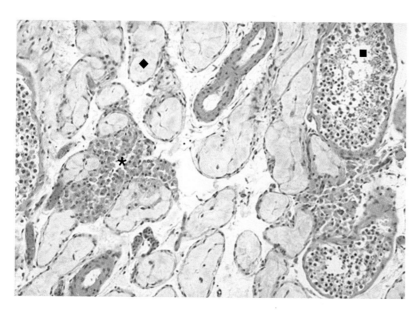

FIGURE 12-12 Testis, atrophy, microscopic

Here is focal atrophy (◆) of seminiferous tubules along with normal Leydig cells (*) and residual normal tubules (■) with active spermatogenesis. Mumps virus infection may be complicated by orchitis in one fourth to one third of cases. In general, the orchitis is unilateral and patchy, so that sterility following infection is uncommon. Other infectious causes of orchitis may include echovirus, lymphocytic choriomeningitis virus, influenza virus, Coxsackie virus, and arboviruses. In contrast, epididymitis is a more frequent cause of scrotal pain and swelling in adult males and is most likely to be the result of a sexually transmissible disease such as *Chlamydia trachomatis* or *Neisseria gonorrhoeae* in younger men or gram-negative bacteria from urinary tract infection in older men.

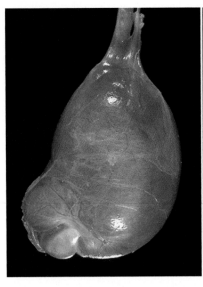 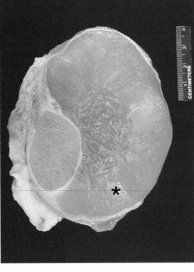

FIGURE 12–13 Hydrocele, gross

Hydroceles are fairly common accumulations of clear fluid within the sac of tunica vaginalis, which is lined by a serosa. It may occur in older men from a variety of inflammatory and neoplastic conditions. The external appearance of a testis with a hydrocele removed from the scrotum at autopsy is seen in the left panel. A cross-section through a frozen hydrocele (∗) removed at autopsy in the right panel shows the relationship of the fluid to the testis. The fluid in a hydrocele is a transudate that accumulates slowly but can produce a mass effect and local discomfort. In many cases, the cause is not determined.

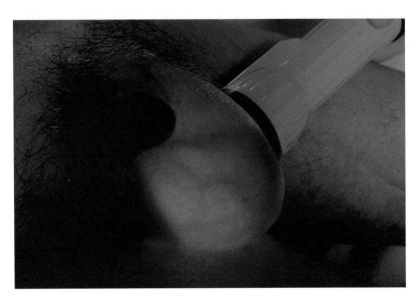

FIGURE 12–14 Hydrocele, gross

One diagnostic technique to detect a hydrocele is transillumination of the fluid-filled space with a light applied to the scrotum. The fluid will transmit the light, while a solid mass will not. This effect shown here resembles a lunar eclipse. A hydrocele must be distinguished from a true testicular mass, and transillumination may help because the hydrocele will transilluminate, but a testicular mass will be opaque to the light. Ultrasound scanning provides a simple, noninvasive way of diagnosing scrotal masses.

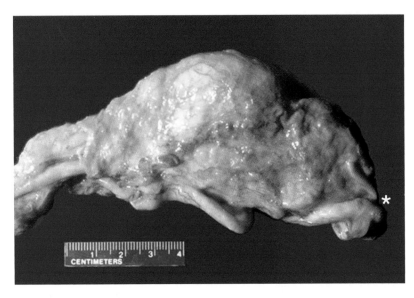

FIGURE 12–15 Testis, varicocele, gross

A common cause of male infertility is a varicocele, a lesion that consists of prominent dilation of the pampiniform plexus of veins (∗) posterior to the testis. The increased blood flow makes this lesion a radiant heat device that raises the temperature of testicular tubules, thus inhibiting normal spermatogenesis.

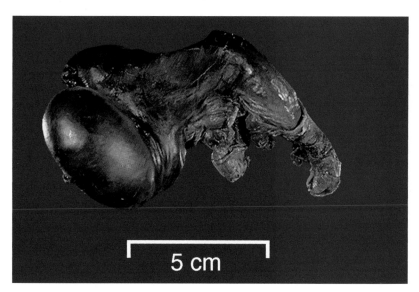

FIGURE 12–16 Testicular torsion, gross

This testis has undergone hemorrhagic infarction after torsion, which is an uncommon condition, but a medical emergency. It occurs when sudden twisting of the spermatic cord cuts off the venous drainage, leading to hemorrhagic infarction. Torsion in adolescents often occurs when there is greater mobility from abnormal incomplete testicular descent or lack of a scrotal ligament. Perinatal torsion occurs rarely and for no apparent reason. Immediate treatment by surgically untwisting and suturing the cord in place to prevent future torsion will prevent infarction and loss of function. Sometimes, just the little appendix testis undergoes torsion to produce acute pain.

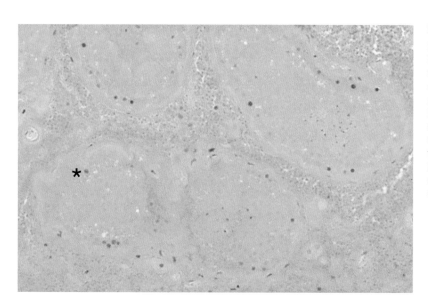

FIGURE 12–17 Testicular torsion, microscopic

In this case, torsion of the testis has proceeded to hemorrhagic infarction with no viable cells within the seminiferous tubules. Note the pale outlines of the residual tubules (∗), but there is loss of nuclear detail, and the interstitium is hemorrhagic. The most common signs and symptoms include a red, swollen scrotum and acutely painful testicle without evidence of trauma. Nausea and vomiting are common. Doppler ultrasound scan be helpful in demonstrating lack of blood flow, confirming the diagnosis.

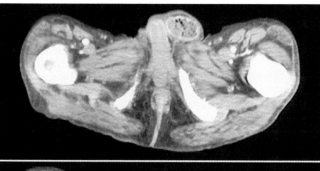
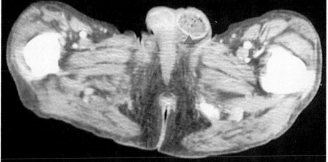

FIGURE 12–18 Inguinal hernia, CT image

These pelvic CT scan views demonstrate a loop of bowel (▲) extending into the scrotum because of a large indirect inguinal hernia. On physical examination, there is a bulging of the scrotum from the loop of bowel that has gone through a hernia in the inguinal region, and bowel sounds may be present on auscultation of this region as well. The bowel may become incarcerated (trapped) within the hernia sac and cause bowel obstruction, or the blood supply to this loop of bowel may become compromised (strangulated), leading to intestinal infarction. Surgical intervention is required when bowel obstruction or ischemia occurs, and surgical repair of the abdominal wall is undertaken to prevent such occurrences.

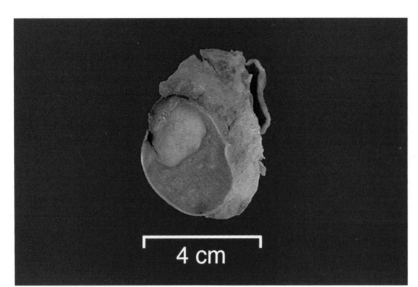

FIGURE 12–19 Seminoma, gross

Germ cell neoplasms are the most common forms of testicular neoplasia. The peak incidence is in the 15- to 34-year age range. They may be a "mixed germ cell tumor" and have more than one histologic component: seminoma, embryonal carcinoma, yolk sac tumor, teratoma, or choriocarcinoma. The germ cell tumor most likely to be a single histologic type is seminoma, shown here as a uniform solid tan mass within the body of the testis. Such a small neoplasm may not increase the size of the testis, but it may be detectable with ultrasonography. Most testicular germ cell tumors arise from a focus of intratubular germ cell neoplasia.

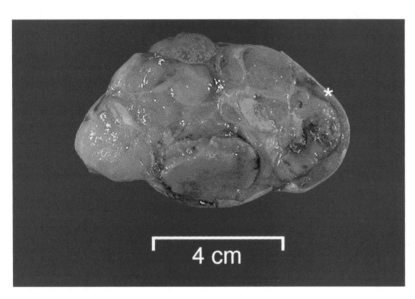

FIGURE 12–20 Seminoma, gross

A small rim (∗) of remaining normal testis appears at the far right. This tumor is composed of lobulated soft tan to brown tissue. At least 95% of testicular neoplasms are germ cell tumors. Half of germ cell tumors are seminomas, which have a uniform lobulated tan to brown appearance as shown. The size this neoplasm attained before treatment demonstrates the factors of fear and denial that occur in many patients, delaying detection and therapy. An i(12p) karyotypic abnormality is found in virtually all testicular germ cell (and ovarian germ cell) neoplasms. Female patients with the androgen insensitivity syndrome ("testicular feminization") are at increased risk for development of seminoma.

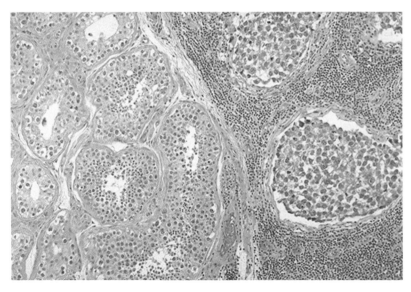

FIGURE 12–21 Seminoma, microscopic

Normal testis appears at the left, and seminoma is present at the right. Note the difference in size and staining quality of the nests of neoplastic cells compared with normal germ cells in seminiferous tubules. The large seminoma cells have vesicular nuclei and pale watery cytoplasm. Lobules of neoplastic cells have an intervening stroma with characteristic T-cell lymphoid infiltrates. This "classic" form of seminoma constitutes 90% of all seminomas, with cells demonstrating positive immunohistochemical staining for human placental lactogen (HPL) but not human chorionic gonadotropin (HCG) or α-fetoprotein (AFP). Occasional syncytial cells may be hCG positive. Many of these seminomas are sensitive to radiation and chemotherapy, with a good prognosis.

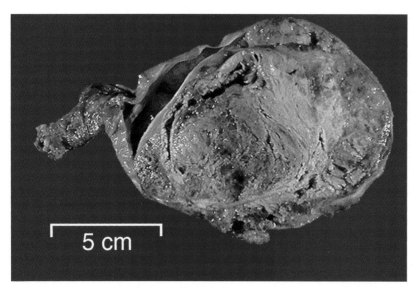

FIGURE 12–22 Embryonal carcinoma, gross

This tumor is soft and much more variegated than the seminoma, with red to tan to brown areas, including prominent foci of hemorrhage and necrosis. There are a few scattered firmer white areas that histologically proved to be teratoma. Thus, this testicular neoplasm is mixed embryonal carcinoma plus teratoma (sometimes called *teratocarcinoma*) or mixed germ cell tumor of the testis. Embryonal carcinoma is the second most common testicular tumor and is more aggressive than seminoma. While most seminomas are stage I at the time of diagnosis, nonseminomatous germ cell tumors, such as embryonal carcinoma, are more likely to be stage II or III at the time of detection.

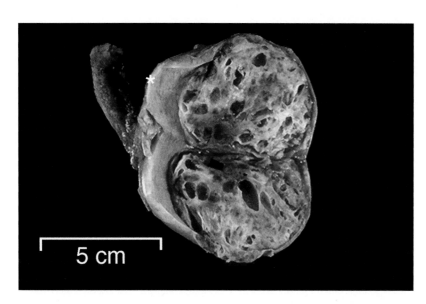

FIGURE 12–23 Embryonal carcinoma and teratoma, gross

Here is an embryonal carcinoma mixed with teratoma in which islands of bluish white cartilage from the teratoma component are present. A rim (∗) of normal pale brown testis appears at the left of the tumor. From a clinical standpoint, it is most useful to know whether nonseminomatous germ cell elements are present because this determines a more aggressive course. Purely seminomatous neoplasms are more likely to be at a low stage at diagnosis, remain localized longer, and be more amenable to chemotherapy and radiation. The *OCT3/4* gene produces a transcription factor in both seminomas and embryonal carcinomas.

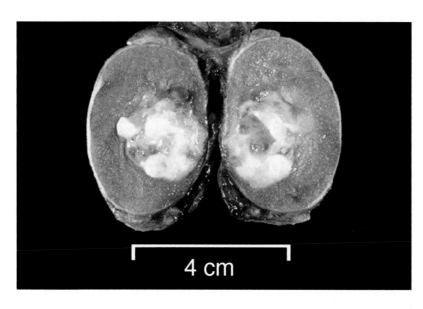

FIGURE 12–24 Teratoma, gross

This small testicular neoplasm has a mixture of bluish cartilage with red and white tumor tissue. This neoplasm microscopically contained mainly teratoma, but areas of embryonal carcinoma were also present. Overall, about 60% of all testicular neoplasms are composed of more than one element. These are "mixed" germ cell tumors. Although rare in children (second in frequency to yolk sac tumor), testicular teratomas at this pediatric age are likely to act in a benign fashion. Germ cell tumors of the testis tend to metastasize first to para-aortic lymph nodes, but hematogenous spread to lungs and other sites occurs. Metastases may have different microscopic germ cell tumor components than the primary.

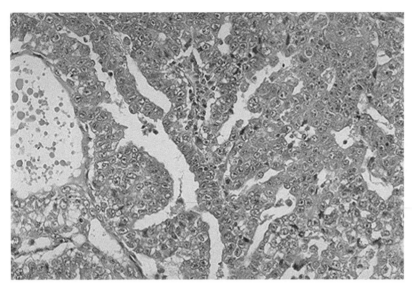

FIGURE 12–25 Embryonal carcinoma, microscopic

The neoplastic cells of this embryonal carcinoma appear more primitive than the seminoma. Sheets of large pale blue cells with indistinct borders are trying to form primitive tubules. Occasional syncytial cells may stain positively for HCG, and some cells with yolk sac differentiation will be positive for AFP. Both hCG and AFP may be elevated in the serum of patients with testicular germ cell tumors.

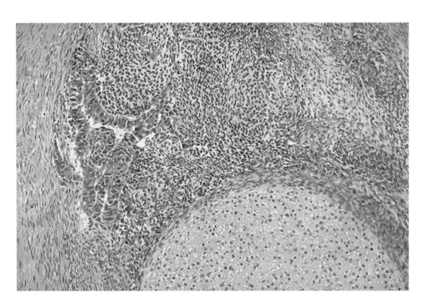

FIGURE 12–26 Embryonal carcinoma and teratoma, microscopic

At the bottom is a focus of primitive but benign-appearing cartilage, representing a teratoma component of a mixed germ cell neoplasm. Above this is a primitive mesenchymal stroma and to the left a focus of primitive cells most characteristic of embryonal carcinoma. This is embryonal carcinoma mixed with teratoma.

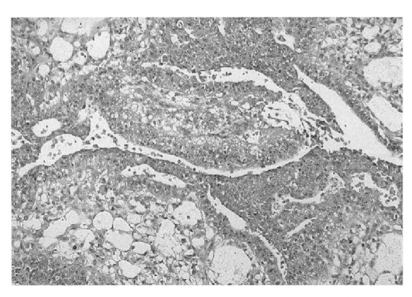

FIGURE 12–27 Yolk sac tumor, microscopic

The endodermal sinus tumor (yolk sac tumor, or infantile embryonal carcinoma) of the testis shown is composed of primitive germ cells that form glomeruloid or embryonal-like structures (Schiller-Duval bodies). These tumors are most frequent in children younger than 3 years, but overall they are a rare type of germ cell neoplasm. The prognosis for most patients is good. The cells of this tumor produce AFP, which can be detected in the serum as a tumor marker. An element of yolk sac differentiation is often present in embryonal carcinomas, so that AFP is often detected in patients with embryonal carcinoma.

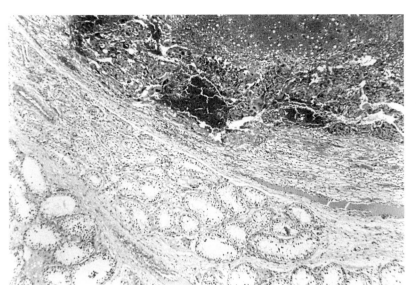

FIGURE 12–28 Choriocarcinoma, microscopic

Pure testicular choriocarcinomas are rare. The primary site in the testis is often small at the time of detection because they are aggressive and metastasize early. Some cases may exhibit the phenomenon of the "disappearing primary" tumor, when the rapidly growing tumor outgrows its blood supply and infarcts with hemorrhage and necrosis, eventually leaving only a small scar, although the metastases continue to grow. Both syncytiotrophoblastic cells (positive for hCG) and cytotrophoblastic cells are present. Shown here is the tumor with large bizarre cells and extensive hemorrhage and necrosis, with uninvolved testis below and to the left.

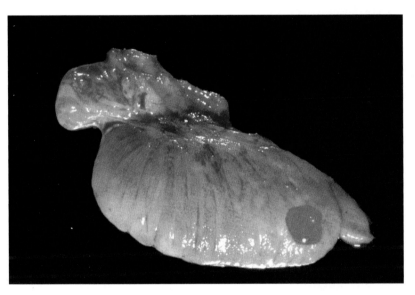

FIGURE 12–29 Leydig cell tumor, gross

The cut surface of this normal-sized adult testis reveals a small discrete brown mass. Most of these interstitial (Leydig) cell tumors arise in men 20 to 60 years of age. They may elaborate androgens, estrogens, or other steroid hormones such as glucocorticoids. Although often less than 1 cm in diameter, some may reach several centimeters in size, enough to produce palpable testicular enlargement. Significant hormone production may lead to gynecomastia in adults. In prepubertal children, such a neoplasm could be a cause of sexual precocity.

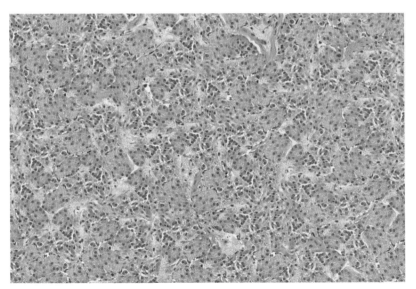

FIGURE 12–30 Leydig cell tumor, microscopic

The small round cells of this tumor are found in nests or clusters, and there are many intervening capillaries, typical of endocrine tissue. A distinctive electron microscopic feature is the cytoplasmic rod-shaped crystalloid of Reinke. About 10% of these neoplasms act in an aggressive fashion, with local invasion or metastases. However, most, like the one shown here, are benign.

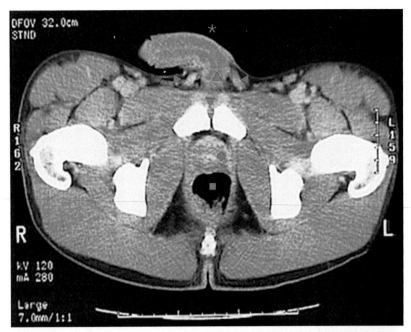

FIGURE 12–31 Normal prostate, CT image

This pelvic CT scan shows the normal penis (∗) and penile urethra (▲), right spermatic cord (▶), left spermatic cord (◀), pubic symphysis (▼), prostate (◆), and rectum (■). The prostate lies below the bladder, and the prostatic portion of the urethra traverses the prostate gland. The prostate is derived embryologically from epithelial evaginations along the urethra. There is little increase in size of the prostate until puberty when, under the influence of testosterone, growth and differentiation occur. The enzyme 5α-reductase in nuclei of prostatic cells converts testosterone produced by Leydig cells of the testes to dihydrotestosterone (DHT), which promotes prostatic growth.

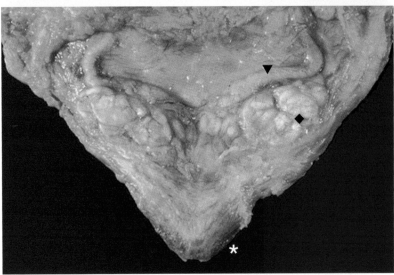

FIGURE 12–32 Normal prostate, gross

The normal prostate (∗) is seen here from a posterior view. Anterior to the rectum and posterior and superior to the prostate are the paired seminal vesicles (◆) that produce about 70% of the secretions constituting seminal fluid. The vas deferens (▼) from each testis is seen to extend to the prostate as well. The seminal vesicles are rarely a site at which pathologic lesions arise. They can on occasion be infiltrated by carcinomas from surrounding organs such as the prostate.

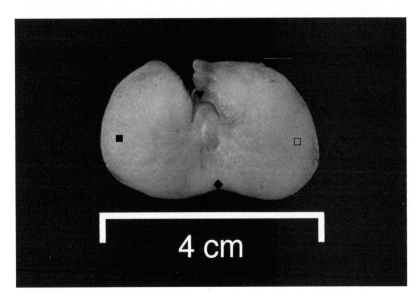

FIGURE 12–33 Normal prostate, gross

This is a transverse (axial) section through a normal prostate. There is a central urethra (▼) at the depth of the cut made to open this prostate anteriorly at autopsy, with the left lateral lobe (■) and the right lateral lobe (□) and the posterior lobe (◆). The consistency is uniform, without nodularity. The normal prostate is 3 to 4 cm in diameter and weighs 20 to 30 gm. About 75% of the prostate is composed of the peripheral zone, or what is traditionally described as lateral and posterior lobes. The small anterior zone contains mostly fibromuscular stroma. The central zone lies between the ejaculatory ducts. A transitional zone lies anterior to the central zone around the internal urethral sphincter.

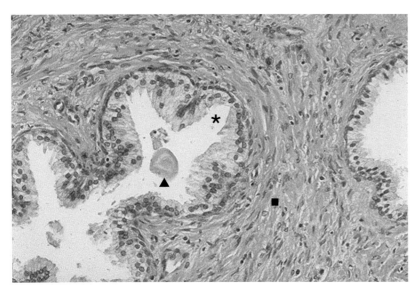

FIGURE 12–34 Normal prostate, microscopic

The normal histologic appearance of prostate glands (∗) and surrounding fibromuscular stroma (■) is shown here at high magnification. A small pink concretion (▲) (typical of the corpora amylacea seen in benign prostatic glands of older men) appears in the gland just to the left of center. Note the well-differentiated glands with double layer of inner tall columnar epithelial lining cells and basal low cuboidal cells. These cells normally do not have prominent nucleoli. The peripheral, central, and transitional zones typically have this appearance. By immunohistochemical staining, prostate-specific antigen (PSA) can be identified within the glandular epithelial cell cytoplasm, and small amounts of PSA can normally be detected in the serum.

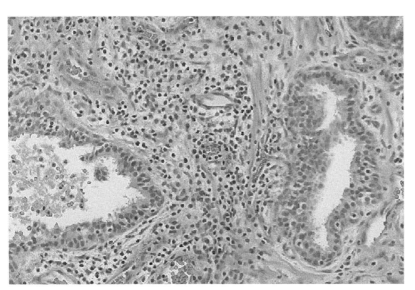

FIGURE 12–35 Prostatitis, microscopic

Numerous small round dark blue lymphocytes are seen in the stroma between the glands. There may be a bacterial agent accompanying this inflammation, and urinary tract infection with cystitis or urethritis may also be present. However, more commonly in men older than 50 years, chronic prostatitis is abacterial, with no history of urinary tract infection, with negative cultures, but with at least 10 leukocytes per high-power field in prostatic secretions. Patients with prostatitis often have perineal or back pain with dysuria, although some are asymptomatic. The serum PSA may be slightly elevated, typically up to twice the upper limit of the normal range. Acute prostatitis is caused by bacteria from urinary tract infections.

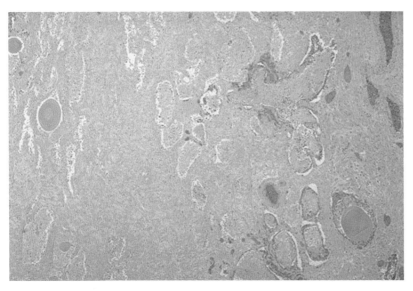

FIGURE 12–36 Prostatic infarction, microscopic

Seen at the left is an area of prostatic infarction, which does not occur often. Such infarcts are typically small but may cause discomfort and may increase the serum PSA, similar to prostatitis or prostatic adenocarcinoma. There can be squamous metaplasia of the glands surrounding such an infarct. Note also the corpora amylacea.

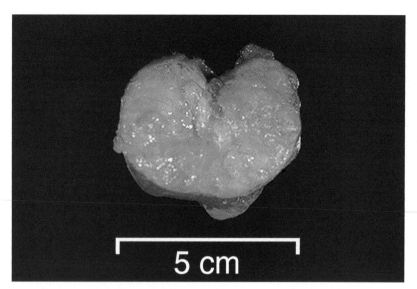

FIGURE 12–37 Prostatic hyperplasia, gross

This prostate is enlarged and nodular as a result of prostatic hyperplasia. Thus, this condition is termed either *benign prostatic hyperplasia* (BPH) or *nodular prostatic hyperplasia*. The hyperplasia is most pronounced in the lateral lobes. This is a process that occurs gradually over many years, typically after age 50, and by age 70, more than 90% of men have some degree of BPH, although a minority are symptomatic. An enlarged prostate can obstruct urinary outflow from the bladder and lead to an obstructive uropathy. BPH is detected as diffuse prostatic enlargement on digital rectal examination. Symptoms relate to inability to void completely, with residual urine causing increasing urinary frequency, along with difficulty starting and stopping the urinary stream.

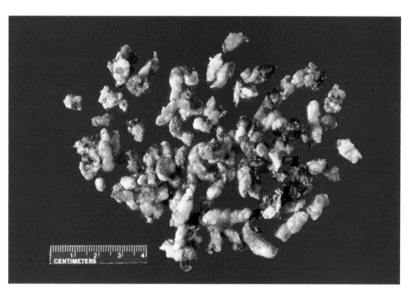

FIGURE 12–38 Prostatic hyperplasia, gross

A frequently performed operation for symptomatic nodular prostatic hyperplasia is a transurethral resection, which yields the small "chips" of rubbery prostatic tissue seen here. Prostatic hyperplasia is the result of increased sensitivity of the prostatic glands and stroma to DHT because there are increased numbers of androgen receptors induced by increasing estradiol levels with aging. The enzyme 5α-reductase type 2, found mainly in prostatic stromal cells, converts circulating testosterone to DHT. Pharmacotherapy for BPH is aimed at blocking either this enzyme or α_{1a}-adrenoreceptors to relax the smooth muscle of the bladder neck and improve urine flow, affording a greater, earlier effect on symptoms, but not reducing prostate size.

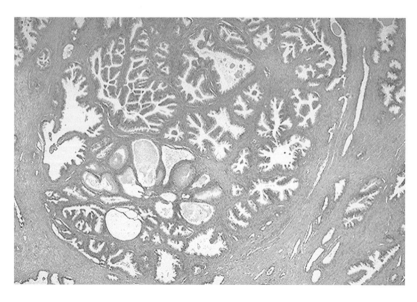

FIGURE 12–39 Prostatic hyperplasia, microscopic

Prostatic hyperplasia can involve both glands and stroma, although the former are usually more prominent. Here, a large hyperplastic nodule with numerous glands is present. There is still stroma between the glands. The glands are larger than normal, with more complex infoldings, but still lined by a double layer of uniform columnar cells and basal cuboidal cells that show no atypia. The transitional zone often gives initial rise to these hyperplastic nodules, although the bulk of prostatic enlargement often comes later from pronounced nodular growth in the peripheral zone.

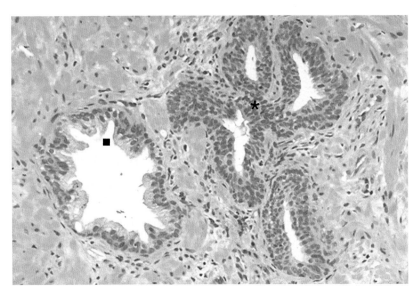

FIGURE 12–40 Prostatic intraepithelial neoplasia, microscopic

Prostatic intraepithelial neoplasia (PIN) is a precancerous cellular proliferation found in a single acinus or small group of prostatic acini. A normal prostatic gland (■) is seen at the left for comparison, with the acini showing PIN (∗) at the right. The PIN can be low grade or high grade (as seen here). The finding of PIN suggests that prostatic adenocarcinoma may also be present, and an adenocarcinoma accompanies high-grade PIN about half the time. Androgen receptor gene mutations that shorten CAG repeat sequences increase androgen sensitivity, which plays a role in driving prostatic neoplasia. Germ line mutations may also be present.

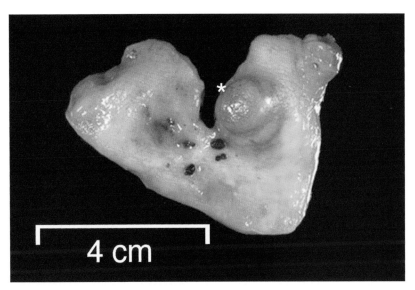

FIGURE 12–41 Adenocarcinoma, gross

This axial section reveals a single prominent nodule (∗) that proved to be adenocarcinoma. Such a nodule may be palpable by digital rectal examination or may be detected on an ultrasound scan. Some small dark glandular concretions are also seen here in the adjacent normal prostate. Note that this prostate is not significantly enlarged, and no nodularity is present. Although the incidence of both BPH and adenocarcinoma increases with age, BPH is not a risk factor for carcinoma. Prostate cancer is the most common nonskin malignancy in elderly men. It is rare before the age of 50, but autopsy studies have found prostatic adenocarcinoma in more than half of men older than 80 years.

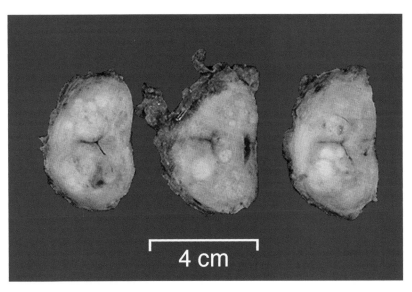

FIGURE 12–42 Adenocarcinoma, gross

These sections through a prostate removed by radical prostatectomy reveal irregular yellowish nodules of adenocarcinoma, mostly in the posterior region. Prostate glands containing adenocarcinoma are not necessarily enlarged. Adenocarcinoma may also coexist with BPH. Staging of prostatic adenocarcinoma is based on how extensive the tumor is. Many of these carcinomas are small and clinically insignificant. However, some, such as the one seen here, are more extensive, and prostatic adenocarcinoma is second only to lung carcinoma as a cause of tumor-related deaths among men. More than 90% of prostatic carcinomas show hypermethylation of the glutathione S-transferase (*GSTP1*) gene promoter.

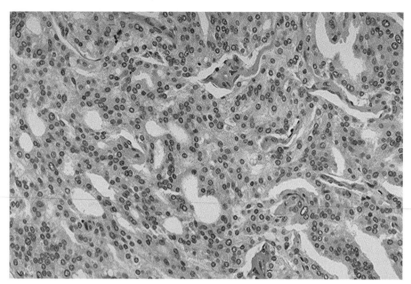

FIGURE 12–43 Adenocarcinoma, microscopic

Note how the glands of the carcinoma are small, irregular, and crowded, with no intervening stroma. Prostatic adenocarcinomas are given a histologic grade. The Gleason grading system is used most often and includes a score of 1 to 5 (increasing as the carcinoma becomes less differentiated) for the most prominent component, added to a score of 1 to 5 for the next most common pattern. For example, this adenocarcinoma could be given a Gleason grade of 3/3. The grade gives an indication of prognosis and how aggressive therapy should be. In general, a combined score of less than 6 suggests that the neoplasm will be indolent. Advanced cancers tend to have scores of 8 and above.

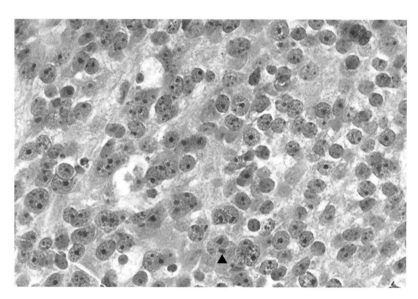

FIGURE 12–44 Adenocarcinoma, microscopic

Prominent nucleoli (▲) are a characteristic histologic feature of prostatic adenocarcinoma. Prostate cancers may be detected by screening with a blood test for PSA. PSA is a glycoprotein produced almost exclusively in the epithelium of the prostate glands. The PSA level tends to rise gradually with age. A mildly increased PSA (4 to 10 ng/mL) in a patient with a very large prostate can be due to nodular hyperplasia, or to prostatitis, rather than carcinoma. A rising PSA is suspicious for carcinoma, even if the PSA is in the normal range. However, a small focus of cancer confined to the prostate may not be accompanied by a rise in PSA. Transrectal needle biopsy is useful to confirm the diagnosis.

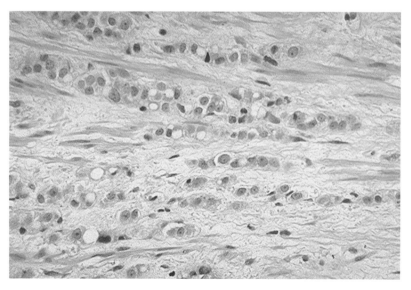

FIGURE 12–45 Adenocarcinoma, microscopic

This adenocarcinoma is so poorly differentiated (Gleason grade 5) that no glandular structure is recognizable, only individual cells infiltrating in rows. Advanced prostatic adenocarcinomas typically cause urinary obstruction and metastasize to regional (pelvic) lymph nodes and to the bones, causing osteoblastic (bone forming) metastases in most cases. The most typical site of bone metastases is the vertebral column, with accompanying chronic back pain. Metastases to the lungs and liver are seen in a minority of cases.

CHAPTER 13

The Female Genital Tract

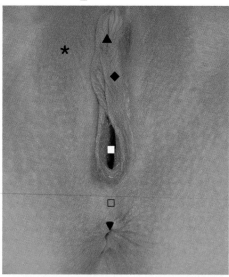
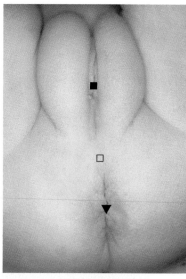

FIGURE 13–1 Normal external genitalia, gross

Adult external genitalia at the left include the labia majora (∗), labia minora (◆), clitoris (▲), vaginal orifice (■), and perineum (□) extending to the anus (▼). At the right, the appearance of the genitalia at birth illustrates the relationship of the vaginal orifice (■), perineum (□), and anus (▼) The external genitalia are covered by keratinizing stratified squamous epithelium.

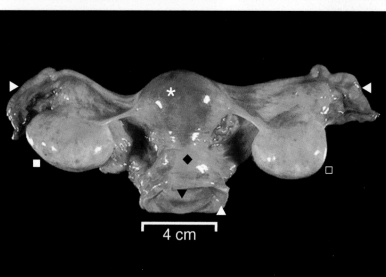

FIGURE 13–2 Normal internal genitalia, gross

Here is the gross appearance of a normal uterus with fundus (∗), lower uterine segment (◆), cervix (▼), vaginal cuff (▲), right fallopian tube (▶), left fallopian tube (◀), right ovary (■), and left ovary (□) from a young woman. In the developing embryo, primordial germ cells from the yolk sac wall migrate to the urogenital ridge to become ovarian germ cells within the epithelium and stroma derived from urogenital ridge mesoderm. The unfused portions of the müllerian (paramesonephric) ducts form the fallopian tubes, and the fused portions become the uterus and vagina, while the distal fused ducts contact the urogenital sinus to become the vestibule of the external genitalia.

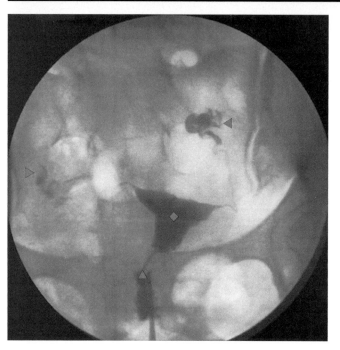

FIGURE 13–3 Normal internal genitalia, radiograph

This is a hysterosalpingogram in which a catheter is introduced through the cervix (▲) to fill the endometrial cavity (◆) with contrast material. Contrast extends into the right fallopian tube and left fallopian tube, eventually spilling out through the fimbriated ends of the fallopian tubes (oviducts) at both the right adnexal (▶) and left adnexal (◀) regions, thus indicating normal tubal patency. Some contrast material here has also backfilled into the vagina. This radiographic study may be undertaken as part of an infertility work-up.

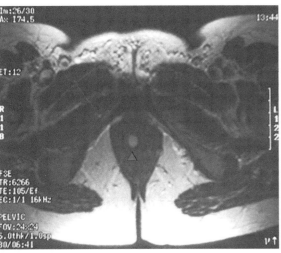
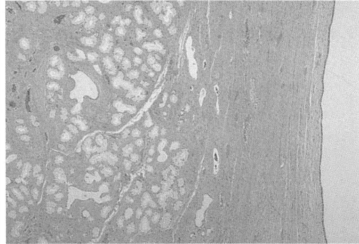

FIGURES 13–4 and 13–5 Bartholin gland cyst, MRI and microscopic

A small, bright, cyst (▲) of the Bartholin gland is seen in the left panel. These paired glands produce mucinous secretions and have ducts that empty into the vaginal orifice. The duct to a gland can become obstructed, leading to cystic glandular enlargement with inflammation and infection, producing pain and discomfort. A Bartholin cyst can reach 3 to 5 cm in size. In the right panel, the cyst with flattened transitional or squamous lining is at the far right, with remaining adjacent normal glands.

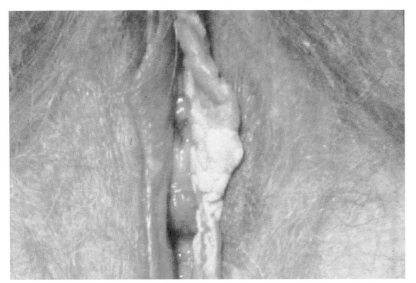

FIGURE 13–6 Lichen sclerosus, gross

The pale white patches of leukoplakia seen here on the vulva with atrophy and fibrosis can narrow the introitus and produce discomfort. This process can develop slowly and involve progressively more labial skin surface in adult women, particularly after menopause. Lichen sclerosus increases the risk for secondary infection.

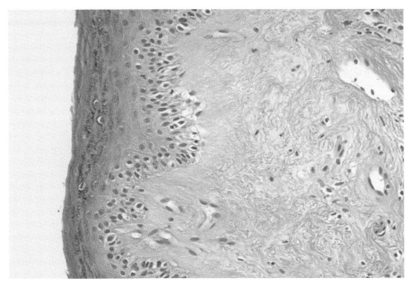

FIGURE 13–7 Lichen sclerosus, microscopic

There is atrophy of the vulvar squamous epithelium with thinning, loss of rete pegs, hydropic degeneration of basal keratinocytes, dermal dense band collagenous fibrous thickening, and sometimes a bandlike infiltrate of lymphocytes. These findings suggest an autoimmune process. A vulvar squamous cell cancer will eventually develop in less than 4% of these women.

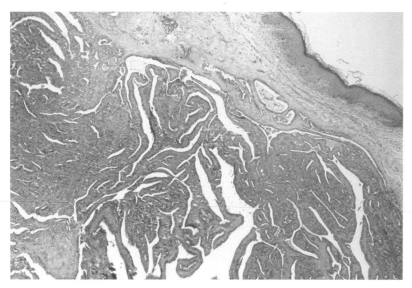

FIGURE 13-8 Papillary hidradenoma, microscopic

The vulva has modified apocrine sweat glands from which a papillary hidradenoma may arise. It forms a sharply circumscribed nodule, most commonly in the labia majora or interlabial folds. A vulvar carcinoma may be suspected because the hidradenoma tends to ulcerate. It has a histologically similar appearance to an intraductal papilloma of the breast. As shown here, there is a regular papillary growth pattern with tubular ducts lined by a single or double layer of nonciliated columnar cells, with a layer of flattened "myoepithelial cells" underlying the epithelium. Myoepithelial elements are characteristic of sweat glands and sweat gland tumors.

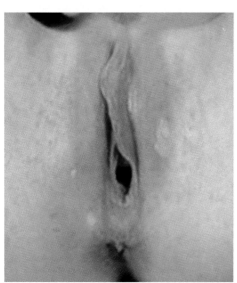

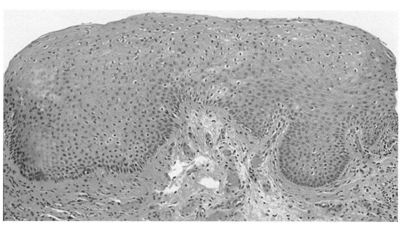

FIGURES 13-9 and 13-10 Condyloma acuminata, gross and microscopic

Shown are warty (verrucous) excrescences on the perineum, vulva, and perianal region, typical of sexually transmitted human papillomavirus (HPV) infection, often HPV subtypes 6 and 11. The lesions can be solitary or multiple. The squamous epithelium becomes thickened, and there is perinuclear vacuolization to produce the characteristic cytologic "koilocytotic atypia." Condylomata are benign and do not progress to malignancy. They may remain the same in size, may regress spontaneously, or enlarge slowly.

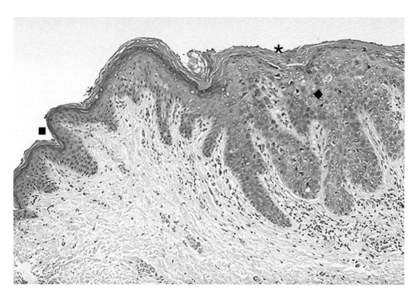

FIGURE 13-11 Vulvar dysplasia, microscopic

Dysplasia (◆) may involve the vulvar epithelium as a consequence of HPV infection. Note the overlying hyperkeratosis (∗) (which produces a grossly visible area of leukoplakia), with more normal (but atrophic) keratinizing squamous epithelium (■) at the left. Most cases of vulvar intraepithelial neoplasia (VIN) do not progress to invasive cancer, but the risk is greater with HPV subtypes 16 and 18. Many lesions are multicentric, and some occur in association with cervical or vaginal squamous carcinoma. In older women, vulvar carcinomas may be preceded by lichen sclerosus, not HPV infection.

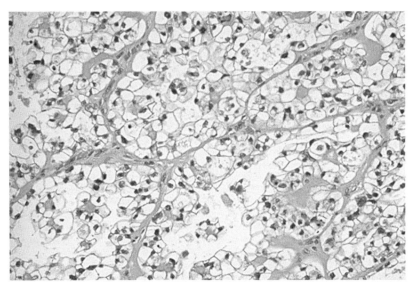

FIGURE 13–12 Clear cell carcinoma, microscopic

Neoplasms of the vagina are rare. Note the vacuolated cells forming irregular clusters with ill-defined glandular lumens. Red, granular foci that appear on the vaginal mucosa and are called *adenosis* and may precede clear cell carcinoma, a lesion most likely to occur in a young woman whose mother was given diethylstilbestrol (DES) during pregnancy. These cancers are rare, even in women with this history. DES exposure increases the risk for clear cell carcinoma arising in the upper vagina and cervix of adolescents and young adults. Clear cell carcinoma often becomes invasive before detection and is difficult to cure.

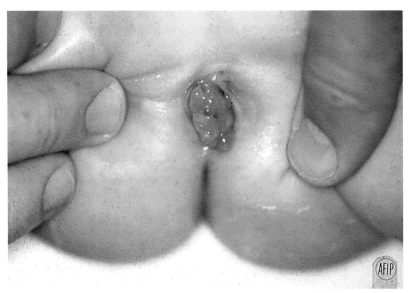

FIGURE 13–13 Sarcoma botryoides, gross

Note the polypoid mass filling the vagina and extending as grapelike masses out the vaginal orifice. Called *sarcoma botryoides*, this is a rare form of embryonal rhabdomyosarcoma, found most often in female infants and children younger than age 5.

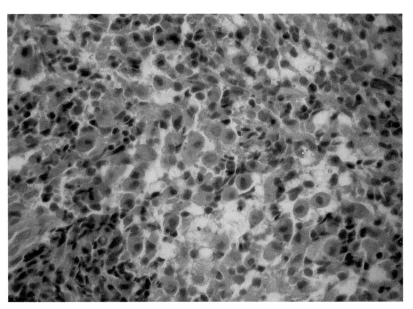

FIGURE 13–14 Sarcoma botryoides, microscopic

This neoplasm is a form of embryonal rhabdomyosarcoma with small, primitive cells within a fibromyxomatous stroma and having variable amounts of pink cytoplasm. These tumors often invade locally. Larger tumors may cause urinary tract obstruction.

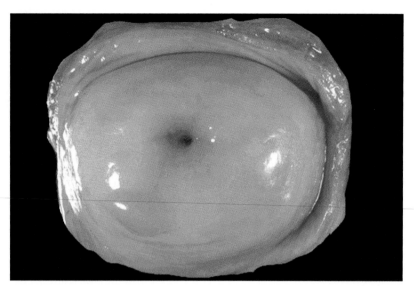

FIGURE 13–15 Normal cervix, gross

The normal cervix has a smooth, glistening mucosal surface. There is a small rim of vaginal cuff seen here from this hysterectomy specimen. The cervical os shown is small and round, typical of a nulliparous woman. The os will attain a fish-mouth shape after one or more pregnancies.

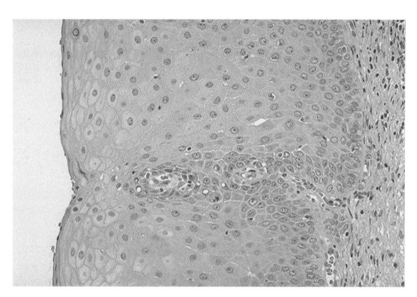

FIGURE 13–16 Normal cervix, microscopic

This is normal cervical nonkeratinizing squamous epithelium. The squamous cells show maturation from the basal layer to the overlying surface. A Pap smear is obtained by scraping or brushing the surface of the cervix (and sometimes the vagina) to obtain cells that are placed in a fixative solution and stained. The maturation pattern of these cells gives an indication of the woman's hormonal status and will change during the normal menstrual cycle. Inflammatory cells and infectious agents such as *Candida albicans*, trichomonads, and "clue cells" of bacterial vaginosis (such as *Gardnerella vaginalis*) can also be seen on a Pap smear. Of course, dysplastic changes can also be detected.

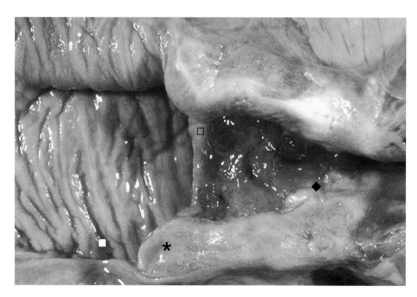

FIGURE 13–17 Normal cervix and vagina, gross

The normal adult vaginal mucosa (■) in women of reproductive years has a wrinkled appearance. The cervix (*) has been opened anteriorly here at autopsy to reveal an endocervical canal leading to the lower uterine segment (◆) at the right that has an erythematous appearance extending to the cervical os (□), consistent with chronic inflammation. The cervix has an underlying dense fibromuscular stroma that appears white on cut section.

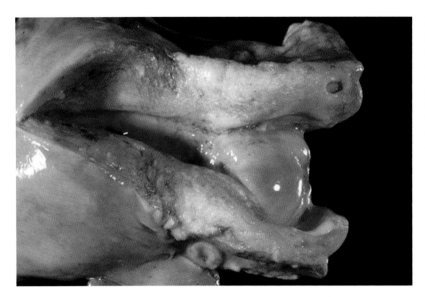

FIGURE 13–18 Nabothian cyst, gross

Seen here is a large translucent nabothian cyst extending from the stroma around the outer endocervical canal in an exophytic manner into the canal. Inflammation with cervicitis may produce submucosal gland obstruction so that glandular cystic dilation occurs. These cysts are filled with a clear, mucoid fluid. These are common lesions, generally ranging from a few millimeters to 1 cm in size. They are benign.

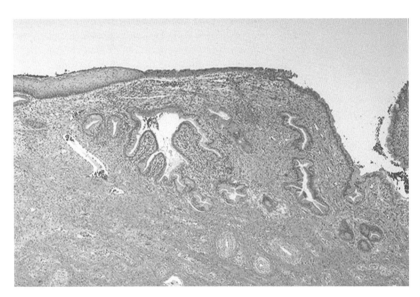

FIGURE 13–19 Normal cervical transformation zone, microscopic

Normal cervix with stratified nonkeratinizing squamous epithelium merges at the transformation zone (squamocolumnar junction) to endocervix lined by tall mucinous columnar cells, as seen here at low magnification. The endocervix has underlying endocervical glands in the stroma that are also lined by tall mucinous columnar cells.

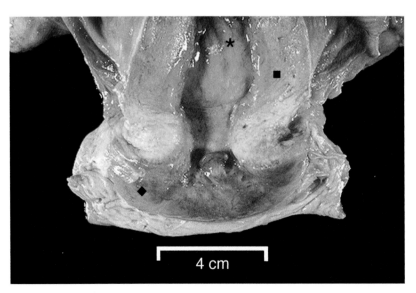

FIGURE 13–20 Chronic cervicitis, gross

Chronic cervicitis typically begins at the squamocolumnar junction of the cervix and can extend to involve the ectocervical squamous epithelium. The uterus has been opened anteriorly here to reveal the endocervical canal (∗) and lower uterine segment (■). Note the erythematous appearance (◆) of this inflamed cervical epithelium. During reproductive years, estrogen levels promote maturation with glycogen uptake of cervical and vaginal squamous epithelium, and this glycogen provides a substrate for the normal vaginal bacterial flora that keeps the pH low to inhibit proliferation of pathogenic organisms.

4 cm

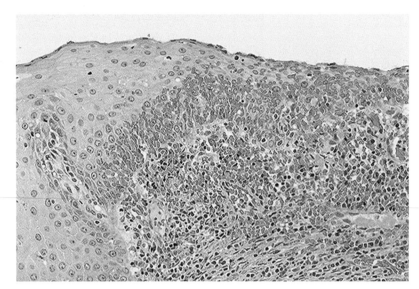

FIGURE 13–21 Chronic cervicitis, microscopic

Chronic cervicitis seen here at the squamocolumnar junction of the cervix has small, round, dark blue lymphocytes in the submucosa, and there is also hemorrhage. Chronic cervicitis is quite common. Common bacterial organisms including streptococci, staphylococci, enterococci, and coliforms, as well as the fungus *Candida* and the protozoan *Trichomonas vaginalis,* may contribute to both cervicitis and vaginitis, which typically have a clinical course marked by episodes of acute inflammation that blend into chronic inflammation. The repair reaction to the inflamed and eroded epithelium may produce mildly atypical-appearing cells ("inflammatory" atypia) on a Pap smear.

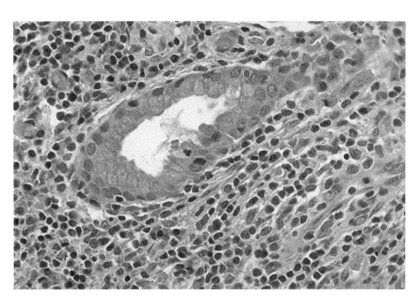

FIGURE 13–22 Chronic cervicitis, microscopic

A predominantly lymphocytic infiltrate extends around this endocervical gland in the stroma of the cervix beneath the epithelium. Epithelial erosion, ulceration, and repair may accompany this inflammation. There is some degree of cervicitis in nearly all adult women, but the amount of inflammation is minimal, and there are usually no significant health problems because of it.

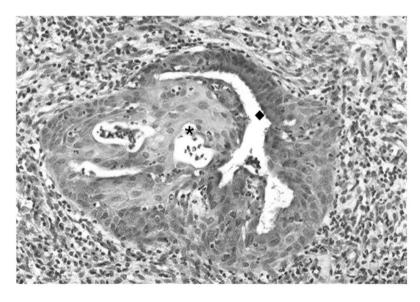

FIGURE 13–23 Cervical squamous metaplasia, microscopic

In this endocervical gland, the normal columnar epithelium (◆) is transforming to a squamous-appearing epithelium (∗) as a consequence of the ongoing inflammatory process. Metaplasia is a potentially reversible process in which one type of epithelium is exchanged for the normal epithelium. Metaplasia may be the first step in epithelial cellular alteration leading to dysplasia.

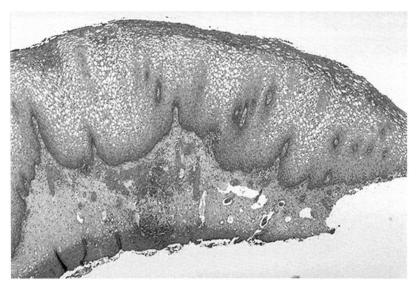

FIGURE 13–24 Human papillomavirus effect, microscopic

This cervical biopsy specimen demonstrates a thickened squamous epithelium, and the squamous cells have a vacuolated appearance. This is koilocytotic change. A condyloma acuminatum of the external genitalia would have a similar appearance. These are changes that typically result from HPV infection. Most healthy adult women will clear an HPV infection after several years. HPV can be subtyped into high-risk and low-risk varieties. High-risk varieties include HPV subtypes 16 and 18. The E6 and E7 oncoproteins in these HPV subtypes bind to p53 and promote its degradation, while E7 binds to RB and up-regulates DNA synthesis.

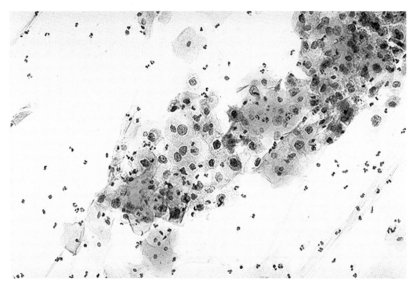

FIGURE 13–25 Cervical squamous dysplasia, Pap smear

Pap smear screening has reduced the incidence of and death rate from cervical carcinoma because dysplasias and early carcinomas can be detected and treated to prevent invasive carcinomas. The cytologic features of normal squamous epithelial cells can be seen at the center top and bottom, with orange to pale blue platelike squamous cells that have small pyknotic nuclei. The dysplastic cells in the center extending to the upper right are smaller overall with darker, more irregular nuclei. Dysplastic lesions are classified as grades I, II, or III cervical intraepithelial neoplasia (CIN).

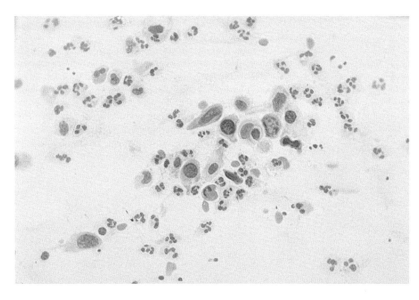

FIGURE 13–26 Cervical squamous carcinoma, Pap smear

In this Pap smear are seen more pleomorphic, darker and larger cells indicative of a carcinoma. The inflammation and hemorrhage in the background are characteristic of a more aggressive, ulcerative, and invasive lesion. Following up an abnormal Pap smear showing CIN or carcinoma with a biopsy and treatment is essential. Risk factors for cervical neoplasia include early age at first intercourse, multiple sexual partners, increased parity, male sexual partners with multiple previous sexual partners, and exposure to high-risk HPV subtypes 16 and 18.

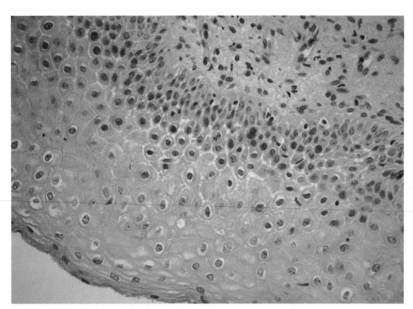

FIGURE 13–27 Cervical intraepithelial neoplasia grade I, microscopic

In this biopsy sample, the dysplastic, disordered cells occupy less than one third of the squamous epithelial thickness above the basal lamina, so this is CIN I. Note the koilocytotic change in some cells, consistent with HPV effect. The term *atypical squamous cells of undetermined significance* (ASCUS) may be applied in some Pap smear reports when there are abnormal cells, but a CIN classification is not possible, and further follow-up is warranted. The term *squamous intraepithelial lesion* (SIL) may also be used in Pap smear reports, and CIN I typically correlates with a low-grade squamous intraepithelial lesion (LSIL).

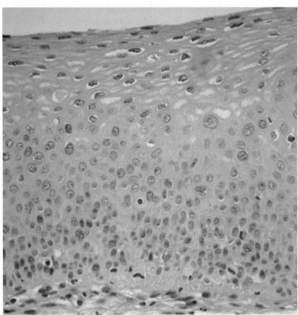

FIGURE 13–28 Cervical intraepithelial neoplasia grade II, microscopic

In this cervical biopsy sample, the dysplastic, disordered cells occupy about one third to one half the thickness of the epithelium, and the basal lamina is still intact, so this is CIN II. Moderate to severe dysplasias (CIN II and III) tend to correlate with a high-grade squamous intraepithelial lesion (HSIL) and infection with more aggressive forms of HPV. There is continued expression of *E6/E7* oncogenes with destabilizing influences on the cell cycle. There is up-regulation of *p16/NK4* with increased expression of *p16*, a cyclin-dependent kinase inhibitor. Nevertheless, dysplasias tend to progress over many years, giving plenty of opportunity to find the early lesions with periodic Pap smear screening and treatment by excising the dysplastic areas. Colposcopy may aid in detection of the abnormal areas for removal.

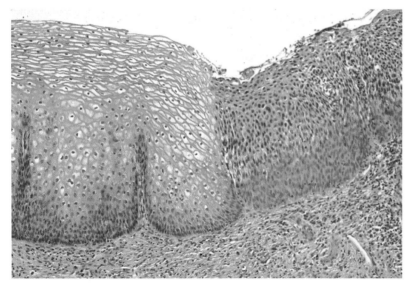

FIGURE 13–29 Cervical intraepithelial neoplasia grade III, microscopic

In this biopsy sample, there is severe cervical squamous dysplasia extending from the center to the right. The nondysplastic epithelium is at the left. Note how the dysplastic cell nuclei are larger and darker, and the dysplastic cells have a disorderly arrangement within the epithelium. This dysplastic process involves the full thickness of the epithelium, but the basal lamina is intact, so this is CIN III. Designations of both severe dysplasia and carcinoma *in situ* (CIS) fall under the CIN III heading. Such lesions are HSILs and have the greatest risk for progression to invasive carcinoma.

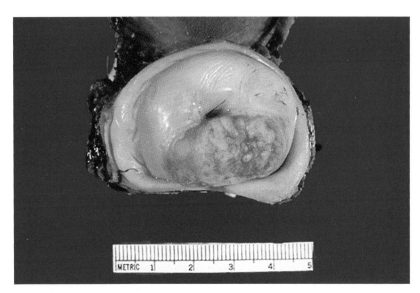

FIGURE 13–30 Squamous cell carcinoma, gross

This hysterectomy specimen shows the gross appearance of a cervical squamous cell carcinoma that is still limited to the cervix (stage I). The 5-year survival rate for CIN is essentially 100%, and it is more than 95% for microinvasive carcinomas (stage Ia). Five-year survival rates of 80% to 90% occur when the neoplasm is more invasive but still confined to the cervix (stage Ib). The tumor seen here from 3 to 7 o'clock around the cervical os is a red to tan to yellow mass that is exophytic (growing outward and extending above the surrounding normal smooth tan epithelium). There is a natural history of progression of dysplasia to carcinoma. Cervical carcinomas may begin appearing as early as the second decade, but the peak incidence is in the fifth decade.

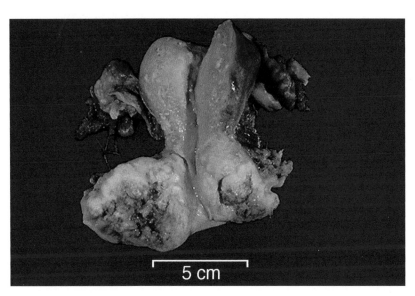

FIGURE 13–31 Squamous cell carcinoma, gross

This is a larger, more advanced cervical squamous cell carcinoma that has spread to the vagina. A total abdominal hysterectomy with bilateral salpingo-oophorectomy (TAH-BSO) was performed as treatment for this stage II cervical carcinoma, which extended beyond the cervix, but not to the pelvic side wall. The 5-year survival rate is 75%. In stage III, the carcinoma has spread to the pelvic side wall, and the 5-year survival is less than 50%.

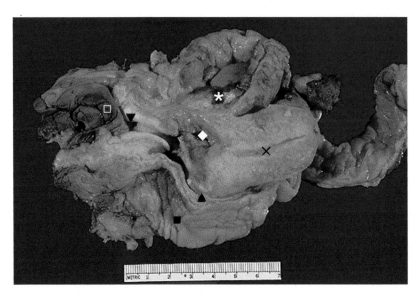

FIGURE 13–32 Squamous cell carcinoma, gross

This is a pelvic exenteration done for stage IV cervical carcinoma, which involves bladder or rectum or extends beyond the true pelvis. At the left, dark vulvar skin (□) leads to the vagina (▼) and to the cervix (▲) in the center, where an irregular tan tumor mass (◆) is seen infiltrating upward into the bladder (*). A slitlike endometrial cavity is surrounded by myometrium at the mid-right. The rectum (■) and sigmoid colon are at the bottom extending to the right. The 5-year survival rate approaches 5%, but that is still 1 in 20, and the quality of life with a reconstructed ileal bladder and colostomy (or Koch pouch) after exenteration is adequate for an active life style. Advanced cancers require a realistic, but not futile, approach.

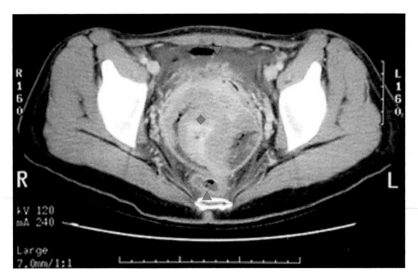

FIGURE 13–33 Squamous cell carcinoma, CT scan

This CT scan of the pelvis shows a large mass (◆) with heterogenous attenuation from necrosis and air-filled spaces arising in the cervix and extending anteriorly to the bladder (▼) and posteriorly to the rectum (▲). This squamous cell carcinoma of the cervix has invaded both rectum and bladder and is thus stage IV.

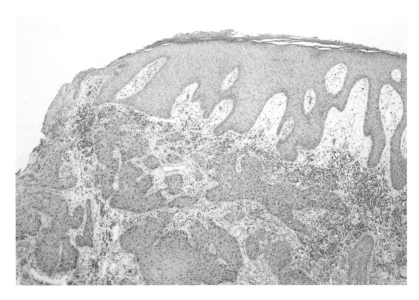

FIGURE 13–34 Squamous cell carcinoma, microscopic

Nests of squamous cell carcinoma are invading downward and undermining the mucosa. There is loss of the epithelial surface from ulceration at the left. Most cervical carcinomas are composed of large pink keratinizing or non-keratinizing squamous cells. Less than 5% are composed of small undifferentiated cells or neuroendocrine cells. Adenocarcinomas arising in the cervix are uncommon. Clear cell carcinomas are rare except in the setting of maternal DES exposure.

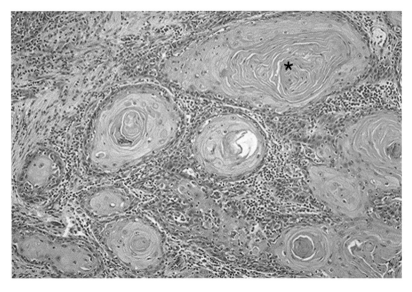

FIGURE 13–35 Squamous cell carcinoma, microscopic

At high magnification, nests of neoplastic squamous cells are invading through a chronically inflamed stroma. This cancer is well differentiated, as evidenced by the formation of keratin pearls (∗) within nests of tumor cells. However, most cervical squamous carcinomas are nonkeratinizing.

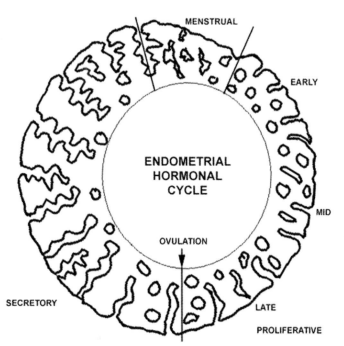

FIGURE 13–36 Endometrial hormonal cycle, diagram

The normal endometrial hormonal cycle is diagrammed here. The average cycle is 28 days. The proliferative (follicular) portion of the cycle is variable among women, but tends to remain the same for any one woman. The time from ovulation to menstruation in the secretory (luteal) portion of the cycle is a constant 14-day period. The menstrual portion of the cycle averages 3 to 7 days. The menstrual cycle is controlled by follicle-stimulating hormone (FSH) and luteinizing hormone (LH) secretion from the adenohypophysis, which is under negative feedback control by ovarian steroids, mainly estradiol, and by inhibin (which selectively suppresses FSH). FSH secretion is inhibited as estrogen levels rise about 8 to 10 days before ovulation. In the latter half of the follicular phase, LH begins to rise, reaching a peak, along with estradiol secretion, that is driven by positive feedback from rising progesterone levels, to trigger ovulation. The luteal phase is marked by decreasing FSH and LH with increasing progesterone and estrogen levels. If fertilization does not occur, estrogen and progesterone levels fall to trigger menses with sloughing of the stratum functionalis layer of endometrium.

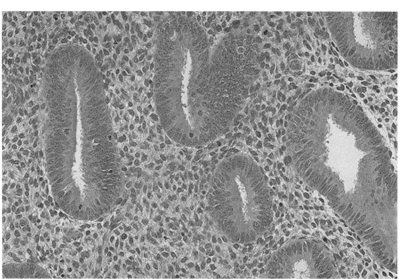

FIGURE 13–37 Endometrium, proliferative, microscopic

The proliferative (follicular) phase is the variable part of the menstrual cycle, but averages about 14 days. In this phase, tubular endometrial glands lined by tall columnar cells and surrounded by a dense stroma are proliferating to build up the amount of functional endometrium after the previous cycle with shedding from menstruation. Mitoses within these proliferating glands can be seen.

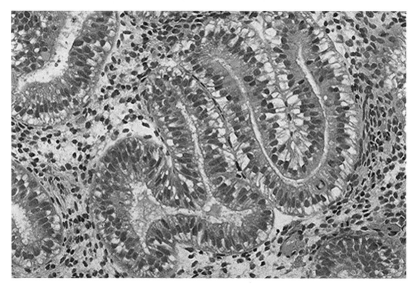

FIGURE 13–38 Endometrium, early secretory, microscopic

This appearance with prominent subnuclear vacuoles in the tall columnar cells lining these larger endometrial glands is consistent with postovulatory day 2 of the luteal phase of the menstrual cycle. The histologic changes after ovulation are quite constant over the next 14 days to menstruation and can be used to date the endometrium with biopsy for diagnostic purposes.

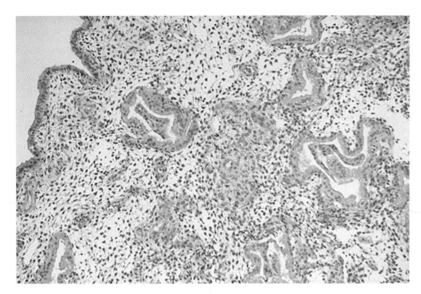

FIGURE 13–39 Endometrium, mid-secretory, microscopic

The mid-secretory endometrium of the normal menstrual cycle shows prominent stromal edema. The endometrial glands are becoming larger and more tortuous as well. Some of the stromal cells have pink cytoplasm, representing the decidualizing effect of the increasing estrogen and progesterone levels in the luteal phase of the cycle after the LH surge with ovulation.

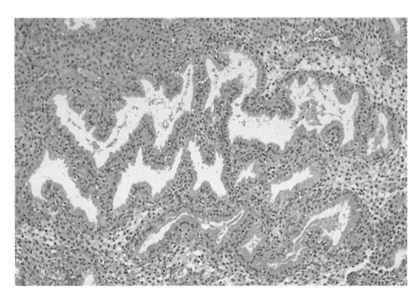

FIGURE 13–40 Endometrium, late secretory, microscopic

The tortuosity of the endometrial glands is apparent in this late secretory endometrium of the luteal phase of the normal menstrual cycle, and there are intraluminal secretions within the glands. There is more pronounced pink decidualization of the surrounding stroma. Such an endometrium is now able to support implantation of a fertilized ovum.

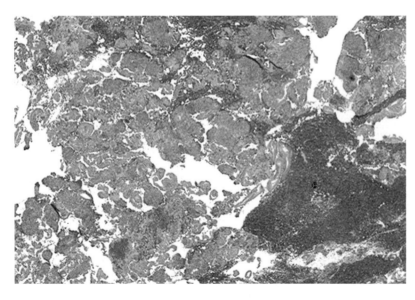

FIGURE 13–41 Endometrium, menstrual, microscopic

The menstrual phase endometrium is marked by breakdown of the glands and stroma from apoptosis triggered by falling estrogen and progesterone levels. There is hemorrhage and leukocyte infiltration. The upper two thirds of the endometrium, the functionalis layer, is shed. From the lower third, the basalis layer, which does not respond in similar manner to the ovarian hormones, will arise a new endometrial lining in the next cycle.

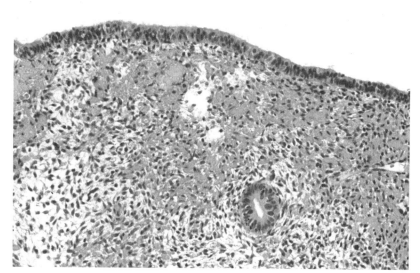

FIGURE 13–42 Endometrium, anovulatory cycle, microscopic

Dysfunctional uterine bleeding is most often due to anovulatory cycles, which are most apt to occur during the reproductive years just after menarche and just before menopause. Endocrine abnormalities of the pituitary or ovary may also be implicated, as may marked obesity or any chronic disease state. The failure of ovulation leads to an inadequate luteal phase with prolonged estrogenic stimulation without the progestational phase. This produces a persistent proliferative endometrial pattern and eventual stromal breakdown with bleeding. The biopsy sample seen here, on what should be postovulatory day 8, shows minimal glandular development and stromal hemorrhage.

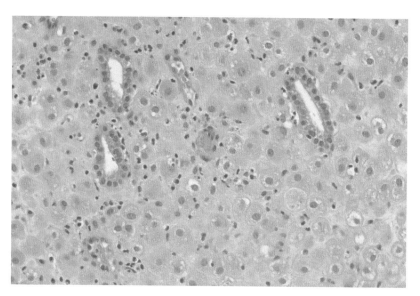

FIGURE 13–43 Endometrium, oral contraceptive effect, microscopic

The endometrial stroma here is markedly decidualized, with large cells having abundant pink cytoplasm, while the few endometrial glands are small and inactive. These changes prevent successful implantation of the blastocyst, but the primary effect of contraceptive agents is prevention of ovulation. The effect on the endometrium is not permanent, and the endometrium will return to normal cyclical changes once the oral contraceptives are discontinued.

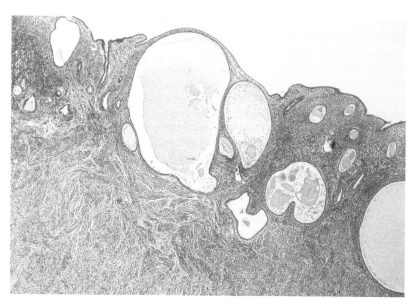

FIGURE 13–44 Endometrium, postmenopausal, microscopic

Note the thin endometrial layer with dense stroma containing small tubular endometrial glands scattered amid other glands that are cystically dilated and lined by flat, atrophic-appearing epithelial cells. After menopause, which typically occurs in the late 40s to early 50s, there is reduced ovarian function with subsequent loss of regular hormonal cycles and decreased ovarian output of the estrogen and progesterone necessary to drive endometrial growth and cycling. Levels of FSH and LH from the pituitary increase as a result of the loss of the feedback loop through the ovary.

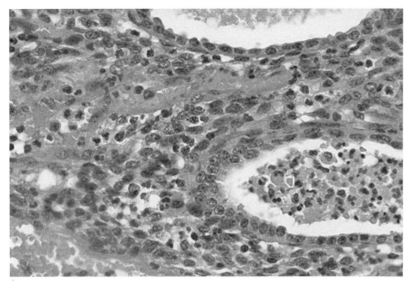

FIGURE 13–45 Acute endometritis, microscopic

There are scattered neutrophils within these endometrial glands and stroma, indicative of acute endometritis, a condition that is most often a complication of childbirth ("puerperal sepsis" or "post-partum fever"), with causative organisms such as group B streptococcus and *Staphylococcus aureus*. Retained products of conception after delivery increase the risk for endometritis. With good obstetrical care, this condition is uncommon, but throughout human history, it has accounted for significant maternal mortality. In addition, chlamydial infections may produce an acute or chronic endometritis.

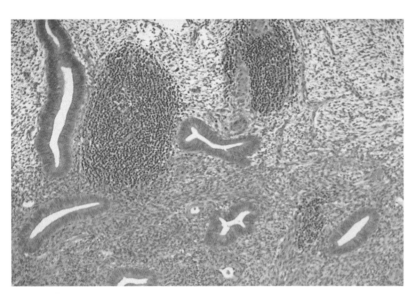

FIGURE 13–46 Chronic endometritis, microscopic

Shown are collections of lymphocytes within the endometrial stroma. At higher magnification, plasma cells would be identified. Chronic endometritis is present to a milder degree when an intrauterine device is present (the low-grade inflammation induced by some of these devices, designed to create a spermicidal environment, secondarily prevents implantation). The more marked inflammation seen here can be present postpartum, typically with retained products of conception, postabortion, or with chronic pelvic inflammatory disease. In one sixth of patients, there is no definable cause of chronic endometritis. These women can have pelvic pain, fever, vaginal discharge, and infertility.

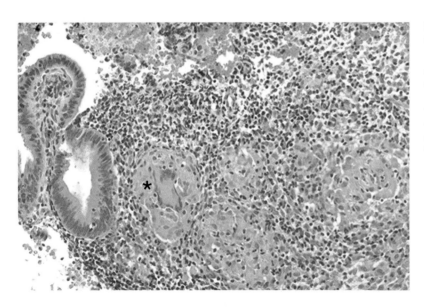

FIGURE 13–47 Granulomatous endometritis, microscopic

In this biopsy sample, note that the endometrial stroma contain ill-defined granulomas (*) with epithelioid cells having abundant pink cytoplasm. Note the Langhans giant cell. The granulomatous form of chronic endometritis shown is due to drainage of tuberculous salpingitis into the endometrial cavity. This can occur in a patient with disseminated tuberculosis.

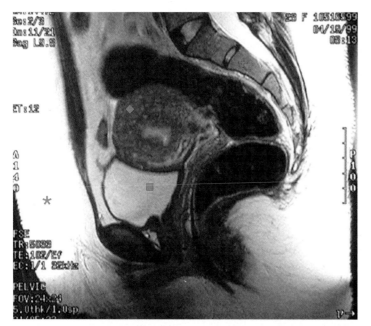

FIGURE 13–48 Adenomyosis, MRI

In this T2-weighted MRI of the pelvis in sagittal view, the uterus shows abnormally low T2 signal intensity with obliteration of the junctional zone, consistent with adenomyosis (◆). The uterus is enlarged by this process. The bladder anteriorly (■) is filled with bright contrast, while the sigmoid (□) and rectum posteriorly appear dark. Note the normal appearance of the sacrum (+). This obese patient has abundant subcutaneous adipose tissue (*).

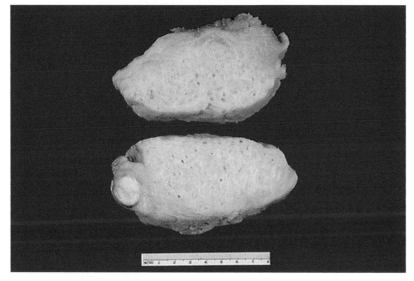

FIGURE 13–49 Adenomyosis, gross

The thickened and spongy-appearing myometrial wall of this sectioned uterus is typical of adenomyosis, a condition in which endometrial glands with (or without) stroma are located within the myometrium. Up to 20% of uteri examined in surgical pathology after hysterectomy have some degree of adenomyosis, usually not as florid as this case. The uterus may be enlarged, usually symmetrically, and there may be menorrhagia, dyspareunia, or pelvic pain. (Shown here is also an incidental small round white leiomyoma.)

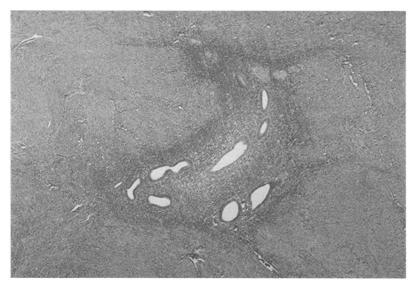

FIGURE 13–50 Adenomyosis, microscopic

Down-growth of the endometrium more than 2 mm from the stratum basalis into the myometrium may account for adenomyosis. In this section through the myometrium can be seen a cluster of endometrial tissue with glands and stroma, typical of adenomyosis. Since these foci are derived from the endometrial stratum basalis, there is usually no significant bleeding within the foci themselves. This condition can lead to uterine enlargement and menorrhagia, dysmenorrhea, and pelvic pain.

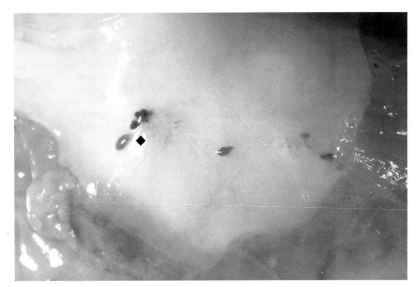

FIGURE 13–51 Endometriosis gross

When endometrial glands and stroma are found outside the uterus, the condition is known as *endometriosis*. Up to 10% of women may have endometriosis. It can be very disabling and painful, even when just a few of these small foci are present. Clinical features include dysmenorrhea, dyspareunia, pelvic pain, and infertility. In these foci of endometriosis, there is bleeding, and the blood is dark (from deoxygenation and from breakdown to hemosiderin), giving the small foci the gross appearance of powder burns. The nodular foci are seen here just beneath the serosa of the posterior uterus in the pouch of Douglas (◆). Such areas of endometriosis can be found and obliterated by cauterization using laparoscopy.

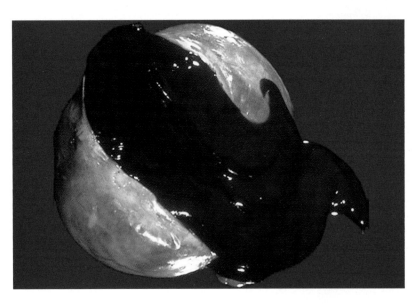

FIGURE 13–52 Endometriosis, gross

Typical locations for endometriosis include ovaries, uterine ligaments, rectovaginal septum, pelvic peritoneum, and laparotomy scars. Endometriosis may even be found at more distant locations such as appendix and vagina. This is a section through an enlarged 12-cm ovary to demonstrate a cystic cavity filled with old blood typical of endometriosis with formation of an endometriotic, or "chocolate," cyst. The chocolate cyst is so named because the old blood in the cystic space formed by the hemorrhage is broken down to produce much hemosiderin that has a brown to black color.

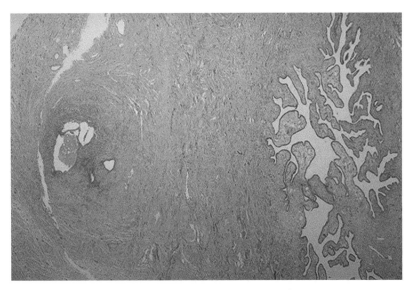

FIGURE 13–53 Endometriosis, microscopic

A focus of endometriosis with a small cluster of endometrial glands and stroma with hemorrhage is seen at the left near the surface of this fallopian tube. The lumen of the tube is at the right. Theories for the origin of endometriosis include regurgitation of menstrual tissue out the fallopian tube with implantation onto the peritoneum, metaplasia of the coelomic epithelium, or vascular dissemination of endometrial tissues through veins or lymphatics. There is an increased risk for development of carcinoma (typically an endometrioid carcinoma) in foci of endometriosis.

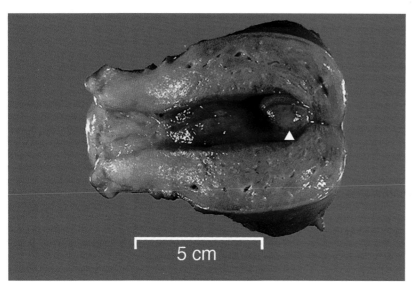

FIGURE 13–54 Endometrial polyp, gross

This uterus from a simple hysterectomy has been opened anteriorly through the cervix and into the endometrial cavity. High in the fundus and projecting into the endometrial cavity is a small endometrial polyp (▲). Such benign polyps may cause uterine bleeding. They are typically between 0.5 and 3 cm in size. Some polyps may be composed of functioning endometrium, but most are associated with endometrial hyperplasia. Rarely, an endometrial carcinoma may arise within such a polyp. There is an increased incidence of endometrial polyps in women treated with tamoxifen for estrogen receptor–positive breast cancer.

FIGURE 13–55 Endometrial hyperplasia, gross

This normal-sized uterus is opened, and the endometrial cavity is filled with lush fronds of hyperplastic endometrium. Endometrial hyperplasia, also known as *endometrial intraepithelial neoplasia*, usually develops under conditions of prolonged estrogen excess in conjunction with relative or absolute decreased progesterone. Hyperplasia can lead to metrorrhagia (uterine bleeding at irregular intervals), menorrhagia (excessive bleeding with menstrual periods), or menometrorrhagia. Predisposing factors include menopause, prolonged administration of estrogenic agents, estrogen-producing ovarian neoplasms, and polycystic ovary syndrome.

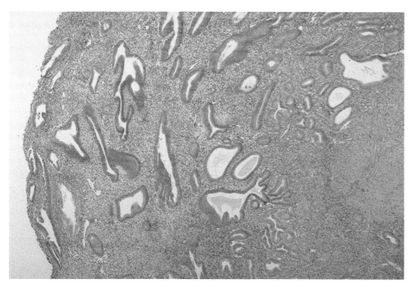

FIGURE 13–56 Endometrial hyperplasia, microscopic

This is endometrial hyperplasia in which the amount of endometrium is abnormally increased and not cycling as it should. The glands are enlarged and irregular, with columnar cells that have some atypia. Some glands are cystic. This is the pattern of simple, non-atypical hyperplasia. Simple endometrial hyperplasias can cause bleeding, but these are not thought to be premalignant. However, adenomatous hyperplasia is premalignant. Estrogen excess can lead to hyperplasia. Inactivation or deletion of the *PTEN* tumor suppressor gene makes endometrial cells more sensitive to estrogenic stimulation, driving this proliferative process.

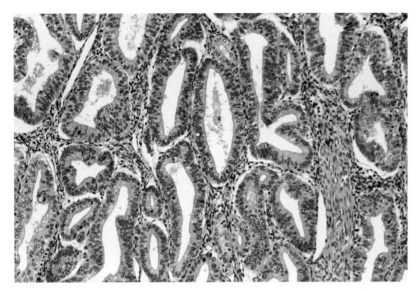

FIGURE 13–57 Endometrial adenomatous (complex) hyperplasia, microscopic

There is crowding of these endometrial glands, which are irregularly shaped and lined by columnar cells with crowded, hyperchromatic nuclei, indicating that the hyperplasia of the endometrium has atypical features. The presence of these changes increases the risk for subsequent development of endometrial carcinoma. Both complex hyperplasia and endometrial carcinomas often have inactivation of the *PTEN* tumor suppressor gene. This condition can be treated by hysterectomy.

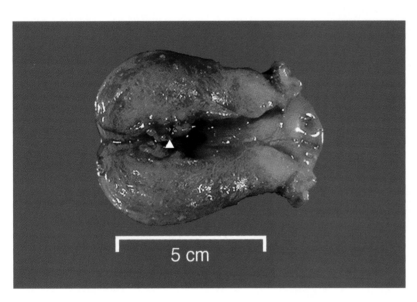

FIGURE 13–58 Endometrial carcinoma, gross

This uterus is not enlarged, as is often the case with many early endometrial carcinomas when signs such as vaginal bleeding first appear. Note the subtle irregular mass (▲) in the upper fundus that proved to be endometrial adenocarcinoma on biopsy. These carcinomas are more likely to occur in postmenopausal women, with a peak incidence from 55 to 65 years. They are rare before age 40. Thus, any postmenopausal bleeding should raise concern about the possibility of endometrial carcinoma. Any condition that increases the exposure to estrogen is associated with an increased risk for endometrial carcinoma. Although the overall risk for cancer increases with obesity, the strongest association occurs with endometrial carcinoma.

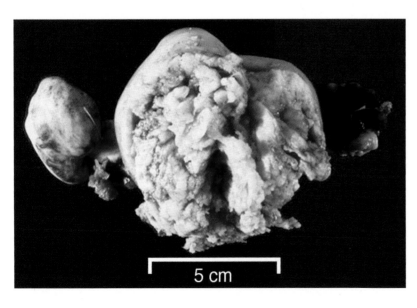

FIGURE 13–59 Endometrial carcinoma, gross

This total abdominal hysterectomy specimen with uterus opened anteriorly shows a more advanced adenocarcinoma of the endometrium that enlarges the entire uterus. This enlarged uterus was no doubt palpable on physical examination. Irregular masses of white tumor are seen filling and expanding the endometrial cavity and extending into the uterine wall. The cervix is at the bottom of the picture. Such a neoplasm often presents with abnormal bleeding. Endometrial carcinomas often develop in the setting of prior complex endometrial hyperplasia, driven by relative estrogen excess. A less common subset of endometrial carcinomas arises from the surface epithelium, has *p53* mutations, and resembles serous peritoneal carcinoma.

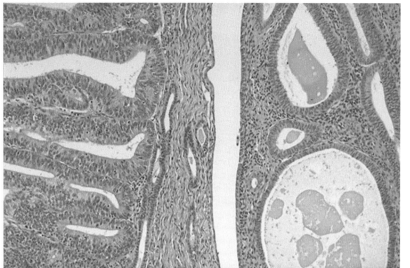

FIGURE 13–60 Endometrial carcinoma, microscopic

The adenocarcinoma at the left is moderately differentiated since a glandular structure can still be discerned. Note the glandular architectural atypia, cellular crowding with hyperchromatism, and pleomorphism of the cells, compared with the underlying endometrium with cystic hyperplasia at the right. More than 85% of endometrial carcinomas have this adenocarcinoma pattern. The diagnosis is most often made with endometrial biopsy, since exfoliated cells are unlikely to be present or diagnostic on a Pap smear. Most of these cancers are detected while confined to the uterus (stage I) so that the 5-year survival is about 90%.

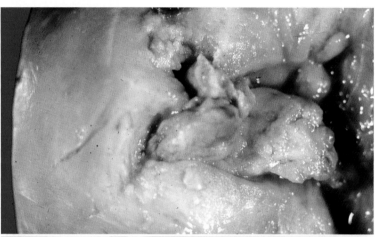

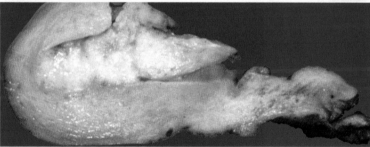

FIGURE 13–61 Carcinosarcoma (malignant mixed müllerian tumor), gross

This irregular, infiltrative neoplasm involves both the endometrium and myometrium. These neoplasms form bulky, polypoid masses that have a fleshy cut surface. They may be so large as to protrude through the cervical os. The typical clinical presentation is similar to that of endometrial carcinoma, with postmenopausal bleeding. Some patients have had prior radiation therapy to the pelvis.

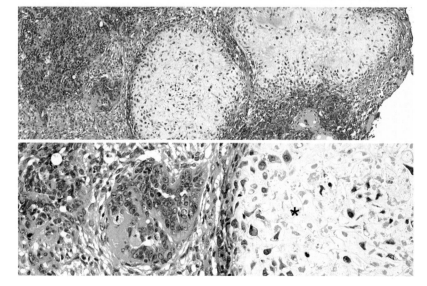

FIGURE 13–62 Carcinosarcoma (malignant mixed müllerian tumor), microscopic

There are carcinomatous elements along with "heterologous" sarcomatous elements (here resembling chondrosarcoma (*)). The malignant mesodermal components can have muscle, bone, adipose tissue, and cartilage differentiation. Most of these neoplasms act in an aggressive fashion. Metastases are most likely to have the microscopic appearance of adenocarcinoma.

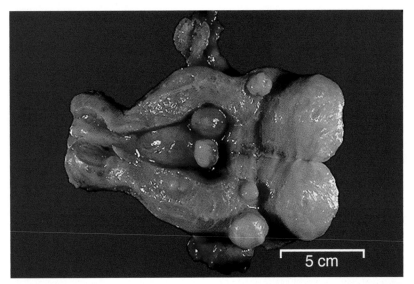

FIGURE 13–63 Leiomyomata, gross

Benign smooth muscle tumors of the uterus are very common and often multiple—perhaps up to 75% of women have one. These neoplasms are sharply circumscribed, firm, and white on cut section. They are uncommon in the genital tract outside of the myometrium. Shown here are submucosal, intramural, and subserosal leiomyomata. Such benign tumors of the myometrium may be the cause of irregular bleeding or infertility, if present in a submucosal location. Larger leiomyomas may also produce bleeding or pelvic discomfort, and they may cause spontaneous abortion. However, most are asymptomatic.

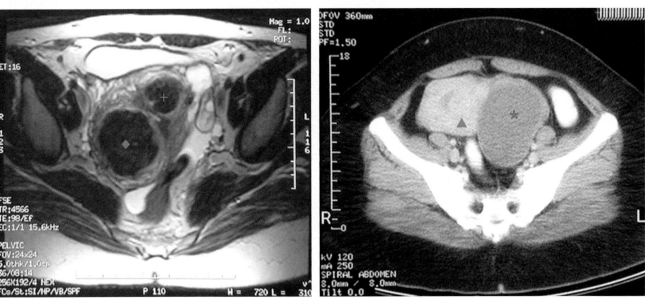

FIGURES 13–64 and 13–65 Leiomyomata, MRI and CT image

The pelvic axial T1-weighted MRI in the left panel shows a large, nodular uterus containing a larger (◆) and smaller (+) leiomyoma of the uterus. The CT scan in right panel shows another patient with an enlarged uterus in which there is a submucosal leiomyoma (▲), and the fluid-filled structure (*) displacing the uterus to the left is an endometrioma of the left ovary.

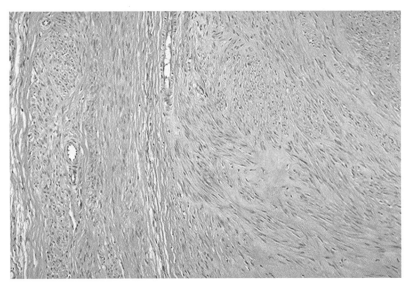

FIGURE 13–66 Leiomyoma, microscopic

Interlacing bundles of uniform spindle cells resembling smooth muscle compose this benign leiomyoma. Mitoses are not seen here (and are rare in leiomyomas). Normal myometrium is at the left, and the neoplasm is so well differentiated that the leiomyoma hardly appears different from the normal myometrium. Leiomyomas may undergo enlargement during the reproductive years, then regress after menopause. Larger leiomyomas may have central softening with hemorrhage (red degeneration). Although a variety of cytogenetic abnormalities can be identified within these tumors, malignant transformation is quite rare, which is fortunate, given their prevalence.

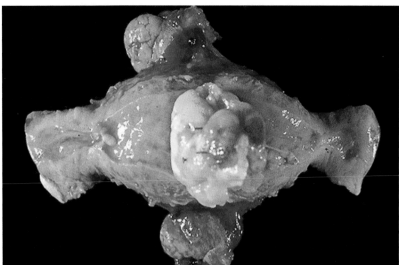

FIGURE 13–67 Leiomyosarcoma, gross

This total abdominal hysterectomy specimen has been sectioned to reveal a large, bulky, polypoid, exophytic mass protruding from the myometrium into the endometrial cavity. (The other growth pattern is endophytic with extensive myometrial invasion.) This uterus has been opened laterally so that the halves of the cervix appear at right and left. Fallopian tubes and ovaries project from top and bottom. The irregular nature of this mass suggests that is not just an ordinary leiomyoma. Leiomyosarcomas are much less common than leiomyomas, and they do not tend to arise from leiomyomas. Their biologic behavior is somewhat unpredictable, but the larger and less differentiated tumors tend to recur or metastasize.

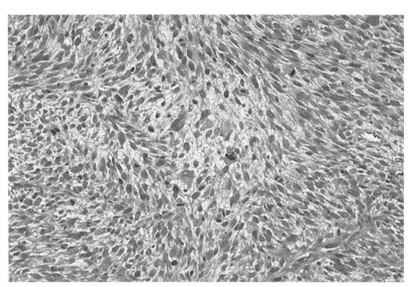

FIGURE 13–68 Leiomyosarcoma, microscopic

A leiomyosarcoma is much more cellular than a leiomyoma, and the cells shown here display both pleomorphism and hyperchromatism. An irregular mitosis is seen in the center. The degree of cellular atypia, the number of mitoses (5 per 10 high-power microscopic fields), and the presence of zonal necrosis aid in making this diagnosis. These neoplasms arise most commonly in the fifth to seventh decades. They have a tendency to recur and metastasize.

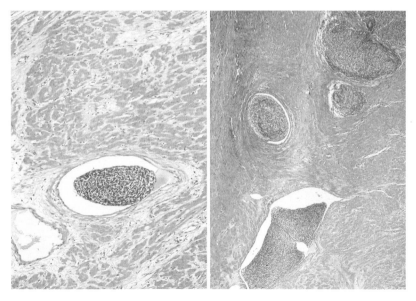

FIGURE 13–69 Endometrial stromal myosis and stromal sarcoma, microscopic

In the left panel is a dilated myometrial lymphatic space containing stromal cells, a process termed *endometrial stromal myosis*. At the right there is more extensive stromal proliferation within lymphatic spaces, with invasion into surrounding myometrium, typical of endometrial stromal sarcoma, which tends to be a low-grade malignancy.

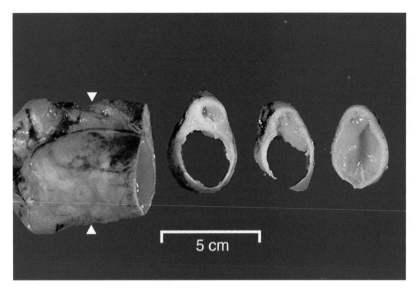

FIGURE 13–70 Tubo-ovarian abscess, gross

This condition resulted from *Neisseria gonorrhoeae* infection, although other organisms, including *Chlamydia trachomatis*, can also cause this disease. Gonorrhea leads to several complications in the female genital tract, including acute inflammation with abscess formation as well as chronic inflammation with tubal scarring (and a greater likelihood of ectopic pregnancy) and pelvic inflammatory disease (PID). Here, there is no clear boundary between tube (▼) and ovary (▲), and the dilated ovary on sectioning is shown filled with purulent material.

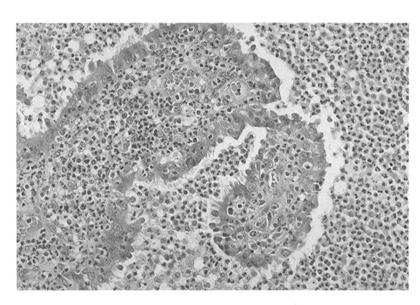

FIGURE 13–71 Acute salpingitis, microscopic

A remnant of tubal epithelium is seen here surrounded and infiltrated by numerous neutrophils. *Neisseria gonorrhoeae* was cultured. The next most likely organism to cause these findings is *Chlamydia trachomatis*. However, multiple pyogenic bacterial species may be present with acute salpingitis that evolves to PID, including enteric bacteria, staphylococci, streptococci, and clostridia. Clinical findings include pelvic pain and fever. Infertility may result from this process. Laboratory findings include leukocytosis with a left shift.

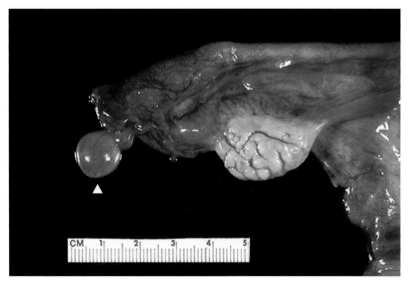

FIGURE 13–72 Paratubal cyst, gross

Here is a common incidental finding: a benign paratubal cyst (▲), an embryologic remnant of the müllerian duct. Sometimes such simple cysts are found adjacent to ovary and are called *parovarian cysts*. They are filled with clear serous fluid and lined by flattened cuboidal epithelium. They can range from barely visible to about 2 cm in size. This one at the fimbriated end of the tube may also be designated as a *hydatid of Morgagni*.

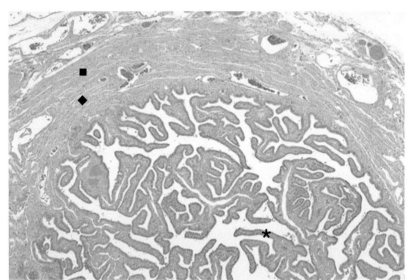

FIGURE 13–73 Normal fallopian tube, microscopic

Normal adult fallopian tube has a thin outer smooth muscular coat composed of ill-defined inner circular (◆) and outer longitudinal (■) layers, and an inner complex branching pattern of finger-like projections (*) of connective tissue lined by a tall columnar epithelium. Some epithelial cells have cilia. Some of the cilia beat upward to help sperm ascend, while others beat downward to conduct ova toward the uterus. Some epithelial cells have a secretory function and are called *peg cell*s. The secretion products of peg cells function in "capacitation" of spermatozoa, which causes them to mature and become capable of fertilizing any ovum lurking in the tube. Few sperm get this far, because, being male, they don't ask for directions.

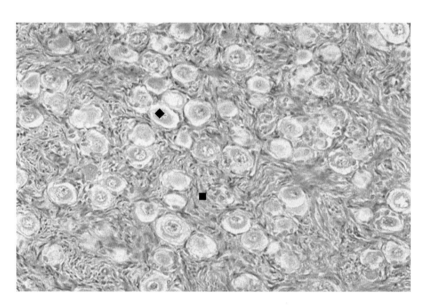

FIGURE 13–74 Normal fetal ovary, microscopic

At high magnification, numerous primordial follicles (◆) and little intervening stroma (■) are seen in this ovary from a late-term gestation. The number of follicles will begin to decrease even before birth. Beginning in late gestation and throughout childhood, ova disappear, until at the time of reproductive maturity at menarche, less than a couple of hundred ova remain in each ovary, which can be released during each menstrual cycle throughout the next 30 or so reproductive years.

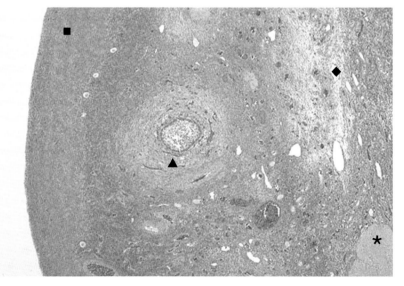

FIGURE 13–75 Normal adult ovary, microscopic

The adult ovary consists of a cortex (■) and a medulla (◆). A mesothelium, also known as the *germinal epithelium*, surrounds the ovary. The outer cortex consists mainly of a stroma, or interstitium, composed of small fusiform cells that can transform under hormonal influence to support the developing ova. The normal adult cortex contains only scattered ova and consists mainly of stroma. A primordial follicle (▲) consists of just the oocyte surrounded by a flattened layer of stromal cells. Seen here at low magnification is ovarian cortex with abundant dense stroma and few follicles. A developing primary follicle with prominent granulosa cells is seen near the center. At the lower right is a pink cloudlike corpus albicans (*).

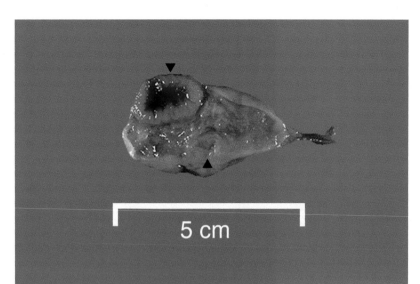

FIGURE 13–76 Corpus luteum, gross

This is an adult ovary with two prominent yellow corpora lutea. The larger one (▼) at the top bulging from the surface is a hemorrhagic corpus luteum of menstruation, and the smaller one (▲) at the bottom is involuting after a previous menstrual period. If implantation of a fertilized ovum occurs, then the corpus luteum will persist because of HCG elaborated from the developing placenta. Of 400,000 ovarian follicles present at birth, only about 400 will mature to the point of ovulation during childbearing years.

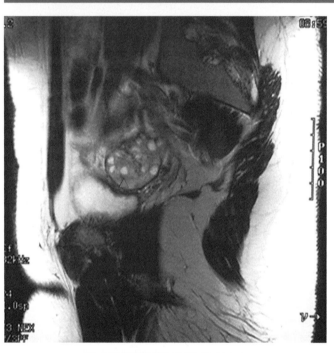

FIGURE 13–77 Polycystic ovary, MRI

This MRI of the pelvis in T1-weighted sagittal view demonstrates multiple small peripheral fluid-filled cysts (▲) of an enlarged ovary consistent with polycystic ovarian disease (PCOD). The cysts average 0.5 to 1 cm in size. Clinical findings include anovulatory cycles with oligo or amenorrhea, acne, and hirsutism. PCOD may be related to insulin resistance, and half of patients are obese, often with type 2 diabetes mellitus. An increased LH pulse frequency results in increased LH secretion and decreased FSH (altered LH/FSH ratio), driving androgen production by follicles with elevated serum testosterone. The decreased FSH is not enough to adequately convert testosterone to estradiol and does not sustain follicular maturation, but because FSH is not totally depressed, new follicular growth occurs, but not to the point of full maturation and ovulation. Multiple cysts result. There is an increased risk for hyperlipidemia and heart disease, endometrial cancer, and pregnancy loss.

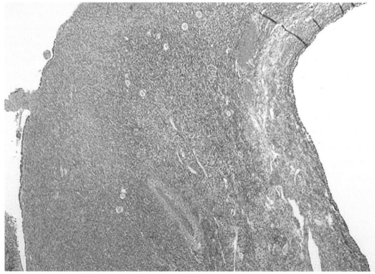

FIGURE 13–78 Polycystic ovarian disease, microscopic

PCOD is characterized by ovarian enlargement with thickening of the outer cortex (at left) and many follicle cysts (one is at the right).

A variation of this syndrome is known as *stromal thecosis*, or *cortical stromal hyperplasia*, and there are no cysts, but only a cortex up to 7 cm thick containing many luteinized stromal cells.

A physiologic response to elevated gonadotropins in pregnancy can lead to theca lutein hyperplasia of pregnancy.

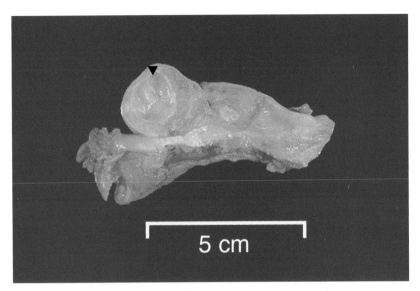

FIGURE 13–79 Follicle cyst, gross

Here is a benign follicular cyst (▼), which is larger than a normal developing cystic follicle. Such cysts can be multiple. They contain clear fluid. Occasionally such cysts may reach several centimeters in size and, if they rupture, can cause abdominal pain.

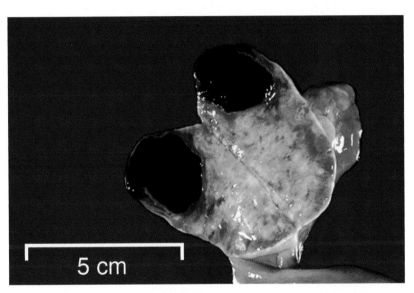

FIGURE 13–80 Hemorrhagic corpus luteum, gross

A normal adult ovary has been sectioned here to reveal a hemorrhagic corpus luteum. Note the dark red-black hemorrhagic region surrounded by a thin rim of yellow corpus luteum. This appearance may be present after ovulation. The hemorrhage may produce lower abdominal or pelvic pain. Larger luteal cysts that persist may resemble the chocolate cysts of endometriosis.

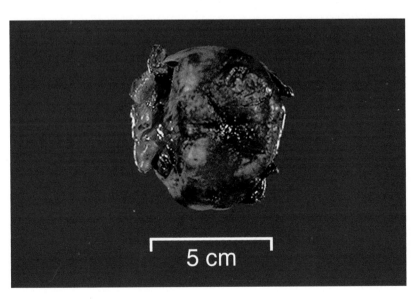

FIGURE 13–81 Ovarian torsion, gross

This ovary is dark and enlarged from hemorrhage after torsion on its ligament. Torsion of the ovary is uncommon but may occur in adults in conjunction with benign ovarian cysts or neoplasms, and in children or infants spontaneously. It leads to a presentation like that of acute appendicitis, but an adnexal mass may be palpable on examination. The disruption of the blood supply results in hemorrhagic infarction and loss of ovarian function.

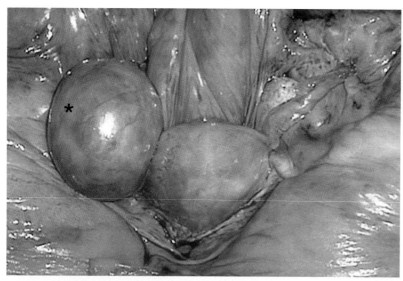

FIGURE 13–82 Serous cystadenoma, gross

Seen here in the pelvis adjacent to the uterus in the midline is a smooth-surfaced tumor (∗) arising from ovarian müllerian surface epithelium—a serous cystadenoma—of the right ovary. Such tumors can reach a large size because they grow slowly and do not impinge on surrounding structures until they are quite large. They may cause some local discomfort. They are typically unilocular cysts filled with serous fluid. Benign serous tumors most often occur between the ages of 20 and 50. The left ovary here is atrophic, consistent with a normal postmenopausal state. The uterus is also normal in size.

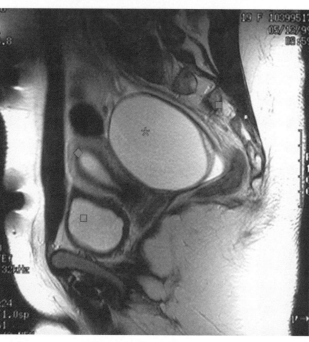

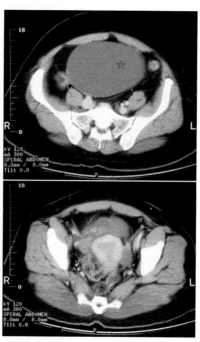

FIGURES 13–83 and 13–84 Serous cystadenoma, MRI and CT image

The sagittal T1-weighted pelvic MRI at the left shows a large fluid-filled mass (∗). The uterus, (◆) bladder (□), and sacrum (■) are visualized as well. A large, unilocular, cystic, fluid-filled mass (∗) fills much of the pelvis in the upper CT panel at the right. The inferior margin of the mass can be seen in the lower panel to attach (▶) to the right ovary next to the bladder, where the wall is somewhat thickened and irregular.

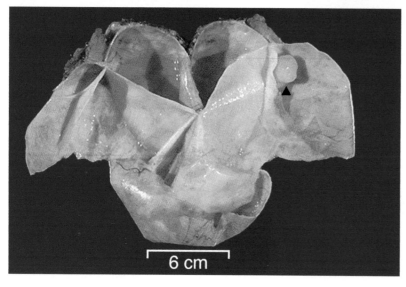

FIGURE 13–85 Multiloculated ovarian tumor, gross

This ovary has been sectioned to reveal multiple fluid-filled cavities, which are smooth surfaced with a rare nodular excrescence (▲). This proved to be a benign mucinous cystadenoma, and 85% of all mucinous tumors are benign. Both serous and mucinous tumors of the ovary are derived from müllerian epithelium. Although slightly less common overall than serous tumors, mucinous tumors of the ovary are more likely to be multiloculated and reach a larger size. Together, serous and mucinous tumors constitute more than half of all ovarian neoplasms (30% are serous, 25% mucinous).

6 cm

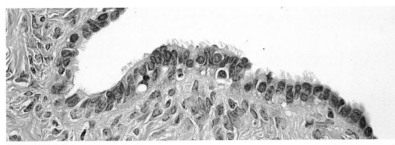

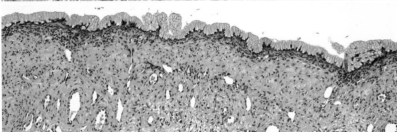

FIGURE 13–86 Cystadenoma, serous, mucinous, microscopic

In the top panel is a thin epithelial lining of tall, ciliated cuboidal cells with minimal infolding and complexity overlying a fibromuscular wall that is not invaded by these epithelial cells. Such a serous ovarian neoplasm is benign and tends to form a unilocular cyst. In the bottom panel, the epithelium lining a neoplastic cyst cavity is mucinous, resembling endocervical mucosa, and thus is termed a *mucinous cystadenoma*, and it would likely have a grossly multilocular appearance.

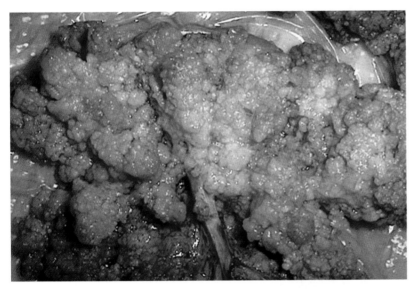

FIGURE 13–87 Borderline tumor, gross

This ovarian mass had a smooth surface, but upon opening revealed the papillary appearance shown here. Borderline tumors have increased numbers of papillary excrescences, larger masses of solid tumor, and greater irregularity or nodularity, and microscopically have a multilayered epithelial lining with cells having some nuclear atypia. However, invasion is absent. Such borderline tumors are not clearly malignant, and conservatively just the ovary can be resected. Some borderline tumors may be accompanied by implants on peritoneal surfaces, but such implants still do not invade, although they may enlarge slowly.

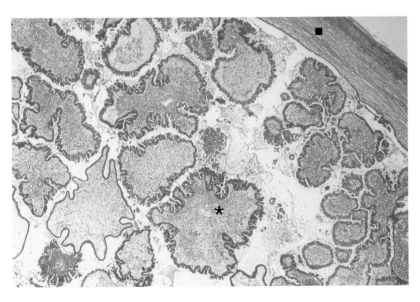

FIGURE 13–88 Borderline tumor, microscopic

Here are papillations (∗) with complex borders, but with one or two cell layers and minimal atypia. Note that there is a thick collagenous capsule (■) that has not been invaded. A borderline tumor must be removed completely, but is very unlikely to metastasize or to recur. *BRCA* mutations, present in about 10% of sporadic ovarian cancers, are unlikely to be present in borderline tumors.

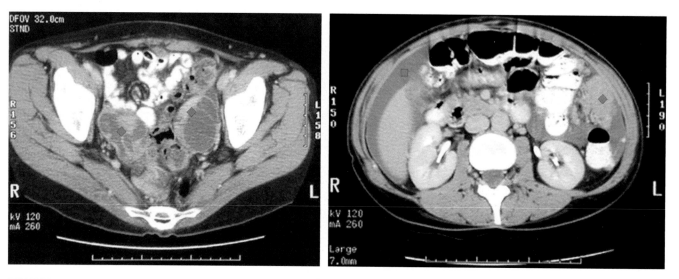

FIGURES 13–89 and 13–90 Cystadenocarcinoma and peritoneal metastases, CT images

The bilateral pelvic masses (♦) seen in the left panel have both cystic and solid components, and they arise in the region of the ovaries. These proved to be bilateral ovarian serous cystadenocarcinomas. In the right panel, the CT scan shows a mass lesion (♦) on the left lateral abdominal wall from seeding of an ovarian serous cystadenocarcinoma. Often, the first sign is abdominal enlargement with ascites. Note the ascitic fluid (■) around the liver and elsewhere in the peritoneal cavity.

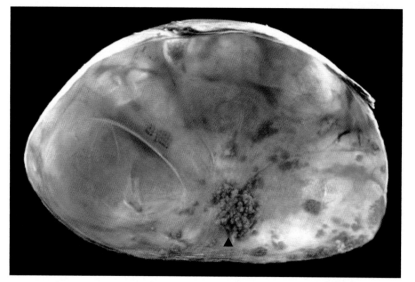

FIGURE 13–91 Cystadenocarcinoma, gross

There are papillations (▲) on the surface of the wall of this neoplasm. These invade through the wall. Cystadenocarcinomas have often spread by seeding the peritoneal surfaces by the time they are detected, giving them a higher stage and poorer prognosis. The ovary can expand considerably in size before symptoms or signs, such as abdominal enlargement with ascites, occur. A serum tumor marker for ovarian serous and endometrioid tumors is CA-125.

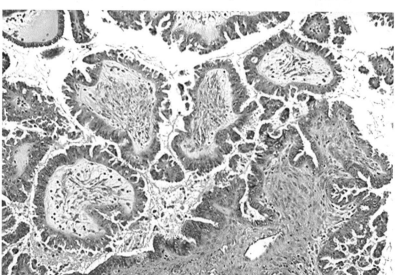

FIGURE 13–92 Cystadenocarcinoma, microscopic

The cystadenocarcinoma shown has more pronounced papillary growth, more complex infolding, more layers of cells, and cells with more hyperchromatism and pleomorphism than a borderline tumor. Invasion is also likely to be present into the underlying stroma or through the capsule of the ovary.

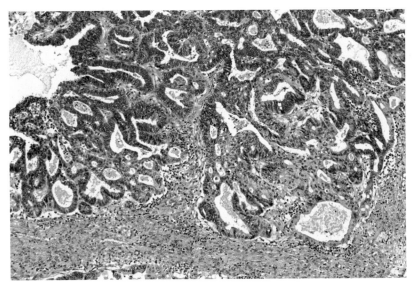

FIGURE 13–93 Endometrioid tumor, microscopic

This neoplasm, although arising in the ovary, resembles an endometrial carcinoma. Endometrioid tumors make up 20% of all ovarian cancers. In about 15% to 30% of cases, there is synchronous occurrence of an endometrial carcinoma. About 15% of cases are associated with preexisting endometriosis. Grossly, they tend have both solid and cystic components.

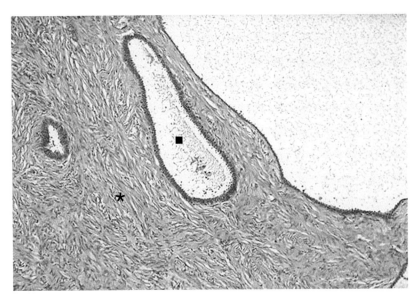

FIGURE 13–94 Cystadenofibroma, microscopic

An uncommon variant of a serous cystadenoma is this cystadenofibroma, or adenofibroma, which is also benign and just has a larger component of stroma, as shown. Note the abundant fibrous stroma (*) between the smaller cystic areas (■) lined by a variety of epithelia, including serous, mucinous, and transitional (Brenner).

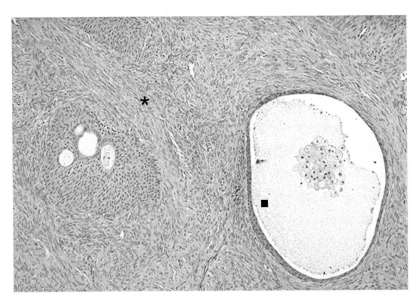

FIGURE 13–95 Brenner tumor, microscopic

This uncommon benign ovarian tumor, a variant of an adenofibroma, has nests of cells resembling transitional epithelium of the urinary bladder. These epithelial nests (■) lie within a fibrous stroma (*) resembling the stroma of a normal ovary. Grossly, they can be solid or cystic. Most are unilateral, and they range from no more than a centimeter to 20 cm in size. There may be a Brenner component within a malignant cystadenocarcinoma.

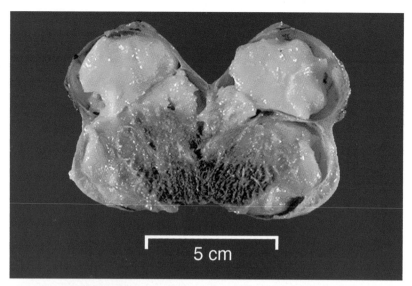

FIGURE 13–96 Mature cystic teratoma, gross

The cystic nature of a mature ovarian teratoma is seen here. A variety of mature, well-differentiated tissue elements may be found from all three embryologic germ layers (ectoderm, mesoderm, endoderm). Often called *dermoid cysts* because they are mostly cystic and mostly contain ectodermal elements, their most frequently found tissue element is skin, so that large amounts of hair and sebum are produced, leading to a challenging cleanup problem in surgical pathology after dissection of these tumors. If these tumors are mostly solid, then they are often "immature" teratomas with less differentiated tissue and may behave more aggressively. Rarely, there are frankly carcinomatous areas.

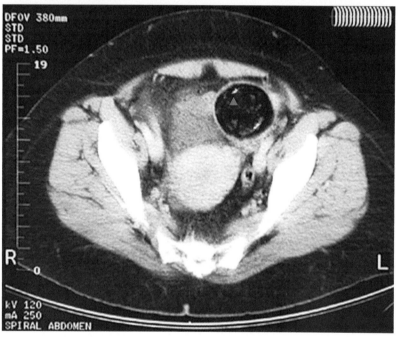

FIGURE 13–97 Mature cystic teratoma, CT image

There is a large but sharply circumscribed, rounded mass involving the left adnexal region of the pelvis adjacent to the uterus and next to the urinary bladder. This mass has variegated contents, including soft tissue densities with low (dark) attenuation as well as bright calcification (▲). This is a mature cystic teratoma (dermoid cyst) of the left ovary. Most of the contents have the same attenuation as the abdominal fat, indicative of the fact that a dermoid cyst contains mostly oily fluid elaborated by sebaceous glands. Most teratomas contain only mature (benign) tissue elements. Immature teratomas have malignant elements, occur in adolescence, grow rapidly, and can metastasize. About 1% of the time, a mature teratoma can undergo malignant degeneration, typically with development of squamous cell carcinoma.

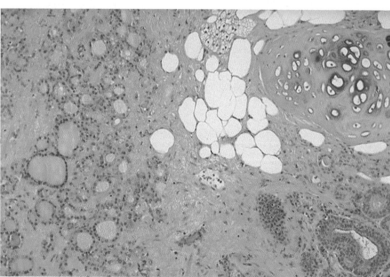

FIGURE 13–98 Mature cystic teratoma, microscopic

Histologically, teratomas contain tissues with differentiation that resembles all three embryonic germ layers (mesoderm, endoderm, and ectoderm). In most benign teratomas, the ectodermal elements predominate. The benign teratoma shown here contains cartilage, adipose tissue, and intestinal glands at the right, while at the left, there are a lot of thyroid follicles. This is a specialized form of teratoma termed *struma ovarii*. Rarely, struma ovarii can even be a cause of hyperthyroidism.

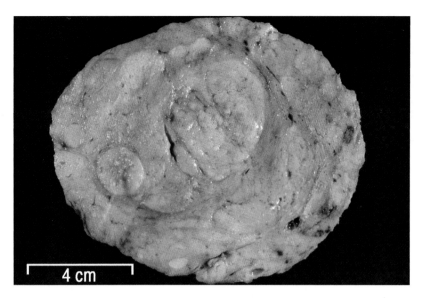

FIGURE 13–99 Dysgerminoma, gross

This dysgerminoma is another form of ovarian germ cell tumor, which is the female counterpart of the male testicular seminoma. This tumor has been sectioned, and the cut surface reveals a lobulated tan appearance. Such tumors are usually solid. Only 10% to 20% are bilateral. They occur most often in young women in their second and third decades. Dysgerminomas account for only about 2% of all ovarian cancers.

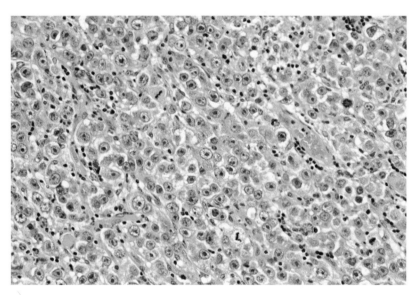

FIGURE 13–100 Dysgerminoma, microscopic

This neoplasm is composed of sheets and cords of large polyhedral cells with large nuclei and pale pink to watery cytoplasm. There is a scant lymphoid infiltrate and virtually no fibrous stroma. Although not seen here, there may by syncytiotrophoblastic cells producing HCG. Although classified as malignant, only one third behave in an aggressive manner. They are radiosensitive.

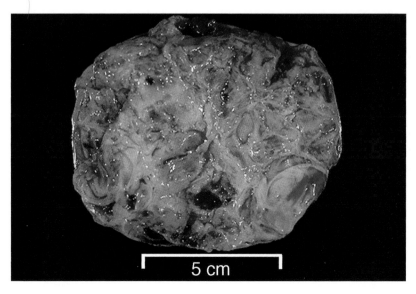

FIGURE 13–101 Granulosa-theca cell tumor, gross

This tumor has a variegated cut surface with both solid and cystic areas. These tumors are derived from the ovarian stroma and have varying amounts of both granulosa cell differentiation and a component of thecoma. They are often hormonally active, with grossly yellowish areas from increased lipids, and can produce large amounts of estrogen such that the patient may initially present with bleeding from endometrial hyperplasia or endometrial carcinoma. On occasion, androgens are produced in excess, leading to virilization. Their biologic behavior is not possible to predict from histologic characteristics, and some may have an aggressive granulosa component.

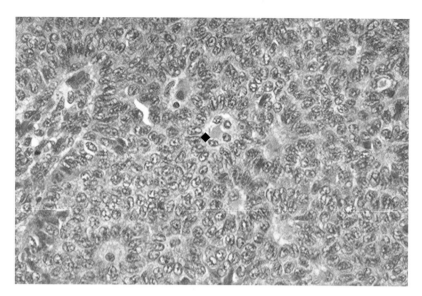

FIGURE 13–102 Granulosa-theca cell tumor, microscopic

Microscopically, the granulosa cell tumor attempts to form structures that resemble primitive follicles. At higher magnification here, the tumor has nests of cells, which are forming primitive follicles filled with an acidophilic material, called Call-Exner bodies (◆). Most of these tumors are histologically benign, but some act in a malignant fashion. There is often an elevated serum inhibin and positive immunohistochemical staining of the tumor cells with antibody to inhibin.

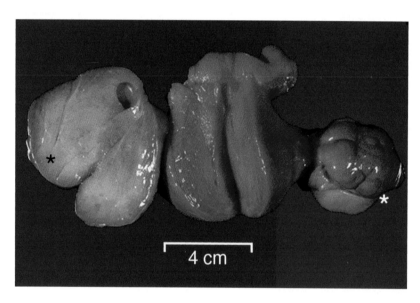

FIGURE 13–103 Thecoma-fibroma, gross

Here are bilateral, solid, sharply circumscribed, benign ovarian tumors (∗). These proved to be fibrothecomas. The thecoma component of the neoplasm gives the tumor a yellowish cast (shown on cut surface of the neoplasm at the left) because of the lipid content. They can also produce abundant estrogen that leads to endometrial hyperplasia and to endometrial carcinoma. These are tumors that arise from the ovarian stroma. They are bilateral in only about 10% of cases. Ascites accompanies about 40% of cases, and the additional finding of a right-sided hydrothorax in association with this tumor is known as *Meigs syndrome*. They can also be associated with basal cell nevus syndrome.

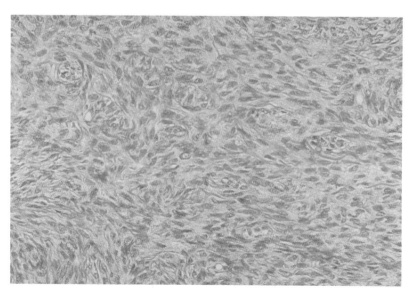

FIGURE 13–104 Thecoma-fibroma, microscopic

The elongated fibroblastic-appearing cells of the fibroma component are fairly uniform. In contrast, the thecoma component is composed of clusters or sheets of plump cuboidal to polygonal cells. The pale to clear cytoplasmic appearance of the thecoma cells is a consequence of the amount of lipid present, and there can be elaboration of estrogens. Fibromas are hormonally inactive. If more collagenous stroma were present, then it would be more fibroma-like. In either case, this neoplasm acts in a benign fashion. Clinical findings include pelvic pain, palpable adnexal mass, and ascites.

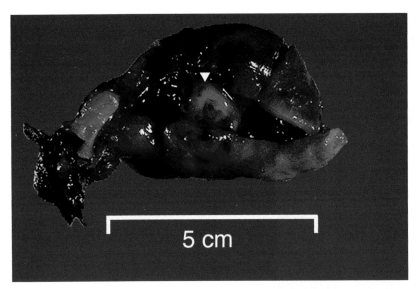

FIGURE 13–105 Ectopic pregnancy, gross

Note the small embryo (▼) in the blood clot emanating from the point of rupture in this resected fallopian tube. This is a medical emergency because of the sudden rupture with hemoperitoneum. Ectopic pregnancy should be considered in the differential diagnosis of severe acute abdominal pain in a woman of childbearing age. About half of ectopic pregnancies occur because of an identifiable lesion such as chronic salpingitis from PID or from adhesions following appendicitis, endometriosis, or previous laparotomy. However, in half of cases, no cause can be found.

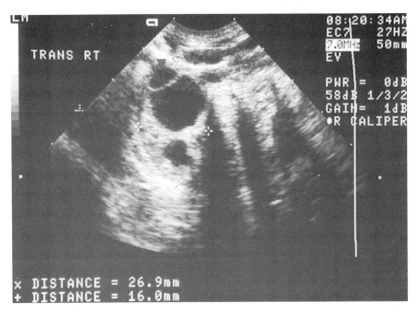

FIGURE 13–106 Ectopic pregnancy, ultrasound

By transvaginal ultrasound, a ringlike structure (▼) is present in the right adnexal region, highly characteristic of an ectopic pregnancy because no gestational sac was present in the uterine cavity, only a thickened endometrium. The β-HCG was also elevated, indicative that a pregnancy had occurred. A culdocentesis may yield blood in cases of ruptured ectopic pregnancy. Isthmic tubal pregnancies tend to rupture at 6 to 8 weeks' gestation, ampullary pregnancies usually rupture at 8 to 12 weeks' gestation, and interstitial pregnancies rupture at 12 to 16 weeks' gestation.

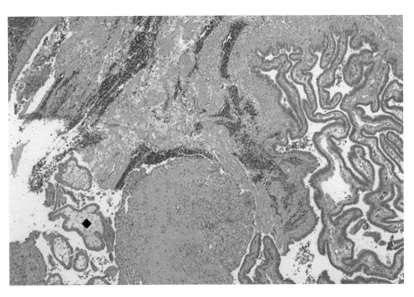

FIGURE 13–107 Ectopic pregnancy, microscopic

A positive pregnancy test (from presence of HCG), ultrasound examination, and culdocentesis with presence of blood are helpful in making the diagnosis of ectopic pregnancy. Seen here is normal tubal epithelium at the right, with rupture site and chorionic villi (◆) at the lower left. These chorionic villi are characteristic of an early pregnancy. If an endometrial biopsy were performed, it would show decidualized endometrium, but no implantation site, fetal parts, or chorionic villi.

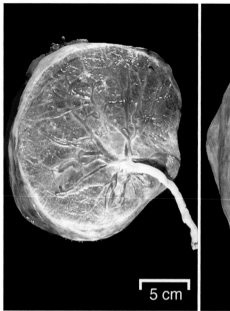
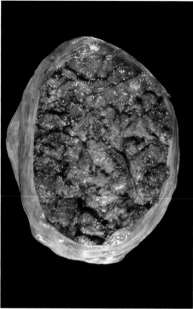

5 cm

FIGURE 13–108 Normal placenta, gross

The umbilical cord inserts into the fetal surface of the placenta, as seen in the left panel. Note the vessels radiating out from the cord over the fetal surface in this normal term placenta. The insertion point is typically just a bit off-center (paracentral). Any insertion onto the disc, including the margin, is of no consequence. If the vessels separate in the membranes before reaching the disc (velamentous insertion), there is a risk for vascular damage and hemorrhage. The maternal surface of this normal term placenta is seen in the right panel. Note that the cotyledons that form the placenta are reddish brown and indistinct.

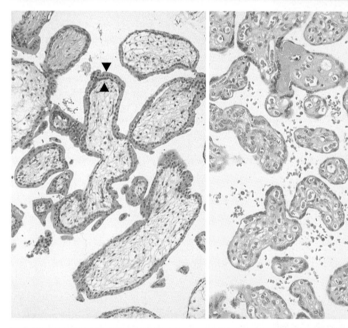

FIGURE 13–109 Normal placenta, microscopic

In the first trimester, as seen in the left panel, the chorionic villi are large and covered by two layers of cells—cytotrophoblast (▲) and syncytiotrophoblast (▼)—and the blood vessels in the villi are not prominent. As the placenta matures in the second trimester, the villi become smaller and more vascular. The syncytiotrophoblast cell layer draws up into "syncytial knots," (▼) which are small clusters of cells, leaving a single cytotrophoblast layer. Clumps of pink fibrin (◆) begin to appear between the villi. A mature placenta in the third trimester, as seen in the right panel, has small and highly vascularized chorionic villi to support the blood gas and nutrient exchange of maternal–fetal circulation required by the growing fetus approaching term gestation. Syncytial knots and intervillous fibrin are prominent.

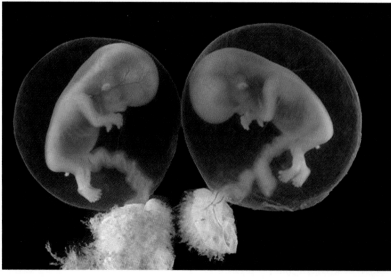

FIGURE 13–110 Twinning, gross

The process of twinning may be monozygous (identical twins derived from one fertilized ovum) or dizygous (separate fertilizations). The former may have one or two amniotic cavities, while the latter always has two. A histologic section through the dividing membranes is useful to help determine these possibilities. A dividing membrane that is monochorionic implies monozygous twinning. However, a dichorionic twin placenta could result from either dizygous or monozygous twinning (the former more likely). These dizygous twin boys are at 9 weeks' gestational age, and each has his own amnionic cavity. These amnions will eventually fuse to form a diamnionic dividing membrane.

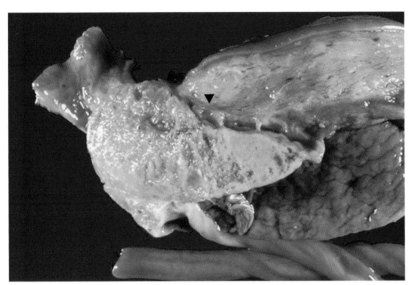

FIGURE 13–111 Placenta accreta, gross

The portion of placenta seen here has invaded (▼) into the myometrial wall in the region of the endocervical canal. These placental villi interdigitate directly with uterine myometrium, without an intervening decidual plate. This will result in lack of normal separation at delivery, leading to marked hemorrhage necessitating emergent hysterectomy. Note that this is also a low-lying placenta previa, which is present in 60% of such cases. The classification of these disorders is as follows: placenta accreta—superficially into myometrium; placenta increta—deep into myometrium; placenta percreta—through the myometrium.

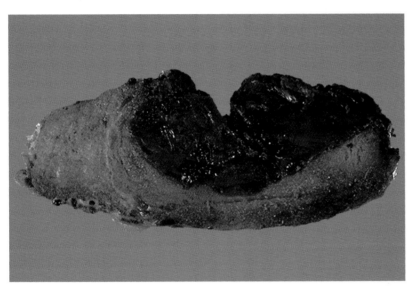

FIGURE 13–112 Abruptio placenta, gross

Placental abruption occurs from premature separation of the placenta in late pregnancy, with formation of a retroplacental blood clot. Such a blood clot is shown here in cross-section of the placenta. Of course, the larger the abruption, the more likely that the vascular supply to the fetus will be compromised. Such abnormal hemorrhage before delivery can lead to sudden onset of severe lower abdominal pain in the mother. Ultrasonography is useful to demonstrate the separation. Emergent delivery is required.

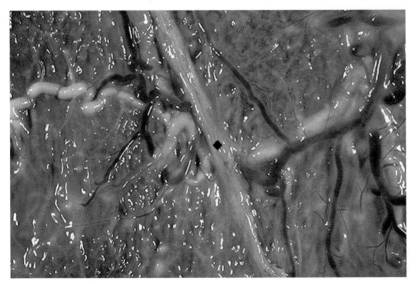

FIGURE 13–113 Twin–twin transfusion syndrome, gross

A twin–twin transfusion syndrome occurs from a vascular anastomosis in a monochorionic placenta between the two fetal circulations that leads to diminished blood flow to one twin (the "donor") and increased blood flow to the other twin (the "recipient"). The donor may die from lack of blood, or the recipient may die from congestive heart failure. The placental blood vessels shown here have been injected with a white fluid to reveal the anastomosis across the dividing membranes (◆) on the placental fetal surface. In general, this syndrome can be suspected when one twin is at least 25% larger than the other. With survival, the size differential eventually disappears.

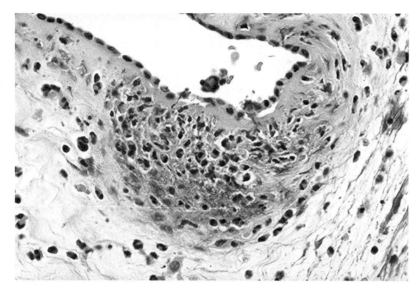

FIGURE 13–114 Chorioamnionitis, microscopic

Note the neutrophilic infiltrates beneath the amnion in these fetal membranes. Premature or prolonged rupture of fetal membranes increases the risk for an ascending infection because bacteria in the vaginal canal can then pass into the normally sealed amniotic cavity. Transplacental spread hematogenously is also possible. This leads to acute inflammation and premature labor with premature birth. The fetus may become infected *in utero* and suffer intrauterine fetal demise.

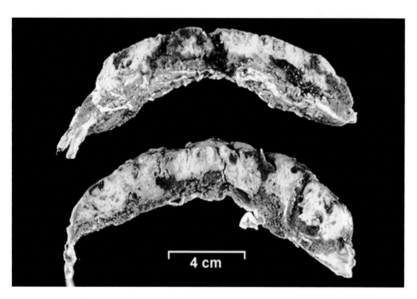

FIGURE 13–115 Placental infarction, gross

Here is a placenta cut in cross-sections to reveal pale yellow areas of infarction involving more than half of the parenchyma. This was so extensive that fetal demise resulted from these infarctions. Small infarcts are common and are of no consequence to the fetus, but if more than one third or one half of the placental parenchyma is infarcted or lost in some fashion, then blood supply to the fetus becomes severely compromised.

4 cm

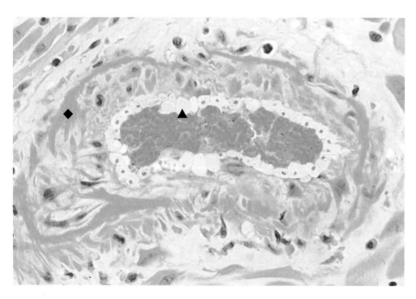

FIGURE 13–116 Placental atherosis, microscopic

This decidual arteriole shows atherosis consisting of prominent intimal macrophage (▲) proliferation along with fibrinoid necrosis (the irregular pink strands (◆) in the arteriolar wall) and edema. This decidual arteriopathy can be seen with pregnancy-induced hypertension (PIH) and with maternal antiphospholipid antibody. Altered placental perfusion can underlie cases of toxemia of pregnancy, manifested in about 6% of pregnancies by hypertension, proteinuria, and edema, called *preeclampsia*; presence of convulsions in addition to these defines *eclampsia*.

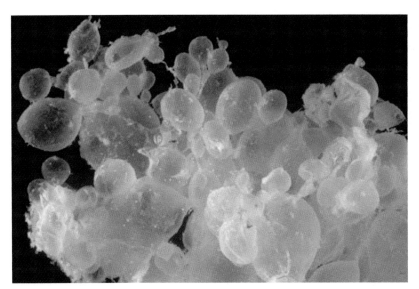

FIGURE 13–117 Hydatidiform mole, gross

Molar pregnancies occur when there is fertilization of an ovum by a sperm but subsequent loss of maternal chromosomes (or less commonly, fertilization of an empty ovum by two sperm), leaving a 46, XX karyotype with only paternal chromosomes, enough to form placental tissue, but not a fetus The grapelike villi typical of the complete hydatidiform mole are seen here. With molar pregnancy, the uterus is enlarged, but no fetus is present. HCG levels are markedly elevated. Patients with a hydatidiform mole are often large-for-date and have hyperemesis gravidarum more frequently. Patients may present with bleeding and may pass some of the grapelike villi.

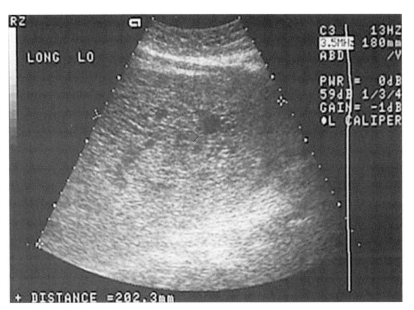

FIGURE 13–118 Hydatidiform mole, ultrasound

This ultrasound view of the pelvis demonstrates a large cystic mass in the uterine cavity, giving a snowstorm (◆) appearance without a fetus present, which is consistent with a complete hydatidiform mole. The uterus is typically large for gestational age. Ultrasound confirms the diagnosis before curettage is done to evacuate this tissue. After evacuation, the patient is followed with serial HCG levels to determine whether an invasive mole or choriocarcinoma has occurred as a complication. About 10% of complete moles develop into invasive moles, whereas choriocarcinoma follows only 2.5% of complete moles.

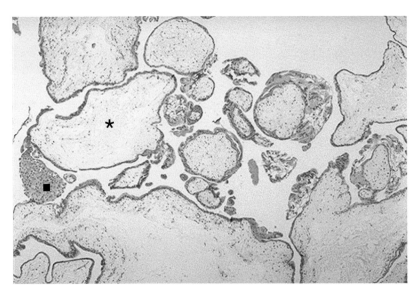

FIGURE 13–119 Hydatidiform mole, microscopic

The complete hydatidiform mole has large avascular chorionic villi (*) and areas of cytotrophoblastic proliferation (■). This must be distinguished from spontaneous abortion with passage of the fetus and retained products of conception with hydropic degeneration of villi. The normal placental villi have immunohistochemical staining for *p57*, a cell cycle inhibitor that is paternally imprinted. Thus, villi of a complete mole, with only paternal X chromosomes, will be *p57* negative.

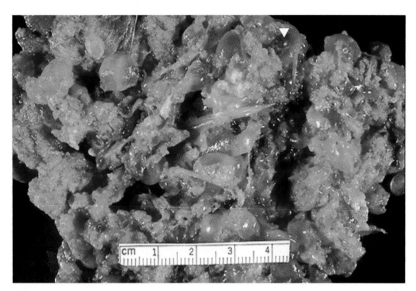

FIGURE 13–120 Partial hydatidiform mole, gross

A partial mole occurs and is diandric when two sperms fertilize a single ovum (or is digynic when the polar body of the last meiotic division is not lost). The result is triploidy (69 chromosomes). Only some of the villi are grapelike (▼), and a growth-retarded fetus with anomalies is typically present but rarely survives past 15 weeks. Note the scattered grapelike masses seen here, with intervening normal-appearing spongy pale red placental tissue. However, the grapelike masses are not as large as those seen with a complete mole. When triploidy is digynic (two haploid sets are maternally derived), the placenta is unlikely to have partial mole features, but the fetus will still exhibit anomalies, and fetal loss occurs.

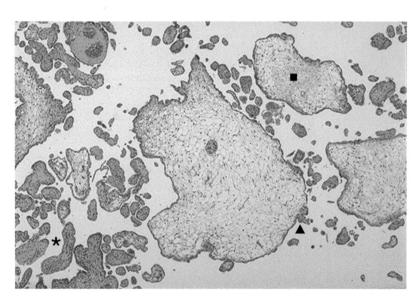

FIGURE 13–121 Partial hydatidiform mole, microscopic

In partial moles, some villi (as seen here at the lower left) appear normal (*), whereas others are swollen and grapelike (■). There is minimal trophoblastic proliferation (▲). The likelihood of subsequent development of invasive mole or choriocarcinoma is much lower for a partial mole than for a complete mole. A characteristic fetal anomaly with triploidy is 3,4 syndactyly of the digits of the hands.

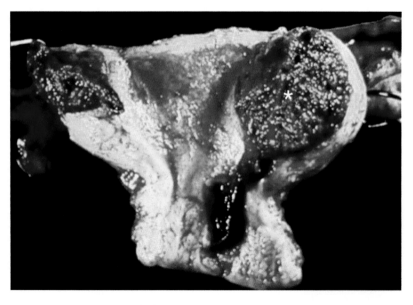

FIGURE 13–122 Choriocarcinoma, gross

The uterus has been opened anteriorly to reveal a hemorrhagic mass (*) lesion in the upper fundus. A choriocarcinoma is the most aggressive of the molar pregnancies. The serum HCG level can be markedly elevated. The patient may not have much uterine enlargement, and vaginal bleeding may be the first clue to its presence. These neoplasms have a propensity to spread locally to the vagina. Distant metastases are most commonly seen in lungs. Brain, liver, and kidneys are also potential sites of metastases.

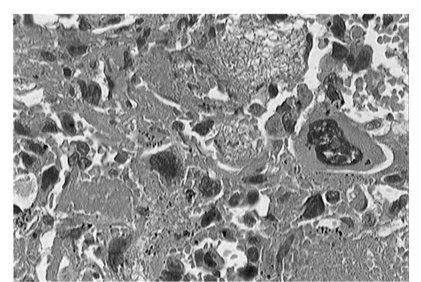

FIGURE 13–123 Choriocarcinoma, microscopic

Villi are not present with choriocarcinoma, but only a proliferation of bizarre trophoblastic cells with loose cohesion and interstitial hemorrhage. These tumors are very aggressive and are associated with very marked HCG levels. Half of them arise in preceding hydatidiform moles. Metastases are common, particularly to the lungs. Chemotherapy results in a nearly 100% cure rate.

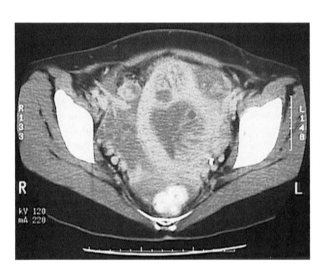

FIGURE 13–124 Choriocarcinoma, CT image

The CT scan of the pelvis demonstrates an irregular solid and cystic mass (♦) in the region of the uterus extending into the pelvis. There is bright contrast in the rectum.

CHAPTER 14

The Breast

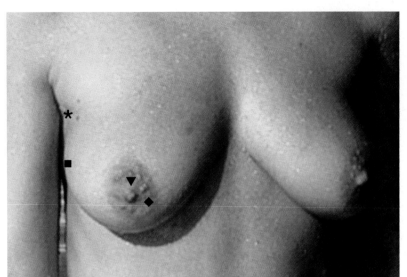

FIGURE 14–1 Normal breast, gross

The normal appearance of female breasts is shown here. The nipple (▼) is surrounded by a darker areola (◆). Some breast tissue extends into the axillary tail of Spence (■). Breast size is primarily determined by the amount of adipose tissue. There may be some asymmetry in development. Macromastia may occur unilaterally or bilaterally with increased sensitivity to hormonal stimulation, and may be called *juvenile hypertrophy* when it occurs at the time of puberty. Rarely, a supernumerary breast may produce a subcutaneous mass anywhere from the axilla (*) to the perineum.

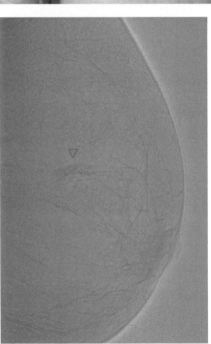

FIGURE 14–2 Breast, mammogram

A mammogram uses a small amount of x-rays to visualize the breast parenchyma. This mammogram demonstrates the normal pattern of lactiferous sinuses and ducts. However, there is one suspicious density (▽) that could be a carcinoma or just an area of pronounced sclerosis with fibrocystic changes. A mammogram is a useful screening tool to find such lesions and determine the need for further work-up. A mammogram may detect lesions that are not palpable. Women in their 30s begin to have some involution of lobules and adjacent stroma, and the breast tissue becomes more radiolucent from an increased composition of adipose tissue replacing fibrous stroma and lobules.

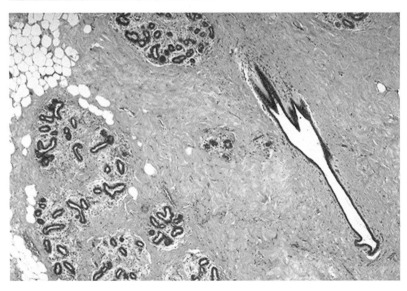

FIGURE 14–3 Normal breast, microscopic

The normal microscopic appearance of female breast tissue is shown here. There is a larger duct to the right and lobular units to the left. A collagenous stroma extends between the structures. A variable amount of adipose tissue can be admixed with these elements. During the normal menstrual cycle, after ovulation under the influence of estrogen and rising progesterone levels, lobular acini increase, epithelial cells become vacuolated, and the interlobular stromal edema increases, leading to increased breast fullness. With menstruation and a decrease in hormone levels, apoptosis of epithelial cells and a reduction in stromal edema occur.

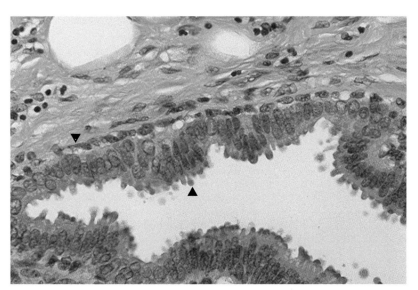

FIGURE 14–4 Normal breast, microscopic

At high magnification, the appearance of a normal breast acinus is shown here. The epithelial cells lining the lumen demonstrate apocrine secretion with snouting, or cytoplasmic extrusions (▲), into the lumen. A layer of myoepithelial cells (▼), some of which are slightly vacuolated, is seen just around the outside of the acinus.

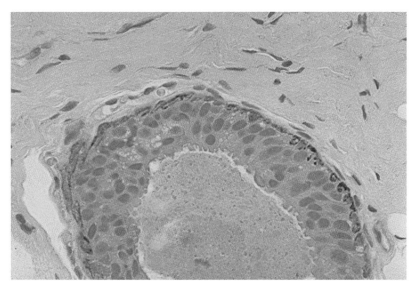

FIGURE 14–5 Normal breast, microscopic

An immunoperoxidase stain with antibody to actin demonstrates the myoepithelial cell layer around the breast acinus. The myoepithelial cells are contractile and are very sensitive to oxytocin. After pregnancy and delivery of the infant, suckling by the infant results in release of oxytocin, from where it is stored in the posterior pituitary gland. The oxytocin induces myoepithelial cell contraction with expression of milk. Breast secretory activity is driven by prolactin from the anterior pituitary. The initial peripartum secretions low in lipid but high in protein, including maternal immunoglobulins, are known as *colostrum*.

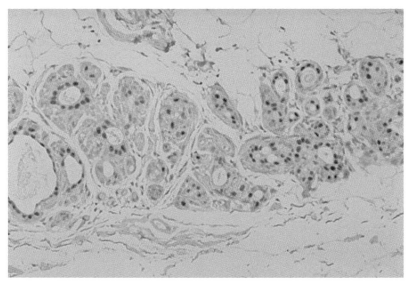

FIGURE 14–6 Normal breast, microscopic

The normal microscopic appearance of female breast tissue is shown here with a terminal duct lobular unit. Note the cluster of lobules lined by epithelial cells that show focal positivity for estrogen receptor (ER) by immunohistochemistry. Note that this steroid hormone receptor is located in the nucleus. Normal breast tissue is responsive to both estrogen and progesterone. Assessment of both estrogen and progesterone receptors is done on tissues removed by biopsy or surgery to evaluate the biologic characteristics of breast carcinomas. Carcinomas that are hormone sensitive may respond to therapy with agents such as tamoxifen.

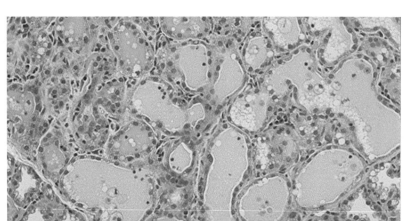

FIGURE 14–7 Normal lactating breast, microscopic

The female breast during pregnancy undergoes hyperplasia and hypertrophy, so that after birth, lactation can occur. Under the influence of estrogen, terminal ducts and ductal epithelium proliferate, while progesterone promotes development of increased acini in the lobular units. Seen here are lobules filled with pink-appearing secretions. The breast, which histologically is a modified sweat gland, secretes by budding off of portions of cell cytoplasm (apocrine secretion) to form breast milk with a high lipid content. After delivery, both estrogen and progesterone levels fall, increasing the lactogenic effect of prolactin. The acinar epithelial cells become vacuolated with increased secretions.

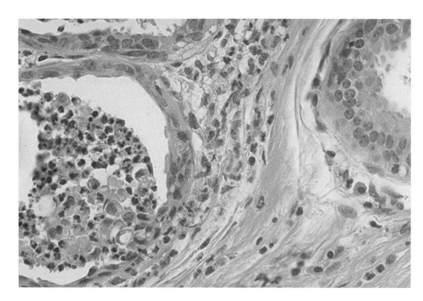

FIGURE 14–8 Acute mastitis, microscopic

While breast-feeding the baby, the skin of the breast may become irritated and inflamed. This skin may fissure, predisposing to infection with entry of microorganisms into underlying breast tissue. Acute mastitis typically involves just one breast and is most often caused by bacterial organisms such as *Staphylococcus aureus*, although streptococci can produce this condition, with neutrophilic infiltrates seen microscopically. If untreated by antibiotic therapy, spread of infection and abscess formation can occur.

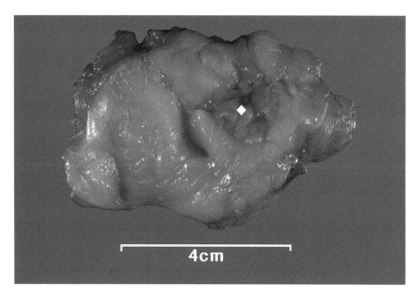

FIGURE 14–9 Breast abscess, gross

During lactation, or at other times with dermatologic conditions that allow cracks and fissures to form in the skin of the nipple, infectious organisms can invade into breast and result in acute inflammation, and this may progress to breast abscess (◆) formation. The most common organism is *Staphylococcus aureus*. Organization with fibrous scar formation around the abscess can form a firm mass that can mimic a carcinoma on physical examination, by mammography, and grossly in the resected tissue specimen.

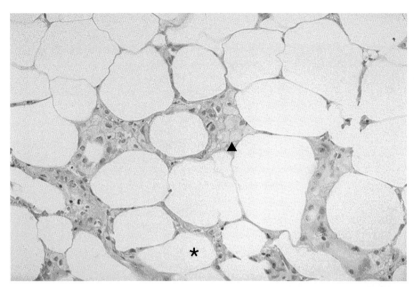

FIGURE 14–10 Fat necrosis, microscopic

The most common etiology of fat necrosis of breast is trauma. The resulting lesion can be a localized, firm area with scarring that can mimic a breast carcinoma. Microscopically, however, fat necrosis consists of irregular steatocytes with loss of their peripheral nuclei and intercellular pink amorphous necrotic material and inflammatory cells, including macrophages and foreign body giant cells responding to formation of the necrotic debris. In this view of fat necrosis at high magnification, some lipid-laden macrophages (▲) are seen among the necrotic adipocytes (∗).

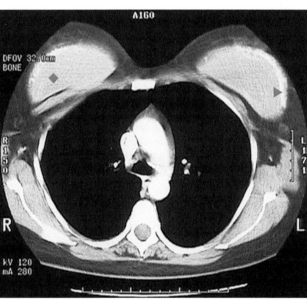
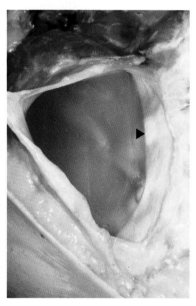

FIGURES 14–11 and 14–12 Breast implant, CT and gross

The chest CT scan in the left panel reveals bilateral silicone breast implants (◆). These implants have resulted in the formation of a fibrous capsule that has partially calcified (▷). The thin connective tissue capsule (▶) around a silicone breast implant is shown grossly in the right panel. Note the overlying skin and adipose tissue at the upper left with the chest wall below the implant and to the right. This is a typical capsule that is pliable and nondeforming, without scarring.

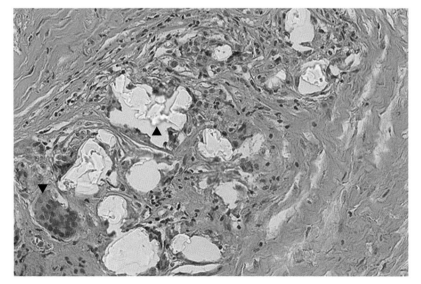

FIGURE 14–13 Breast implant capsule, microscopic

Microscopic examination of the fibrous capsule from a silicone breast implant will often reveal the refractile silicone material (▲) as shown here because this material gradually leaks out from the implant into surrounding connective tissues. This process induces a foreign-body granulomatous response. This is a localized reaction not associated with systemic disease, such as autoimmune disease. The fibrosis with scar formation around a breast implant may produce deformity and pain in some women. Rupture of an implant is uncommon.

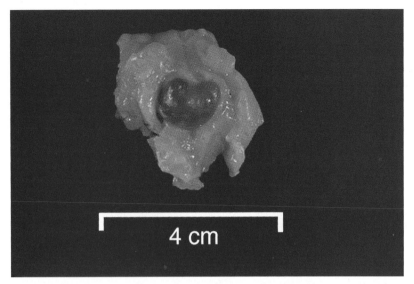

FIGURE 14–14 Fibrocystic changes, gross

A 1.5-cm parenchymal breast cyst is noted here. Its presence led to palpation of an ill-defined but focal "lump" in the breast to be distinguished from other lesions, including carcinoma. Sometimes, fibrocystic changes in the breast, particularly in women of childbearing age, produce a more diffusely lumpy breast. One or more mammographic densities, with or without calcifications, is present. Fine-needle aspiration of fluid from a cyst found in conjunction with fibrocystic changes will typically yield benign-appearing cells seen on cytologic preparations, and the cyst may disappear after aspiration.

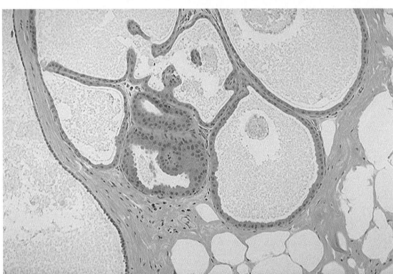

FIGURE 14–15 Fibrocystic changes, microscopic

The appearance of fibrocystic changes in breast includes irregular, cystically dilated ducts and intervening stromal fibrosis. The cysts are lined by uniform benign cuboidal to columnar epithelial cells. This is a "nonproliferative" breast change. Fibrocystic changes account for most breast lumps that are found in women of reproductive years, particularly between the age of 30 and menopause.

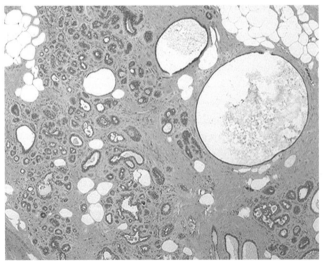 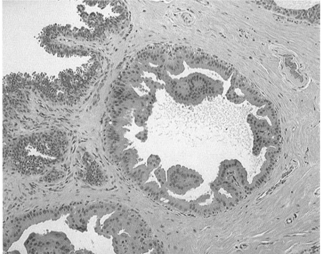

FIGURES 14–16 and 14–17 Fibrocystic changes, microscopic

Additional fibrocystic changes are seen here. Note the irregular duct and lobule size in the left panel. There is prominent apocrine change (abundant pink-staining cytoplasm) of tall columnar epithelial cells lining the cysts in the right panel. These appearances are benign.

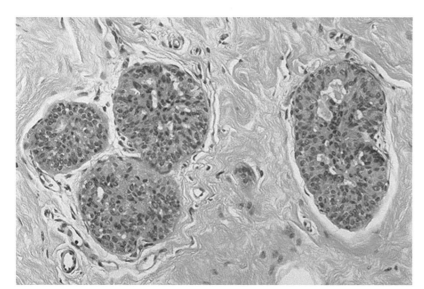

FIGURE 14–18 Epithelial hyperplasia, microscopic

Proliferative breast disease includes the florid ductal epithelial hyperplasia shown here. This can occur within areas of fibrocystic changes. The epithelial cells are multilayered, filling and expanding the ducts or acini. However, there is no epithelial cell atypia. There is a slightly increased risk (1.5 to 2 times normal) for development of breast carcinoma when such changes (more than four layers of epithelial cells) are present.

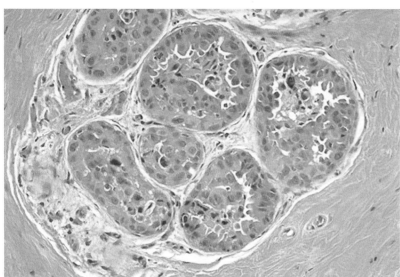

FIGURE 14–19 Atypical ductal hyperplasia, microscopic

Proliferative breast disease with atypia is shown by this cluster of ductular structures, which has irregular proliferation of epithelial cells that show variation in size and shape. Some of the epithelial cell nuclei are enlarged and slightly hyperchromatic. These atypical changes are indicative of an increased risk for subsequent malignancy, although atypical hyperplasia itself is not yet malignant, remaining confined to the ducts, and closely resembles ductal carcinoma *in situ* (DCIS) or lobular carcinoma *in situ* (LCIS). However, atypical ductal hyperplasia does not fill the entire ductal space and lacks the monomorphism seen in the *in situ* carcinomas.

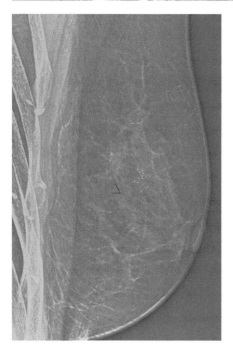

FIGURE 14–20 Atypical ductal hyperplasia, mammogram

This mammogram demonstrates a suspicious dense area (▲) with microcalcifications that could be a carcinoma, proliferative breast disease, or just an area of fibrocystic changes. On biopsy, this lesion had areas of fibrocystic changes along with atypical epithelial hyperplasia. Microcalcifications can be seen in either benign or malignant breast lesions. There are no pathognomic criteria on radiologic imaging for either benign or malignant breast lesions, but imaging serves to confirm the presence and extent of palpable lesions, find nonpalpable lesions as part of screening for breast disease, and provide an index of suspicion for the nature of the lesions to determine further work-up.

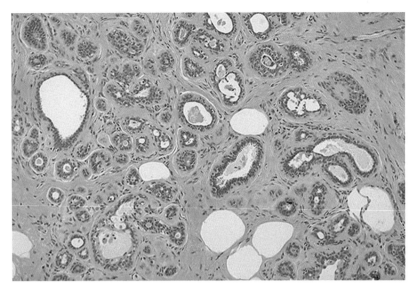

FIGURE 14–21 Sclerosing adenosis, microscopic

Prominent sclerosing adenosis, one of the proliferative breast diseases and a feature that is often seen in association with fibrocystic changes, is demonstrated by the appearance of a proliferation of small ducts in a fibrous stroma. Although not seen here, calcifications can be numerous. The number of acini per terminal duct is more than double the normal found in normal lobules. This lesion may produce a palpably firm and irregular mass. Although it is benign, the gross and mammographic appearance may mimic carcinoma, and it can be difficult to distinguish from carcinoma on frozen section of a biopsy specimen.

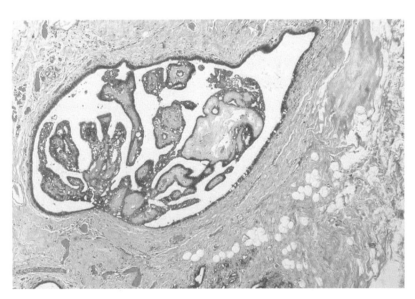

FIGURE 14–22 Intraductal papilloma, microscopic

A small benign intraductal papilloma appears here in a breast duct, typically in one of the main lactiferous ducts beneath the areola, where it can be palpated as a lump. Note that the epithelial cells show no atypia and that there is a fine pink collagenous stroma in branching fibrovascular cores within the papilloma. There can be associated proliferative and nonproliferative breast changes. An intraductal papilloma may be associated with a serous or bloody nipple discharge, or it may cause some nipple retraction. There is a slight (1.5 to 2 times normal) risk for carcinoma when a papilloma is present.

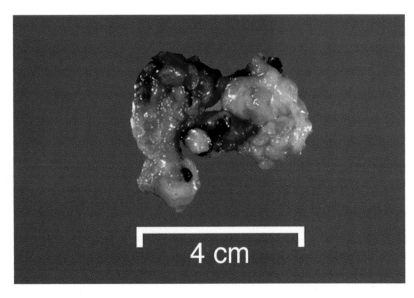

FIGURE 14–23 Fibroadenoma, gross

Here is a surgical excision of a small mass from the breast. This mass is well-circumscribed. On physical examination, it felt firm and rubbery and was movable. The blue dye around this fibroadenoma was used to mark the lesion during needle localization in radiology so that the surgeon could find this small mass within the breast tissue. Fibroadenomas are common causes of breast lumps and the most common benign breast tumor in women. During reproductive years, they may gradually increase in size, then regress after menopause. During menstrual cycles, they may cause some pain with transient enlargement in response to increasing estrogen levels.

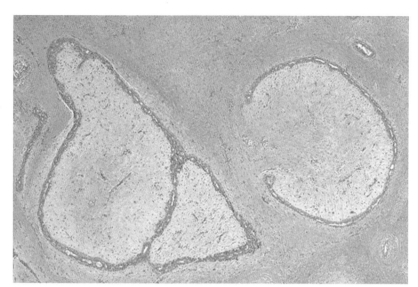

FIGURE 14–24 Fibroadenoma, microscopic

This solid mass is composed of a proliferating fibroblastic stroma in which are located elongated compressed ducts lined by benign-appearing cuboidal epithelium. These lesions are most likely to be found as a breast lump on examination in young women. They are palpably discrete, firm, rubbery masses that are freely movable. After menopause, they become more dense and may calcify. Some fibroadenomas are true neoplasms, while others represent polyclonal proliferations.

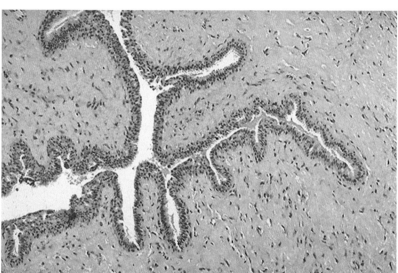

FIGURE 14–25 Phyllodes tumor, microscopic

A phyllodes tumor of the breast arises from the interlobular stroma, but unlike fibroadenomas, it is not common and is often much larger in size. Phyllodes tumors are low-grade neoplasms that rarely metastasize but can recur locally after excision. Microscopically, they are more cellular than fibroadenomas. Projections of stroma between the ducts create the leaflike pattern for which these tumors are named (from the Greek word *phyllodes* meaning "leaflike").

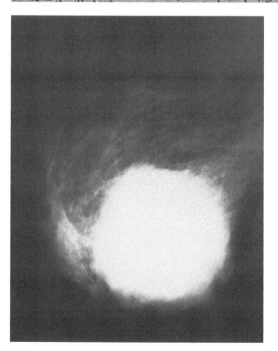

FIGURE 14–26 Phyllodes tumor, mammogram

This mammogram demonstrates a bright, solid 10-cm rounded mass lesion consistent with a phyllodes tumor. It still has discrete margins, similar to a fibroadenoma, but is much larger. The biologic behavior of a phyllodes tumor is difficult to predict, and it may recur locally, but rarely are there high-grade lesions that can metastasize. These neoplasms tend to occur at an older age than do fibroadenomas, most commonly in the sixth decade.

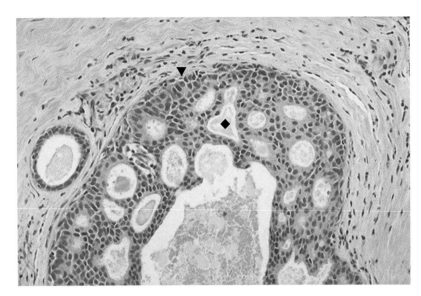

FIGURE 14–27 Intraductal carcinoma, microscopic

The classic cribriform pattern of intraductal carcinoma of the breast is shown here. The neoplastic epithelial cells within the duct are monomorphous, with minimal hyperchromatism and pleomorphism, but they surround irregular spaces with sharp margins (◆), as though punched out by a cookie cutter. This neoplasm is limited to the duct, confined by the basement membrane (▼). DCIS may produce an ill-defined lump on palpation or an irregular density on mammogram, but it may be found incidentally on biopsy. Excision is curative in more than 95% of cases.

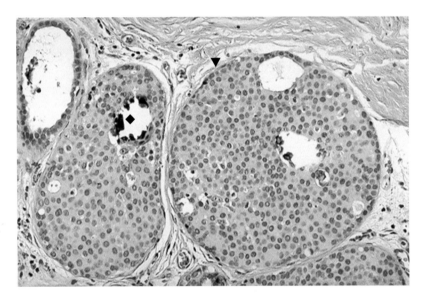

FIGURE 14–28 Intraductal carcinoma, microscopic

The intraductal carcinoma seen here has a solid pattern with neoplastic cells that fill and expand the duct lumens but are still within the ducts and have not broken through the basement membrane (▼) into the adjacent stroma. Note that the two large ducts in the center contain microcalcifications (◆), a form of dystrophic calcification in response to focal necrosis in the neoplasm. Such microcalcifications can appear on mammography. However, microcalcifications may also appear in benign breast lesions, including fibrocystic changes and proliferative breast diseases. DCIS makes up about 15% to 30% of all cancers in women receiving screening for breast cancer.

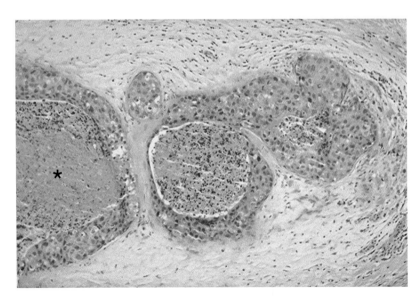

FIGURE 14–29 Comedocarcinoma, microscopic

A comedocarcinoma pattern of intraductal carcinoma is characterized by the presence of rapidly proliferating, high-grade malignant cells. Note the prominent central necrosis (∗) in these ducts. There is prominent periductal fibrosis with minimal chronic inflammation. This central necrosis leads to the gross characteristic of extrusion of cheesy material from the ducts with pressure (comedone-like). This pattern is not common, but the overall prognosis for patients with comedocarcinoma is generally good.

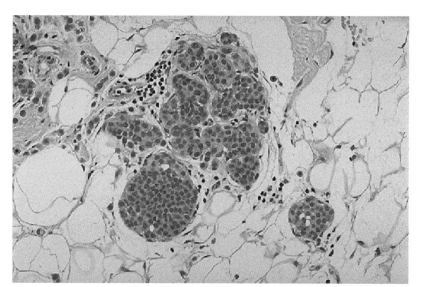

FIGURE 14–30 Lobular carcinoma *in situ*, microscopic

LCIS is unlikely to form a palpable mass or radiologic density, but it is frequently bilateral and multicentric. LCIS does not form microcalcifications. LCIS consists of a neoplastic proliferation of monomorphic epithelial cells within the terminal breast ducts and acini. These epithelial cells are small and round. Although these lesions are low grade, there is a 25% to 35% risk for development of invasive carcinoma in the same or the opposite breast (greater for the ipsilateral breast). LCIS constitutes 1% to 6% of all breast carcinomas.

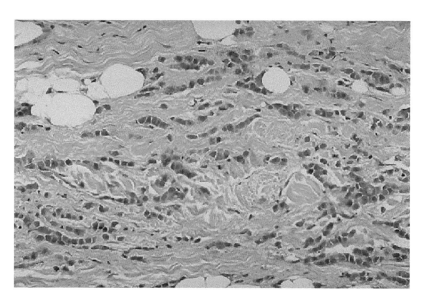

FIGURE 14–31 Infiltrating lobular carcinoma, microscopic

This neoplasm arises in the terminal ductules of the breast. The characteristic "Indian file" strands of infiltrating lobular carcinoma cells are seen here within the fibrous stroma. Pleomorphism of these neoplastic cells is not marked. About 5% to 10% of breast cancers are of this type. There is about a 20% chance that the opposite breast will also be involved, and many of these neoplasms arise multicentrically in the same breast.

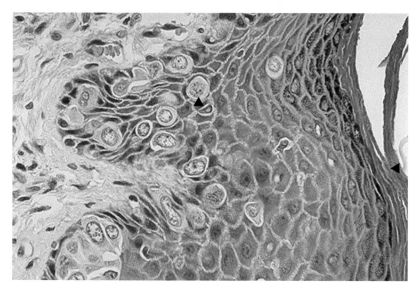

FIGURE 14–32 Paget disease of breast, microscopic

Note the overlying hyperkeratosis (◄) of the skin seen here, which contributes to the rough, red, scaling appearance seen grossly, and there is often skin ulceration. The large cells (▲) infiltrating into the epidermis represent intraepithelial extension of an underlying DCIS or invasive ductal carcinoma. The large Paget cells of Paget disease of the breast have abundant clear cytoplasm and appear within the epidermis either singly or in clusters. The nuclei of the Paget cells are atypical and, although not seen here, often have prominent nucleoli.

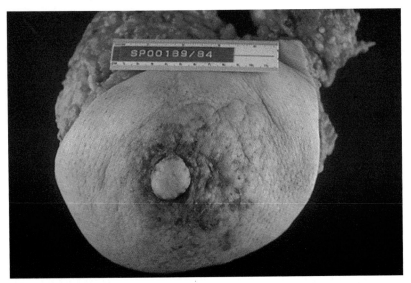

FIGURE 14–33 "Inflammatory" carcinoma, gross

This mastectomy specimen demonstrates the gross findings of an "inflammatory" carcinoma of the breast. This is not a specific histologic type of breast cancer; rather, it implies dermal lymphatic invasion by some type of underlying breast carcinoma (usually invasive ductal carcinoma). Such involvement of dermal lymphatics gives the grossly thickened, erythematous, and rough skin surface with the appearance of an orange peel (*peau d'orange*, for you Francophiles). There may not be an obvious underlying mass lesion.

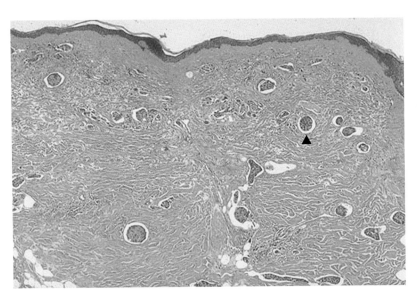

FIGURE 14–34 "Inflammatory" carcinoma, microscopic

The skin overlying this breast shows prominent dermal lymphatic spaces (▲) filled with small clusters of metastatic cells from an underlying breast carcinoma. Carcinomas typically metastasize first to lymphatics. Breast cancers most often metastasize to the axillary lymph nodes, and these nodes can be sampled or removed at the time of surgery for breast cancer. Rarely, a metastasis is detected first because the primary site is "occult" and not detectable by physical examination or radiographic imaging techniques.

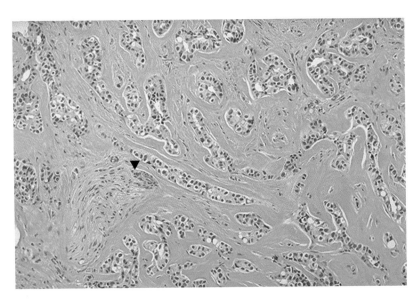

FIGURE 14–35 Invasive ductal carcinoma, microscopic

Note the small nests and infiltrating strands of neoplastic cells with prominent bands of collagen between them in this invasive ductal carcinoma of the breast. Ductal carcinoma here is not confined to the ducts but infiltrates outward into the surrounding stroma. As it does so, it is the marked increase in the dense fibrous tissue stroma that produces the characteristic hard "scirrhous" appearance of the typical infiltrating ductal carcinoma. Note the nerve surrounded by the neoplasm (▼) at the lower left. Perineural invasion is a frequent feature of invasive carcinoma and can account for the dull but constant character of "neoplastic" pain.

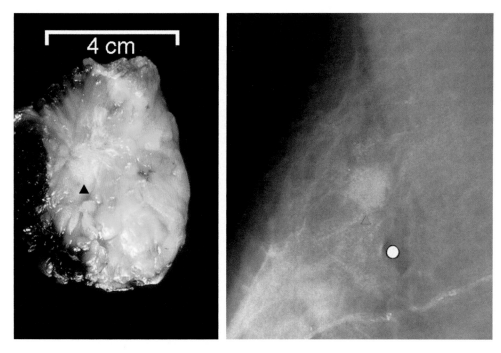

FIGURES 14–36 and 14–37 Invasive ductal carcinoma, gross and mammogram

Note the grossly irregular margins and varied cut surface of this breast carcinoma (▲) in the left panel. This lesion felt firm on physical examination with palpation and was not freely movable. The cut surface of this excised lesion felt gritty because of desmoplasia and microcalcifications. The margins of the specimen were inked with green dye after removal to assist in determining whether cancer extends to the margins once histologic sections are made. The mammogram in the right panel shows tiny peripheral calcifications within a lesion (▲) consistent with a neoplasm in the upper portion above and just to the left of the white dot marking the point the patient felt some pain on palpation.

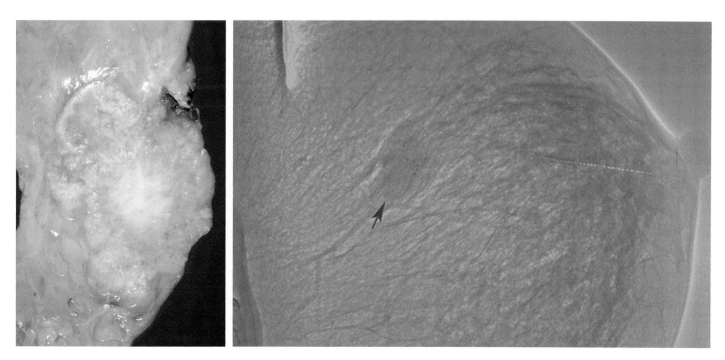

FIGURES 14–38 and 14–39 Infiltrating ductal carcinoma, gross and mammogram

The grossly irregular mass lesion seen in the left panel is an infiltrating ductal carcinoma of breast. The center is very firm (scirrhous) and white because of the desmoplasia. There are areas of yellowish necrosis in the portions of neoplasm infiltrating into the surrounding breast and adipose tissue. Such tumors are very firm and nonmobile on physical exam. The mammogram in the right panel demonstrates a large, irregular mass lesion (*arrow*).

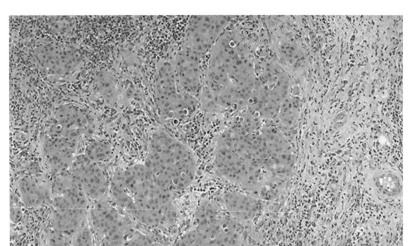

FIGURE 14–40 Medullary carcinoma, microscopic

Medullary carcinomas account for less than 5% of breast cancers. These tumors can sometimes be large, fleshy masses up to 5 cm in size. Medullary carcinoma is composed of cells with pleomorphic nuclei that have prominent nucleoli. Although not seen here, foci of necrosis and hemorrhage can be found. Shown here at low power, sheets and nests of cells are surrounded by a lymphoid stroma with little desmoplasia. Some of these tumors occur in association with *BRCA1* gene mutations. *HER2/neu* overexpression is not observed. The prognosis with medullary carcinoma is better than for infiltrating ductal or lobular carcinoma.

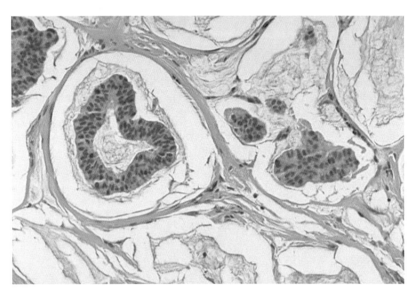

FIGURE 14–41 Colloid carcinoma, microscopic

This variant of breast cancer is known as *colloid*, or *mucinous*, carcinoma. Note the abundant bluish mucin. The carcinoma cells appear to be floating in the mucin. This mucinous matrix gives the tumor a grossly soft, blue to gray appearance. Some of these tumors occur in association with *BRCA1* gene mutations. This variant tends to occur in older women as a small, circumscribed mass. It is slow growing, and if it is the predominant histologic pattern present in a breast cancer, then the prognosis is better than for nonmucinous, invasive carcinomas.

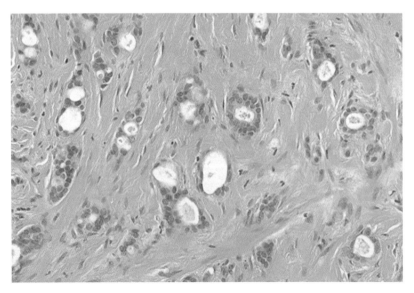

FIGURE 14–42 Tubular carcinoma, microscopic

This variant of breast cancer accounts for only about 2% of all cases. These cancers tend to be small and often detected only mammographically. These well-differentiated neoplastic cells form a single cuboidal layer in small round to teardrop-shaped ductules widely spaced in a fibrous stroma. The prognosis tends to be better than for an intraductal carcinoma, despite the multifocal nature and bilaterality that are more common with this variant, because of the well-differentiated nature of the cells and the younger average age at onset (40s).

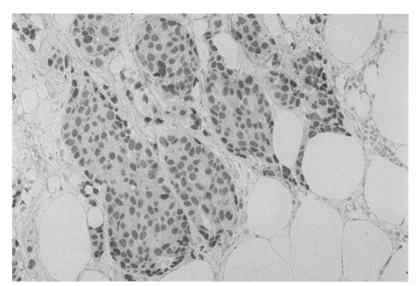

FIGURE 14–43 Estrogen receptor–positive breast carcinoma, microscopic

The cells of this breast carcinoma are highly positive for ER with this immunoperoxidase stain. ER positivity often correlates with a better prognosis because such positive neoplastic cells are better differentiated and more amenable to hormonal manipulation, including use of the drug tamoxifen. The use of the immunoperoxidase technique shown here allows determination of the degree of ER positivity within the nuclei of just the neoplastic cells, without interference from other cells.

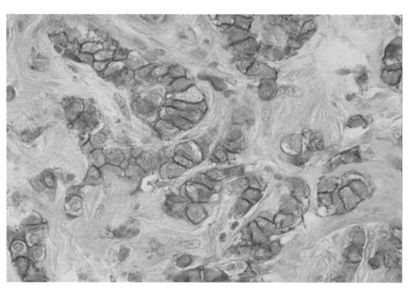

FIGURE 14–44 *HER2*–positive breast carcinoma, microscopic

This is positive immunoperoxidase staining for *C-erb B-2* (*HER2/neu*) gene product in a breast carcinoma. Note the membranous staining of the neoplastic cells with the antibody directed against the *HER2* gene product (normal cells do not make this product). This gene encodes for an epithelial growth factor receptor on the cell membrane that stimulates cellular proliferation. There is a correlation between *HER2* positivity and high nuclear grade and aneuploidy. The drug trastuzumab is a monoclonal antibody directed against *HER2*-positive breast cancer cells.

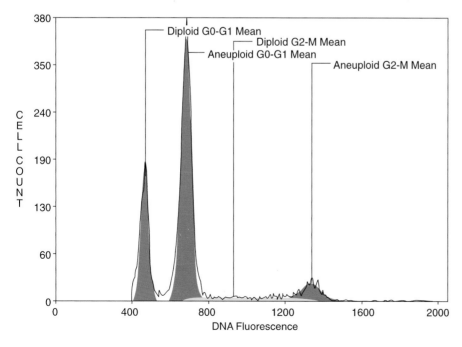

FIGURE 14–45 Breast carcinoma, flow cytometry

Flow cytometry performed on cells obtained by fine-needle aspiration, excisional biopsy, or resection from a breast cancer can be analyzed to determine the characteristics of the DNA content. The presence of an increased proliferative rate (high S phase) and aneuploidy, as shown in this flow cytometric pattern of this breast carcinoma, suggest a worse prognosis.

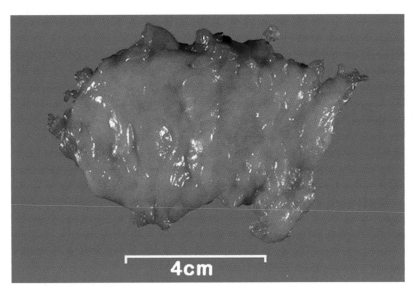

FIGURE 14–46 Gynecomastia, gross

An increased amount of breast tissue in a male is known as *gynecomastia*. This condition is not common. In pubertal males, it may be idiopathic and resolve spontaneously, or persist and require surgical removal, as in this case seen here. In older males, it results from hyperestrinism and may be the result of cirrhosis of the liver (from decreased hepatic clearance of estrogenic substances), from pharmacologic agents, Klinefelter syndrome (47, XXY), or neoplasms such as a Leydig cell tumor of the testis.

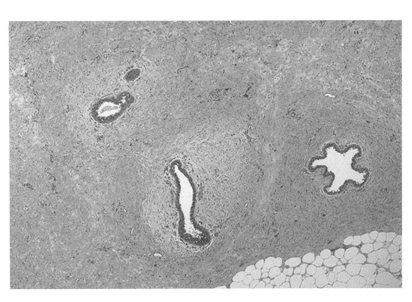

FIGURE 14–47 Gynecomastia, microscopic

The normally small amount of male breast tissue consists of just a few ducts, without lobules, in a fibrous stroma. With gynecomastia, this stromal and ductular tissue is increased, and there can be ductal epithelial hyperplasia, or prominent periductular edema as seen here. However, lobule formation does not occur. Gynecomastia can be unilateral or bilateral.

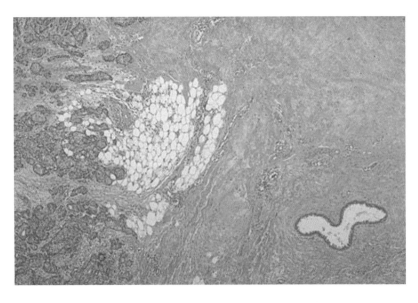

FIGURE 14–48 Male breast carcinoma, microscopic

Male breast cancers are much less common than female breast cancers, perhaps by a ratio of 100:1. Most occur as a subareolar mass with nipple discharge in elderly men and have spread to contiguous structures, giving them a high stage at diagnosis. Some are related to the *BRCA1* and *BRCA2* gene mutations. The same diagnostic techniques, such as mammography can be utilized for screening and diagnosis. At low power at the right can be seen a duct in a fibrous stroma, with absence of lobules, typical of male breast. At the left is an infiltrating carcinoma. Most male breast cancers are of the infiltrating ductal carcinoma variety. More than 80% are ER positive.

CHAPTER 15

The Endocrine System

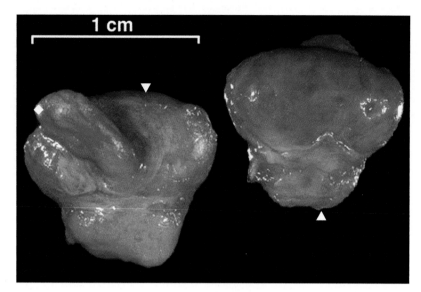

FIGURE 15–1 Normal pituitary gland, gross

The normal adult pituitary, situated in the sella turcica, weighs about 1 gm. Embryologically, the anterior pituitary (▼) (adenohypophysis) is derived from an upward evagination of the oral cavity, called *Rathke pouch*. The posterior pituitary (▲) (neurohypophysis) is derived from the diencephalon and consists of modified glial cells (pituicytes) and their axons extending down the pituitary stalk (◆) (seen here superiorly) from supraoptic and paraventricular hypothalamic nuclei. The adenohypophysis has a dual blood supply, with a hypophyseal portal system as well as small perforating arteries. Seen inferiorly at the right, the neurohypophysis appears at the bottom.

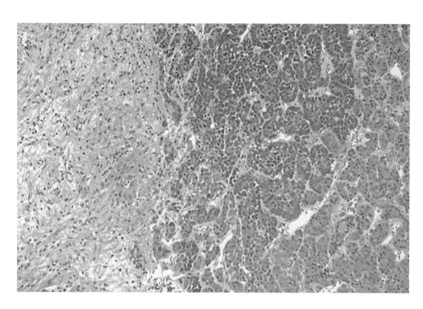

FIGURE 15–2 Normal pituitary, microscopic

The neurohypophysis, which resembles neural tissue because it is composed of modified glial cells along with the axons of hypothalamic nerve cells bodies, appears at the left. The highly vascularized adenohypophysis appears at the right. The neurohypophyseal hormones oxytocin and vasopressin (antidiuretic hormone, or ADH) are synthesized in the hypothalamus and transported along axons to the neurohypophysis, from where they are released into the bloodstream and carried systemically to act on cells in target organs.

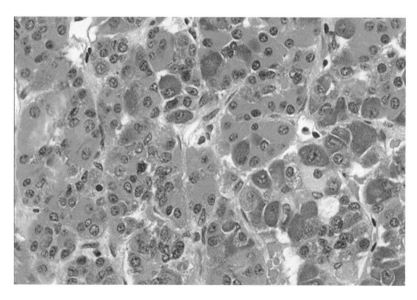

FIGURE 15–3 Normal pituitary, microscopic

In the adenohypophysis at higher magnification can be seen the pink acidophils that produce prolactin (lactotrophs) and growth hormone (somatotrophs). The dark purple basophils can produce luteinizing hormone, or LH, and follicle-stimulating hormone, or FSH (gonadotrophs); thyroid-stimulating hormone, or TSH (thyrotrophs); and adrenocorticotropic hormone, or ACTH (corticotrophs). The paler cells are the chromophobes. As in all endocrine glands, there is prominent vascularity with many capillaries into which the hormones are secreted for distribution throughout the body. The secretions of these cells are under control of hypothalamic-releasing factors, which are all positive acting, except for dopamine, which inhibits lactotrophs.

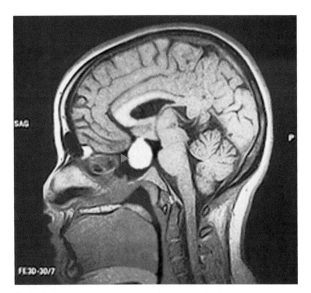

FIGURE 15–4 Pituitary macroadenoma, MRI

In this T1-weighted sagittal MRI can be seen a large bright pituitary macroadenoma (▶) larger than 1 cm. Pituitary adenomas arise in the adenohypophysis. They may be null cell adenomas producing a mass effect but without detectable hormonal secretion, or they may be composed of either acidophils or basophils secreting an excess of one hormone (or less commonly, several hormones). Overall, the most common types of pituitary adenomas (and their clinical outcomes) include prolactinoma (amenorrhea-galactorrhea in women, decreased libido in men), followed by null cell adenoma, corticotroph adenoma (Cushing disease), gonadotroph adenoma (paradoxic hypogonadism), and somatotroph adenoma (acromegaly in adults and gigantism in children). About 3% of pituitary adenomas are associated with multiple endocrine neoplasia type 1 (MEN 1).

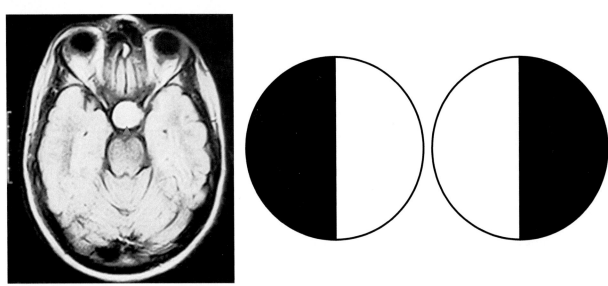

FIGURE 15–5 Pituitary macroadenoma, MRI

This T1-weighted MRI in axial view demonstrates a bright pituitary macroadenoma (▲). Macroadenomas by their size can erode the sella turcica to produce headaches and impinge on the optic chiasm to produce visual field defects, most commonly bitemporal hemianopsia, as demonstrated by the diagram to the right of the figure.

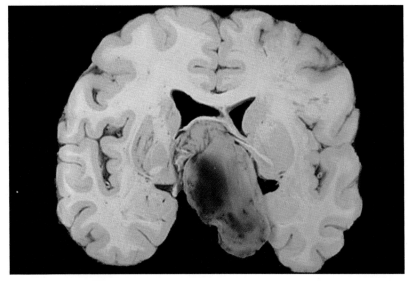

FIGURE 15–6 Pituitary macroadenoma, gross

This large pituitary adenoma (macroadenoma) impinges on the ventricular system, as seen here, with subsequent elevation in intracranial pressure producing symptoms of headache, nausea, and vomiting. Occasionally, there can be acute hemorrhage into the adenoma to increase the mass effect. Some pituitary adenomas have mutations in *GNAS1* that result in activation of the α subunit of a G-stimulatory protein, increasing cyclic adenosine monophosphate (AMP) production that drives cellular proliferation. Mutations in *RAS* and c-*MYC* genes may also be present in more aggressive adenomas such as the one seen here.

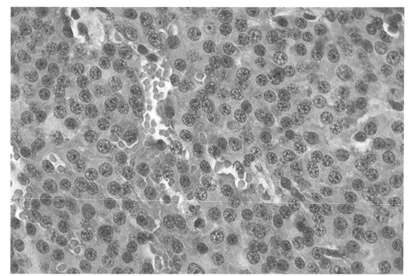

FIGURE 15–7 Pituitary adenoma, microscopic

This pituitary adenoma has a monotonous pattern of fairly uniform, rounded cells and capillary channels. The H+E staining pattern can vary, The most common pituitary adenoma (25% of cases) in adults secretes prolactin, while 20% are null cell adenomas that do not secrete a hormone, but can exert a mass effect, diminish pituitary function (hypopituitarism), or even have a "stalk section" effect to disrupt prolactin-inhibiting factor release into the anterior pituitary, leading to hyperprolactinemia. Growth hormone–secreting adenomas are most common in children, but are not common in adults.

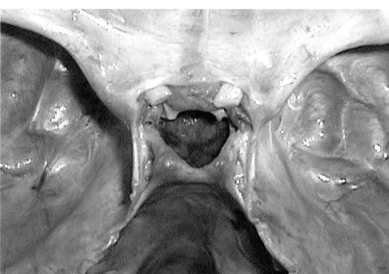

FIGURE 15–8 Empty sella syndrome, gross

At autopsy, the brain has been removed, and the base of the skull is seen with the sella turcica in the center. Just a remnant of flattened pituitary is present at the base of the sella. This most often results from herniation of arachnoid through the diaphragma sellae, resulting in a slow pressure atrophy of the pituitary, eventually leading to hypopituitarism. Other causes of hypopituitarism include a null cell adenoma, ischemic necrosis (Sheehan syndrome), and surgical or radiation therapy. In children, the first manifestation is growth failure, while in adults, lack of gonadotropins leads to loss of secondary sex characteristics, infertility, and decreased libido. This is followed by hypothyroidism and hypoadrenalism.

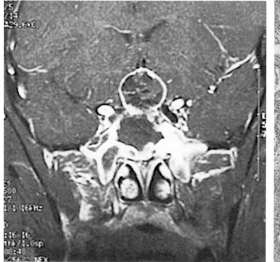 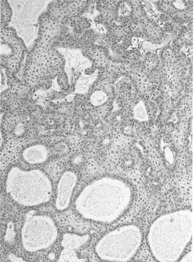 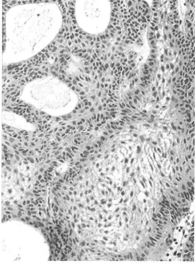

FIGURES 15–9 and 15–10 Craniopharyngioma, MRI and microscopic

The coronal MRI shows an expansile suprasellar mass (▶) derived from Rathke pouch remnants eroding surrounding structures. Microscopically, there are cystic spaces, and nests of squamoid cells are surrounded by columnar cells. Although histologically benign, these neoplasms are difficult to eradicate because of their location and their extension.

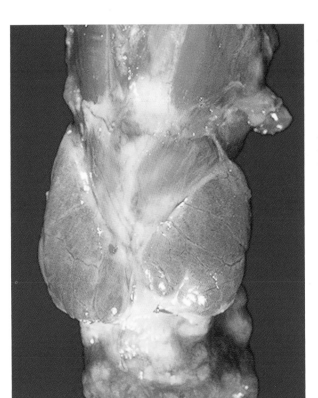

FIGURE 15–11 Normal thyroid *in situ*, gross

The thyroid gland is present over the anterior trachea. It normally has a reddish brown, firm appearance and is difficult to palpate on physical examination. The normal adult thyroid gland weighs 10 to 30 gm. There is a right lobe, a left lobe, and an isthmus (from which a small pyramidal lobe may project superiorly along the track of the embryologic thyroglossal duct). The thyroid in embryogenesis is derived from an evagination from the foramen cecum of the tongue that migrates downward along the thyroglossal duct to a position over the thyroid cartilage in the anterior neck. The C cells are derived from the fifth branchial pouches. The thyroid produces the thyroid hormones triiodothyronine (T_3) and tetraiodothyronine (T_4). A small amount of dietary iodine is required for thyroid hormone synthesis, and in the past, many cases of adult goiter with myxedema were due to a diet lacking in iodine, while in infants and children, this manifested as cretinism. Mostly T_4 is released, but peripherally T_4 is deiodinated within cells to the more biologically active T_3. Both T_3 and T_4 increase the basal metabolic rate, including both anabolic and catabolic processes.

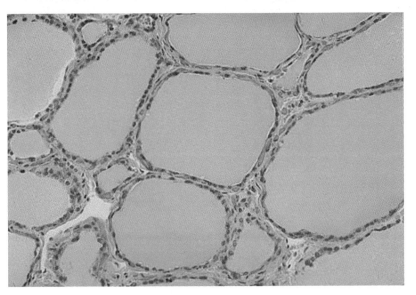

FIGURE 15–12 Normal thyroid, microscopic

The normal thyroid gland is composed of round follicles lined by cuboidal epithelial cells and filled with colloid, a storage product containing thyroglobulin, that is metabolized to release thyroid hormones (T_4 and T_3) under the influence of TSH released from the anterior pituitary thyrotrophs, which sense levels of circulating thyroid hormone. Thyroid hormone acts on nuclear thyroid hormone receptor in target cells to up-regulate transcription of proteins that drive carbohydrate and lipid metabolism while stimulating protein synthesis.

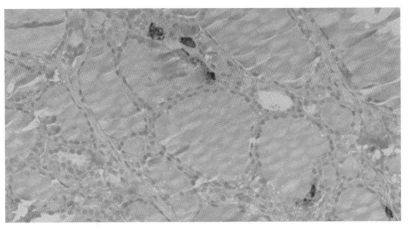

FIGURE 15–13 Normal C cells, microscopic

This immunohistochemical stain of normal thyroid with antibody to calcitonin identifies the C cells by the brown reaction product. The C cells (parafollicular cells) of the thyroid interstitium are located between the follicles, adjacent to the epithelium of follicles. The C cells secrete calcitonin, which can inhibit resorption of bone by osteoclasts and lower the serum calcium, but has a much lesser role to play in calcium hemostasis than parathyroid hormone.

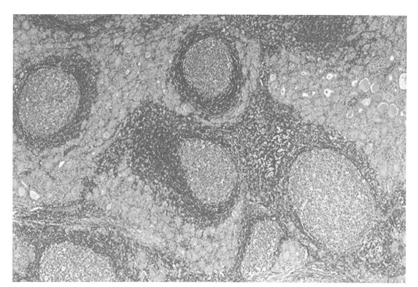

FIGURE 15–14 Hashimoto thyroiditis, microscopic

This autoimmune disease can be associated with HLA-DR3 and HLA-DR5 alleles. It results in chronic inflammation characterized by infiltrates of CD8+ and CD4+ T lymphocytes forming much of the lymphoid follicles seen here. The B cells in the germinal centers produce anti-TSH receptor antibodies blocking the action of TSH. The remaining thyroid follicles become atrophic, and the epithelial cells undergo Hürthle cell change, with abundant pink cytoplasm. Initially, there can be painless enlargement of the thyroid. Laboratory findings can include antithyroglobulin and antimicrosomal (thyroid peroxidase) antibodies detected in serum.

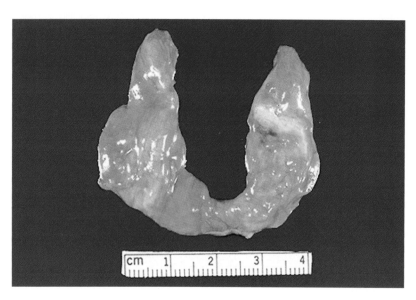

FIGURE 15–15 Hashimoto thyroiditis, gross

There is relentless destruction of thyroid follicles over the years, with eventual atrophy, so that the thyroid is often not palpable when a patient presents with myxedema from hypothyroidism, and the serum TSH is elevated. Early in the course of this disease, there may be transient hyperthyroidism from excessive release of thyroid hormones from damaged follicles. Other autoimmune diseases, such as Addison disease or pernicious anemia, may also occur in patients with Hashimoto thyroiditis. There is an increased risk for subsequent development of B-cell non-Hodgkin lymphoma.

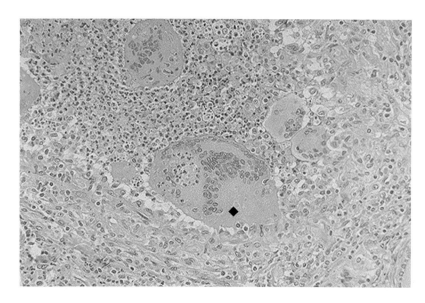

FIGURE 15–16 Subacute thyroiditis, microscopic

Also known as *granulomatous thyroiditis*, or *de Quervain disease*, this uncommon form of thyroiditis begins with diffuse painful thyroid enlargement. It most often occurs from the fourth to the sixth decades and is more common in women, similar to the demographic pattern of other thyroid diseases. Note the marked acute inflammation along with lymphocytes, macrophages, and prominent giant cells (♦). There is destruction of thyroid follicles. This condition typically follows a viral infection. It usually follows a course of 1 to 3 months during which transient hyperthyroidism or hypothyroidism along with fever can occur. Most patients completely recover within months and remain euthyroid.

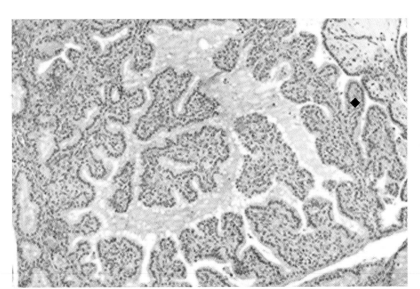

FIGURE 15–17 Graves disease, microscopic

At low magnification, this thyroid hyperplasia is characterized by many papillary infoldings (◆) within follicles. This is an autoimmune disease in which autoantibodies to TSH receptors both stimulate growth of follicular epithelial cells and stimulate adenylate cyclase to increase thyroid hormone output. There is an association with the HLA-DR3 allele. The entire thyroid gland becomes diffusely enlarged to double or triple normal size. Patients with Graves disease can have fever, diarrhea, heat intolerance, tachycardia, weight loss, tremor, and nervousness. Exophthalmos and infiltrative dermopathy (pretibial myxedema) are clinical features characteristic of Graves disease.

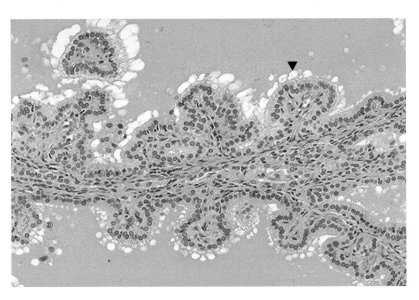

FIGURE 15–18 Graves disease, microscopic

At higher magnification, the tall columnar appearance of the hyperplastic follicular epithelial cells is evident. Small, clear vacuoles (▼) appear next to each cell, indicating increased processing of colloid to produce increased output of thyroid hormone leading to hyperthyroidism. The feedback on the adenohypophyseal thyrotrophs decreases the serum TSH, while the serum T_4 is high. Antithyroid antibodies may be present. An uncommon but serious complication is "thyroid storm" with malignant hyperthermia. Graves disease can be treated by propranolol to diminish β-adrenergic effects, by antithyroid drugs such as propylthiouracil, and by subtotal thyroidectomy.

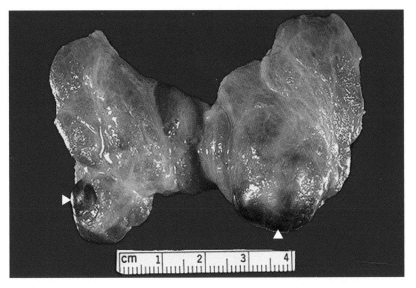

FIGURE 15–19 Thyroid with colloid cysts, gross

One of the most common lesions to produce a palpable nodule of the thyroid gland is a colloid cyst. The cyst is filled with colloid and surrounded by flattened cuboidal epithelium. It is just an exaggerated follicle in an otherwise normal thyroid. Patients are euthyroid. Seen here is a larger colloid cyst (▲) anteriorly and inferiorly in the left lower lobe and a smaller cyst (▶) laterally in the right lower lobe. Such nodules can mimic a neoplasm on physical examination or imaging studies. They can mimic a nodular goiter, although the overall size of the thyroid is not enlarged here. By radionuclide imaging, this would be a "cold" nodule, as are most neoplastic and non-neoplastic thyroid nodules.

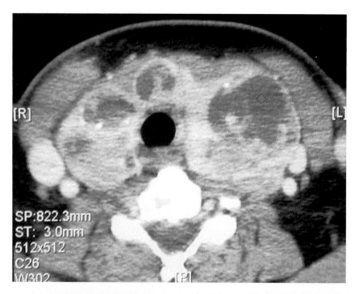

FIGURE 15–20 Thyroid, multinodular goiter, CT scan

This large thyroid surrounds the trachea and contains several nodular areas (◆) with diminished attenuation (brightness). This is a multinodular goiter in a patient who is euthyroid, the most typical clinical picture accompanying goiter. The painless enlargement produces discomfort and cosmetic deformity to the neck. Multinodular goiters usually arise from simple goiters after many years. Simple goiters may be endemic in populations with decreased dietary iodine intake. Sporadic goiters can be due to goitrogens in foods such as Brussels sprouts, cauliflower, cassava, and turnips (favorites of mine, but perhaps not yours) that interfere with thyroid hormone synthesis and promote development of goiter. Most patients with goiters remain euthyroid. Inborn errors of metabolism that interfere with thyroid hormone production are rare but can lead to goiter with cretinism in children.

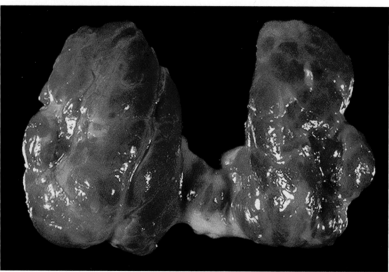
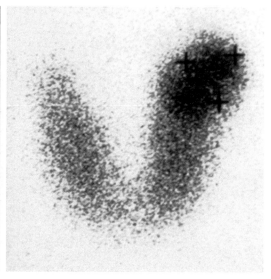

FIGURE 15–21A and B Thyroid, multinodular goiter, gross and scintigraphic scan

Multinodular goiters are often asymmetric, although both lobes become enlarged. Most patients remain euthyroid, bothered only by the mass effect. In some patients, a hyperfunctioning nodule (Plummer syndrome) causes hyperthyroidism. The nodule (◀) is "hot" with increased activity on radionuclide scintigraphic scanning, as shown in the right panel.

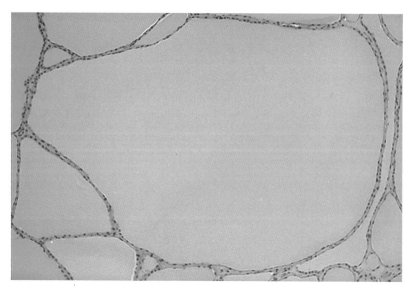

FIGURE 15–22 Thyroid, goiter, microscopic

Shown here from a goiter are enlarged thyroid follicles lined with inactive, flattened epithelial cells and filled with abundant stored colloid. The process starts as a simple, diffuse, nontoxic goiter. Over time, there can be irregular nodular enlargement with fibrosis, hemorrhage, and calcification in areas of cystic change. The irregular growth and enlargement may mimic thyroid carcinoma. Mutations in TSH-signaling pathway proteins may lead to autonomous growth and function of a nodule within a goiter.

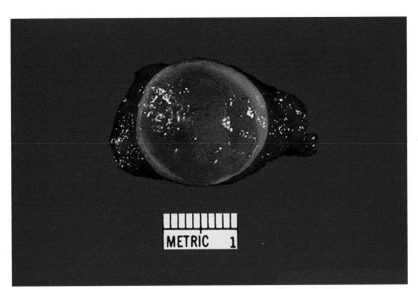

FIGURE 15–23 Thyroid, follicular neoplasm, gross

This cross-section through a resected lobe of thyroid gland reveals an encapsulated round neoplasm with uniform brown appearance, surrounded by a rim of normal thyroid. This is a follicular adenoma, which typically presents as a painless mass. This lesion is often diagnosed on microscopic examination as a "follicular neoplasm" because, in up to 10% of cases, although it is benign histologically, such a lesion proves to act in a malignant fashion. A follicular neoplasm forms a palpably firm nodule and is more common in women in middle age. Most are hypofunctioning "cold" nodules on radionuclide scanning.

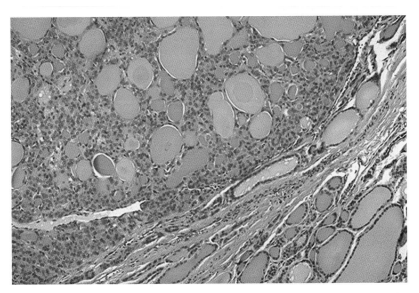

FIGURE 15–24 Thyroid, follicular neoplasm, microscopic

This well-differentiated follicular neoplasm is composed of recognizable follicles that are small and packed closely, while the adjacent normal thyroid has compressed and flattened follicles at the lower right. There is no invasion seen here, so this neoplasm is more likely to act in a benign fashion. Most follicular neoplasms do not function, but a rare hyperfunctioning adenoma, or "toxic" adenoma, can be a cause of hyperthyroidism. Some toxic adenomas have a G-protein–coupled receptor mutation encoding the stimulatory α subunit (*GNAS1*) that up-regulates adenyl cyclase and cyclic AMP to drive thyroid hormone output.

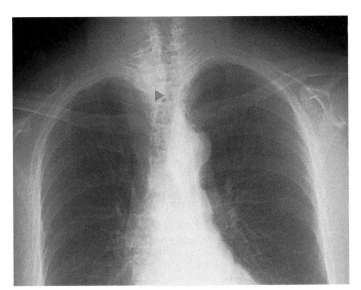

FIGURE 15–25 Thyroid, neoplasm, chest radiograph

The subtle evidence of a mass involving the thyroid is seen here as tracheal deviation (▶) to the right as a consequence of displacement by the mass effect. Thyroid neoplasms may be palpable on physical examination, although less so in corpulent individuals. Radiologic procedures including CT imaging can help document the size, extent, and consistency of the thyroid, while scintigraphic scans can determine the amount and distribution of isotopic uptake into the thyroid parenchyma. Fine-needle aspiration with cytologic examination of the aspirated cells is a useful tool to determine the histologic nature of thyroid lesions. Removal of part (subtotal) or all (total) of the thyroid (thyroidectomy) may be undertaken for diagnostic and therapeutic purposes.

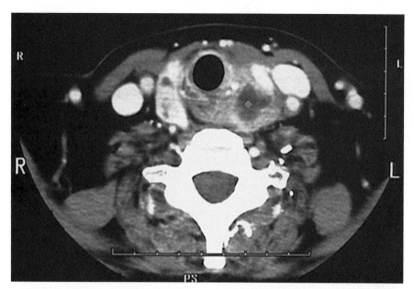

FIGURE 15–26 Thyroid, papillary carcinoma, CT image

This CT scan of the neck reveals a left thyroid lobe mass with an irregular cystic area (◆) of decreased attenuation within the mass. This neoplasm often presents as a painless palpable thyroid nodule. In some cases, the carcinoma is not palpable, but metastasis results in a nearby enlarged cervical lymph node (called a *Delphian node*, after the ancient Greek Oracle of Delphi, who predicted future events). Underlying molecular mechanisms for development of this neoplasm include chromosomal rearrangement of the tyrosine kinase receptors *RET* (with formation of the *ret/PTC* fusion gene) or *NTRK1*, *BRAF* oncogene–activating mutations, and *RAS* mutations.

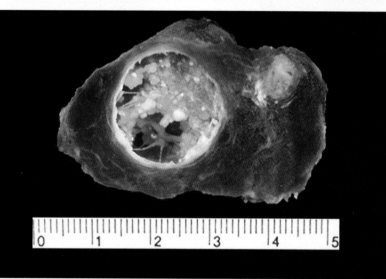

FIGURE 15–27 Thyroid, papillary carcinoma, gross

Papillary carcinoma can be multifocal, as seen here, because of the propensity to invade lymphatics within thyroid, and metastases to adjacent lymph nodes not only are common but also may be the presenting feature. The larger mass shown here in this cross-section through an excised thyroid gland is cystic and contains papillary excrescences. Papillary carcinoma, which constitutes 80% of all thyroid carcinomas, invariably produces a "cold" nodule by radionuclide scanning.

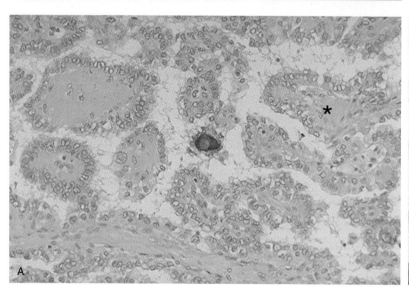
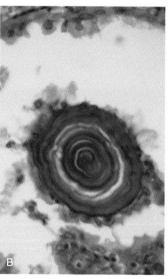

FIGURE 15–28*A* and *B* Thyroid, papillary carcinoma, microscopic

This papillary carcinoma in the left panel has fronds of tissue with thin fibrovascular cores (*) that form a papillary pattern with papillations lined by cells with nuclei that appear clear (empty) on H+E staining after formalin fixation. Another microscopic feature, seen at high magnification in the right panel, is the round laminated concretion, a psammoma body. Papillary carcinomas are indolent tumors that have a long survival, even with metastases.

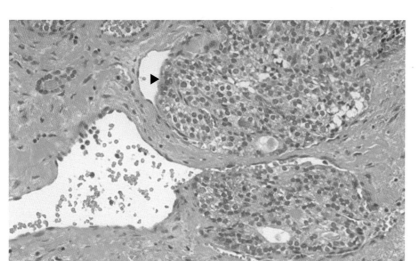

FIGURE 15–29 Thyroid, follicular carcinoma, microscopic

Vascular invasion (▶) here is evidence of malignancy in a neoplasm that is vaguely follicular, with absence of microscopic features of papillary carcinoma. Often, cells of thyroid neoplasms, whether benign or malignant, are not highly pleomorphic or hyperchromatic. *RAS* gene mutations are common. Somatic rearrangements of the tyrosine kinase portion of the *RET* proto-oncogene with fusion of other genes such as *PAX8* and *PPARγ1* can result in the *RET/PTC* oncogene that is present in many follicular carcinomas. It is the second most common thyroid malignancy, accounting for about 15% of all cases. It tends to be indolent and metastasizes hematogenously to locations such as lung or liver.

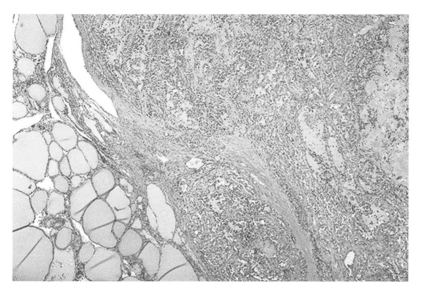

FIGURE 15–30 Thyroid, medullary carcinoma, microscopic

The carcinoma cells are at the top and right, with adjacent normal thyroid follicular tissue seen at the lower left. At the far right is pink hyaline material with the appearance of amyloid (it will stain positively with Congo red). These neoplasms are derived from the thyroid C cells and, therefore, have neuroendocrine features such as secretion of calcitonin (but without hypocalcemia). Medullary carcinomas can be sporadic or familial. The familial form has a better prognosis and can be multifocal and associated with MEN syndromes. *RET* gene mutations are present in all familial and half of sporadic medullary carcinomas.

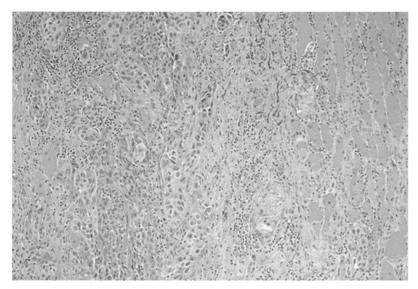

FIGURE 15–31 Thyroid, anaplastic carcinoma, microscopic

This is the least common thyroid malignancy but the most aggressive, rapidly growing, and invasive to involve adjacent esophagus with dysphagia or trachea with dyspnea. Seen here are highly irregular cells infiltrating into adjacent skeletal muscle at the right. Half of cases arise in the setting of a multinodular goiter. Foci of papillary or follicular carcinoma can be present in 20% to 30% of cases, suggesting origin from a prior differentiated carcinoma. They occur in elderly people. Clinical findings caused by invasion of adjacent structures include dyspnea, dysphagia, hoarseness, and cough. A mutated *p53* gene is often present.

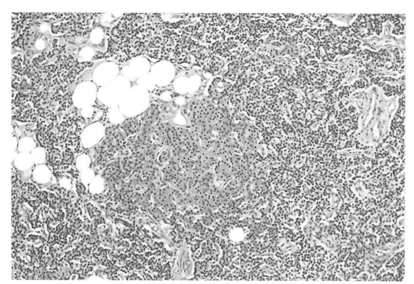

FIGURE 15–32 Parathyroid gland, normal

In the normal parathyroid gland, there are variable numbers of adipocytes, seen here mostly at the left, that are mixed with the small nests of chief cells that secrete parathyroid hormone. There are typically small nodules of pink oxyphil cells whose function is obscure. There is a rich vascular supply, as in all endocrine tissues secreting hormonal products directly into the bloodstream. Embryologically, parathyroids are derived from the third and fourth pharyngeal pouches and are present on the posterior aspect of the thyroid gland as superior and inferior pairs. Occasionally, an ectopic parathyroid is located substernally in thymus. Parathormone is released inversely to ionized calcium and magnesium levels in the blood.

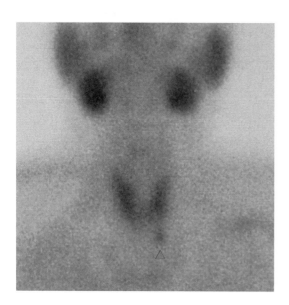

FIGURE 15–33 Parathyroid, adenoma, scintigraphic scan

This parathyroid scan after intravenous administration of technetium-99m demonstrates, in addition to radiotracer uptake in both thyroid lobes and salivary glands, a small area of increased activity inferior to the left lobe of the thyroid, consistent with a left lower parathyroid adenoma (▲). Clinical findings with hyperparathyroidism include bone pain, nephrolithiasis, constipation, peptic ulcer disease, pancreatitis, cholelithiasis, depression, weakness, and seizures. Metastatic calcification of tissues such as lung, kidney, and gastric mucosa is rare. Surgical exploration to find the adenoma can be difficult, and a second adenoma may be present, or there may be parathyroid hyperplasia with asymmetric enlargement of the parathyroids. Parathyroid surgery is the most common cause of hypoparathyroidism, so serum calcium levels are checked postoperatively. Clinical findings with hypoparathyroidism include neuromuscular irritability, behavioral changes including either anxiety or depression, papilledema, cataract formation, and cardiac dysrhythmias with prolonged QT(corrected) interval.

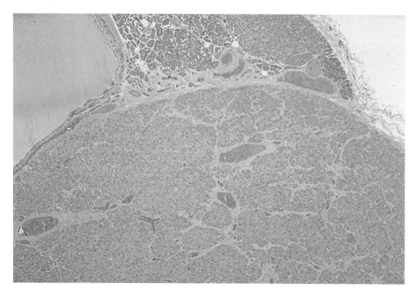

FIGURE 15–34 Parathyroid adenoma, microscopic

Adjacent to this parathyroid adenoma is a rim of normal parathyroid (with a pink oxyphil cell nodule at the upper right) and a small benign parathyroid cyst (an incidental finding) filled with pink proteinaceous fluid at the upper left. Adenoma accounts for nearly 80% to 90% of all cases of primary hyperparathyroidism. In addition to elevated serum ionized calcium with hypophosphatemia, a parathormone (PTH) assay reveals a high-normal to elevated level of PTH. Overexpression of the *cyclin D1* gene (*PRAD1*) is present in some cases. Twenty to 30% of these adenomas occur in association with MEN 1.

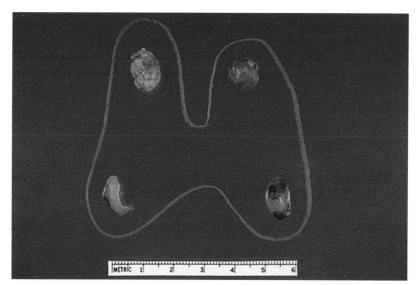

FIGURE 15–35 Parathyroid hyperplasia, gross

Three and one half hyperplastic parathyroid glands have been removed (only half the gland at the lower left is present) from this patient. Although all these glands are enlarged, they may be asymmetrically enlarged. Microscopically, there is most often chief cell hyperplasia, but other parathyroid cell types may proliferate, too. Parathyroid hyperplasia is the second most common form of primary hyperparathyroidism, accounting for 10% to 20% of cases. Parathyroid hyperplasia is less commonly seen in association with MEN 1 or MEN 2A).

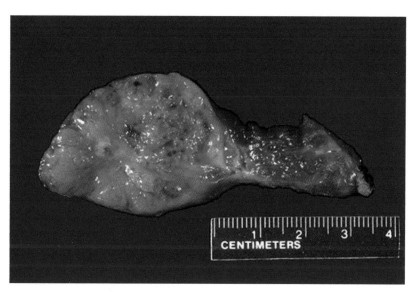

FIGURE 15–36 Parathyroid carcinoma, gross

Shown here is an irregular tan mass invading into adjacent red-brown thyroid tissue. Parathyroid carcinoma is the least common form of primary hyperparathyroidism, accounting for less than 1% of cases. These carcinomas tend to invade into surrounding tissues in the neck, complicating their removal. The serum calcium level is often quite high. Markedly elevated serum calcium levels can also be seen in association with nonparathyroid malignancies elsewhere, particularly those that produce a paraneoplastic syndrome from elaboration of parathormone-related peptide.

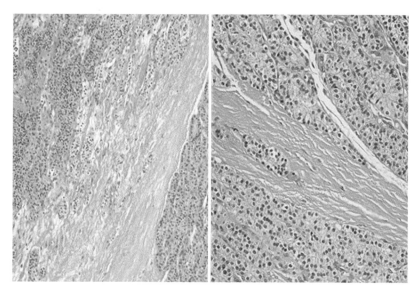

FIGURE 15–37 Parathyroid carcinoma, microscopic

This parathyroid carcinoma, seen at medium power on the left and higher power on the right, shows distinctive bands of fibrous tissue between the nests of carcinoma cells. The nests of neoplastic cells are not very pleomorphic, so invasion and metastases are the only reliable indicators of malignancy. The high serum PTH levels with parathyroid carcinomas, as well as adenomas and hyperplasia, can increase bone osteoclast activity and bone remodeling to produce osteitis fibrosa cystica and "brown tumor" of bone.

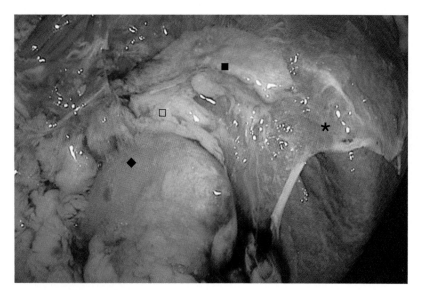

FIGURE 15–38 Normal adrenal gland, gross

This normal right adrenal gland (■) is positioned between the liver (∗) and the kidney (◆) in the retroperitoneum. There is surrounding retroperitoneal adipose tissue (□). Each normal gland weighs 4 to 6 gm. Embryologically, the adrenals develop from induction of coelomic epithelial cell proliferation by the ureteric bud, forming fetal adrenal cortex, which eventually becomes the zona reticularis. This is invaded by neural crest forming neuroblasts to become adrenal medulla. Another proliferation of coelomic epithelium surrounds the fetal cortex to become the adult cortical zona glomerulosa and zona fasciculata.

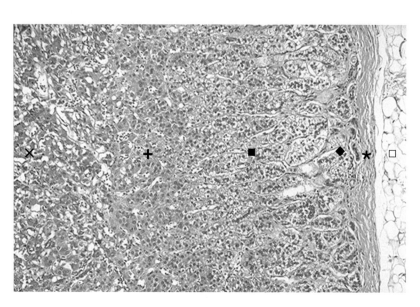

FIGURE 15–39 Normal adrenal gland, microscopic

The normal layers of the adrenal gland are not that distinctive. At the far right is the surrounding adipose tissue (□). Next, moving left in the image, is the fibrous tissue capsule (∗). Adjacent to the capsule is the zona glomerulosa (◆), whose cells produce mineralocorticoids such as aldosterone. Then comes the zona fasciculata (■) in the center of this image, whose cells produce glucocorticoids, mainly cortisol. Next is the zona reticularis (+), composed of darker and slightly smaller pink cells producing sex steroid hormones. At the far left is the medulla (×), which produces catecholamines, mainly norepinephrine and some epinephrine and dopamine.

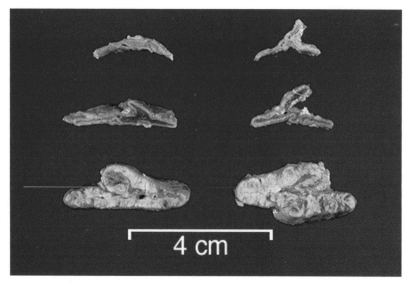

FIGURE 15–40 Comparison of atrophic, normal, and hyperplastic adrenal glands

The topmost pair of adrenal glands are atrophic, characteristic of either idiopathic Addison disease or chronic use of corticosteroids. The normal adrenals at the center have a well-defined rim of golden cortex and a center of reddish medulla. The hyperplastic pair of adrenals at the bottom are typical of increased ACTH secretion with ectopic production either from a neoplasm such as a small cell lung carcinoma, which results in Cushing syndrome, or from a pituitary adenoma, resulting in Cushing disease. The adrenals may become hyperplastic from enzymic defects in steroidogenesis or, rarely, without the stimulus of ACTH, as a primary idiopathic process.

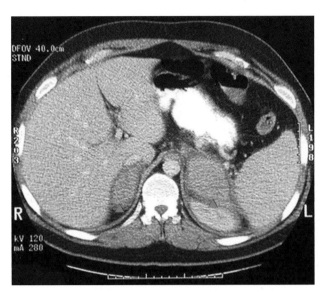

FIGURE 15–41 Waterhouse-Friderichsen syndrome, CT

This abdominal CT scan demonstrates the typical locations of the adrenal glands (▲), but these glands are enlarged because of bilateral adrenal gland hemorrhage from the Waterhouse-Friderichsen syndrome with *Neisseria meningitidis* (meningococcal) infection. Less commonly, infection with other organisms, such as *Pseudomonas aeruginosa*, *Streptococcus pneumoniae*, or *Haemophilus influenzae*, may lead to this condition. This condition causes acute adrenal insufficiency along with endotoxin-induced vasculitis and disseminated intravascular coagulopathy (DIC).

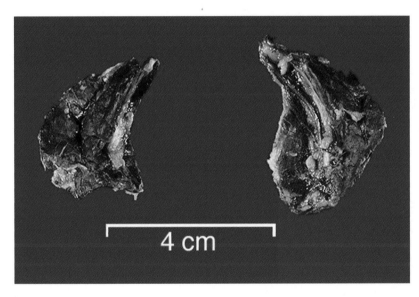

FIGURE 15–42 Waterhouse-Friderichsen syndrome, gross

These adrenals have a dark red to black color from extensive hemorrhage with DIC as a consequence of endotoxin release from *Neisseria meningitidis* organisms causing septicemia. This is known as Waterhouse-Friderichsen syndrome and is more likely to complicate infections in children. Infection with *N. meningitidis* can start initially as a mild pharyngitis, but become a florid septicemia with hypotension and shock within hours. Destruction of more than 90% of the adrenal cortex leads to adrenal cortical insufficiency.

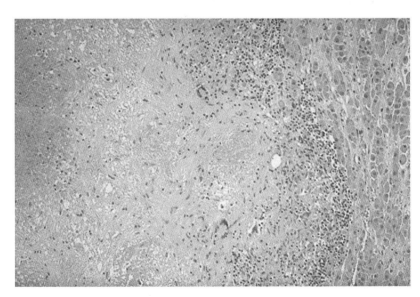

FIGURE 15–43 Tuberculous adrenalitis, microscopic

Although most cases of Addison disease are now idiopathic (presumably autoimmune in etiology), there are still cases resulting from disseminated *Mycobacterium tuberculosis* infection. Seen here is a caseating granuloma with central pink areas of caseous necrosis and surrounding inflammation with lymphocytes, epithelioid cells, and Langhans giant cells. Some residual adrenal is present at the right. This infection proceeds over months to years and leads to adrenal cortical destruction with chronic adrenal insufficiency. The decreased plasma cortisol leads to increased ACTH and precursors that can stimulate melanocytes, leading to skin hyperpigmentation.

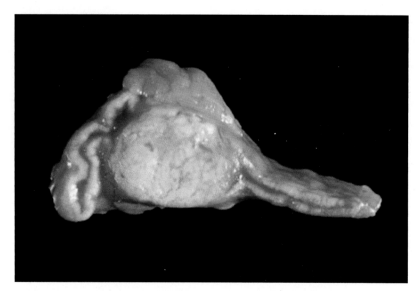

FIGURE 15–44 Adrenal adenoma, gross

This circumscribed uniformly yellow-tan mass is a 1.3-cm adrenal adenoma found in a patient with hypertension and hypokalemia. Further work-up revealed high serum aldosterone and low plasma renin activity, findings consistent with an aldosterone-secreting adenoma (Conn syndrome). This lesion accounts for about two thirds of primary hyperaldosteronism cases. Such adenomas are typically smaller than 2 cm and have a yellow hue on cut surface. If such an adenoma were secreting cortisol, the patient would have Cushing syndrome.

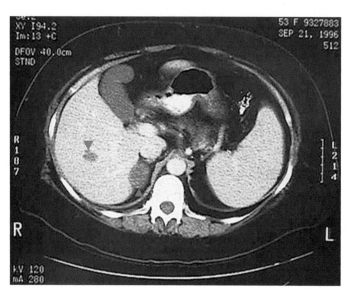

FIGURE 15–45 Adrenal adenoma, CT

This abdominal CT scan demonstrates a small adrenal adenoma (▲) with decreased attenuation adjacent to the liver on the right. There is also an incidental simple cyst (▼) of the liver. Some adrenal adenomas are incidental findings on an abdominal CT scan performed for other indications, and those smaller than 2 cm without signs or symptoms of adrenal hyperfunction may be left alone (as in fishing—catch and release).

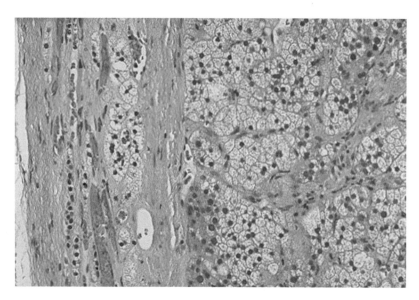

FIGURE 15–46 Adrenal adenoma, microscopic

This adrenal cortical adenoma at the right is well differentiated and resembles normal adrenal fasciculata. It appears histologically nearly the same as the compressed normal adrenal at the left, just outside the capsule of the adenoma. There may be minimal cellular pleomorphism within these adenomas. If such an adenoma does not function, it may not be detected except by imaging studies done for other reasons.

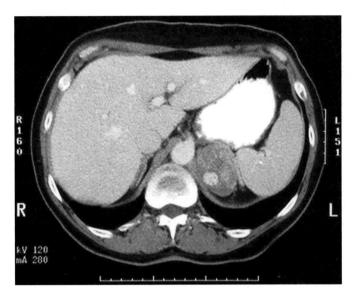

FIGURE 15–47 Adrenal cortical carcinoma, CT image

This large mass arising in the left adrenal gland is an adrenal cortical carcinoma (◆). Such carcinomas tend to be larger than adrenal adenomas and more variegated in their radiographic and gross pathologic appearance, typically from areas of hemorrhage and necrosis. Most weigh more than 100 gm. They can occur over a wide age range. After administration of intravenous contrast, there is a focus of brighter attenuation seen here in the posterior aspect of the mass that corresponds to an area of hemorrhage. The major differential diagnosis for this mass, in the absence of clinical or laboratory evidence of endocrine function, is a metastasis, most often from a lung primary. Metastases to both adrenals may lead to adrenal cortical insufficiency, while many cortical carcinomas function hormonally.

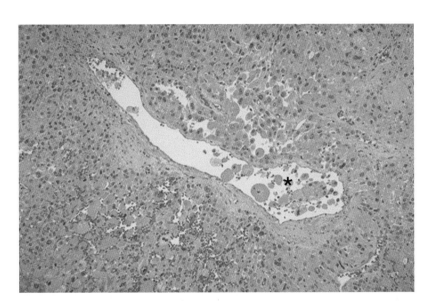

FIGURE 15–48 Adrenal cortical carcinoma, microscopic

This adrenal cortical carcinoma has a microscopic appearance that closely resembles normal adrenal cortex. It is difficult to determine malignancy in endocrine neoplasms based on cytologic features alone. Thus, invasion (as seen here in a vein (∗)) and metastases are the most reliable indicators of malignancy. Adrenal cortical carcinomas often are hormonally functional and can lead to Cushing syndrome from glucocorticoid secretion, or there can be sex steroid hormone secretion with clinical features of masculinization in a woman or femininization in a man. These carcinomas rarely produce mineralocorticoids in excess.

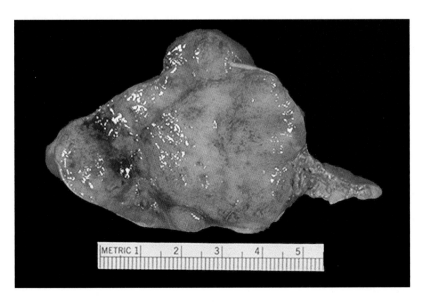

FIGURE 15–49 Pheochromocytoma, gross

Note the gray-tan color of this neoplasm arising from the adrenal medulla, and compare that with the yellow color of the residual cortex of normal adrenal stretched around it, and a small remnant of remaining adrenal gland at the lower right. This patient had episodic hypertension from secretion of catecholamines (norepinephrine and epinephrine) acting on α- and β-adrenergic receptors in various cells. Although most pheochromocytomas occur sporadically, they may be associated with MEN 2A or 2B, neurofibromatosis type I, Sturge-Weber disease, and von Hippel-Lindau (VHL) disease. Pheochromocytomas follow the 10% rule—10% are either bilateral, malignant, pediatric, familial, or extra-adrenal in location.

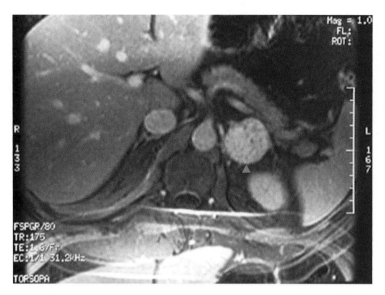

FIGURE 15–50 Adrenal pheochromocytoma, MRI

The abdominal axial MRI is a postgadolinium T1-weighted scan with fat saturation that demonstrates diffuse contrast enhancement (because of this neoplasm's vascularity) in a pheochromocytoma (▲) that is replacing the left adrenal gland. This patient had hypertension, tachycardia, palpitations, headache, tremor, and diaphoresis, along with an elevated plasma norepinephrine level. The hypertension is most often sustained and less often of the more suggestive episodic variety. The patient also had increased free urinary catecholamines, vanillylmandelic acid, and metanephrines. Cardiac dysrhythmias may lead to sudden death. The anesthesiologist can report elevation of the blood pressure when the surgeon manipulates this tumor during removal.

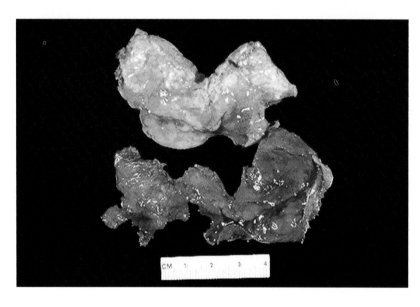

FIGURE 15–51 Adrenal pheochromocytoma, chromaffin reaction, gross

It is a traditional pathology "magic trick" to display the chromaffin reaction in which the tissues of a pheochromocytoma turn from tan to brown when placed in a freshly made solution of potassium dichromate. This occurs because large amounts of biogenic amines (catecholamines) in the cytoplasm of the neoplastic cells are oxidized by this solution. In addition to catecholamines, these neoplasms may also secrete ACTH (leading to Cushing syndrome) or somatostatin.

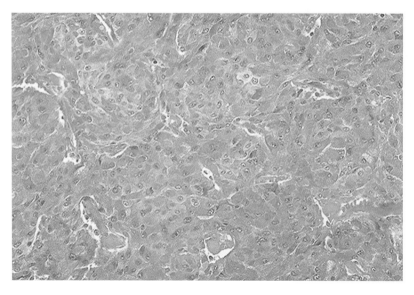

FIGURE 15–52 Pheochromocytoma, microscopic

This pheochromocytoma is composed of large polygonal to spindle chromaffin (chief) cells that have pink to mauve cytoplasm. The cells are arranged in nests ("*Zellballen*") with adjacent smaller sustentacular cells, surrounded by abundant intervening capillaries. The microscopic appearance gives no reliable clue to biologic behavior, so malignancy determination is based on presence of invasion or metastases. Laboratory findings with pheochromocytomas include increased urinary catecholamines, vanillylmandelic acid, and metanephrines. The symptoms can be treated with adrenergic-blocking agents before surgical removal.

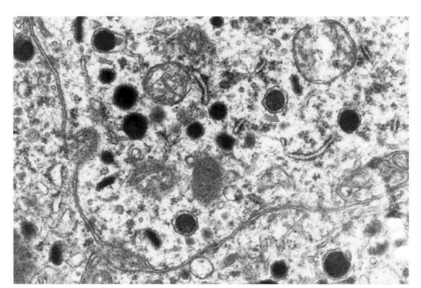

FIGURE 15–53 Adrenal pheochromocytoma, electron microscopy

By electron microscopy, these chromaffin (chief) cells of a pheochromocytoma, like those of other neoplasms with neuroendocrine differentiation, contain dark round membrane-bound neurosecretory granules (▲) in their cell cytoplasm. These granules contain the catecholamines in a pheochromocytoma. Immunohistochemical staining for chromogranin and synaptophysin is present in chief cells, while the sustentacular cells are positive for S-100, a calcium-binding protein. Persistently elevated catecholamine levels can produce a catecholamine cardiomyopathy complicated by congestive heart failure and arrhythmias.

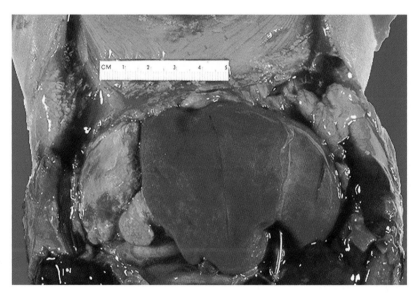

FIGURE 15–54 Adrenal neuroblastoma, gross

Abdominal enlargement palpated in this neonate resulted from a congenital neuroblastoma arising within the right adrenal gland. This irregular tan mass with focal hemorrhage is a neuroblastoma large enough to displace the liver to the left. Most of these neoplasms arise during the first 3 years of life, and despite the higher stage seen here, neuroblastomas arising in infancy have a better overall prognosis. *N-myc* gene amplification is often present. Like adult pheochromocytomas, they may also arise in extra-adrenal paraganglia.

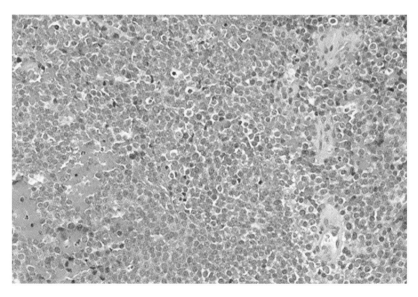

FIGURE 15–55 Adrenal neuroblastoma, microscopic

The neuroblastoma is one of the "small round blue cell" tumors most typically seen in children. Note the population of round blue cells resembling embryonic neuroblasts. These neoplasms can reach a large size in the retroperitoneum before they are detected. They often contain focal areas of necrosis and calcification. They may be detected because they secrete homovanillic acid, a precursor in catecholamine synthesis, as well as vanillylmandelic acid, dopamine, and norepinephrine, although not in as large quantities as pheochromocytomas. Hypertension may be present in some cases.

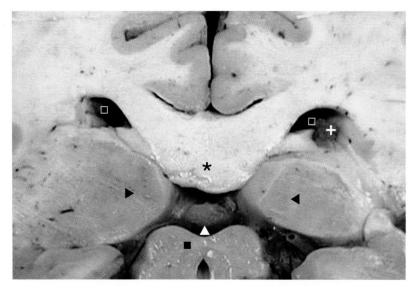

FIGURE 15–56 Normal pineal gland, gross

The normal pineal gland (▲) is present in the third ventricle above the superior collicular plate (■), beneath the splenium (∗) of corpus callosum, and between right (▶) and left (◀) pulvinar of the thalami. The posterior horns (□) of the lateral ventricles have choroid plexus (+). The pineal elaborates the hormone melatonin, which plays a role in maintenance of normal circadian rhythms.

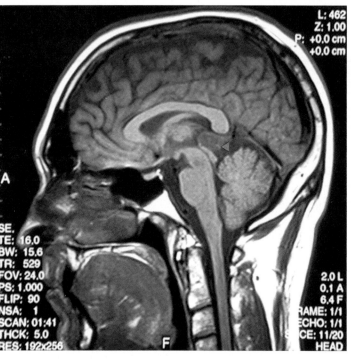

FIGURE 15–57 Pineocytoma, MRI

In the sagittal T1-weighted MRI scan, there is mass lesion (◀) in the region of the pineal gland. This is a pineocytoma, which most often occurs in adults as a slowly enlarging, circumscribed lesion that can compress, but not invade, surrounding structures. The enlarging mass can occlude the aqueduct of Sylvius and lead to hydrocephalus. It is challenging to remove because of its location. In contrast, pineoblastomas arise in children and spread by seeding into the cerebrospinal fluid.

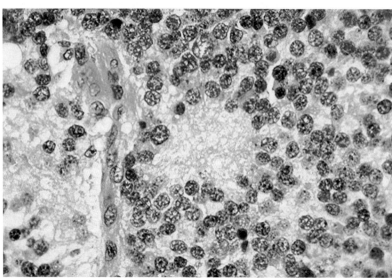

FIGURE 15–58 Pineocytoma, microscopic

This pineocytoma demonstrates large Homer Wright rosettes with central acellular areas composed of tumor cell cytoplasmic processes that are surrounded by well-differentiated cells having round to oval nuclei. Histologically, these tumors resemble a normal pineal gland with nests of well-differentiated cells.

CHAPTER 16

The Skin

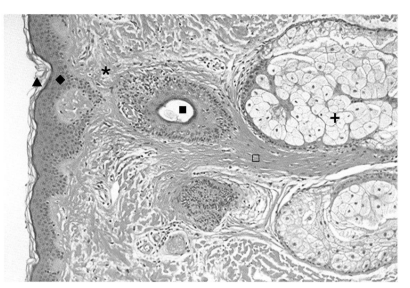

FIGURE 16–1 Normal skin, microscopic

The normal histologic appearance of the skin is shown here. At the left is the epidermis. A thin layer of keratin (▲) overlies this epidermis. This keratinized layer is thicker on the palms and soles and over areas of the body surface where the skin is persistently rubbed or irritated. Beneath the epidermis (◆) is the dermis (*) containing connective tissue with collagen and elastic fibers. At the center can be seen a hair follicle (■) with surrounding sebaceous glands (+). Associated with the hair follicle is a small bundle of smooth muscle (□) known as the *arrector pili* that can cause the hair to "stand on end" and dimple the skin to form "goose bumps" when exposed to a cold environment.

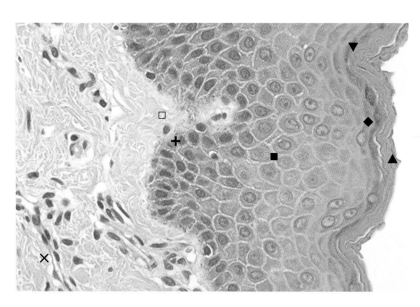

FIGURE 16–2 Normal skin, microscopic

At high magnification, the skin has an overlying acellular keratin layer called the *stratum corneum* (▲) that continually desquamates. Beneath this is the nearly indistinguishable thin, darker red stratum lucidum (▼). The outer layer of epidermal cells has prominent purplish cytoplasmic granules and is called the *stratum granulosum* (◆). Below this is the thickest layer, the *stratum spinosum* (■), with polyhedral cells that have prominent intercellular bridges. A basal layer (+) of cells rests on a basement membrane. In this case there is also prominent brown melanin pigmentation in the basal region. The upper papillary dermis (□) has small capillary blood vessels (×) that play a role in temperature regulation.

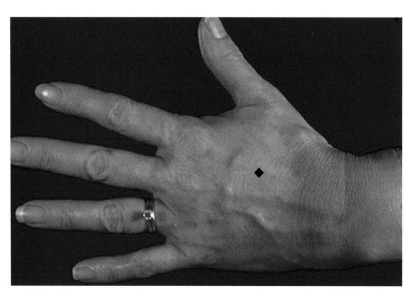

FIGURE 16–3 Vitiligo, gross

Irregular areas of hypopigmentation (◆) of the skin are shown here on the hand. This is a localized form of hypopigmentation (as contrasted with the diffuse form known as *oculocutaneous albinism*). Many localized cases are idiopathic, although sometimes a systemic disease may be present. Microscopically, melanocytes are absent in the areas of vitiligo. The degree of skin pigmentation is related to melanocyte activity through the enzyme tyrosinase, with formation of pigmented melanin granules, which are passed off to adjacent keratinocytes by long melanocyte cytoplasmic processes.

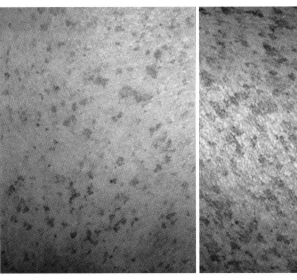

FIGURE 16–4 Freckles, gross

Ephelis is a fancy word for a freckle. These freckles represent hyperpigmentation that can occur in some fair-skinned people, particularly those with red hair. The onset occurs in childhood, and the extent is related to the amount of sun exposure. Microscopically, the number of melanocytes in the skin is normal, but there is focally increased melanin production from each melanocyte. There is no increased risk for malignancy.

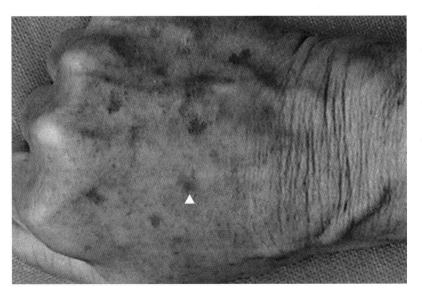

FIGURE 16–5 Age spots, gross

Seen on the hand are age spots or "liver" spots, termed *senile lentigines* (▲), which are common on areas of sun-exposed skin of older adults. Perhaps 90% of white people older than 70 years have one or more of them. They are flat lesions with irregular borders, can be pinpoint to 1 cm in size, and are often multiple. They have no significance except for their cosmetic appearance. They do not change in response to sun exposure.

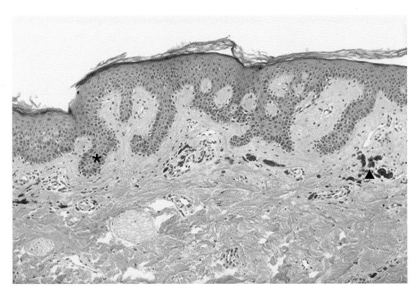

FIGURE 16–6 Lentigo senilis, microscopic

This is the microscopic appearance of lentigo senilis, commonly known as an age or "liver" spot. The rete ridges (∗) of the epidermis are elongated and appear club shaped or tortuous. Melanocytes are increased in number along the basal layer of the epidermis, and melanophages (▲) filled with brown melanin granules appear in the paler pink lower papillary dermis, just above the darker pink reticular dermis. This process is localized and benign.

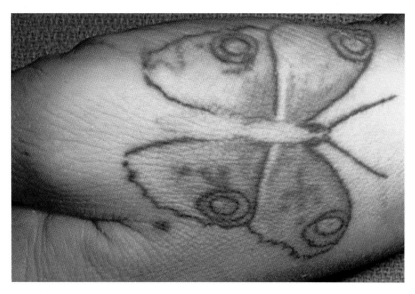

FIGURE 16–7 Tattoo, gross

Tattooing is a practice that is thousands of years old. In many human cultural groups, tattoos have great significance. Rituals can have usefulness for social groups, as long as no one gets hurt. The pigment in tattoos is transferred into the dermis with a needle, so there can be a risk for infection from the tattooing procedure. The tattoo itself over time tends to lose sharpness and intensity of color. Removal of a tattoo can be difficult; a laser light can be used to vaporize the pigment granules beneath the epidermis, but this is a laborious, time-consuming process. Removal at a later date is more likely to be undertaken when the blood ethanol level was high at the time of the tattooing procedure.

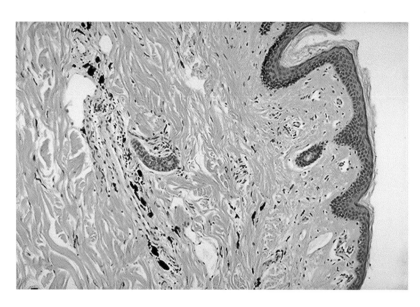

FIGURE 16–8 Tattoo, microscopic

The tattoo pigment (seen here as black granules) is introduced into the dermis with a needle. Note that this pigment is well within the dermis; therefore, removing or changing a tattoo is difficult. Over time, the pigment can be taken up into dermal macrophages, which can concentrate it or redistribute it, blurring the pattern, particularly on intricate designs. Different tattoo pigments account for different colors. Some pigments, such as those creating a green color, can impart photosensitivity. At the time of tattooing, the needle may introduce infectious agents.

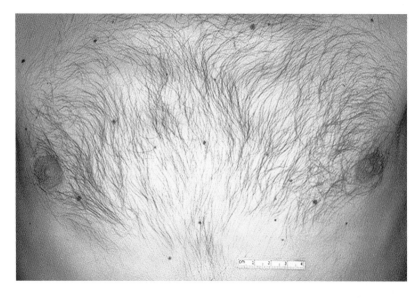

FIGURE 16–9 Melanocytic nevi, gross

Note the discrete brown lesions on the skin of the anterior chest. A melanocytic nevus is a small, brown, flat to slightly raised lesion with sharp borders that is quite common in light-skinned people. Such lesions are commonly called *moles*. These nevi are usually less than 0.6 cm in diameter, and they tend to grow very slowly and retain the same uniform degree of pigmentation and same sharp outlines, so that they seem hardly to change over time. Such nevi are benign, with no risk for subsequent malignancy, but they must be distinguished from more aggressive lesions.

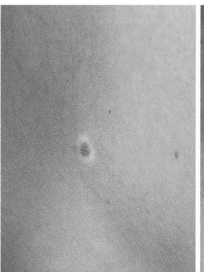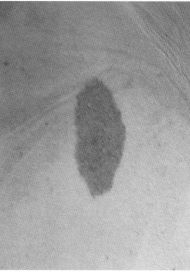

FIGURE 16–10 Melanocytic nevi, gross

Seen in the left panel is a halo nevus, so called because the central pigmented area is surrounded by a lighter zone. Nevi can show considerable variation in appearance: flat to raised and pale to darkly pigmented. However, most are small, well-circumscribed lesions that hardly seem to change at all, or change very slowly over time. In the right panel is a larger, flat, pigmented nevus on the upper back that can sometimes be termed a *café-au-lait spot*. Larger nevi are often congenital, and they may extend into the deep dermis. Very large congenital nevi have an increased risk for malignant melanoma.

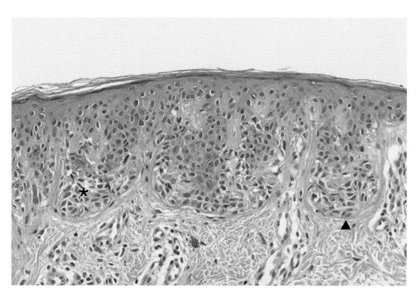

FIGURE 16–11 Junctional nevus, microscopic

This is the early stage of a junctional, or nevocellular, nevus. It is termed a *junctional nevus* because there are nevus cells in nests (*) in the lower epidermis. As nests of cells continue to "drop off" (▲) into the upper dermis, the lesion could then be termed a *compound nevus*. Unlike a melanoma, there is no significant atypia of the nevus cells and no adjacent dermal inflammation. In addition, there is a maturation effect, so that the nevus cells in the lower epidermis tend to be larger, with pigment, while those that extend deeper into the dermis are smaller, with little or no pigment. This microscopic maturation with differentiation to smaller cells helps distinguish this lesion from a malignant melanoma.

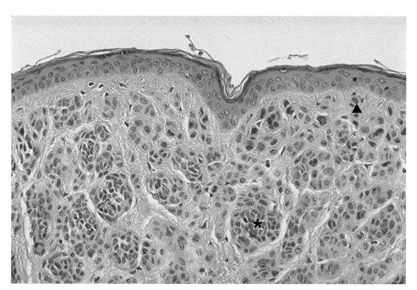

FIGURE 16–12 Intradermal nevus, microscopic

This lesion is termed an *intradermal nevus* because the nevus cells (melanocytes that are transformed to rounded cells that proliferate as aggregates or nests (*)) are found solely within the dermis, although close to (▲) the overlying epidermis. This is considered to be a later stage of a junctional (nevocellular) nevus in which the connection of the nevus cells to the epidermis has been lost. The benign nature of the nevus cells is confirmed by their small, uniform appearance. The cells form small aggregates in nests and cords, which are not encapsulated and may interdigitate with adnexal structures. The nevus cells (derived from melanocytes) have clear cytoplasm and small round blue nuclei without prominent nucleoli or mitoses.

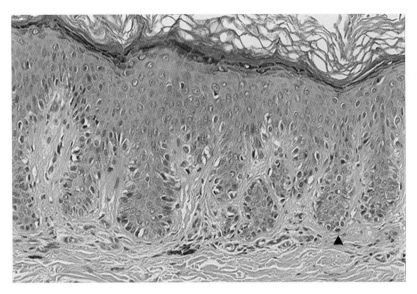

FIGURE 16–13 Dysplastic nevus, microscopic

This atypical melanocytic hyperplasia is histologically "in between" a clearly benign melanocytic nevus and a malignant melanoma. There are an increased number of melanocytes, some with atypical features such as enlarged, irregular nuclei, at the dermal–epidermal junction (▲). They are generally larger than 0.5 cm and have an irregular distribution of pigment. A familial, inherited condition in which such lesions occur frequently is the dysplastic nevus syndrome (or familial melanoma syndrome), which carries an increased risk for development of malignant melanoma. There is a *CDNK2* gene mutation leading to production of an abnormal p16INK4A cyclin-dependent kinase inhibitor.

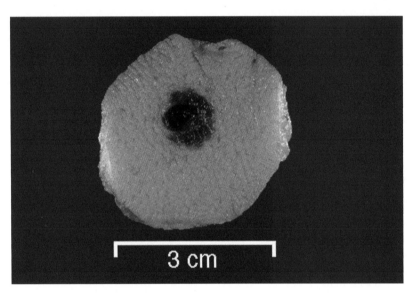

FIGURE 16–14 Malignant melanoma, gross

This malignant melanoma has been excised with a wide margin. Although this lesion is only about a centimeter in size, it shows irregular borders, variable pigmentation, and an irregular surface, all worrisome signs. Melanomas begin with a radial growth phase, but then over time start a vertical growth phase, invading down into the dermis and developing the potential for metastases to distant sites. The prognosis for patients with a malignant melanoma correlates best with the microscopic depth of invasion, as assessed in the resected lesion. Larger lesions are more likely to have invaded further. Sun exposure in light-skinned people leads to an increased risk for malignant melanoma formation.

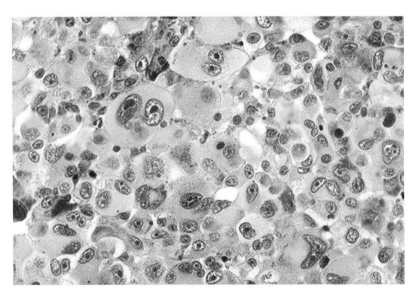

FIGURE 16–15 Malignant melanoma, microscopic

This neoplasm is composed of large polygonal cells (or spindle cells in some other cases) that have very pleomorphic nuclei that contain prominent nucleoli. The neoplasm here is making brown melanin pigment. Melanoma cells can make variable amounts of melanin pigment, even within the same lesion (leading to the characteristic variability in pigmentation, which helps distinguish it from a benign nevus). Some melanomas may make so little pigment that grossly they appear "amelanotic."

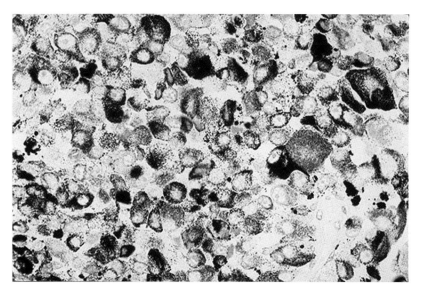

FIGURE 16–16 Malignant melanoma, microscopic

This Fontana-Masson silver stain (melanin stain) shows a fine black dusting of melanin pigment within the cytoplasm of the neoplastic cells of this malignant melanoma. Both familial and sporadic malignant melanomas can have the *CDKN2A* (*p16INK4A*) gene mutation, a cyclin-dependent kinase inhibitor. Mutations in the *BRAF* and *CDK4* genes are also seen.

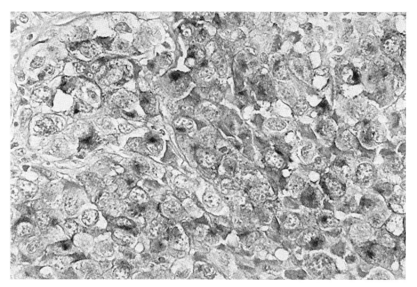

FIGURE 16–17 Malignant melanoma, microscopic

A variety of immunohistochemical stains are helpful in distinguishing a metastatic lesion as a melanoma, particularly when the cells are poorly differentiated to anaplastic. The polygonally shaped neoplastic cells shown here stain positively with HMB-45, suggesting that the primary neoplasm is a melanoma. A melan-A stain also has high specificity for melanoma.

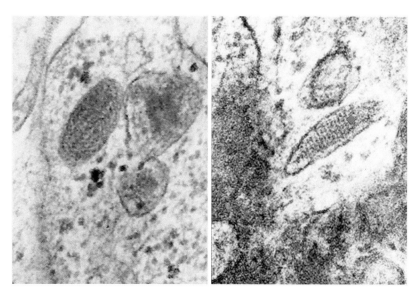

FIGURE 16–18 Malignant melanoma, electron microscopy

Sometimes a melanoma will not be well differentiated enough to show the typical melanin pigmentation either grossly or by light microscopy. By electron microscopy, it may be possible to prove the neoplasm is a melanoma if premelanosomes are seen. Two examples of premelanosomes (◆) are shown here as oval structures with a faint barred pattern, looking like miniature snowshoes.

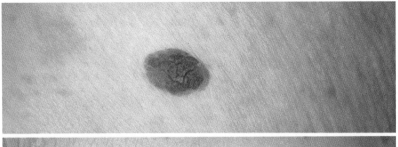

FIGURE 16–19 Seborrheic keratosis, gross

Seen here are examples of a very common lesion of older adults—seborrheic keratoses. Seborrheic keratoses are usually distributed over the skin of the face, neck, and upper trunk. They develop into rough-surfaced, coinlike plaques that vary from a few millimeters in size to several centimeters. They slowly enlarge over time. They are usually pigmented brown, but the amount of pigmentation can vary from one lesion to the next. On close inspection of a lesion, keratin appears to erupt out of small pores on the surface of the lesion.

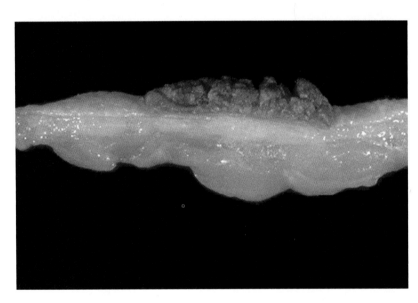

FIGURE 16–20 Seborrheic keratosis, gross

A seborrheic keratosis has an appearance as though it had just been pasted or "stuck on" the skin, as seen here in cross-section in this excised lesion where the brownish nodular, rough-surfaced lesion extends above the level of the surrounding epidermis. In some cases, they can have a downward growth phase, in which case they are termed *inverted follicular keratoses*. Seborrheic keratoses enlarge slowly over time. Their unsightliness is their only real consequence. They are never malignant.

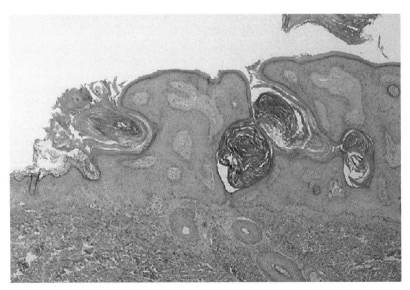

FIGURE 16–21 Seborrheic keratosis, microscopic

Note how this seborrheic keratosis is formed of benign-appearing, well-differentiated squamous epithelium and how the lesion extends above the level of the surrounding epidermis seen at the left, giving it the raised appearance as though it were "stuck on" to the skin surface. Broad bands of normal-appearing epidermal cells have large keratin-filled "horn cysts" within them. When irritated by scratching or rubbing, they can enlarge from inflammation with swelling.

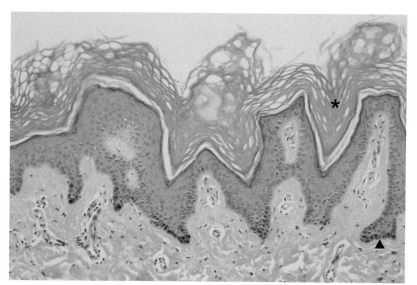

FIGURE 16–22 Acanthosis nigricans, microscopic

These hyperpigmented lesions occur most commonly in areas of flexure such as at the elbow, axilla, neck, or groin. Their hyperpigmentation is due to increased melanin granules in the epidermal basal layer. Seen here is epidermal papillomatosis with hyperkeratosis (∗) and patchy hyperpigmentation (▲) of the basal cell layer. Most cases occur in childhood and are the result of either an autosomal dominant condition or a manifestation of obesity or an endocrinopathy. The appearance of acanthosis nigricans in adults may presage signs and symptoms of an underlying malignancy.

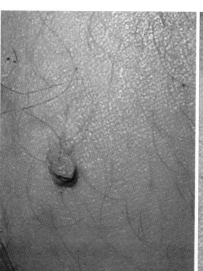 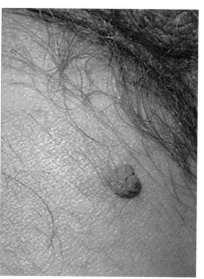

FIGURE 16–23 Fibroepithelial polyp, gross

Here are two examples of fibroepithelial polyps, also known as *skin tags*, each about 0.6 cm long. These are also termed *soft fibromas* or *acrochordons*. They appear as papules or baglike pedunculated growths connected by a narrow pedicle to the skin of the neck, trunk, or extremities. They are covered by epidermis and composed centrally of a loose overgrowth of connective tissue from the reticular dermis. They can be a nuisance when they appear at the belt line or axillary line, where rubbing and irritation can occur. Similar to hemangiomas and nevi, they may become more numerous during pregnancy.

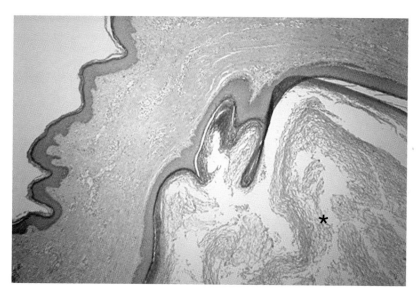

FIGURE 16–24 Epithelial cyst, microscopic

An epithelial cyst (also known as a *wen*, or *sebaceous cyst*) is palpably fluctuant and freely movable. It becomes filled with soft keratinaceous debris. A wen forms when there is down-growth of the overlying epidermis or epithelium of a hair follicle into the underlying dermis. There is continued desquamation of keratin into the center of the expanding cyst (∗). These lesions are common. Larger cysts may become traumatized and rupture, inducing a surrounding inflammatory reaction that can include acute, chronic, and granulomatous elements.

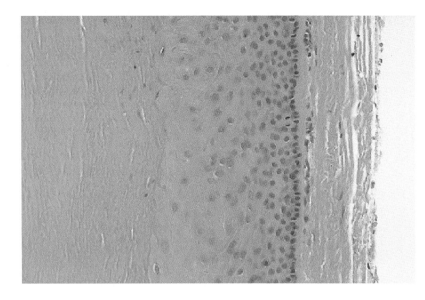

FIGURE 16–25 Epithelial cyst, microscopic

This epithelial cyst was excised from beneath the skin surface, with a rim of dermal connective tissue at the right. These cysts are seen most frequently on face, scalp, neck, and trunk. They are about 1 to 5 cm in size. They have a wall of epidermis that desquamates keratin, seen here as the laminated pink material at the left, which forms the soft cyst contents that give it characteristics that lead to the clinical description *sebaceous cyst*. The cyst can rupture and lead to marked foreign-body inflammation. The lack of a granular cell layer in this example is most characteristic of the variant known as a *pilar cyst* beneath the scalp.

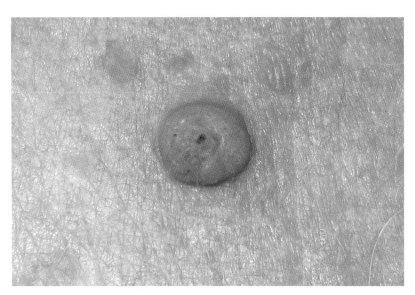

FIGURE 16–26 Keratoacanthoma, gross

This lesion can grow rapidly over weeks to months, reaching a size of 1 cm to several centimeters, suggesting a more aggressive behavior. The presence of *p53* gene mutations suggests that this lesion is a variant of a squamous cell carcinoma. However, a keratoacanthoma can be a self-limited lesion that may even spontaneously heal after a few months. They are most often seen on sun-exposed skin in men older than 50 years. Grossly, the lesion seen here appears as a symmetric dome-shaped nodule with a central keratin-filled crater.

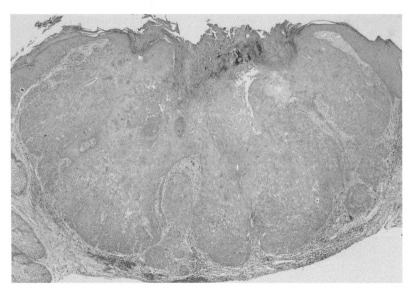

FIGURE 16–27 Keratoacanthoma, microscopic

Note the endophytic crater-like lesion with a proliferation of well-differentiated squamous epithelium extending downward in tongues and nests into the dermis, with a central keratin plug. The abundant keratin production results in the central collection of keratinaceous material that appears to erupt outward. It resembles a well-differentiated squamous cell carcinoma. The large cells have prominent glassy pink cytoplasm and minimal atypia.

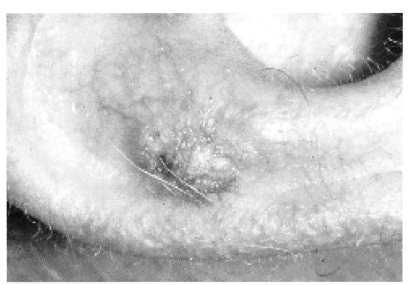

FIGURE 16–28 Actinic keratosis, gross

The irregular tan to red, plaquelike lesion with a rough surface seen here in a sun-exposed area (the ear) may enlarge over time. These lesions are usually less than 1 cm in size. This is a potentially premalignant lesion that can give rise to squamous cell carcinoma *in situ*, which can evolve into an invasive squamous carcinoma. It is not uncommon for patients to have more than one such lesion in sun-exposed areas of skin. If such a lesion appears on the lips, it is termed *actinic cheilitis*. Since squamous cell carcinomas often arise in areas of actinic keratosis, removal of these lesions is recommended.

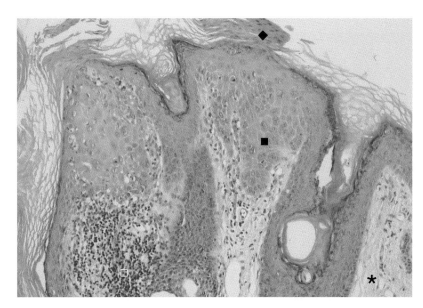

FIGURE 16–29 Actinic change, microscopic

Actinic damage from increased skin exposure to ultraviolet light (exposure to sunlight) is seen here. There is parakeratosis (◆) along with keratinocyte atypia (■) limited to the lower epidermal layers. The damaged collagen and elastic fibers appear as homogenous pale blue areas (∗) in the dermis, termed *solar elastosis*. With more extensive solar damage, there can be dermal inflammation (□), as seen here. Fair-skinned people are at greater risk for development of this condition. This actinic damage is cumulative and nonreversible. The loss of dermal elastic fibers contributes to skin aging with wrinkling.

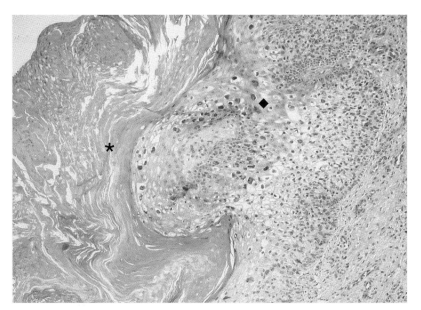

FIGURE 16–30 Carcinoma *in situ*, microscopic

This actinic keratosis has marked overlying hyperkeratosis with a dense layer of keratin (∗) at the left. Sometimes the hyperkeratosis is so pronounced that there is formation of a "cutaneous horn" of projecting keratin. Actinic keratoses are predisposed to progress to squamous cell carcinomas. Note the epithelial atypia (◆) here involving the full thickness of the epidermis, which qualifies this lesion as a squamous cell carcinoma *in situ*.

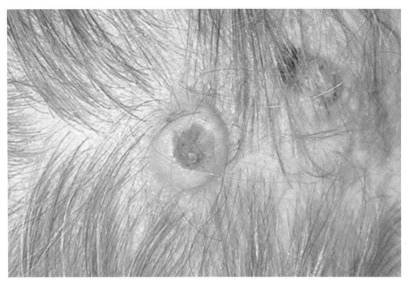

FIGURE 16–31 Squamous cell carcinoma, gross

This small nodule on the scalp proved to be a squamous cell carcinoma, although a basal cell carcinoma could have a similar appearance. Such small tumors are often noticed by the patient before reaching a larger size, and the smaller, more localized lesions are unlikely to have invaded far or metastasized. This is why the "cure" rate for nonmelanoma skin cancers is very high. Squamous cell carcinomas of the skin are related to the amount of past sun exposure, and UVB rays are the most damaging. The surrounding skin may show actinic keratoses (premalignant actinic change from sun damage to the epidermis). Human papillomavirus (HPV) infection may play a role in development of some of these cancers.

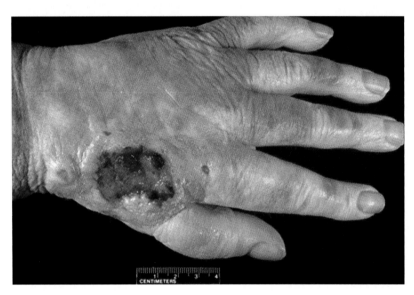

FIGURE 16–32 Squamous cell carcinoma, gross

This is an ulcerated squamous cell carcinoma that arose on the dorsum of the hand. Besides sun exposure, risk factors for squamous cell carcinoma of skin include carcinogens such as tars, chronic ulcers, burn scars, arsenic poisoning, and radiation exposure. In this case, there was a history of both sun exposure and exposure to carcinogens. Patients with the rare autosomal recessive disorder xeroderma pigmentosum have defects in nucleotide excision and repair (*NER*) genes so that pyrimidine dimers formed in cellular DNA from ultraviolet light exposure lead to a 2000-fold increased risk for squamous cell carcinomas, which can arise even in childhood.

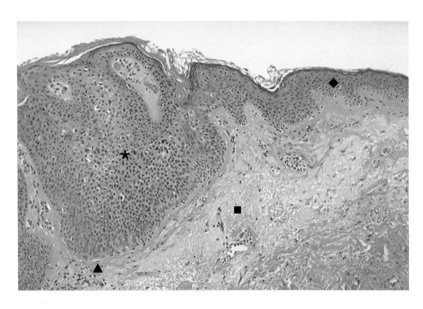

FIGURE 16–33 Squamous cell carcinoma, microscopic

Since this neoplasm does not extend below the basement membrane (▲), this lesion is termed a *squamous cell carcinoma* in situ. This condition is sometimes called *Bowen disease*. Note the normal skin (◆) on the right adjacent to the thicker carcinoma (∗) at the left with more cellular pleomorphism and hyperchromatism. There is also extensive solar elastosis (■), marked by the pale blue homogenous appearance of the underlying dermal collagen, a result of chronic sun damage. Loss of normal *p53* tumor suppressor gene function in such lesions is common, and *RAS* mutations may also be present. The cells of these neoplasms are often aneuploid.

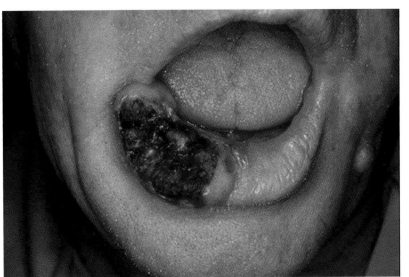

FIGURE 16–34 Basal cell carcinoma, gross

This large basal cell carcinoma of the lower lip has a pearly pink papular border and an ulcerated center. These lesions rarely metastasize, but they are slow growing and progressively infiltrative over time (a "rodent ulcer" that keeps eating away at normal tissues). Leaving them to get larger just makes the plastic surgeon's job that much harder, with more disability to the patient, so early detection and excision are a must. Most basal cell carcinomas occur in the head and neck area of adults. There is an increased risk for development of basal cell carcinoma with prolonged sun exposure, specifically damaging UVB rays.

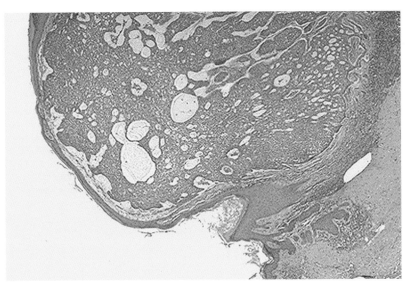

FIGURE 16–35 Basal cell carcinoma, microscopic

Basal cell carcinoma and squamous cell carcinoma are the most common skin malignancies. Note here the densely packed dark blue cells expanding in a nodular growth pattern beneath the thin overlying epidermis. This tumor can grow quite large and invade surrounding tissues, but it virtually never metastasizes. The lesion shown here is growing as a nodular mass. Basal cell carcinomas around the eye present a challenge to the surgeon to remove and retain functionality of the eyelid. Therefore, it is best to detect these tumors early and treat them when they are small.

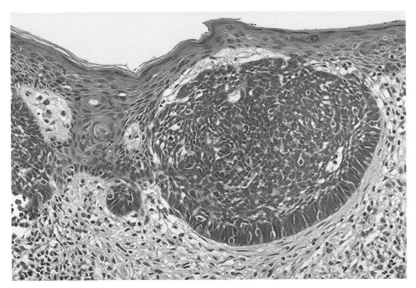

FIGURE 16–36 Basal cell carcinoma, microscopic

The cells of a basal cell carcinoma are dark blue and oblong with scant cytoplasm, resembling the cells along the basal layer of normal epidermis. These cells are arranged into nests or trabeculae that infiltrate downward into the dermis. A nest of tumor often has a pallisaded arrangement of cells around its periphery. These tumor cell nests have an intervening fibrous stroma with variable inflammatory cell component. Shown here are nests of basaloid cells dropping off into the upper dermis. These neoplasms can often be multifocal in areas of chronic sun exposure. They also occur frequently in patients with xeroderma pigmentosum and in patients with immunosuppression.

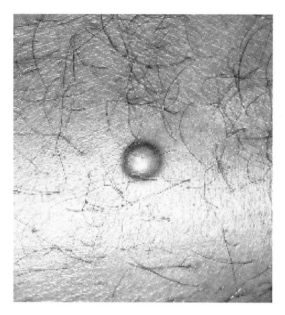

FIGURE 16–37 Benign fibrous histiocytoma, gross

Here is a very discrete, dome-shaped mass on the skin of the leg. This benign proliferation of fibroblasts with collagen is also called a *dermatofibroma*. These lesions may represent an abnormal but localized response to trauma. They can occur singly or as multiple small nodules only a few millimeters in size on the skin of the extremities in adults. On occasion they can exceed 1 cm in size, and they may increase or decrease in size over time, but they rarely grow rapidly and are not invasive. There may be some overlying hyperkeratosis and hyperpigmentation, giving them a reddish brown color. They tend to dimple inward upon lateral compression.

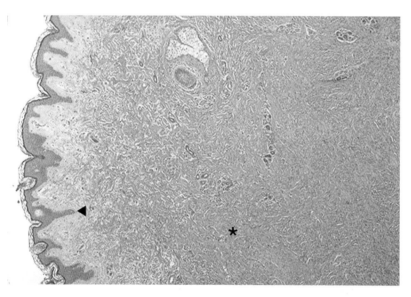

FIGURE 16–38 Benign fibrous histiocytoma, microscopic

At low magnification, beneath the epidermis at the left, there is a dense proliferation (∗) of cells in the lower dermis to form a nodule. In some cases, a prior history of trauma is present, suggesting that this lesion is an abnormal but localized response to injury, like a keloid, but more localized. The overlying epidermis is often hyperplastic, with downward elongation of rete ridges (◀), as shown here. In contrast, a malignant fibrous histiocytoma is a type of sarcoma arising in soft tissues that acts very aggressively.

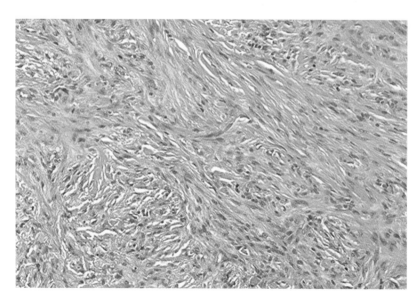

FIGURE 16–39 Benign fibrous histiocytoma, microscopic

At high magnification, the whorling fibroblastic cells with abundant collagen bundles are seen in this tumor. They may extend into subcutaneous fat. These lesions often grow slowly and are generally just an annoying "bump" beneath the skin surface. They may be tender to palpation. Curiously, some of the cells of these dermatofibromas can express coagulation factor XIIIa.

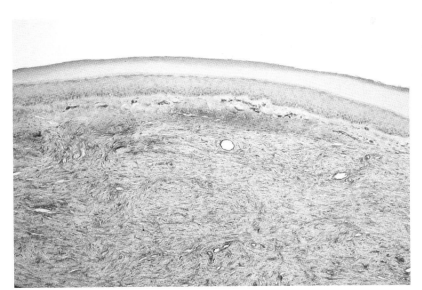

FIGURE 16–40 Dermatofibrosarcoma protuberans, microscopic

This rare sarcoma produces a slow-growing solid dermal nodule or nodules, often on the trunk. This nodular growth protrudes and may ulcerate when large. There is often invasion into underlying soft tissues, but metastases are rare. The overlying skin may become thinned and ulcerate. The microscopic spindle cell pattern, with swirling (storiform) pattern, is shown here with positivity by immunohistochemical staining with antibody to CD34.

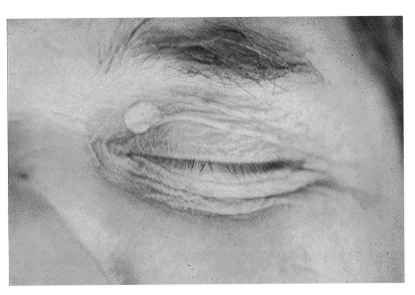

FIGURE 16–41 Xanthoma, gross

Xanthomas are collections of lipid-laden (foamy) histiocytes (macrophages) within the dermis, producing a grossly visible yellowish nodule or plaque. This little yellow plaque on the upper eyelid seen here on a patient (who did not have any abnormality of blood lipids) is called a *xanthelasma*. Eruptive xanthomas, in contrast, may appear in patients who have familial or acquired forms of hyperlipidemia. Xanthomas tend to increase or decrease in proportion to blood lipid levels.

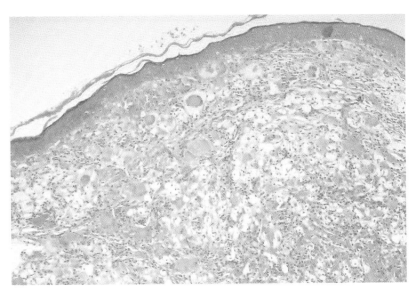

FIGURE 16–42 Xanthoma, microscopic

There are numerous foamy macrophages (histiocytes) with a pale appearance to their cytoplasm seen here within the dermis. The foamy appearance results from extensive lipid deposition, including cholesterol, phospholipids, and triglycerides, contained within the macrophage cytoplasm.

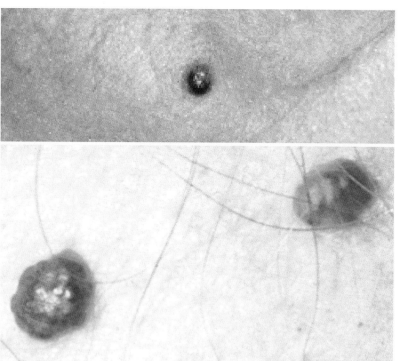

FIGURE 16–43 Hemangioma, gross

The nodules seen here are benign neoplasms with sharp borders composed of proliferations of small blood vessels. Some of these lesions may be present from birth, suggesting that they are hamartomas rather than true neoplasms. In any case, they are so slow growing that they seemingly never change. They can range in color from blue to reddish blue to purple to bright red. They generally average a few millimeters to several centimeters in size, although some congenital lesions (typically cavernous hemangiomas) can be more extensive ("port wine stain"). Some "juvenile" hemangiomas may grow rapidly in the first few months of infancy but then regress by the age of 5.

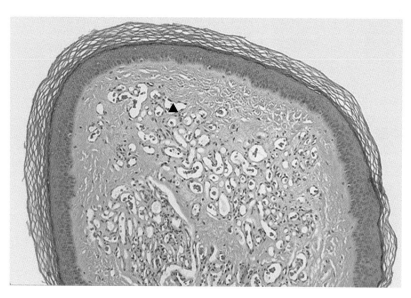

FIGURE 16–44 Hemangioma, microscopic

A reddish "mole" that is small, round, and raised may represent a hemangioma, seen here to be composed of small vascular spaces in the upper dermis. These small vascular channels, which may vary in size and shape, are lined by flattened endothelial cells (▲). These lesions appear to change slowly, if at all, over time and seem to have been present as long as the patient can remember. In a capillary hemangioma, the vascular spaces are small or collapsed, as seen here, and the intervening loose connective tissue stroma may contain larger arterioles or venules. In contrast, a cavernous hemangioma has large, dilated vascular spaces that may extend into the underlying adipose tissue.

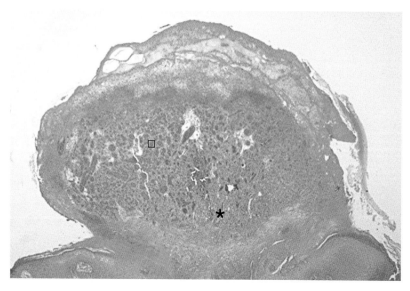

FIGURE 16–45 Pyogenic granuloma, microscopic

Also known as a *lobular capillary hemangioma*, a pyogenic granuloma is a lesion that can grossly resemble a hemangioma, but it is characteristically rapidly growing, arising and then receding within weeks to months, rather than persisting for years unchanging, as a typical hemangioma would. They may develop during pregnancy, then disappear after delivery. Local inflammation or irritation may result in formation of a nodule of granulation tissue (*) with prominent capillaries (□), as seen here. Around the capillaries are inflammatory cell infiltrates. The lesion often ulcerates. Similar lesions can appear on the gingiva.

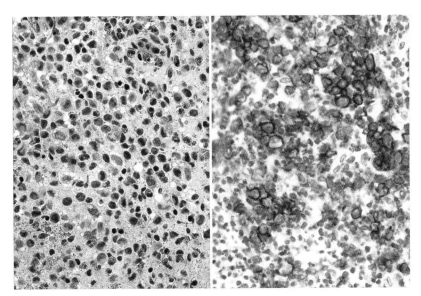

FIGURE 16–46 Histiocytosis X, microscopic

Multisystem Langerhans cell histiocytosis (Letterer-Siwe disease) most often appears before the age of 2. Skin lesions may be solitary or multiple, ranging from papules to nodules to scaling erythematous plaques resembling seborrheic dermatitis, particularly on the trunk and scalp. Most patients also have hepatosplenomegaly, lymphadenopathy, pulmonary lesions, and destructive osteolytic bone lesions. Marrow involvement can lead to pancytopenia. The most common microscopic pattern of skin involvement is that of a diffuse dermal infiltrate of large, round to ovoid cells and scattered eosinophils. Immunohistochemical staining for CD1a antigen is positive.

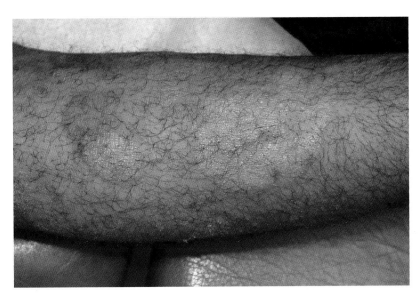

FIGURE 16–47 Mycosis fungoides, gross

This cutaneous T-cell lymphoma may evolve into a generalized lymphoma in a small number of cases. Seen here are well-demarcated, erythematous, slightly scaly plaques on the skin of the dorsal arm. These lesions may persist for many years. They may resemble psoriatic or eczematous lesions. Over time, the lesions may become nodular and ulcerate. In some patients with cutaneous T-cell lymphoma, the malignant T-cells seed into the bloodstream, called *Sézary syndrome*, and are distributed diffusely to large areas of the body, leading to erythroderma, characterized by extensive erythema and scaling of skin.

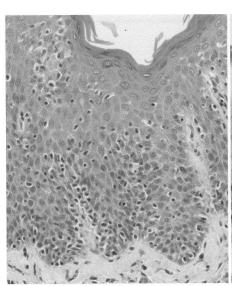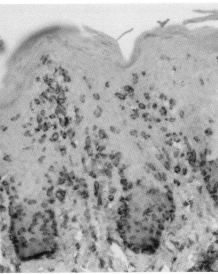

FIGURE 16–48 Mycosis fungoides, microscopic

Seen here is psoriasiform hyperplasia of the epidermis with infiltration by atypical T-cells, shown with H+E staining in the left panel and immunohistochemical staining for CD5 in the right panel, which highlights epidermotropism, where the intraepidermal lymphocytes are aligned along the basal cell layer in short linear arrays. These cells are also CD4 positive, and they have folded "cerebriform" nuclei. They are known as *Sézary-Lutzner cells*, and they can form small epidermal clusters known as *Pautrier microabscesses*.

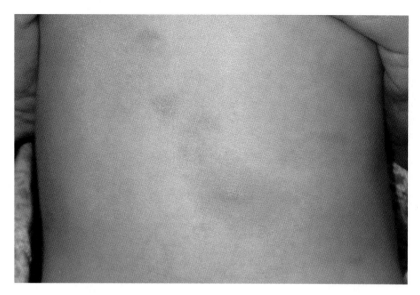

FIGURE 16–49 Mastocytosis, gross

Seen here is a red-brown maculopapular eruption called urticaria pigmentosa resulting from focal dermal infiltration by mast cells, which is a localized form of mastocytosis, accounting for half of all cases of mastocytosis, seen most often in children. These lesions often arise in groups, or they may be solitary, and appear as brown pruritic papules. Rubbing a lesion leads to development of surrounding edema and erythema, from the release of mediators such as histamine from mast cells, called *Darier sign*.

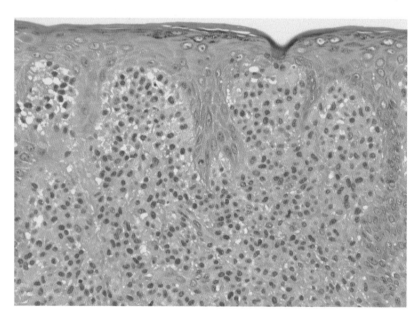

FIGURE 16–50 Mastocytosis, microscopic

The dermis is heavily infiltrated by cells with uniform, round nuclei and abundant pink cytoplasm, typical of mast cells. A mutation in the c-*KIT* proto-oncogene can activate a receptor tyrosine kinase that leads to this mast cell proliferation.

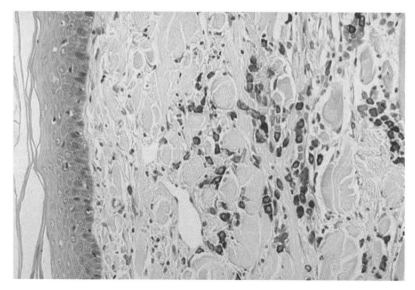

FIGURE 16–51 Mastocytosis, microscopic

A Giemsa stain highlights numerous mast cells within the dermis in this case of urticaria pigmentosa. The mast cells contain numerous purple cytoplasmic granules; the granules contain many substances, including vasoactive amines such as histamine, which are released upon activation and degranulation of the mast cells to cause symptoms such as itching and wheal formation. In systemic mastocytosis, which usually occurs in adults, tissues of the mononuclear phagocyte system, including spleen, liver, lymph nodes, and bone marrow, are often infiltrated by mast cells.

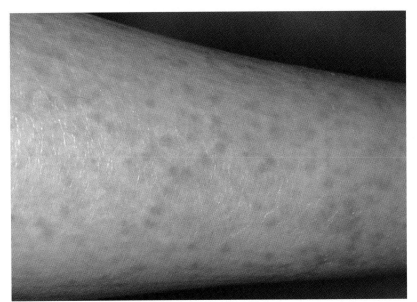

FIGURE 16–52 Ichthyosis, gross

The skin of this lower leg shows mild ichthyosiform change. In this uncommon condition of impaired epidermal maturation, there is marked hyperkeratosis that forms fishlike superficial scales. Inherited forms of ichthyosis are present from birth, while acquired forms in adults may be related to an underlying malignancy. Defective desquamation may underlie this abnormality.

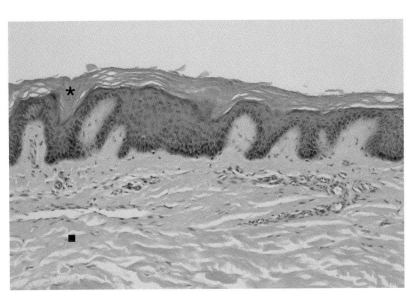

FIGURE 16–53 Ichthyosis, microscopic

There is prominent hyperkeratosis with a thick, compacted stratum corneum (∗) over this epidermal surface. Note the absence of inflammation within the dermis (■). There is diminution of the epidermal granule cell layer. In an X-linked form of ichthyosis, there is a deficiency of steroid sulfatase leading to accumulation of intercellular non-degraded cholesterol sulfate that increases cellular adhesion in the stratum corneum, diminishing epidermal desquamation.

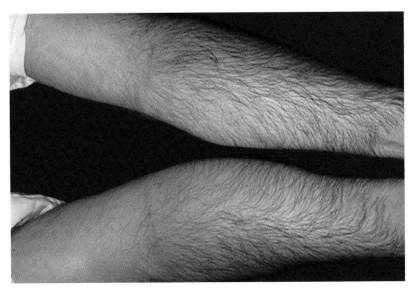

FIGURE 16–54 Urticaria, gross

The skin of the right arm shown here at the bottom is swollen (edematous) from angioedema and reddened (erythematous) from vasodilation, compared with the left arm at the top. The cardinal signs of inflammation are rubor (redness), calor (heat), tumor (swelling), dolor (pain), and loss of function. This urticarial response resulted from an insect sting leading to a systemic allergic reaction with type I hypersensitivity. These manifestations resulted from immunoglobulin E (IgE)–mediated mast cell degranulation with release of vasoactive substances such as histamine. More localized anaphylaxis, typically seen with food allergy, may also result in urticaria (hives). These lesions usually appear and disappear within hours.

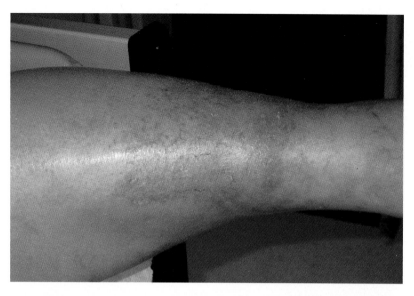

FIGURE 16–55 Acute eczematous dermatitis, gross

Eczema is a generic clinical term for any red, papulovesicular area of skin eruption that can develop oozing of fluid with crusting as well as scaling. Forms of eczematous dermatitis can include reactions to insect bites, contact dermatitis, atopic dermatitis, drug-induced dermatitis, and photodermatitis. Many irritants (those with the fine print on the warning label of the container reading "avoid contact with skin") produce this pattern of skin disease.

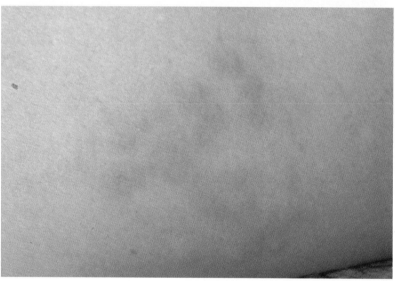

FIGURE 16–56 Contact dermatitis, gross

Focal slightly raised areas of erythema are seen here on the skin exposed to poison oak, a plant containing resin with the compound urushiol. The lesions may produce a burning or itching sensation. Cases of contact dermatitis, a form of eczematous dermatitis, are typically self-limited from focal exposure to an antigen, subsiding in days to a couple of weeks. The irritant antigen is processed by Langerhans cells, presented to CD4 cells that migrate to the site of exposure, releasing cytokines that recruit additional inflammatory cells. More severe forms may progress to papulovesicular lesions with oozing and crusting that can persist as scaling plaques.

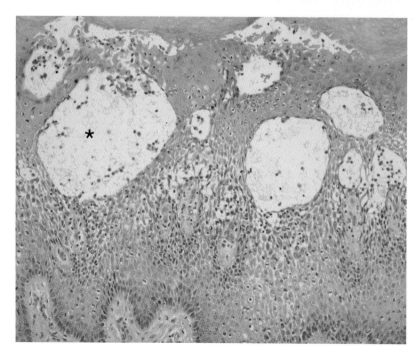

FIGURE 16–57 Acute eczematous dermatitis, microscopic

A key microscopic feature with any form of eczema is spongiosis consisting of edema fluid (∗) that collects within the epidermis, forming vesicles. Many cases of eczema are related to type IV hypersensitivity with initial antigen exposure resulting in formation of memory T cells. Re-exposure to the antigen leads to recruitment of CD4 lymphocytes releasing cytokines that mediate the inflammatory reaction. Classic cases of contact dermatitis appear within 24 to 72 hours after antigen exposure.

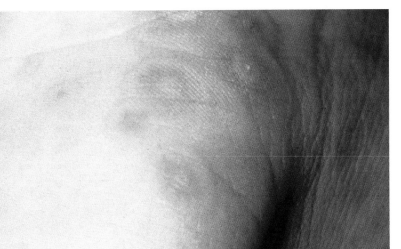

FIGURE 16–58 Erythema multiforme, gross

This condition presents with a variety of skin lesions (multiform) ranging from macules to papules to vesicles to bullae. The classic "target" lesion has a central vesicle surrounded by a zone of erythema and usually appears on the hands after herpes simplex virus infection (such as "cold sores" in the mouth). This uncommon, but usually self-limited, disorder may arise from a hypersensitivity reaction to an infection, drugs, neoplasia, or collagen vascular diseases. It is classified as "minor" with less than 10% total body surface area involvement. More extensive "major" involvement is often seen on the face or symmetrically over the extremities.

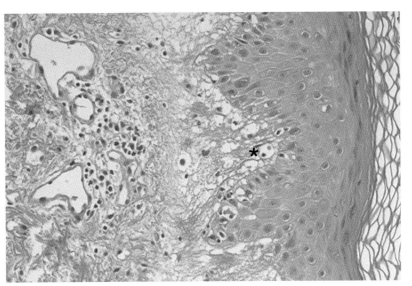

FIGURE 16–59 Erythema multiforme, microscopic

This cytotoxic CD8 cell inflammatory reaction of erythema multiforme is characterized by squamous epithelial cell necrosis (∗) at the dermal–epidermal junction. These lesions are "multiform" because macules, papules, vesicles, and bullae may be seen grossly, with symmetric involvement of the extremities. The Stevens-Johnson syndrome is a febrile illness that is a more severe, generalized form of erythema multiforme, most often occurring in children, that can also involve mucus membranes and typically follows administration of a drug (such as a sulfa drug or an anticonvulsant).

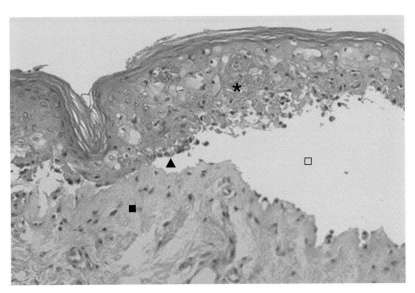

FIGURE 16–60 Erythema multiforme, microscopic

There are few dermatologic emergencies. This is one of them, known as *toxic epidermal necrolysis*. This is a severe febrile disorder with blistering and extensive sloughing of skin and mucosal surfaces as a consequence of full-thickness epidermal necrosis. Seen here is a necrotic epidermis (∗) lifting off (▲) the dermis (■) to form a subepidermal bulla (□). There are several variations on this theme, which may be the result of a reaction inducing keratinocyte apoptosis as a consequence of an infection or administration of a drug.

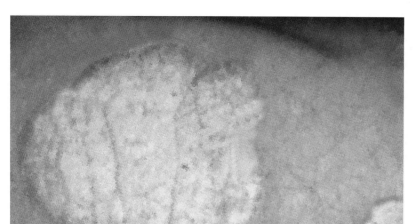

FIGURE 16–61 Psoriasis, gross

As many as 1% to 2% of people at all ages may develop psoriasis. Some may also develop psoriatic arthritis (resembling rheumatoid arthritis), spondylitis, or myopathy. About two thirds of affected people have the HLA-Cw allele. Interaction of CD4 cells with epidermal dendritic cells and CD8 cells leads to cytokine release, including tumor necrosis factor, interleukin-12, and interferon-γ, driving keratinocyte proliferation with inflammation. The thick, silvery, scaling lesions seen here are most often found over bony prominences, scalp, genitalia, and hands. The abnormal proliferation and turnover of epidermis, reduced from a month to only 4 days for a cell to transit from basal layer to surface, accounts for the buildup of these scales.

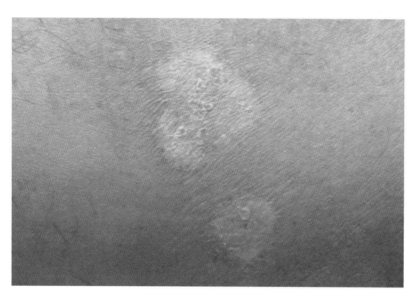

FIGURE 16–62 Psoriasis, gross

This is psoriasis after phototherapy with UVB. Note that the scaling lesions are less florid on the background of this tanned skin. The long-term morbidity from the increased risk for skin cancer with UVB is probably not as great as the morbidity with psoriasis itself. Serious complications of psoriasis include extensive erythema and scaling, termed *erythroderma*, and extensive pustule formation with secondary infection accompanied by fever and leukocytosis, termed *pustular psoriasis*. A minor problem seen in one third of patients is yellow-brown nail discoloration with pitting and separation from the nail bed.

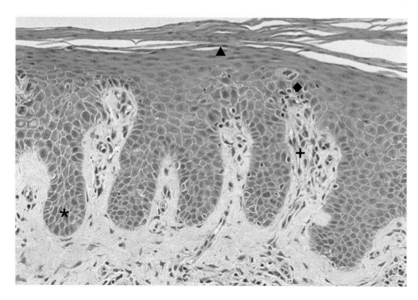

FIGURE 16–63 Psoriasis, microscopic

Microscopically, psoriasis has downward elongation of the rete ridges (*) with thinning to absence of the overlying stratum granulosum, with prominent parakeratosis (▲) above this. Small aggregates of neutrophils (◆) with surrounding spongiform change are seen in the superficial epidermis and parakeratotic region. Capillaries (+) within dermal papillae are brought close to the surface, and lifting the scale from a plaque will produce pinpoint areas of hemorrhage, known as *Auspitz sign*.

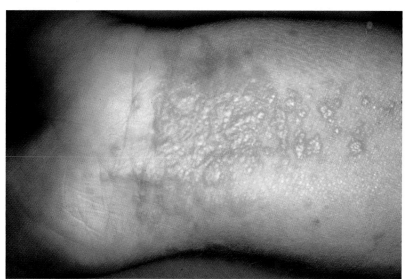

FIGURE 16–64 Lichen planus, gross

The lesions of lichen planus typically spontaneously resolve in 1 to 2 years, leaving hyperpigmented areas where the lesions were present. However, during the course of this disease, there are pruritic papules with a pink to violaceous appearance, as shown here. These lesions are symmetrically distributed, most often at the elbows and wrists, or the glans penis in men.

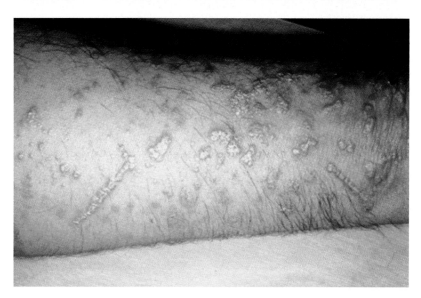

FIGURE 16–65 Lichen planus, gross

The linear arrangement of these lichenoid lesions is an example of Koebner's phenomenon (also seen with psoriasis), in which lesions appear on the skin at the sites of trauma. In addition to skin lesions, oral lesions are common with lichen planus. On the oral mucosa, the lesions appear as white, reticulated, netlike areas, and these may persist for years. White dots or lines known as *Wickham striae* may also appear in papular lesions. The cause of this condition is unknown but is presumably a cell-mediated immune reaction.

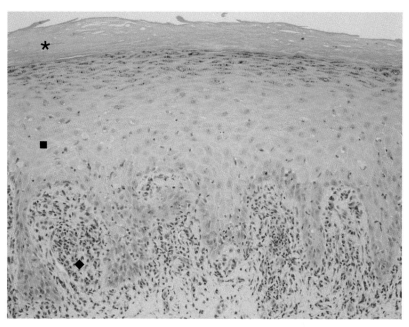

FIGURE 16–66 Lichen planus, microscopic

Seen here is irregular acanthosis (■), orthokeratotic hyperkeratosis (*), and hypergranulosis of the epidermis along with a bandlike upper dermal infiltrate (♦) of T lymphocytes. This lymphocytic infiltrate involves the dermal–epidermal junction, and the basal layer of keratinocytes may undergo degeneration and necrosis, while the stratum granulosum often increases in thickness. The rete ridges take on a sawtooth appearance.

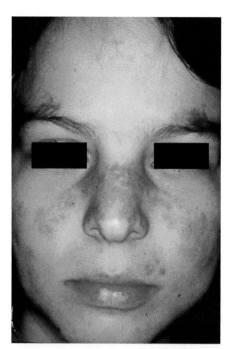

FIGURE 16–67 Lupus erythematosus, gross

This young woman has a malar rash (the so-called butterfly rash because of the shape of the reddened skin across the cheeks). Such a rash suggests lupus. More sharply demarcated "discoid" scaling plaques may also occur. The variant of lupus known as *discoid lupus erythematosus* (DLE) involves mainly just the skin and is, therefore, relatively benign compared with systemic lupus erythematosus (SLE), which typically is a systemic disease that affects internal organs such as the kidney, but may manifest with skin rashes in one third of cases. In either DLE or SLE, sunlight exposure accentuates this erythematous rash. A small number (5% to 10%) of DLE patients go on to develop SLE (usually those DLE patients with a positive antinuclear antibody).

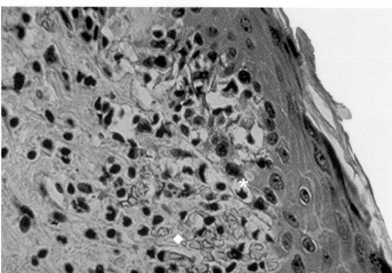

FIGURE 16–68 Lupus erythematosus, microscopic

This is a severe inflammatory skin infiltrate in the upper dermis of a patient with SLE in which the basal layer (∗) is undergoing vacuolization and dissolution, and there is purpura with red blood cells (◆) spilling out of blood vessels into the upper dermis (which is the reason for the rash). A lymphocytic infiltrate is present at the dermal–epidermal junction.

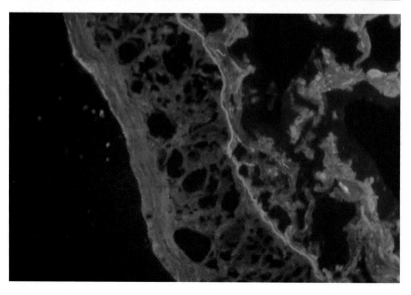

FIGURE 16–69 Lupus erythematosus, immunofluorescence

Immunofluorescence studies can be performed on skin biopsies. Seen here is a bright green fluorescing band from staining with antibody to IgG. The localization at the dermal–epidermal junction is typical of immune complex deposition. These complexes are formed from antigens and antibodies and tend to be trapped along the basement membranes. Complement activation further enhances the inflammatory reaction. Skin diseases with this immunofluorescence pattern may include SLE, DLE, and bullous pemphigoid.

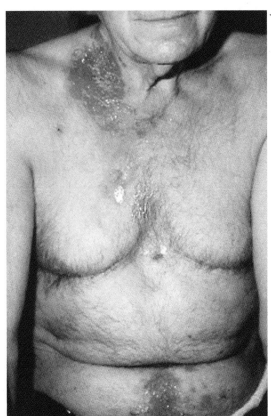

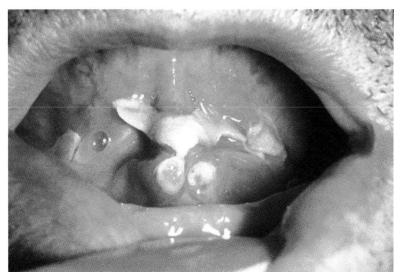

◄FIGURES 16–70 and 16–71 Pemphigus vulgaris, gross

Blistering skin diseases include pemphigus vulgaris. The stratum spinosum separates from the basal layer to form a flaccid bulla that often ruptures, as shown here. Lesions are most common on the scalp, in the periumbilical and intertriginous regions, and on mucous membranes.

FIGURE 16–72 Pemphigus vulgaris, microscopic ▶

The blister is seen forming above (▲) the basal layer within the epidermis, a suprabasal acantholytic blister. These lesions can become progressively larger, and more lesions can appear, leaving considerable skin surface denuded after rupture. Corticosteroid therapy is required to halt progression of the disease, and immunosuppressive therapy may be required for maintenance therapy.

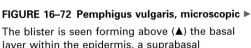

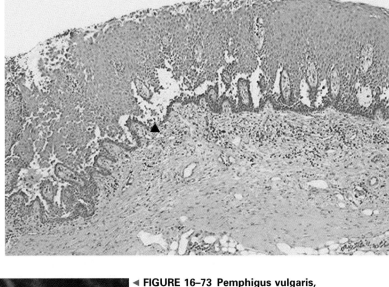

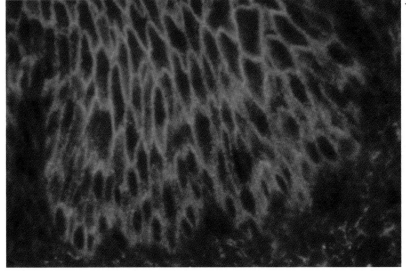

◄ FIGURE 16–73 Pemphigus vulgaris, immunofluorescence

Pemphigus vulgaris is an autoimmune disease produced by antibodies directed against a protein associated with desmosomes of keratinocytes. The antibody is directed against desmoglein 3, a component of desmosomes that aids in keratinocyte binding. With immunofluorescence using antibodies directed against IgG, an intercellular staining pattern is observed here, producing a netlike pattern. Circulating antibody can also be detected.

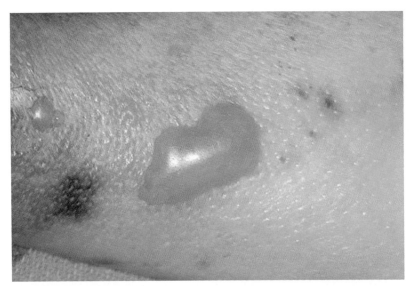

FIGURE 16–74 Bullous pemphigoid, gross

Seen here is a large, tense bulla at the center and a smaller bulla to the left. Bullous skin lesions may occur in association with infections and drugs. The lesions here developed with a condition known as *bullous pemphigoid*, which typically affects older people and involves both cutaneous and mucosal surfaces. These lesions filled with clear fluid may reach several centimeters in size, but they do not rupture as easily as those of pemphigus. Flexural regions of axillae, groin, forearms, and abdomen, as well as the inner thighs, are most often involved.

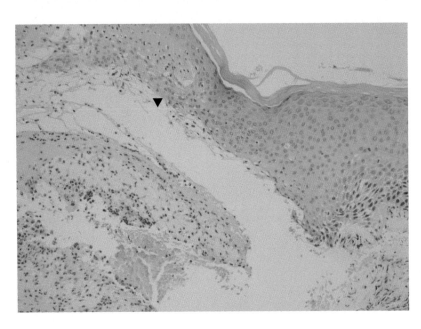

FIGURE 16–75 Bullous pemphigoid, microscopic

This is a subepidermal (▼), nonacantholytic blister. The inflammatory infiltrate can include fibrin along with lymphocytes, eosinophils, and neutrophils. The superficial dermis is edematous. These lesions may heal without scarring. Oral lesions may be seen in 10% to 15% of cases.

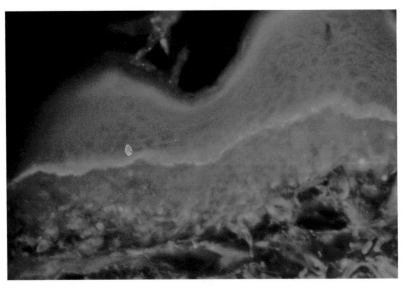

FIGURE 16–76 Bullous pemphigoid, immunofluorescence

Immunoglobulin and complement are usually distributed in a linear fashion along the basement membrane in this blistering disease. The antibody, here IgG, is directed against hemidesmosomes in the squamous epithelium. Autoantibodies to the bullous pemphigoid antigens 1 and 2 in these hemidesmosomes results in complement fixation with recruitment and activation of inflammatory cells.

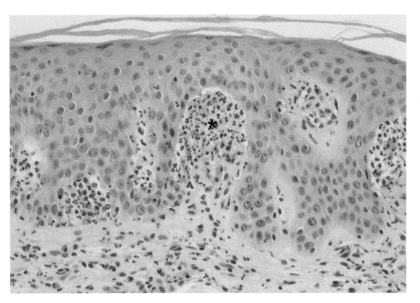

FIGURE 16–77 Dermatitis herpetiformis, microscopic

Grossly, areas of urticaria with vesicle formation can occur. Middle-aged adults are usually affected, mostly men. There is an association with celiac disease involving the small intestine. The IgA and IgG antibodies formed against ingested gliadin protein found in gluten of grains such as wheat, barley, and rye are also directed against reticulin. The reticulin is part of anchoring fibrils that connect epidermal basement membrane to the dermis. The characteristic microscopic finding seen here is collections of neutrophils (*) within the dermal papillae, forming papillary microabscesses. Over time, these areas can coalesce, with blister formation.

FIGURE 16–78 Acne vulgaris, gross

Seen here are mild acne lesions on the skin of the back, with scattered inflammatory papules and occasional pustules. Acne, which is seen in nearly all teenagers and young adults after puberty to some degree, results from increased sebaceous gland sebum production with an increase in androgenous steroid hormone production. Sebum and keratinaceous debris block hair follicles, leading to comedone formation. Bacteria in the comedones, such as *Propionibacterium acnes*, cause inflammation and enlargement to form a pustule or nodule. This can rupture to produce a cystic area, generally a lesion larger than 0.5 cm, in which the purulent lesion extends with inflammation into the surrounding dermis.

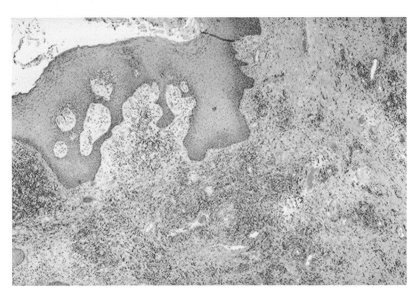

FIGURE 16–79 Acne vulgaris, microscopic

There is marked inflammation, both acute and chronic, extending all the way through the dermis. Acne is most often self-limited and generally abates in young adulthood, but about 10% to 20% of adults may continue to manifest acne. Males are affected more than females, although persistence of acne may be longer in women. A small subset of patients develop the severe lesion seen here. The result of severe acne can be scarring, more likely in males. Androgenic stimulation of sebaceous gland activity, coupled with breakdown of lipids by *Propionibacterium acnes* bacteria to irritating fatty acids, may drive the inflammatory process. Treatment with a synthetic vitamin A derivative (isotretinoin) is often successful.

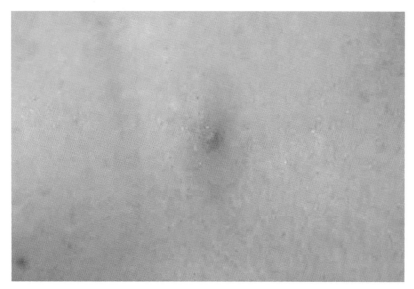

FIGURE 16–80 Erythema nodosum, gross

Erythema nodosum is a type of panniculitis (inflammation of subcutaneous adipose tissue) manifested by a central tender nodule with surrounding zone of erythema. The lesions may reach several centimeters in size over weeks to months and then fade. Lesions are most common on the skin of the anterior leg and thigh. In time, they will become purple, then flat and brown, then fade out. In some cases, an underlying systemic inflammatory condition, such as a granulomatous disease, is present, while other cases occur in association with drug therapy (sulfonamides), malignancies, and inflammatory bowel disease. In many cases, this condition is idiopathic.

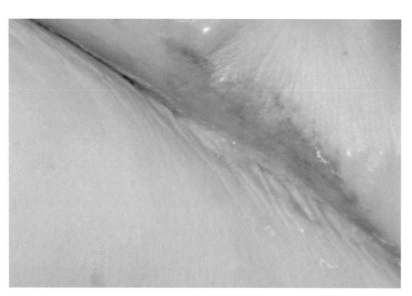

FIGURE 16–81 Intertrigo, gross

The erythematous region present in this lower abdominal skin fold is known as *intertrigo*. The rubbing of skin surfaces in the fold is more prone to chafing of the epidermis, while the warm, moist environment encourages fungal and bacterial growth. Secondary infection may occur. This is most often a complication of obesity.

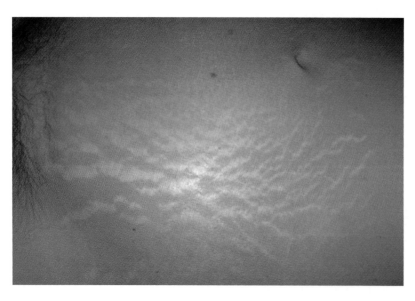

FIGURE 16–82 Abdominal striae, gross

The pale linear depressed white scarlike marks seen here on the lower abdomen are striae (more formally called *striae atrophicae* or *striae distensae*). They can be pink to purple when they first appear. These striae can arise on the abdomen, breasts, buttocks, and thighs in association with weakening of the dermal elastic tissue. Predisposing conditions include pregnancy, obesity, and Cushing syndrome.

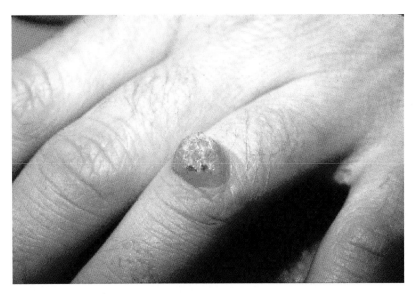

FIGURE 16–83 Verruca vulgaris, gross

A "warty" nodule very common on the skin, particularly in children and adolescents, is a verruca vulgaris. They are most often seen on the hands. They can be solitary or multiple. They have a rough surface and may be grey to tan to brown. These warts are caused by infection with the HPV and occur from direct contact between people or by autoinoculation from one skin site to another. These lesions tend to grow slowly over several years before they begin to regress over the next 6 months to 2 years.

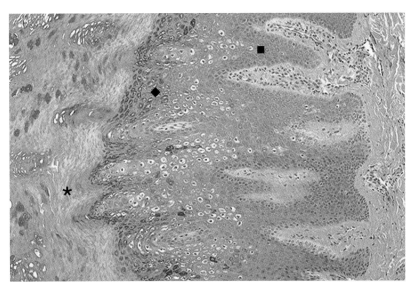

FIGURE 16–84 Verruca vulgaris, microscopic

A common wart, or verruca vulgaris, has prominent epithelial hyperplasia marked by hyperkeratosis (∗) along with papillomatosis (■) to produce the rough, warty gross appearance. The epidermal granular layer (◆) is prominent. These lesions are usually a few millimeters to 1 cm in size and are most often located on the dorsa of the hands. However, such lesions can also appear on the face (verruca plana), on the soles of the feet (verruca plantaris), or on the palms of the hands (verruca palmaris).

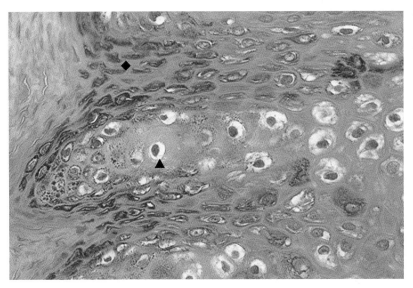

FIGURE 16–85 Verruca vulgaris, microscopic

At higher magnification, the vacuolization (▲) of nuclei along with large basophilic keratohyaline granules (◆) of the epidermal cells (koilocytotic change) in this verruca vulgaris is prominent and indicates the viral origin of this lesion. Viral particles are present within the epidermal cell nuclei. Such warts are usually caused by subtypes of HPV that are not associated with malignant transformation. HPV subtype 16, however, has been associated with development of squamous cell carcinoma.

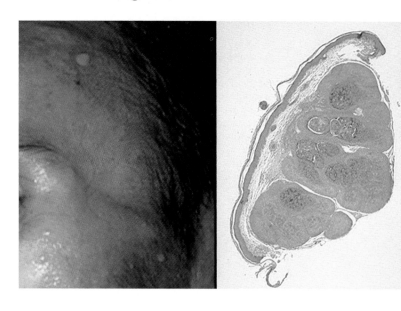

FIGURE 16–86 Molluscum contagiosum, gross and microscopic

Multiple 2- to 4-mm dome-shaped, flesh-colored, firm papules caused by molluscum contagiosum are seen grossly in the left panel. These lesions can also be umbilicated. They are most often found on the skin of the trunk and anogenital region, but may appear elsewhere, as shown here on the face. The biopsy in the right panel shows a cuplike verrucous epidermal hyperplasia. This infection is spread by direct contact between people.

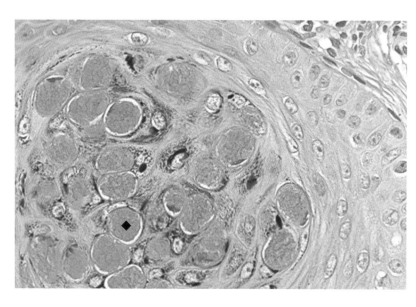

FIGURE 16–87 Molluscum contagiosum, microscopic

At high magnification, there are large pink ovoid inclusions (◆) in epidermal cells. These are the "molluscum bodies" of molluscum contagiosum, which is caused by a large brick-shaped DNA containing poxvirus. These lesions will spontaneously involute over a couple of months. These molluscum bodies may be identified with Giemsa staining of the cheesy material expressed from the center of a lesion.

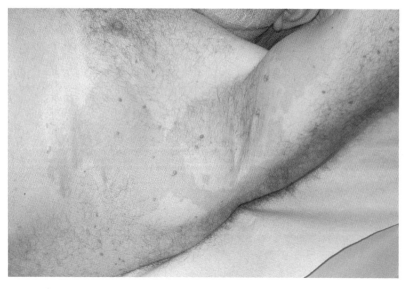

FIGURE 16–88 Superficial fungal infection, gross

Seen here is an irregularly shaped, lightly hyperpigmented confluent patch on the upper trunk characteristic of pityriasis versicolor (*Tinea versicolor*) caused by *Malassezia furfur*. A variety of dermatophytes can produce irregular areas of eczema or irregular pigmentation, crusting, or scaling. Dermatophytes can include the genera *Trichophyton* and *Epidermophyton*. The lesions are called *Tinea* and further described by the location, such as *Tinea corporis* (body), *Tinea capitis* (head), *Tinea cruris* (groin, or "jock itch"), *Tinea barbae* (male beard area), and *Tinea pedis* ("athlete's foot").

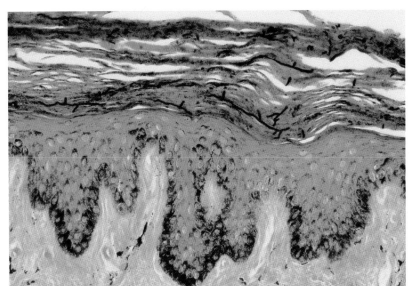

FIGURE 16–89 Superficial fungal infection, microscopic

Note the thin, black, elongated, branching hyphae of fungal organisms within the stratum corneum, seen here with Gomori methenamine silver stain. Warm, moist environments aid in promoting fungal growth. Involvement of the nails is called *onychomycosis*. Viewing the areas with fluorescent light (Woods lamp) may reveal the autofluorescence of these fungi.

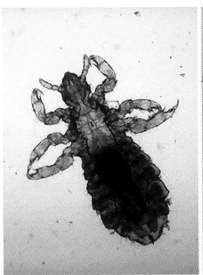
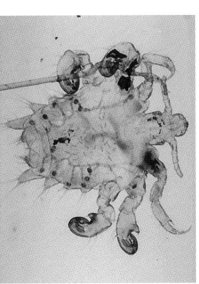

FIGURE 16–90 Pediculosis, microscopic

A "crab" louse is seen in the right panel hanging on to a pubic hair shaft. The more elongated body louse (or head louse, which is similar) is shown in the left panel. These wingless insects (note the six legs) live by biting and sucking on the blood of the human host. They are an annoyance. The focal irritation they cause can lead to scratching and excoriation that may become secondarily infected. The body louse (*Pediculus humanus corporis*) is also the vector for *Rickettsia prowazekii* (epidemic typhus), *Borrelia recurrentis* (relapsing fever), and *Bartonella quintana* (trench fever, bacillary angiomatosis, endocarditis, lymphadenopathy).

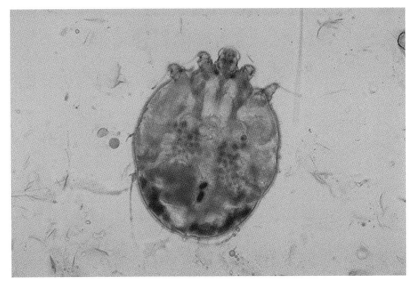

FIGURE 16–91 Scabies, microscopic

A skin scraping from between the fingers on the hand of a patient with linear reddish lesions from 0.2 to 0.6 cm in length that had been excoriated (scratched) yielded this scabies mite (*Sarcoptes scabiei*). The female mite burrows under the stratum corneum, typically on the hands, but also in the genital region of males and periareolar region of females. The lesions itch intensely, and scratching leads to excoriation.

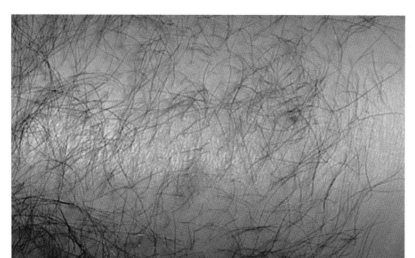

FIGURE 16–92 Bee sting, gross

The focal erythematous area seen here resulted from a bee sting. There is a pale center to the bite, representing an acute necrotic response, and the surrounding skin is edematous and mildly erythematous from the acute inflammation. In a small percentage of people, such stings may elicit a systemic anaphylactic reaction (type 1 hypersensitivity).

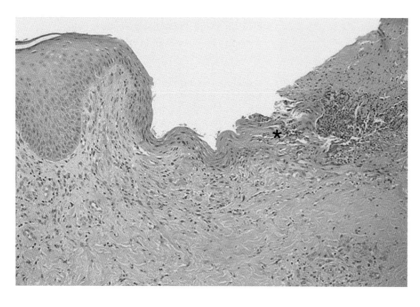

FIGURE 16–93 Brown recluse spider bite, microscopic

The bite of the brown recluse spider (*Loxosceles* spider) initially produces a mild stinging sensation, but within hours, there is intense pain along with erythema and then bulla formation. This can be followed by formation of a deep ulcer with necrotic base (∗). Most of these ulcerative lesions will heal spontaneously, although weeks to months may pass, and some cases require débridement or skin grafting.

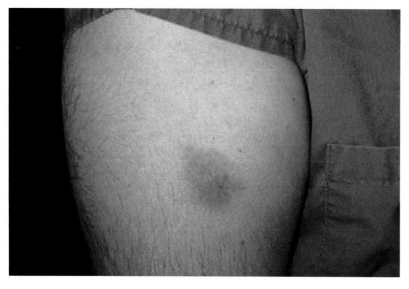

FIGURE 16–94 Contusion, gross

Blunt force injury that does not break the skin can rupture small blood vessels in the dermis and underlying soft tissue, resulting in the extravasation of red blood cells. Initially, the contusion appears dull red to blue, but over time, the red cells are broken down, releasing bilirubin and heme (which is processed by macrophages to hemosiderin), to give the yellow-brown hue seen here a week after the injury to the upper outer arm.

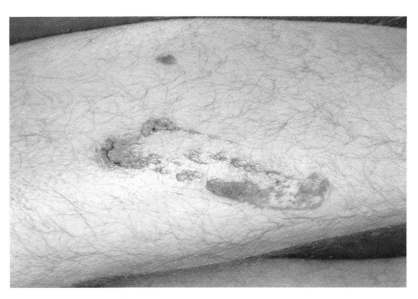

FIGURE 16–95 Abrasion, gross

Abrasions are made by a scraping injury to the skin surface, typically in an irregular fashion, as seen here over the skin of the leg. Note the superficial tearing of the epidermis, but no break in the skin surface. Sometimes the pattern of the abrasion can indicate what kind of surface the skin contacted when the force was applied. Sometimes foreign material can become embedded into the abraded surface.

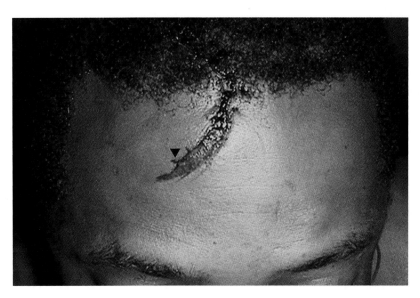

FIGURE 16–96 Laceration, gross

This superficial laceration of the forehead shows that the skin surface is broken. There are some small tags of skin (▼) where the surface was irregularly torn. The tearing may be linear to stellate, depending on the direction and amount of force applied. Lacerations typically occur by contact with an irregular object, either from blunt force or sharp force, with enough force applied to break the skin surface. Lacerations are deeper than abrasions and more irregular than incised wounds.

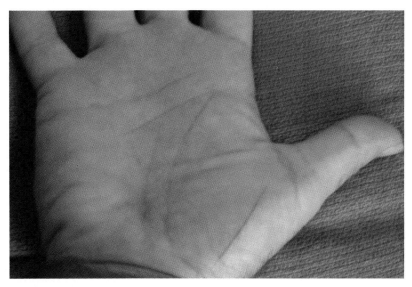

FIGURE 16–97 Incised wound, gross

An incision is defined as a very regular cut made by a sharp object such as a knife. Seen here is an incised wound of the skin of the hand. An incision has clean, straight edges made by the sharp object, in this case a rose thorn. It is easier to approximate the edges of an incision, such as a surgical incision, with sutures so that the wound heals by primary intention and leaves little or no scar.

CHAPTER 17

Bones, Joints, and Soft Tissue Tumors

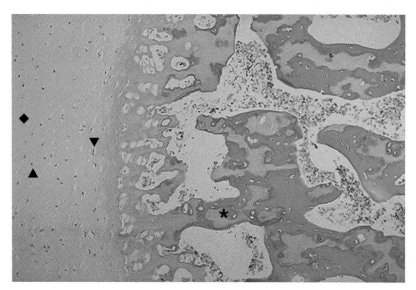

FIGURE 17–1 Normal fetal bone, microscopic

This normal fetal growth plate of long bones shows features of endochondral ossification. Hyaline cartilage (◆) at the left contains chondroblasts that secrete an extracellular matrix with glycosaminoglycans and proteoglycans along with type II collagen fibers and some elastic fibers. The chondroblasts (▲) become chondrocytes (▼) within lacunae defined by a pericellular capsule and surrounded by the cartilaginous matrix. The cartilage template then transforms into bone spicules (∗) of osteoid that become calcified. As this process continues, the bone lengthens. The hyaline cartilage remaining at the ends of long bones forms the articular cartilage of joints.

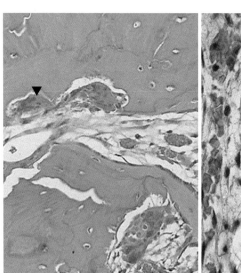
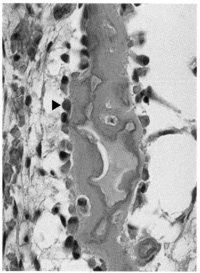

FIGURE 17–2 Normal bone, microscopic

The fetal bone spicule shown in the right panel has numerous osteoblasts (▶) lining the surface and generating new osteoid, or uncalcified organic bone matrix, which is formed of type I collagen upon which hydroxyapatite crystal (hydrated calcium phosphate) is deposited. Osteoblasts have parathormone (PTH) receptors and when stimulated by PTH release RANKL that binds onto pre-osteoclast RANK receptors to initiate osteoclastogenesis. Remodeling of bone is carried out through bone resorption with release enzymes such as carbonic anhydrase and alkaline phosphatase by osteoclasts (▼), the multinucleated cells seen occupying Howship lacunae in the left panel.

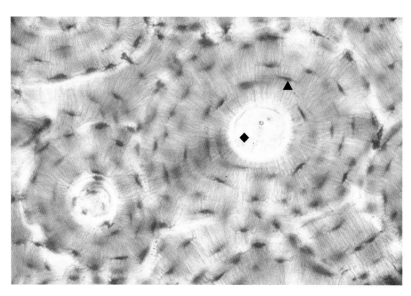

FIGURE 17–3 Normal adult bone, microscopic

This cross-section through unstained adult long compact bone cortex reveals round osteons formed of concentric layers of hydroxyapatite crystal around a central haversian canal (◆) containing the neurovascular supply. Within the crystal are entrapped osteocytes (▲) inside their lacunae. Canaliculi radiate from these lacunae to allow communication between osteocytes. These osteocytes can respond to mechanical forces and can influence local calcium and phosphorus levels to maintain optimum bone structure. In adults, mineralization of osteoid takes about 2 weeks. Bone is a warehouse for body minerals, including 99% of calcium, 85% of phosphorus, and 65% of sodium found in the human body.

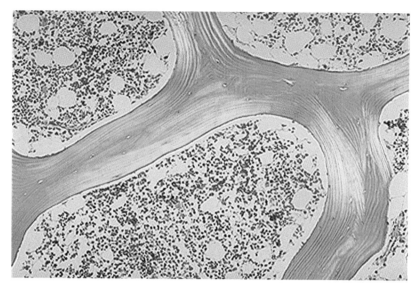

FIGURE 17–4 Normal adult bone, microscopic

Normal trabecular (cancellous) bone, seen here with polarized light, demonstrates a regular lamellar architecture. The lamellae of bone form by remodeling from primitive woven bone into a complex three-dimensional structure in response to stresses of gravity and movement to provide strength and support. Bone is constantly, albeit slowly, remodeling throughout the life span through the actions of osteoblasts and osteoclasts. Children have greater bone growth in size primarily from endochondral ossification with increasing length and girth of long bones until the epiphyses close. Between the bone trabeculae are marrow spaces, seen here with hematopoietic elements as well as adipocytes.

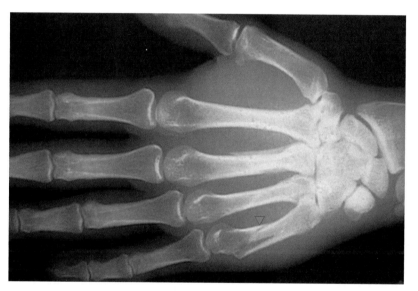

FIGURE 17–5 Bones of hand, fracture, x-ray

The normal radiographic appearance of bone is shown by this left hand. The outer rim of cortical bone is denser and, therefore, appears brighter. Soft tissues have a light to dark gray appearance. Note the appearance of a recent unhealed and displaced fracture (▽) of the fifth metacarpal as a consequence of external trauma.

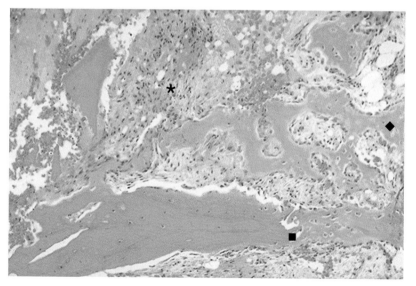

FIGURE 17–6 Fracture callus, microscopic

The region of fracture demonstrates disrupted bony trabeculae (■) at the left and bottom. The paler pink new woven bone (◆) is forming in response to the injury at the right and top in areas of hemorrhage with early granulation tissue (*). In the region of fracture, the new woven bone is called *callus*. After 6 to 8 weeks, enough healing has occurred to support weight and movement. Eventually, over months to years, this new bone is remodeled into more regular lamellar bone that attains original shape and strength. Fracture healing is more complete in children than adults. Orthopedic procedures to stabilize fractures and provide proper alignment with plates and screws are often performed on adults.

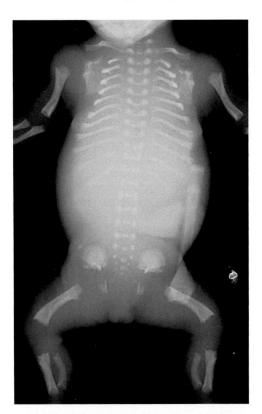

FIGURE 17–7 Thanatophoric dysplasia, radiograph

Congenital malformations involving bone are uncommon but distinctive. Many of them result in dwarfism because the endochondral ossification process is affected, and this leads to shortened long bones. There are many dwarfism syndromes. The most common is achondroplasia, which in the heterozygous state can allow a normal life span, but is lethal *in utero* to homozygotes. The disorder results from a point mutation in the gene encoding for the fibroblast growth factor receptor 3 (FGFR3). About 80% of cases result from spontaneous new mutations. A less common but uniformly lethal malformation occurring in only 1 in 20,000 live births is the one pictured here—thanatophoric dysplasia—which is caused by a different mutation in the *FGFR3* gene. Note the narrow chest with bell-shaped abdomen that is giving the torso an outline similar to a formula-one racing car. Dwarfism syndromes that lead to a small chest cavity cause pulmonary hypoplasia, which becomes the rate-limiting step to survival after birth.

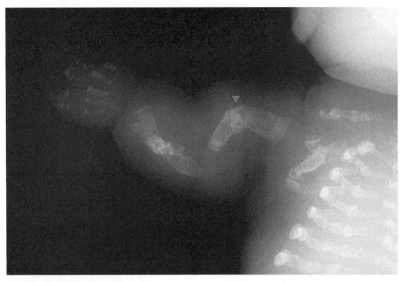

FIGURE 17–8 Osteogenesis imperfecta, radiograph

There are multiple fractures (▼) in these bones that are markedly osteopenic, represented here as diminished brightness. The formation of type I collagen, a major constituent of the bone matrix, is impaired, by either reduced synthesis or production of an abnormal triple helix of collagen. This leads to bone fragility and a propensity for fractures. Shown here is the perinatal lethal form (type II) of osteogenesis imperfecta (OI). Most cases are due to a short pro-α1(1) collagen chain that leads to an unstable collagen triple helix. The chest cavity is poorly formed, leading to pulmonary hypoplasia and respiratory distress upon birth.

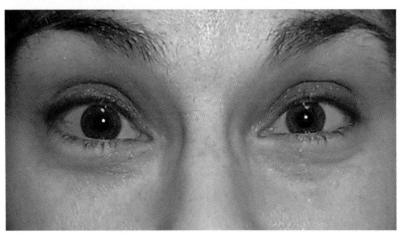

FIGURE 17–9 Osteogenesis imperfecta, gross

There is a bluish-gray appearance to these sclerae, which reflects the deficient collagen structure with abnormal type I collagen synthesis. This condition is most often due to an acquired mutation, but some cases are inherited in an autosomal dominant fashion and may be due to either decreased or abnormal pro-α1(1) or pro-α2(1) collagen chains. OI type I is compatible with normal survival and stature, but affected patients have an increased risk for fractures and have dental and hearing problems.

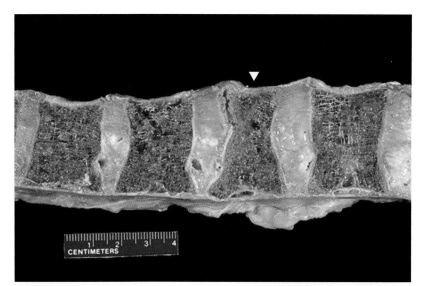

FIGURE 17–10 Osteoporosis, gross

The bone in these vertebral bodies shows marked osteoporosis with thinning of diminished bony trabeculae. One vertebral body shows a greater degree of compression fracturing (▼) than the others. Osteoporosis is accelerated bone loss for age, greater than the usual 0.7% loss per year after the fourth decade. It is most common among postmenopausal women with reduced estrogen levels, putting them at risk for fractures, particularly involving hip, wrist, and vertebrae. Continued physical activity and a good diet help build and maintain bone mass. Vitamin D deficiency in adults can lead to osteomalacia, which has gross and radiographic appearances similar to osteoporosis.

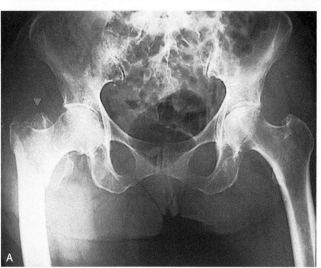
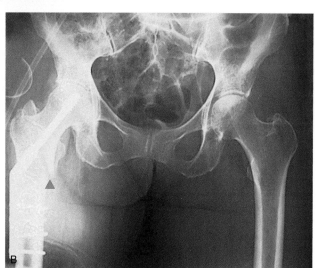

FIGURE 17–11A and B Osteoporosis with fracture, x-rays

There is severe osteoporosis involving the femurs of this elderly woman, and as a consequence a right intertrochanteric fracture (▼) has occurred and has been repaired (▲) surgically. This bone should be much more dense and bright, but instead displays greater lucency in these radiographic views because of the osteopenia.

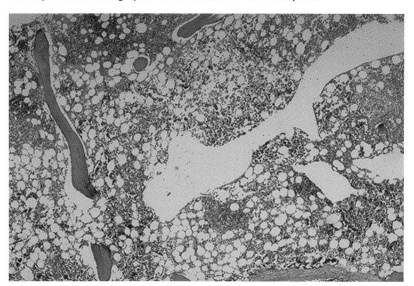

FIGURE 17–12 Osteoporosis, microscopic

Bone trabeculae are thin and sparse in this vertebral body with osteoporosis. The bone structure is normal, there is just less of it. The bone cortex becomes thinner, and trabeculae have less complex branching, providing less three-dimensional support. Laboratory measurements of serum calcium, phosphorus, alkaline phosphatase, and PTH are all within normal ranges. In contrast, PTH levels are high or high normal, calcium is elevated, and phosphorus is decreased with primary hyperparathyroidism. Osteocalcin (bone γ-carboxyglutamate) synthesized by osteoblasts is incorporated into extracellular bone matrix, and circulating levels correlate with bone density.

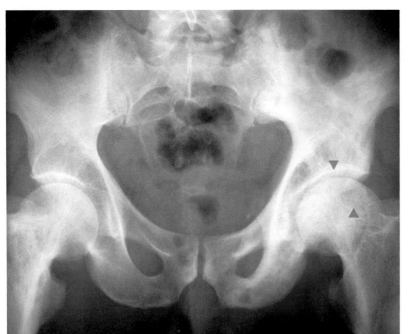

FIGURE 17–13 Paget disease of bone (osteitis deformans), radiograph

The left hip reveals a more irregular appearance to the bone than the right because of both osteosclerosis (▼) with greater density and osteolysis with greater lucency (▲). This is the mixed osteoclastic and osteoblastic stage of Paget disease of bone, which most often occurs in elderly whites of European ancestry. A slow paramyxovirus infection may increase interleukin-6 secretion to drive osteoclast activity. In addition, osteoclasts may become more sensitive to RANKL and vitamin D. The serum alkaline phosphatase is increased, but the serum calcium and parathormone levels are normal. This increased bone proliferation carries an increased risk for malignant neoplasia—a Paget sarcoma, typically an osteosarcoma—in up to 1% of all affected patients.

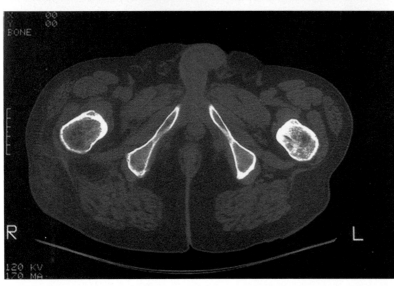

FIGURE 17–14 Paget disease of bone (osteitis deformans), MRI

There is more irregularity to this upper left femur, with increased bony sclerosis along with areas of lucency. Paget disease is mainly seen in older people, and the course of the disease extends over many years. Initially, there may be more osteolysis, but this is followed by the most diagnostic phase—mixed osteolysis and osteosclerosis. Eventually, the final phase results in prominent osteosclerosis. The clinical hallmark of Paget disease is pain with diminished joint range of motion. The abnormally thickened bone is paradoxically weaker and prone to fracture. Skull involvement can lead to cranial nerve entrapment.

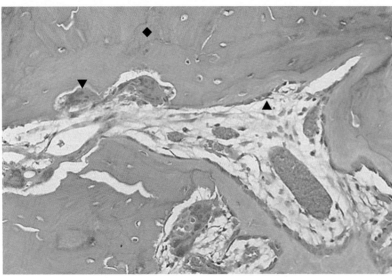

FIGURE 17–15 Paget disease of bone (osteitis deformans), microscopic

There is more bone turnover, with an uncoupling of osteoblast and osteoclast coordination in bone remodeling, leading to a haphazard microscopic appearance. Shown here are both prominent osteoclast (▼) and osteoblast (▲) activity. The result is a thicker but weaker bone that has irregular cement lines (◆), producing a "mosaic" pattern instead of an organized lamellar pattern. This proliferating bone is highly vascularized, and the increased vascular flow can lead to high-output congestive heart failure. Localized disease may require no therapy other than occasional use of analgesics. More extensive polyostotic disease can be treated with osteoclast-inhibiting bisphosphonates.

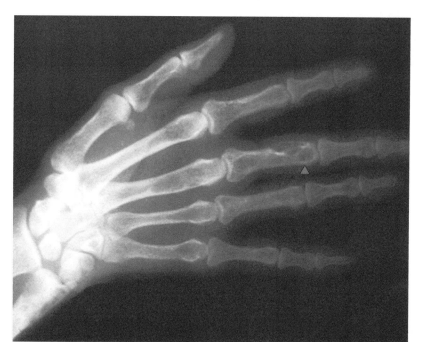

FIGURE 17–16 Hyperparathyroidism, radiograph

This patient has primary hyperparathyroidism with a parathyroid adenoma and an increased serum calcium, decreased phosphorus, and elevated parathormone. This is osteitis fibrosa cystica of bone, with expansile areas of lucency (▲), shown here as deformities involving the metatarsals and phalanges of this right hand. Such lesions can cause pain, but the focal decrease in bone mass also predisposes to fracture. In contrast, secondary hyperparathyroidism is due to chronic renal failure with retention of phosphate that increases serum phosphorus, depresses serum calcium to stimulate parathormone release, and also produces osteitis fibrosa cystica, as well as osteomalacia, osteoporosis, osteosclerosis, and growth retardation, collectively known as *renal osteodystrophy*.

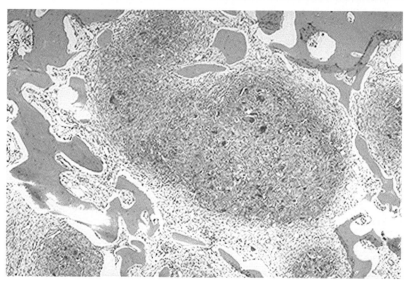

FIGURE 17–17 Hyperparathyroidism, "brown tumor" of bone, microscopic

A focal radiolucent lesion in the category of osteitis fibrosa cystica on a radiograph is seen here. This area of reactive fibrous tissue proliferation with admixed multinucleated giant cells is called a *brown tumor* because of the grossly apparent brown color imparted by the vascularity, hemorrhage, macrophage infiltration, and hemosiderin deposition that often accompany this proliferation. These lesions can undergo cystic degeneration and produce focal pain as well as predispose to fracture.

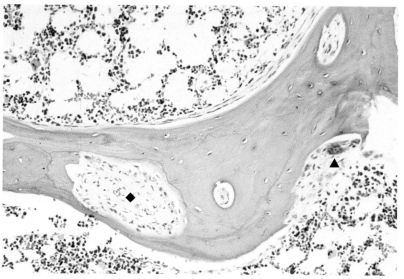

FIGURE 17–18 Hyperparathyroidism, dissecting osteitis, microscopic

Shown here is a bone spicule with pronounced osteoclastic and osteoblastic activity (◆). This is accelerated bone remodeling with osteoclasts (▲) that "tunnel into" the bone trabeculae and form pockets of fibrovascular tissue. The fibrovascular tissue is increased in the peritrabecular spaces as well. In secondary hyperparathyroidism from chronic renal failure, the metabolic acidosis also stimulates bone resorption. Increased circulating β_2-microglobulin with long-term hemodialysis can lead to amyloid deposition in bone.

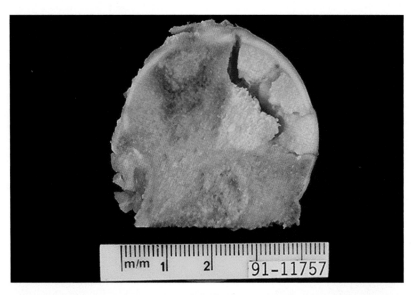

FIGURE 17–19 Avascular necrosis, gross

Beneath the articular cartilage of the femoral head is a pale, wedge-shaped area of osteonecrosis in this patient who had pain in the hip that developed after long-term use of corticosteroids. Additional risk factors include traumatic vascular disruption, thrombosis, barotrauma, vasculitis, sickle cell disease, and radiation therapy. The usual initial symptom is pain with movement, but this progresses to constant pain. Replacement of necrotic bone by new bone (creeping substitution) does not proceed fast enough to prevent focal collapse with disruption of articular cartilage and fracture. Infarction within the medullary cavity is more likely to be clinically silent.

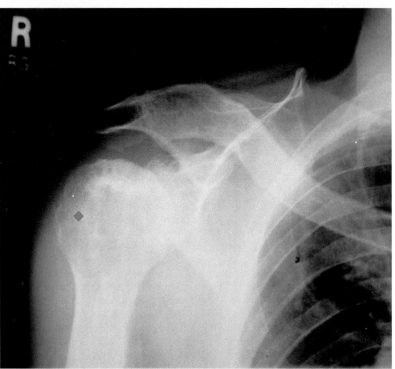

FIGURE 17–20 Avascular necrosis, radiograph

Note the irregular remodeling (♦) of the head of this proximal humerus as a result of avascular necrosis. The bones of both the humeral head and the femoral head have a tenuous blood supply that can be traumatically disrupted. The devitalized bone then undergoes remodeling and bone distortion, and the adjacent joint becomes painful with increased use and decreased function. The remodeling process is inefficient and slow, so that there is eventual collapse with distortion of the overlying articular cartilage, leading to secondary osteoarthritis.

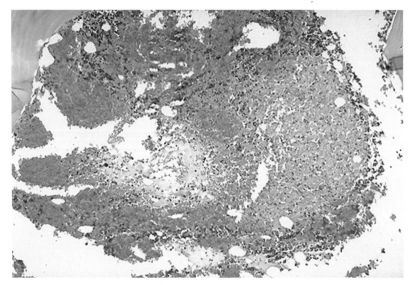

FIGURE 17–21 Bone marrow infarct, microscopic

Seen here is hemorrhage with necrosis involving the marrow of a vertebral body. This lesion occurred in a patient experiencing a sickle cell crisis and severe back pain. Microvascular occlusions by the "sticky" sickled red blood cells leads to release of hemoglobin that binds nitric oxide (NO). Reduced NO favors vasoconstriction and platelet aggregation. These vaso-occlusive crises can affect multiple organs, including acute chest syndrome with pulmonary vascular bed occlusion. The pain of bone infarcts mimics acute osteomyelitis.

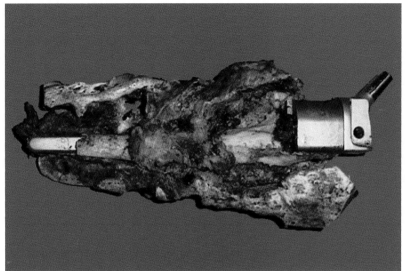

FIGURE 17–22 Chronic osteomyelitis, gross

Extensive bone destruction with irregular remodeling results in the appearance of a lighter-colored necrotic sequestrum (here immediately adjacent to the prosthetic device) surrounded by the darker involucrum that is the new reactive bone. Osteomyelitis may result from penetrating injury with introduction of organisms, typically bacteria, into bone. More commonly, osteomyelitis is acquired by hematogenous dissemination. In growing bones of children, most bone infections begin predominantly in the metaphyseal region, with the greatest blood flow. Osteomyelitis in adults most often begins in epiphyseal and subchondral locations.

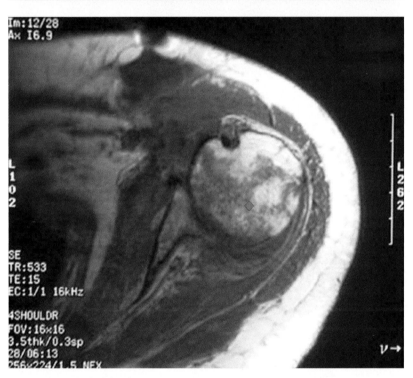

FIGURE 17–23 Chronic osteomyelitis, MRI

This proximal humeral head shows irregularity (◆) from chronic osteomyelitis. An acute osteomyelitis presents with pain, fever, and leukocytosis. A blood culture may be positive. About 5% to 25% of acute cases fail to resolve and go on to chronic osteomyelitis. There may be acute exacerbations. The weakened bone is prone to fracture. A fracture complicated by osteomyelitis may fail to heal, with development of a pseudarthrosis. An uncommon complication is development of a draining sinus tract, and rarer still is development of a squamous cell carcinoma within such a sinus tract.

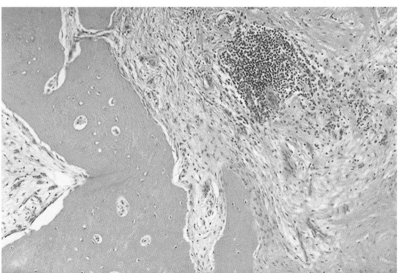

FIGURE 17–24 Chronic osteomyelitis, microscopic

Shown here in the marrow is fibrosis accompanied by chronic inflammatory cell infiltrates. The bony trabeculae have become disorganized, and the bone is devitalized. Osteomyelitis is difficult to treat and may require surgical drainage as well as antibiotic therapy. The most common organism causing osteomyelitis is *Staphylococcus aureus*. Neonates may have *Haemophilus influenzae* and group B streptococcal bone infections. Patients with sickle cell anemia are at risk for *Salmonella* osteomyelitis. Urinary tract infections and injection drug users are at risk for osteomyelitis with *Escherichia coli* and *Pseudomonas* and *Klebsiella* species.

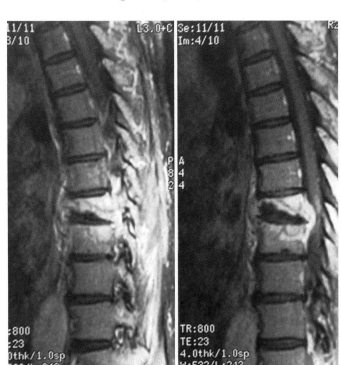
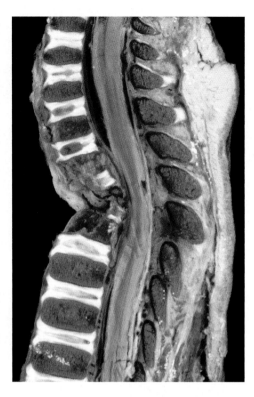

FIGURES 17–25 and 17–26 Tuberculous osteomyelitis, MRI and gross

Extensive bone destruction is seen involving the T8 and T9 mid-thoracic vertebrae in a patient with disseminated *Mycobacterium tuberculosis* infection. This is Pott disease of the spine. The vertebral body destruction seen here has resulted in impingement on the spinal cord.

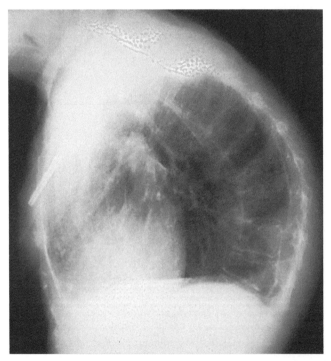

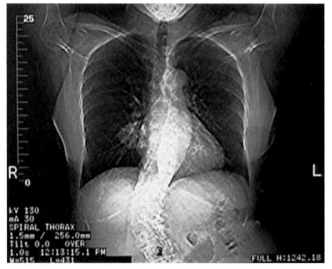

FIGURES 17–27 and 17–28 Kyphosis, radiograph, and scoliosis, CT image

The lateral chest radiograph at the left demonstrates marked kyphosis of the vertebral column, so that the head and neck are bent forward and the total chest volume is markedly reduced. This patient had severe osteoporosis, and a fall with trauma resulted in a fracture of the humerus that required open reduction and internal fixation, evidenced by the bright metal rod seen here. The chest CT scout image in coronal view in the right panel shows marked scoliosis of the lower thoracic vertebral column, with a major curve to the right. Both the superior-inferior axis and the anterior-posterior axis of the vertebral column show rotation. (Note that this patient also has a mass lesion within the right lung—bronchogenic carcinoma).

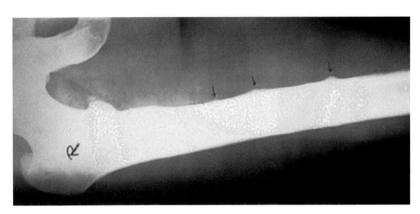

FIGURE 17–29 Osteoma, radiograph

This radiograph of the femur reveals multiple osteomas (*arrows*) in a patient with "Gardner syndrome" caused by *APC* gene mutation. The osteomas are typically the incidental findings. This is one of the original radiographs from one of the first cases diagnosed by Dr. Henry Plenk, a radiologist. Thus, the syndrome is actually Plenk-Gardner syndrome. Solitary osteomas are seen in middle-aged adults as sessile periosteal or endosteal masses. Osteomas are composed of a dense mixture of woven and lamellar bone.

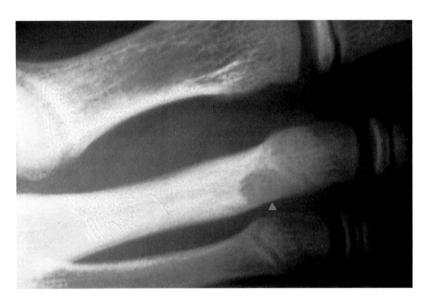

FIGURE 17–30 Osteoid osteoma, radiograph

The discrete round lucency (▲) surrounded by a thin rim of sclerosis in this proximal phalanx is an osteoid osteoma. Despite their size (usually smaller than 2 cm), they can produce considerable pain, owing to their prostaglandin production, which can be blocked by analgesics such as aspirin. They most commonly arise in the second or third decade. They are most often found in the cortex of femur or tibia.

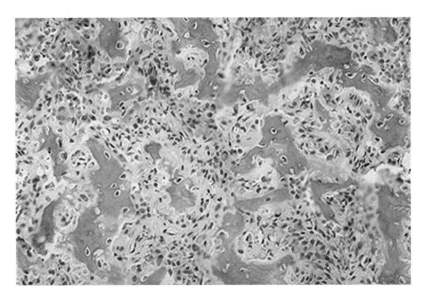

FIGURE 17–31 Osteoid osteoma, microscopic

This is the central nidus, or radiolucent portion, of an osteoid osteoma, composed of irregular reactive new woven bone. Osteoid osteomas usually occur in the bone cortex. An osteoblastoma is a well-circumscribed mass that has an identical microscopic appearance and is just a big osteoid osteoma (defined as larger than 2 cm) that is more likely to be present in vertebrae. These lesions are benign and cured by local resection, but they may recur if not completely resected. However, radiotherapy may induce malignant transformation.

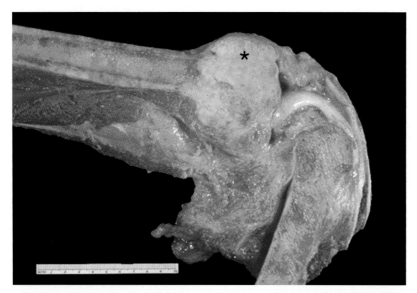

FIGURE 17–32 Osteosarcoma, gross

This irregular mass lesion (∗) is arising within the metaphysis at the upper tibia in this cross-section of the lower extremity. It breaks through the bone cortex and extends into adjacent soft tissue. The tumor tissue is firm and tan-white. The glistening white articular cartilage of the femoral condyle can be seen just to the right of the tumor in the opened joint space. Osteosarcoma is the most common primary malignant bone tumor. Most arise during the first two decades of life. Men are affected more than women. More than half the tumors occur around the knee. Other sites of origin include pelvis, proximal humerus, and jaw. Familial osteosarcomas often have *RB* gene mutations. Most are sporadic and also have *RB* mutations as well as *p53*, *CDK4*, *p16*, and *CYCLIN D1* mutations.

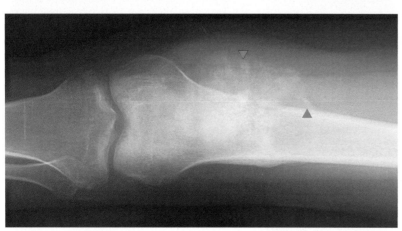

FIGURE 17–33 Osteosarcoma, radiograph

This osteosarcoma (▽) involves the metaphyseal region of the distal femur. Long bones are more often affected in young people, probably because bone growth with mitotic activity increases risk for genetic mutations. This tumor erodes and destroys the bone cortex, extending into soft tissue where irregular reactive bone formation with calcification is seen as brighter areas in the normally dull gray soft tissues. The periosteum here is lifted off (▲) to form a Codman triangle.

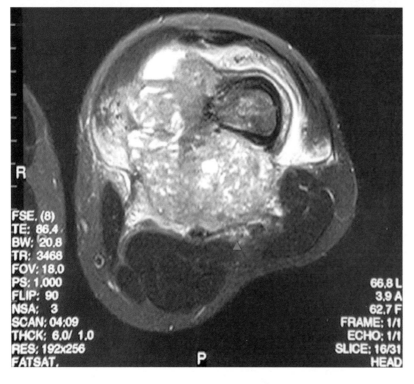

FIGURE 17–34 Osteosarcoma, MRI

An osteosarcoma of the distal femur is seen with axial T2-weighted fast spin echo MRI with fat saturation. There is extensive cortical bone disruption with extension (▲) of the tumor into the adjacent soft tissue. Areas of hemorrhage and cystic degeneration impart the variegation seen here as different areas of brightness. The first clinical manifestation is often pain as the tumor breaks through the bone cortex and lifts off the periosteum. Osteosarcomas, like sarcomas in general, are most likely to metastasize hematogenously, most often to lungs.

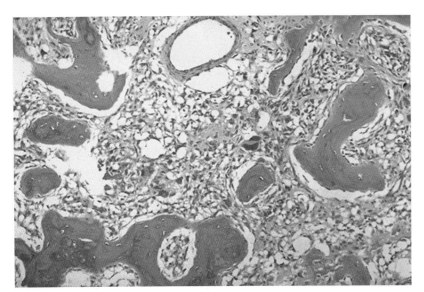

FIGURE 17–35 Osteosarcoma, microscopic

This tumor is composed of very pleomorphic cells, many with a spindle shape. One large, bizarre multinucleated cell with very large nuclei is present. Nuclear hyperchromatism and cellular pleomorphism are features of malignant neoplasms. There are islands of reactive new woven bone forming in response to the infiltration and destruction of normal bone by the tumor.

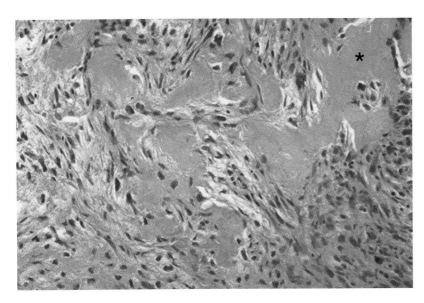

FIGURE 17–36 Osteosarcoma, microscopic

The neoplastic spindle cells of osteosarcoma are seen to be making pink osteoid (∗) here. Osteoid production by a sarcoma is diagnostic of an osteosarcoma. This osteoid matrix vaguely resembles primitive woven bone. Additional microscopic elements of an osteosarcoma may include vascular proliferation, cartilaginous matrix, and fibrous connective tissue. There may be considerable microscopic variation within a single tumor, and metastases may not exactly resemble the primary site microscopic appearance.

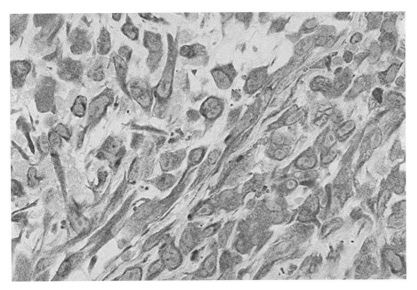

FIGURE 17–37 Osteosarcoma, microscopic

Immunohistochemical staining with antibody to vimentin reveals positive red-brown reaction product within the cytoplasm of these neoplastic cells. Positive vimentin staining is a characteristic of many types of sarcomas. Note the spindle shape of many of these cells, another feature of neoplasms of mesenchymal derivation.

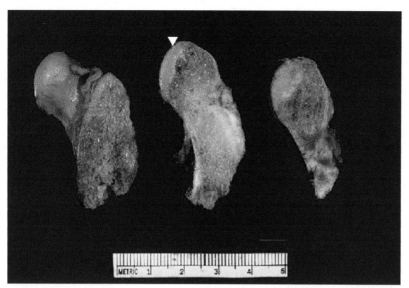

FIGURE 17–38 Osteochondroma, gross

Longitudinal cross-sections through this excised osteochondroma reveal a bluish white cartilaginous cap (▼) overlying a bony cortex. These lesions are probably not true neoplasms but are likely an aberration of endochondral bone formation with lateral displacement of the growth plate. They form a slowly growing mass lesion that extends outward from the metaphyseal region of a long bone—an exostosis. They are typically solitary, arising most often in the metaphyseal region of a long bone before growth plate closure. The knee is the most common site, but pelvis, scapula, and ribs may be involved. Less commonly, more than one lesion can appear at multiple sites, with an onset in childhood.

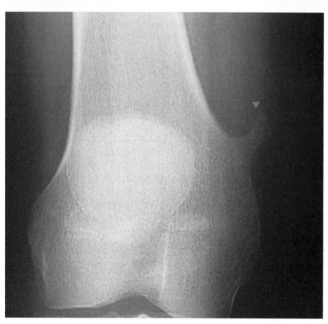

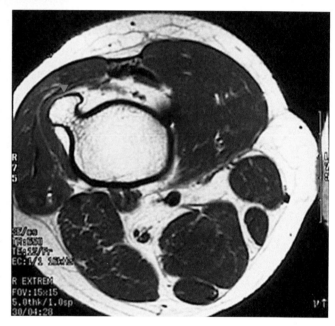

FIGURES 17–39 and 17–40 Osteochondroma, radiograph and MRI

. An osteochondroma (▼) of the metaphyseal region projects laterally from the distal femur in the radiographic coronal view in the left panel and in the axial T1-weighted MRI in the right panel, and has a composition very similar to the normal bone.

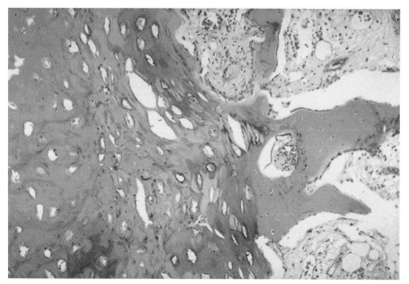

FIGURE 17–41 Osteochondroma, microscopic

The osteochondroma displays a benign cartilaginous cap at the left with underlying bony cortex at the right. This abnormal growth enlarges very slowly and usually stops growing when the epiphyseal plate closes. Although benign, osteochondromas can sometimes cause pain and irritation if the exostosis causes nerve compression, is traumatized, or is fractured. Those that are symptomatic may be surgically removed. Malignant transformation to a sarcoma, such as a chondrosarcoma, is uncommon, although such a risk is greater when multiple osteochondromas are present as part of a hereditary syndrome.

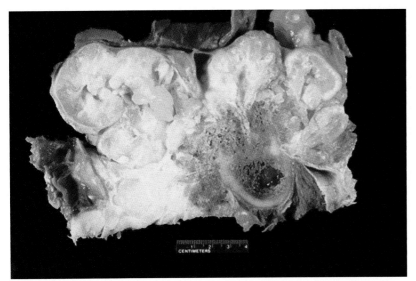

FIGURE 17-42 Chondrosarcoma, gross

This large, irregular mass is arising within the pelvis and extending into soft tissues. Most chondrosarcomas arise in the central skeleton. The more peripheral a cartilaginous tumor, the more likely that it may be benign. Note these extensive nodules of white to bluish white cartilaginous tumor tissue eroding bone and extending outward from the residual bone. Chondrosarcomas can occur over a wide age range, and there is a slight male predominance. Many of them are low grade and slow growing, with symptoms present for a decade or more. Larger tumors are more aggressive than smaller ones. This is the second most common primary bone tumor.

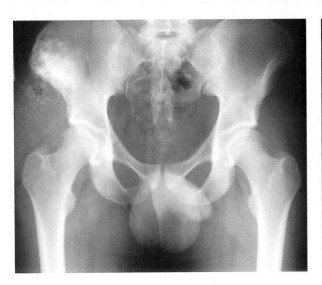

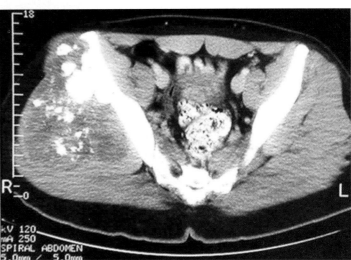

FIGURES 17-43 and 17-44 Chondrosarcoma, radiograph and CT

In the left panel, a chondrosarcoma (∗) arising in the right iliac wing and extending to soft tissues exhibits irregular brightness. In the right panel, the CT image shows extensive soft tissue involvement (∗) with bright calcified areas.

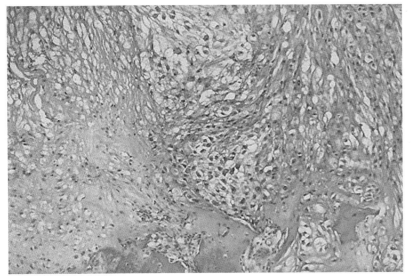

FIGURE 17-45 Chondrosarcoma, microscopic

At low magnification, the chondrosarcoma is still recognizable as cartilage, and there are chondrocytes within lacunae, but there is no orderly pattern, and there is increased cellularity. At the bottom, this neoplasm can be seen invading and destroying bone. Most chondrosarcomas are low grade and indolent, but a focus of high-grade sarcoma may be present in up to 10% of them. A few chondrosarcomas arise within an intraosseous cartilaginous tumor known as an enchondroma, typically when multiple enchondromas (enchondromatosis) are present.

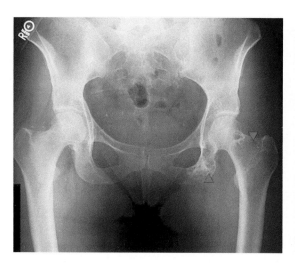
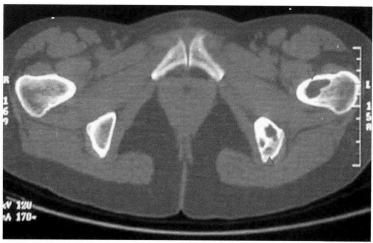

FIGURES 17–46 and 17–47 Fibrous dysplasia, radiograph and CT

A single irregular area of bone lucency is seen in the region of the left femoral neck (▼) as well as in the left ischium (▲) in this case of fibrous dysplasia of bone. Polyostotic (multiple bone site) lesions associated with endocrinopathies and café-au-lait spots on the skin comprise McCune-Albright syndrome, representing about 3% of all cases. Most cases of fibrous dysplasia are monostotic (involve just one bone site) and appear in adolescence. In the pelvic CT image at the right can be seen a lucency in the femoral neck on the left as well as another lucency in the left ischium. This is a condition in which there is progressive replacement of bone by a disorganized proliferation of fibrous tissue and woven bone. Skeletal deformity and fracture can occur.

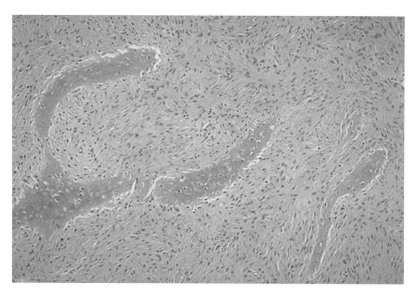

FIGURE 17–48 Fibrous dysplasia, microscopic

Shown here is a proliferative process with irregular spicules of woven bone in a cellular stroma. There is little osteoblastic activity. This localized area of irregular woven bone proliferates but does not develop into solid lamellar bone, leaving a weakened area that can produce deformity or fracture. Transformation of this process into a sarcoma is rare. This lesion arises from a somatic mutation during embryogenesis for a G-protein–coupled receptor activating adenylyl cyclase, leading to excess cyclic adenosine monophosphate that drives cellular proliferation.

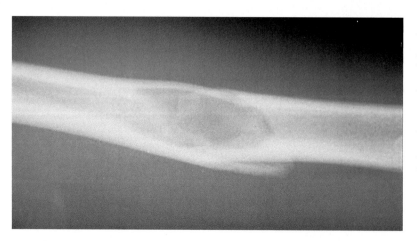

FIGURE 17–49 Solitary bone cyst with pathologic fracture, radiograph

A fracture extends across a radiolucent area in the humeral diaphysis. This area of lucency represents a unicameral bone cyst. The cyst weakened the bone so that a pathologic fracture occurred. Lesions producing a similar radiographic appearance, although more likely in the metaphysis and often multicentric, can include a fibrous cortical defect that can progress to a nonossifying fibroma when 5 to 6 cm in size. These are developmental abnormalities, not neoplasms.

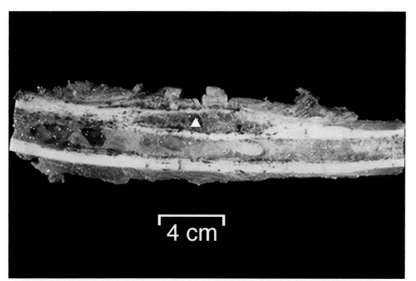

FIGURE 17–50 Ewing sarcoma, gross

This primary bone tumor mainly arises within the medullary cavity in the diaphysis of long bones and pelvis in the first two decades of life, with a slight male predominance. The fibular tumor mass shown here is breaking through (▲) the cortex. The tan tumor tissue has prominent areas of reddish hemorrhage and brownish necrosis. More normal fatty marrow is seen at the far right. Such an enlarging mass may present with local tenderness, warmth, and swelling at the affected site. Some patients have fever and leukocytosis, suggesting an infection.

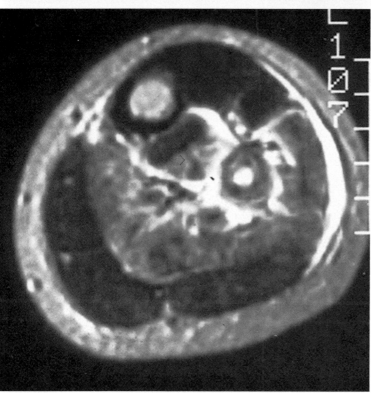

FIGURE 17–51 Ewing sarcoma, MRI

This T2-weighted MRI shows irregular bright tumor (♦) extending from the fibula into surrounding soft tissue. Note that the normal bone cortex of the tibia is dark, while the marrow cavity filled with fatty marrow is bright. With a standard radiograph, this lesion often appears lytic, with cortical destruction.

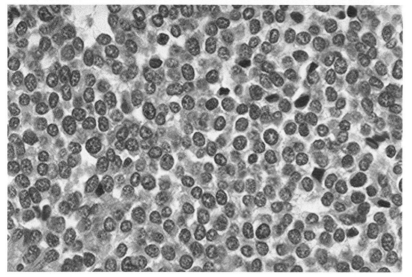

FIGURE 17–52 Ewing sarcoma, microscopic

This is one of the "small round blue cell" tumors of childhood. Note the marked cellularity and the high nuclear-to-cytoplasm ratio of these tumor cells, which are slightly larger than lymphocytes. There is little intervening stroma. Mitoses are present. PAS stain may reveal abundant glycogen within tumor cell cytoplasm. These malignancies often arise when there is a t(11;22) chromosomal translocation that produces the *EWS-FLI1* fusion gene acting as a transcription factor to drive cellular proliferation. Ewing sarcoma and primitive neuroectodermal tumor (PNET) have a similar molecular origin, but the PNET has more neural differentiation.

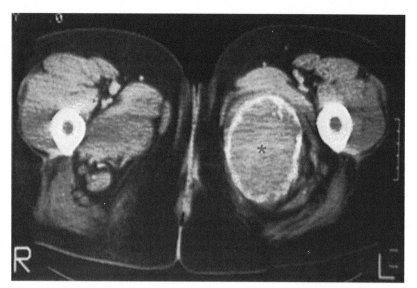

FIGURE 17–53 Giant cell tumor, CT image

Here a giant cell tumor involves the left ischial ramus of the pelvis. The tumor appears as an eccentric, expansile, lytic mass (∗) with extension into adjacent soft tissue. As the tumor expands, it produces a bright rim of overlying reactive new bone. This locally aggressive lesion is most likely to arise in the epiphyseal and metaphyseal regions of bone, most often around the knee, in the third to fifth decades. These tumors are locally aggressive and may recur after local resection. A few of them act in a malignant fashion, with sarcomatous transformation, and can have distant metastases.

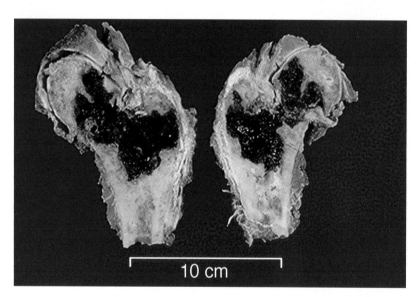

FIGURE 17–54 Giant cell tumor, gross

This proximal femur has been amputated and sectioned longitudinally to reveal an irregular dark red-black hemorrhagic mass arising within the epiphyseal region and extending into the metaphysis. The expansion of this tumor near a joint can produce arthritic pain. The weakened bone may fracture (pathologic fracture) or become deformed.

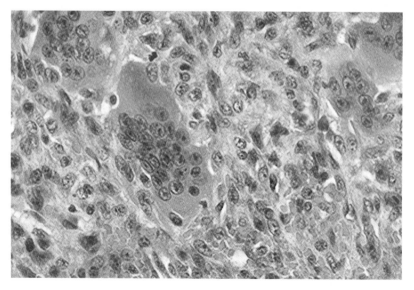

FIGURE 17–55 Giant cell tumor, microscopic

Giant cell tumors of bone are composed of osteoclast-like multinucleated giant cells in a sea of round to oval mononuclear stromal cells. There may also be lipid-laden macrophages along with hemorrhage and hemosiderin deposition within the stroma. These cells have a monocyte-macrophage origin.

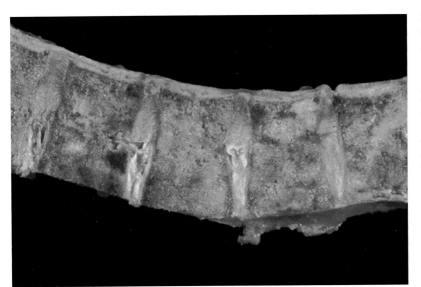

FIGURE 17–56 Metastases, gross

This sagittal section of vertebral bone at autopsy shows multiple foci of pale and irregular metastatic tumor. Overall, the most common neoplasm involving bone is a metastasis. Virtually all bone metastases occur from carcinomas, and the most common primary sites are remembered with the "lead kettle" mnemonic (PBKTL): prostate, breast, kidney, thyroid, lung. Metastases from renal cell carcinomas, and most other carcinomas, tend to be osteolytic (they destroy the bone) and are radiolucent, whereas metastases from prostatic carcinomas tend to be osteoblastic (they initiate prominent new bone formation) and are radiodense.

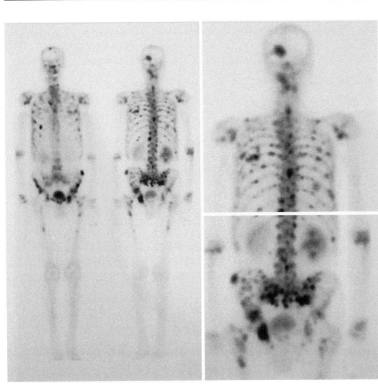

FIGURE 17–57 Metastases, bone scan

This radionuclide bone scan reveals numerous areas of increased uptake—the dark foci, or "hot spots"—from metastases, which are usually multifocal. Note the darker right kidney, which is hydronephrotic from obstruction by the primary tumor—a urothelial carcinoma of the bladder involving the right ureteral orifice. The increased cellularity and vascularity of the metastatic foci compared with normal bone produces this differential uptake of the radioactive compound. Osteolytic lesions can occur when metastases produce parathormone-related peptide (PTHrP)-stimulating osteoclasts. Most metastases have a mixture of osteoclastic and osteoblastic activity since bone lysis often elicits reactive new bone formation, but osteolysis predominates.

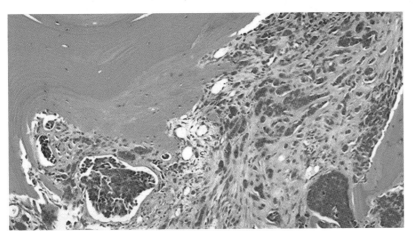

FIGURE 17–58 Metastases, microscopic

Metastatic infiltrating ductal carcinoma of breast is seen within vertebral bone, and it is filling the marrow cavity. There is reactive new bone at the margin of the carcinoma, with pale pink osteoid being laid down next to a bony spicule at the upper left. Metastases may produce pain. They may weaken the bone to an extent that a pathologic fracture occurs. The serum alkaline phosphatase is often elevated with metastatic bone disease.

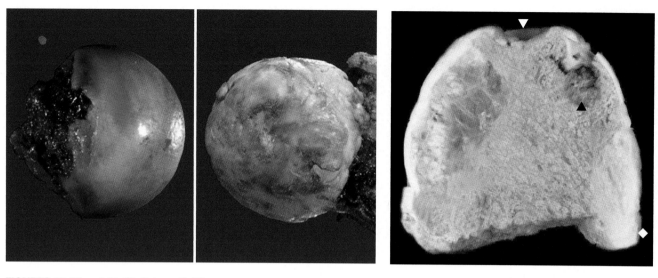

FIGURES 17–59 and 17–60 Osteoarthritis, gross

The changes of osteoarthritis are most often reported by the patient as pain or difficulty with movement. There is often minimal outward deformity. Osteoarthritis has little inflammation. In the panels at the left, the femoral head at the left (removed because of fracture) shows smooth, glistening articular cartilage, while the femoral head at the right shows a rough, eburnated, irregular appearance of eroded articular cartilage typical of osteoarthritis. In the far right panel is surface erosion (▼), a subchondral cyst (▲), and an osteophyte (◆).

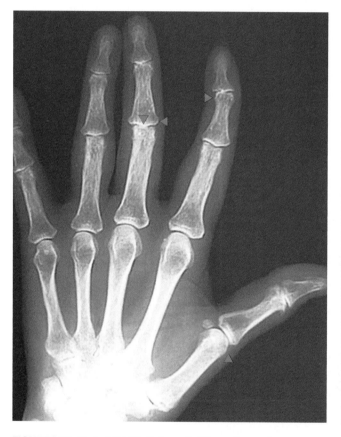

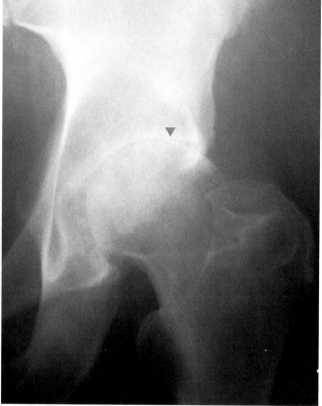

FIGURES 17–61 and 17–62 Osteoarthritis, radiographs

The hand in the left panel shows degenerative osteoarthritis with joint space narrowing (▼) and greater lateral widening (◄) at the distal interphalangeal (DIP) joints than the proximal interphalangeal (PIP) joints. There is subluxation (►) at the DIP joints as well, most marked in the second digit. The base of the thumb (▲) has marked osteoarthritis. The pelvis in the right panel shows joint space narrowing (▼) of the left hip with osteoarthritis. Hip joints are commonly involved because they are heavy weight–bearing joints. These degenerative changes are progressive with aging.

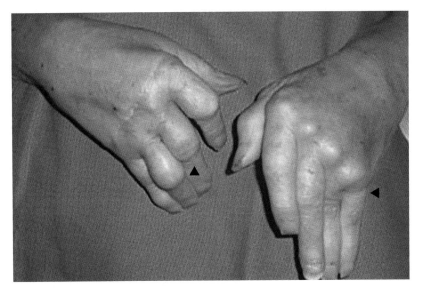

FIGURE 17–63 Rheumatoid arthritis, gross

There is prominent ulnar deviation (◄) of the hands and flexion-hyperextension ("swan neck") deformities (▲) of the fingers. This autoimmune disease leads to inflammation with synovial proliferation (pannus formation) that causes joint destruction, typically in a symmetric pattern that first involves small joints of the hands and feet, followed by wrists, ankles, elbows, and knees. Many patients are HLA-DR4 or -DR1 positive, suggesting a genetic susceptibility. Exposure to an infectious agent may initiate an inflammatory response that continues as an autoimmune reaction to a variety of tissues, principally synovium, but also vasculature and soft tissues. CD4 lymphocyte activation leads to cytokine production, principally tumor necrosis factor and interleukin-1.

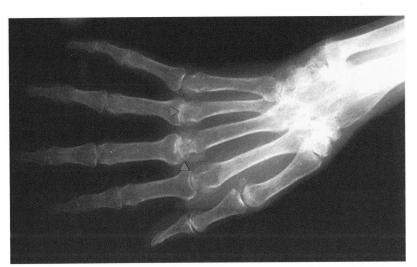

FIGURE 17–64 Rheumatoid arthritis, radiograph

This hand shows joint space narrowing (▶) with marginal erosions (▲) and osteoporosis, mainly involving the proximal PIP joints and metacarpophalangeal joints. Bone loss is primarily juxta-articular. Activated CD4 lymphocytes help B cells produce antibodies, mainly immunoglobulin M (IgM), directed at the Fc portion of IgG, known as *rheumatoid factor*. This disease may begin insidiously with malaise, fever, and generalized aches and pains before joint swelling, warmth, and tenderness appear. Rheumatoid arthritis (RA) tends to follow a course of remissions and exacerbations. Significant "morning stiffness" is often present.

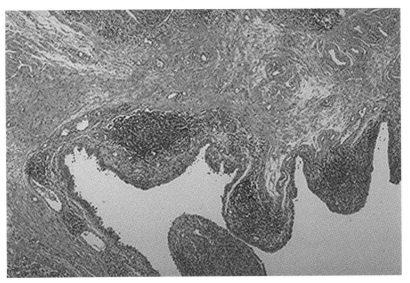

FIGURE 17–65 Rheumatoid arthritis, microscopic

This synovium shows marked chronic inflammation with aggregates of lymphocytes and plasma cells that produce the blue areas seen here within the nodular proliferations of synovium. This process forms a proliferative "pannus" that is destructive through release of collagenases and produces erosion of the adjacent articular cartilage, eventually destroying the joint and leading to deformity and ankylosis. Lymphocytes and fibroblasts produce RANKL that activates osteoclasts to promote bone destruction. An aspirate of joint fluid will typically show increased turbidity, decreased viscosity, increased protein, and leukocytosis with predominance of neutrophils.

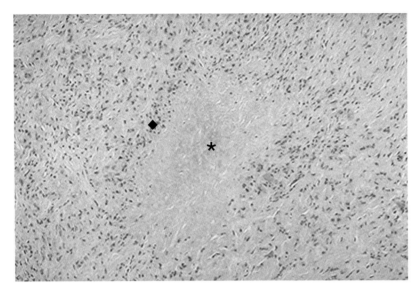

FIGURE 17–66 Rheumatoid nodule, microscopic

These firm, nontender nodules occur in about one fourth of RA patients, typically those with more severe involvement. They can appear in soft tissues beneath the skin over bony prominences such as the elbow. They can occasionally appear in visceral organs, including lungs and heart. The nodule has a central area of fibrinoid necrosis (*) surrounded by palisading epithelioid macrophages (◆) and other mononuclear cells. RA affects about 1% of the population. Women are more often affected than men. The peak incidence is the fifth to eighth decades, but RA occurs over a wide age range.

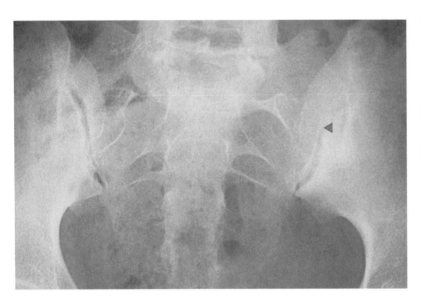

FIGURE 17–67 Ankylosing spondylarthritis, radiograph

This pelvis demonstrates sacroiliitis on the left, with narrowing and sclerosis (◄) of the sacroiliac (SI) joint. The SI joint on the right appears relatively normal by comparison. One third of patients have involvement of other joints, including hips, knees, and shoulders. This is a chronic progressive inflammatory arthritis producing spinal immobility with low back pain. The chronic synovitis leads to loss of articular cartilage with progressive bony ankylosis that limits range of motion. Low back pain is a frequent feature. About 90% of affected patients have the HLA-B27 allele.

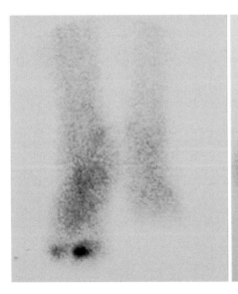
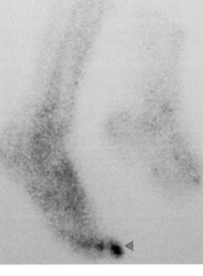

FIGURE 17–68 Suppurative arthritis, bone scan

Note the increased uptake (◄) in the region of the great toe. Suppurative arthritis is marked by intense pain with swelling and reduced range of motion. Fever and leukocytosis are often present. It is typically caused by bacterial infection. *Staphylococcus aureus* is the most common agent past childhood, while *Haemophilus influenzae* is commonly seen in children younger than 2 years of age. Sexually active people are at risk for *Neisseria gonorrhoeae* infection. Patients with sickle cell disease are prone to develop *Salmonella* infections.

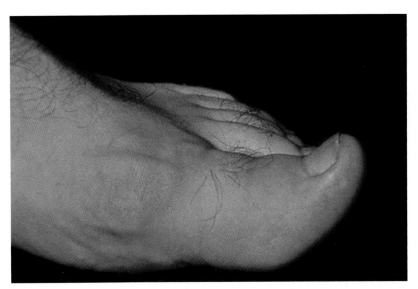

FIGURE 17–69 Gouty arthritis, gross

Gout results from deposition of sodium urate crystals in joints, and sometimes other soft tissues. In most cases, there is hyperuricemia. Uric acid is the end point of purine metabolism, and a decrease in hypoxanthine guanine phosphoribosyl transferase (HGPRT) in the purine salvage pathway increases *de novo* urate pathway production. Increased cell turnover and decreased renal uric acid excretion can also increase the serum uric acid. The first metatarsophalangeal joint (big toe), as seen here, is most often affected, but multiple joints may be involved. Acute attacks of gouty arthritis are characterized by severe pain, swelling, and erythema of the involved joint.

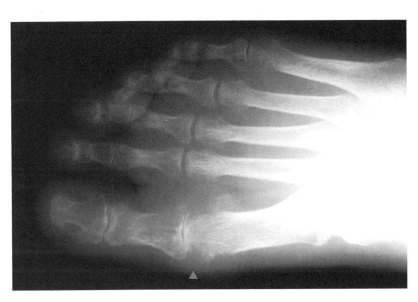

FIGURE 17–70 Gouty arthritis, radiograph

Chronic gout occurs about 12 years after the initial acute attack. It is marked by deposition of urates into a chalky mass known as a *tophus*. Such tophi can appear around a joint and the adjacent bone, as seen here (▲) radiographically. The tophus can erode and destroy adjacent bone. A joint aspirate during an acute gouty attack will show increased turbidity, decreased viscosity, and leukocytosis with many neutrophils. The characteristic microscopic finding is the presence of the needle-shaped birefringent sodium urate crystals in the fluid. The crystals activate complement and attract neutrophils that phagocytize the crystals and then release leukotrienes, prostaglandins, free radicals, and lysosomal enzymes to produce inflammation.

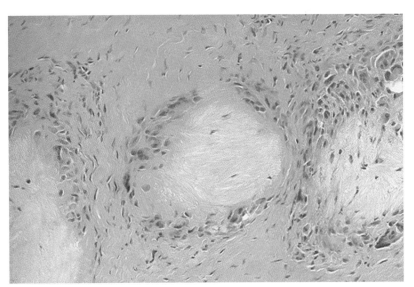

FIGURE 17–71 Gouty arthritis, microscopic

Tophaceous gout results from continued precipitation of sodium urate crystals during attacks of acute gout. The sodium urate crystals incite a surrounding destructive inflammatory response. The pale areas seen here are aggregates of urate crystals surrounded by chronic inflammatory infiltrates of lymphocytes, macrophages, and foreign body giant cells. Tophi are most likely to be found around joints, in soft tissues, including tendons and ligaments, and less commonly in visceral organs. Urate deposition can also occur in the kidneys, and about 20% of patients with gout may eventually develop renal failure.

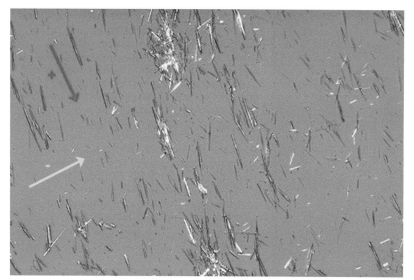

FIGURE 17–72 Gouty arthritis, microscopic

Synovial fluid aspirated from a joint in a patient with gout can be examined for presence of needle-shaped sodium urate crystals. If these crystals are observed under polarized light with a red compensator, they appear negatively birefringent (yellow) like the arrow in the main ("slow") axis of the compensator and blue in the opposite perpendicular direction. Risks for gout include increased alcohol consumption, obesity, drugs such as thiazides, and lead poisoning.

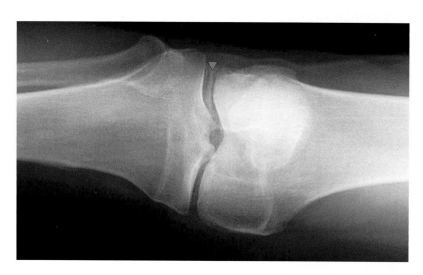

FIGURE 17–73 Calcium pyrophosphate crystal deposition disease (pseudogout), radiograph

Calcium pyrophosphate crystal deposition (CPPD) disease, also called "pseudogout," is more common in people older than 50 years and can lead to acute, subacute, or chronic arthritis of knees, wrists, elbows, shoulders, and ankles. The articular damage is progressive, although in most cases not severe. This knee reveals extensive chondrocalcinosis involving the menisci (▼) and articular cartilage. The relationship to osteoarthritis is not clear, but CPPD can contribute to osteoarthritic changes, and both diseases can be present simultaneously. A joint aspirate may show weakly birefringent rhomboid crystals along with neutrophils.

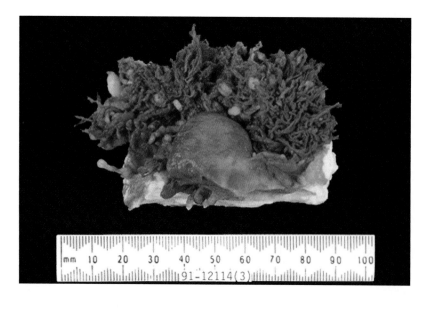

FIGURE 17–74 Pigmented villonodular synovitis, gross

This neoplastic process can develop in the synovium of joints (usually the knee), tendon sheaths, and bursae. Note the tangled mat of red-brown folds and finger-like projections. A related tumor, known as a *giant cell tumor of tendon sheath*, is similar histologically (multinucleated giant cells, macrophages, hemosiderin) but is a localized mass. Most of these lesions arise in the third to fifth decades, and usually a single joint is involved. There is pain, swelling, and reduced range of joint motion. Some more aggressive lesions can erode adjacent bone and recur after resection.

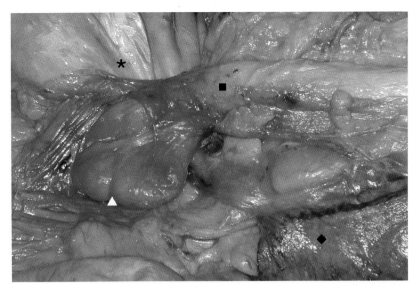

FIGURE 17–75 Lipoma, gross

Here is a yellow mass (▲) on the external surface of the esophagus (■) above the diaphragm (∗) near the right lung (◆), as seen at autopsy. It has the characteristics of a benign neoplasm: it is well circumscribed, slow growing, and resembles the tissue of origin (fat). Lipomas consist of mature adipocytes forming a slowly growing, soft, mobile, localized mass, which is often an incidental finding. Any symptoms may relate to a mass effect on an adjacent structure. Most lipomas are small subcutaneous masses. They can occur anywhere adipose tissue is present. They can easily be excised.

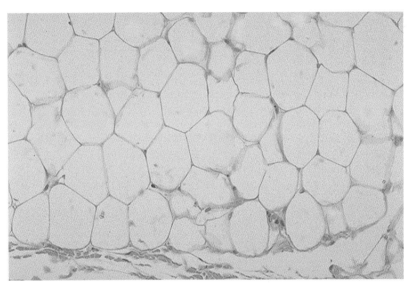

FIGURE 17–76 Lipoma, microscopic

This lipoma is composed of cells that are so well-differentiated that they are indistinguishable from normal adipocytes. Lipomas can be found in many places but rarely reach more than a few centimeters in size. Lipomas are the most common soft tissue tumor.

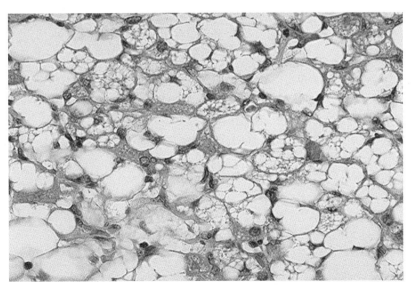

FIGURE 17–77 Liposarcoma, microscopic

Soft tissue sarcomas are not common. They are usually seen in older adults in sites such as retroperitoneum, thigh, and lower extremities. This liposarcoma has enough differentiation to determine the cell of origin, large bizarre lipoblasts, but there is still significant pleomorphism. Sarcomas are best treated surgically because most respond poorly to chemotherapy or radiation. Sarcomas tend to be much larger masses than their benign counterparts. They often invade locally, but there can be distant hematogenous metastases.

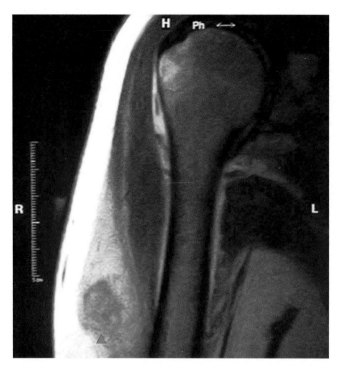
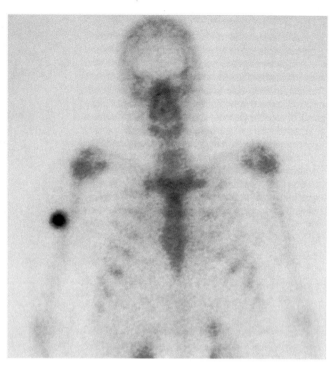

FIGURES 17–78 and 17–79 Myositis ossificans, MRI and bone scan

The rounded lesion (▲) of the upper arm adjacent to the humerus in the T1-weighted MRI at the left is a tumor-like mass within skeletal muscle called *myositis ossificans*. It is a benign form of metaplasia that results from a florid healing response to injury. The lesion appears as a discrete "hot spot" in soft tissue in the bone scan at the right.

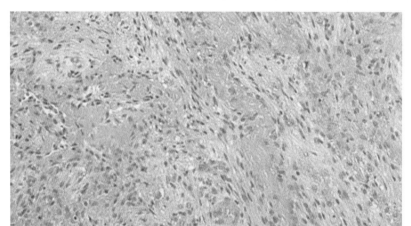

FIGURE 17–80 Myositis ossificans, microscopic

Myositis ossificans is an uncommon condition and occurs not within bone, but in adjacent muscle, and lesions can reach several centimeters in size. There is a central core of exuberant, cellular granulation tissue that can mimic a sarcoma. The correct diagnosis is suggested by radiographs. Unlike a true neoplasm, this lesion will decrease in size over time. It can cause pain and local irritation.

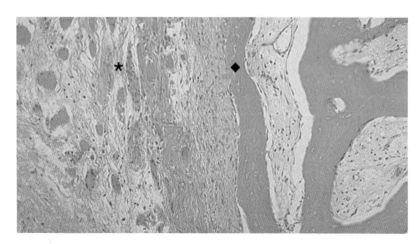

FIGURE 17–81 Myositis ossificans, microscopic

Peripheral to the cellular core (*) of the lesion is a zone of reactive new bone formation with a rim (◆) of dense trabecular bone seen here at the right. This outer shell of bone blends with adjacent muscle fibers seen here at the left. The whole process eventually calcifies and shrinks over weeks to months.

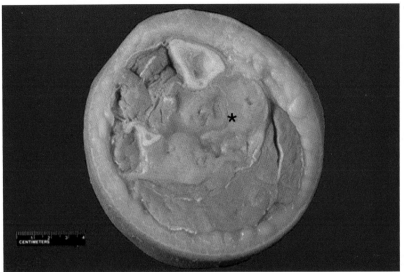

◄ **FIGURE 17–82 Soft tissue sarcoma, gross**

This malignant fibrous histiocytoma (MFH) is a fleshy mass (∗) arising within soft tissues of the lower leg behind the knee, with the tibia and fibula seen here in transverse section. Sarcomas tend to be bulky masses that invade locally, as can be seen here by the ill-defined margins of this mass. Hematogenous metastases are common.

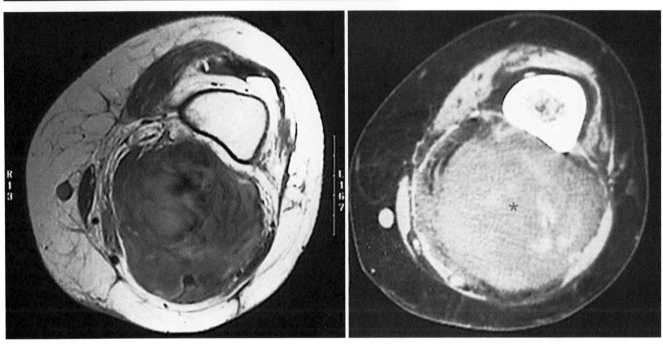

FIGURE 17–83 Sarcoma, MRI and CT image ▲

This sarcoma (∗) posterior to the knee at the lower femur is seen below in the left panel with MRI and in the right panel with CT. This mass is separate from bone.

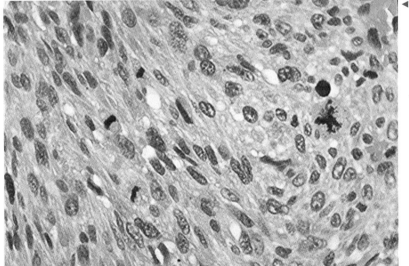

◄ **FIGURE 17–84 Sarcoma, microscopic**

Sarcomas tend to have a spindle cell pattern. Note that some of the cells are very pleomorphic. A very large abnormal mitotic figure is seen at the right. The cell of origin of sarcomas is often difficult to determine because of their tendency to be poorly differentiated or even anaplastic. Immunohistochemical staining can help determine their origin. Most sarcomas are vimentin positive, whereas carcinomas are cytokeratin positive.

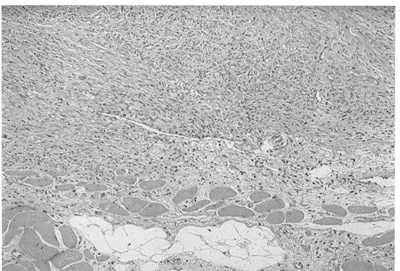

◄ FIGURE 17–85 Fibromatosis (desmoid tumor), microscopic

These aggressive fibroblastic proliferations can occur within the shoulder, chest wall, neck, and thigh. In women during or just after pregnancy, they may appear in the abdominal wall. Desmoid tumors are poorly demarcated and often invade surrounding soft tissues, so they must be excised with a wide margin. Microscopically, they are composed of spindle-shaped fibroblastic cells in a collagenous stroma, seen here at the top, which extend into adjacent skeletal muscle and adipose tissue at the bottom.

FIGURES 17–86 and 17–87 Rhabdomyosarcoma, MRI and CT image

This coronal MRI of a child reveals a soft tissue mass (♦) beneath the cranial cavity and expanding upward. Although rare, rhabdomyosarcomas are one of the more frequent soft tissue malignancies in children. The head and neck area is a common site for a pediatric rhabdomyosarcoma. The pelvis or abdomen may be involved, as shown in the CT image by a large mass (♦) leading to hydronephrosis (+). These masses are often locally infiltrative and difficult to remove completely.

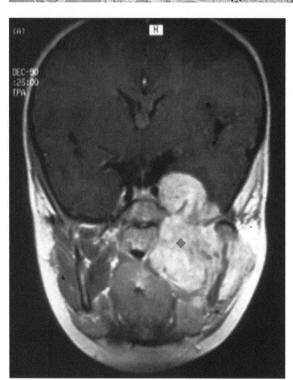

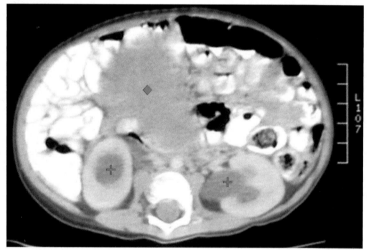

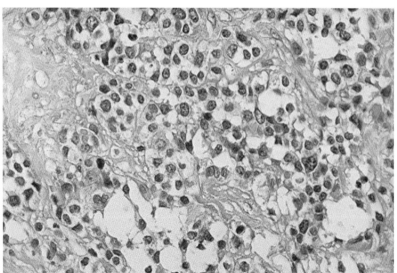

◄ FIGURE 17–88 Rhabdomyosarcoma, microscopic

This alveolar rhabdomyosarcoma is composed of primitive round blue cells (rhabdomyoblasts) arranged in nests with spaces and surrounded by a fibrous stroma. A variant of this neoplasm seen in the genital tract is the sarcoma botryoides. A common genetic alteration is a chromosomal translocation producing a chimeric PAX3-FKHR protein that is involved in muscle differentiation.

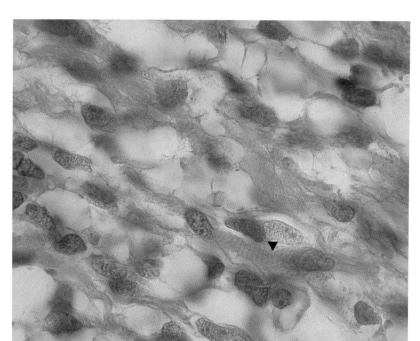

FIGURE 17–89 Rhabdomyosarcoma, microscopic

In adults, rhabdomyosarcomas can arise in large muscles such as those of the thigh. At high magnification, this rhabdomyosarcoma reveals pleomorphism and hyperchromatism of the nuclei, along with variable amounts of pink cytoplasm. Note the appearance of a characteristic "strap cell," which has recognizable cross-striations (▼) mimicking a skeletal muscle fiber.

CHAPTER 18

Peripheral Nerve and Skeletal Muscle

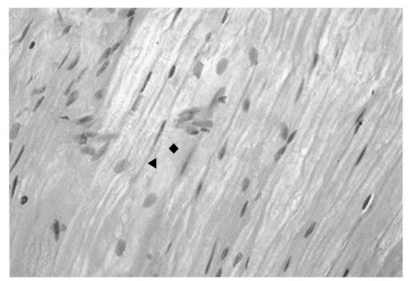

FIGURE 18–1 Normal peripheral nerve, microscopic

This normal peripheral nerve in longitudinal section shows slightly wavy, elongated cell bodies (axons, ◆) of the nerve fibers. A thin connective tissue layer, the endoneurium (◀), surrounds individual nerve fibers. A perineurium encloses a fascicle of nerve fibers and forms a blood-nerve barrier. The epineurium surrounds a whole nerve. Motor fibers are myelinated. Most sensory fibers are unmyelinated, although fibers for fine discriminatory senses such as touch and vibration are myelinated. The major component of an axonal myelin sheath is myelin protein zero, and myelin basic protein is the second most common structural protein.

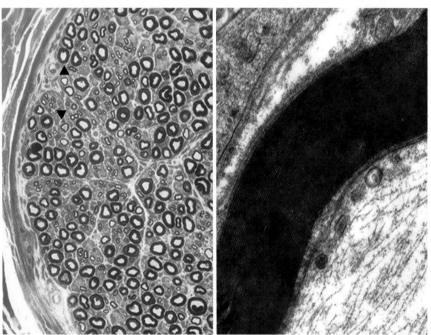

FIGURE 18–2 Normal peripheral nerve, microscopic

This normal peripheral nerve in transverse section with toluidine blue stain in the left panel has blue-black myelin around a normal number and distribution of thickly (▲) and thinly (▼) myelinated fibers. Pale background areas have the unmyelinated fibers. Overall, unmyelinated axons from 0.4 to 2 μm in diameter are more numerous than myelinated axons ranging from 1 to 20 μm in diameter. Myelinated fibers transmit impulses with higher conduction velocity (6 to 120 m/sec) than nonmyelinated fibers (0.5 to 2 m/sec). The larger the fiber, the faster the conduction velocity. Note the even spacing between the dark myelin lamellae around an axon in the electron micrograph in the right panel.

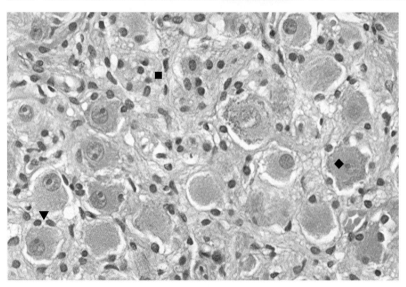

FIGURE 18–3 Normal peripheral ganglion, microscopic

This peripheral ganglion has nerve cell bodies (◆) and surrounding satellite cells (▼) and interstitial fibroblasts (■). The nerve cell bodies have fine pink Nissl granules, and some nerve cells display light brown lipochrome pigment within their cytoplasm. There is no blood-nerve barrier around a ganglion. The sensory and the postganglionic autonomic nerve fibers have neuronal cell bodies located in ganglia associated with cranial nerves, dorsal spinal roots, and autonomic nerves. Ganglia and Schwann cells are embryologically derived from the neural crest.

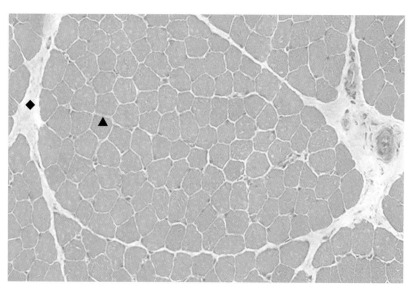

FIGURE 18–4 Normal skeletal muscle, microscopic

Skeletal muscle fibers are seen here in cross-section at low magnification. There are several fascicles. A connective tissue band, the *perimysium* (◆), surrounds each individual fascicle. An individual muscle fiber within the fascicle is invested by the endomysium (▲). The entire muscle is surrounded by a connective tissue band called the *epimysium*. The muscle cell nuclei are located at the periphery of the fibers. Each fiber is bounded by a sarcolemma, which projects into the cytoplasm as T tubules containing a high concentration of calcium ions. A nerve impulse causes depolarization with release of the calcium ions to initiate muscle contraction.

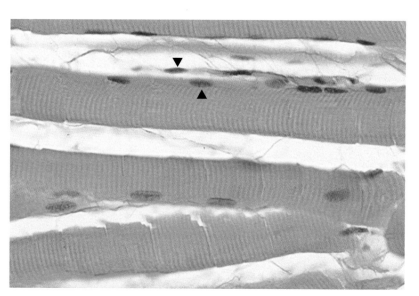

FIGURE 18–5 Normal skeletal muscle, microscopic

In longitudinal section, a skeletal muscle fiber has prominent cross-striations formed by the Z discs. The thin actin filaments are attached to Z discs and interdigitate with the thick myosin filaments to allow muscle contraction. The functional contractile unit is a sarcomere between two Z discs. The additional proteins tropomyosin and troponin complex regulate actin, myosin, and calcium binding. The skeletal muscle fiber is a multinucleated cell with numerous sarcolemmal nuclei (▲) at the periphery of each muscle fiber. Occasional satellite cells (▼) provide for maintenance, repair, and regeneration of injured fibers.

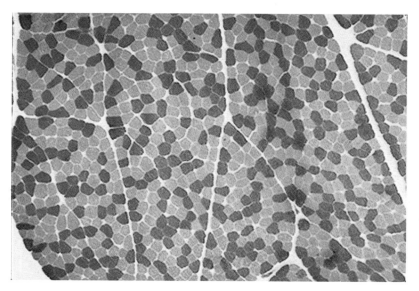

FIGURE 18–6 Normal skeletal muscle, microscopic

In cross-section with adenosine triphosphatase (ATPase) stain at pH 9.4, the normal pattern of type 1 and type 2 skeletal muscle fibers within fascicles is seen. These fibers are intermixed to form a checkerboard pattern. The type 1 fibers (slow twitch, oxidative) are light tan, and the type 2 fibers (mainly glycolytic) stain dark brown at this pH. Type 1 fibers have more mitochondria and more myoglobin for sustained contraction. A lower motor neuron innervates a group of myofibers, known as *motor units*. The motor units are small (less than 50 myofibers) when fine motor control is required (extraocular muscles) and large (hundreds of myofibers) in postural muscles such as the quadriceps femoris.

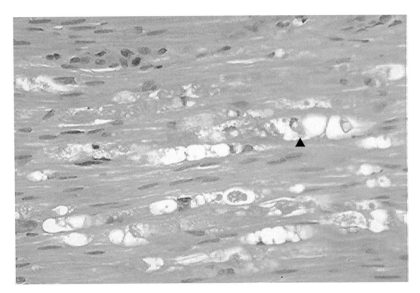

FIGURE 18–7 Wallerian degeneration, microscopic

Wallerian degeneration occurs distal to the site of an injury with traumatic transection of a peripheral nerve. In this distal nerve segment in longitudinal section, small axonal and myelin fragments are shown within the vacuolar digestion chambers (▲). Regeneration is possible because the proximal nerve stump undergoes axonal sprouting, and Schwann cells proliferate to remyelinate the nerve fiber. Regeneration proceeds along the course of the degenerated axon at a rate of about 2 mm per day.

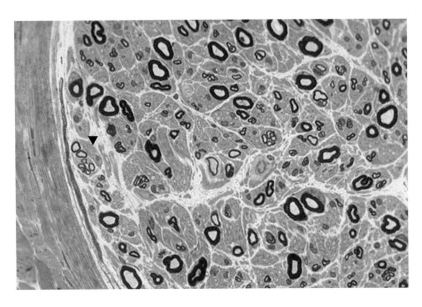

FIGURE 18–8 Peripheral nerve with axonal sprouting, microscopic

Here is axonal regrowth in a plastic-embedded cross-section of a peripheral nerve, with clusters of regrowing axons (▼) surrounded by the basement membrane of a Schwann cell. Small clusters of thinly myelinated fibers represent regrowth (axonal sprouting).

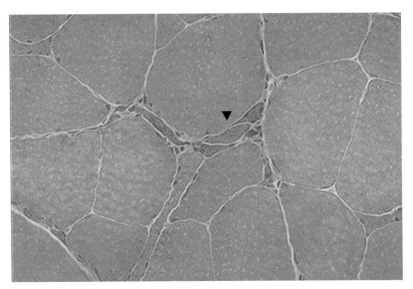

FIGURE 18–9 Denervation atrophy, microscopic

This modified Gomori trichrome stain shows the neurogenic form of skeletal muscle atrophy, with the characteristic pattern of "grouped atrophy" (▼) of muscle fibers that have lost their innervation from a peripheral nerve or motor neuron. These affected muscle fibers do not die, but "downsize" with loss of actin and myosin, becoming small and angular. Grouped atrophy of muscle fibers occurs with denervation and could result from traumatic injury to a nerve, peripheral neuropathy, or a motor neuron disease such as amyotrophic lateral sclerosis.

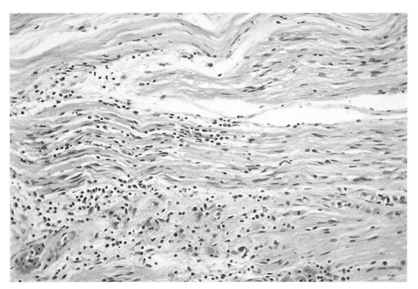

FIGURE 18–10 Guillain-Barré neuropathy, microscopic

Neuritis secondary to an acute inflammatory demyelinating polyradiculoneuropathy (Guillain-Barré syndrome) is shown in a longitudinal section of peripheral nerve with H+E stain. This disease is characterized by an acute ascending paralysis that occurs over a period of days, advancing distally to proximally. Respiratory paralysis is life-threatening. A viral illness may precede the onset of this disease. Note the lymphocytic infiltrates here. This inflammation will damage the nerve, and then macrophages will strip off the myelin lamellae, leading to demyelination with relative preservation of axons in most cases. Recovery occurs in most patients receiving ventilatory support.

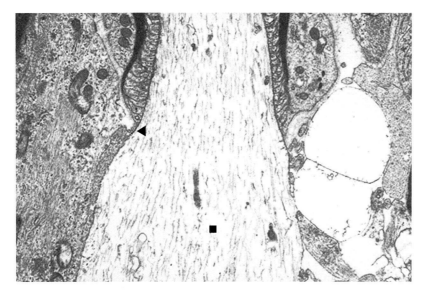

FIGURE 18–11 Demyelination, electron microscopy

This peripheral nerve shows a demyelinated axon next to an internode (◀). The axoplasm in the lower demyelinated portion (■) is swollen. The Schwann cell will be attracted to the demyelinated axon and will remyelinate it. In Guillain-Barré syndrome, there is segmental demyelination between internodes. During recovery from this form of inflammatory neuropathy, these areas will become remyelinated. Examination of the cerebrospinal fluid in Guillain-Barré syndrome shows few inflammatory cells, little or no pleocytosis, but an elevated protein.

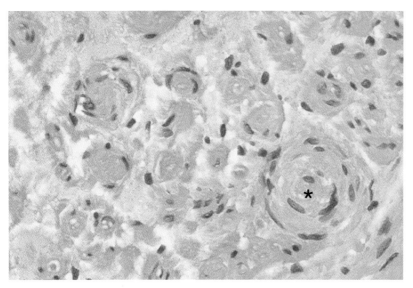

FIGURE 18–12 Demyelination and regeneration, microscopic

In chronic inflammatory demyelinating polyneuropathy, proliferation of Schwann cells around axons may occur. These groups of Schwann cells are called *onion bulbs* (∗) because the layering effect is similar to the layers of a cut onion. The process is called *onion skinning*. It is seen in peripheral nerve diseases that lead to repeated bouts of demyelination and remyelination over several years, with relapses and remissions, and both sensory and motor nerves can be involved.

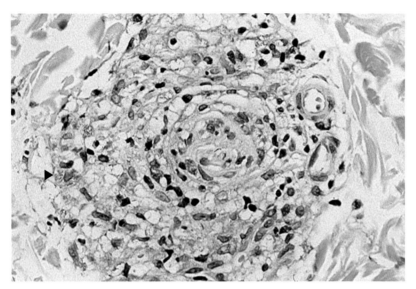

FIGURE 18–13 Leprosy, microscopic

A poorly formed granuloma is seen around a peripheral nerve within the dermis. The lepra bacilli grow best just below body temperature, preferring the cooler skin and peripheral nerves. Hypopigmented patches or macular lesions with decreased sensation are seen on the face, extremities, and trunk. Nodular disfiguring lesions can appear, with the lepromatous form having many macrophages filled with numerous acid-fast bacilli ("globi") (▶). In the tuberculoid form, acid-fast organisms are hard to find. Seen here is the "borderline" form, with some organisms and some epithelioid cells. It is now possible to control leprosy with drug therapy (rifampin as a first-line drug and dapsone second).

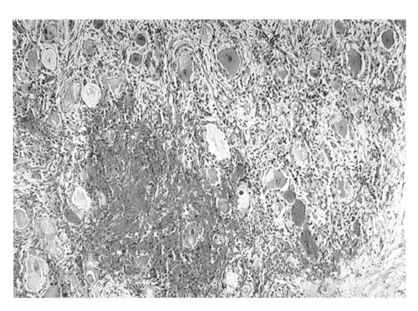

FIGURE 18–14 Varicella-zoster virus, microscopic

Acutely, varicella-zoster virus (VZV) infects the dorsal root ganglia. Shown here is a hemorrhagic lesion with neuronal loss from a reactivated infection in a dorsal root ganglion of an immunosuppressed patient who developed "shingles" (a dermatomal distribution of skin vesicles) 2 weeks before death. The latent form of VZV will remain dormant in the dorsal root ganglia for years after the initial infection with chicken pox, and then can activate into an acute lesion. The virus travels distally down the axon to the periphery, causing the vesicular skin eruption that is shingles. Thus, involvement of a dorsal root ganglion gives rise to the typical dermatomal distribution of the skin lesions.

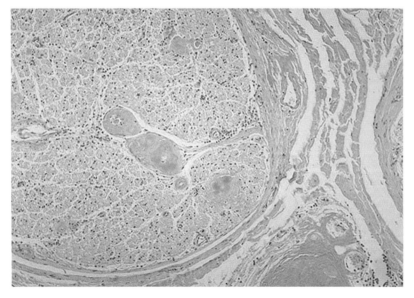

FIGURE 18–15 Amyloid neuropathy, microscopic

Note the thickening of endoneurial vessels from deposition of amorphous material within the vascular walls that appears orange with the Congo red stain for amyloid. Amyloidosis can involve the endoneurial vessels of a peripheral nerve. Axonal degeneration occurs over time in amyloidosis. The amyloid can be derived from the breakdown of a variety of proteins, such as light chains with multiple myeloma, or serum amyloid–associated protein when there is a chronic inflammatory condition such as tuberculosis or rheumatoid arthritis.

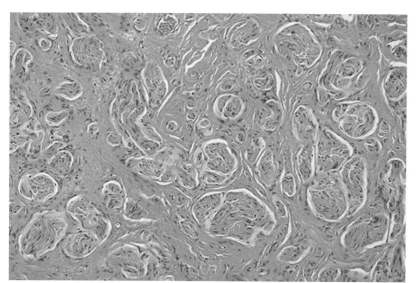

FIGURE 18–16 Traumatic neuroma, microscopic

This disorganized jumble of sprouting neurites or axons that have become embedded within a dense reactive connective tissue stroma is a *traumatic neuroma*. This non-neoplastic lesion occurs when a peripheral nerve is severed or damaged, and the proximal axons try to regrow, but are unable to connect with the distal axonal sheaths, forming the haphazard mass of nerve and fibrous connective tissues. The resulting neuroma can become a painful nodule. A common location for this lesion is between the bases of the second and third digits of the foot, because a characteristic human folly is fashion over function, with choice of footwear such as pointed-toe shoes and high heels that produce compression injury.

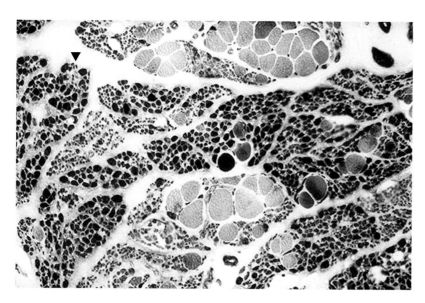

FIGURE 18–17 Spinal muscular atrophy, microscopic

This is grouped atrophy (▼) of rounded infantile muscle fibers, demonstrated with ATPase stain at pH 9.4. This neurogenic atrophy has resulted from Werdnig-Hoffman disease, the most common form of spinal muscular atrophy (SMA), but still a rare condition. It is one of several autosomal recessive disorders resulting from homozygous mutations in the survival motor neuron 1 (*SMN1*) gene. There is severe loss of lower motor neurons during infancy. These "floppy infants" generally die from respiratory failure during infancy or within the first 3 years of life. Other forms of SMA are milder, and affected patients die in childhood.

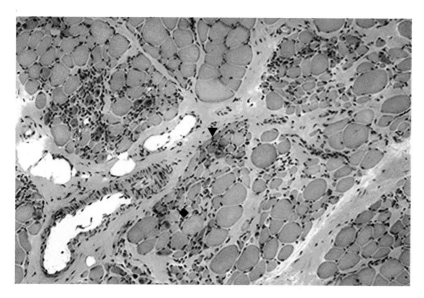

FIGURE 18–18 Duchenne muscular dystrophy, microscopic

Seen here is degeneration (♦) of muscle fibers along with some small purple regenerating fibers (▼), scattered chronic inflammatory cells, fibrosis, adipocytes, and hypertrophy of remaining muscle fibers. Duchenne muscular dystrophy is due to a defective *dystrophin* gene on the X chromosome that leads to an inability to produce the striated muscle sarcolemmal membrane protein dystrophin. Thus, this is an X-linked recessive disorder. About one third of cases arise from spontaneous new mutations rather than maternal inheritance. Progressive muscular weakness begins by age 5 and generally leads to death by age 20.

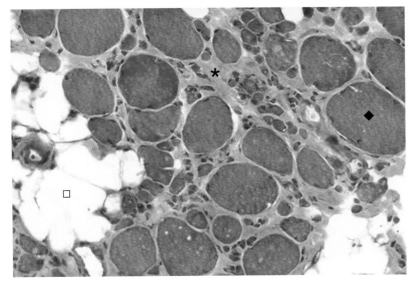

FIGURE 18–19 Duchenne muscular dystrophy, microscopic

Note the adipose tissue (□) and the increased endomysial pale blue-green connective tissue (∗) revealed by this modified Gomori trichrome stain. There are large oval hypertrophic fibers (◆) that are thought to be hypercontracted fibers interspersed with smaller atrophic degenerating or regenerating fibers, typical of a myopathic disease process. Early in the course, such large fibers can lead to "pseudohypertrophy" of calf muscles. Patients with Duchenne muscular dystrophy initially develop more proximal muscle weakness early in childhood by the age of 5, but they are typically wheelchair-bound by age 10 and die from respiratory failure by the second or third decade.

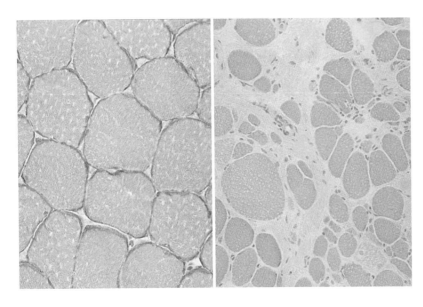

FIGURE 18–20 Duchenne muscular dystrophy, microscopic

This immunohistochemical stain utilizes antibody to the sarcolemmal protein dystrophin, which is seen here to be localized at the periphery of the normal muscle fibers in the left panel, but absent in the atrophic fibers of a patient with Duchenne muscular dystrophy in the right panel. Dystrophin, coded by a gene in the chromosome Xp21 region, appears to stabilize the membrane. Female carriers of this gene may have an elevated serum creatine kinase (CK) but little or no muscular weakness. Affected males have an elevated CK in childhood, but with eventual extensive muscular atrophy, the CK returns to normal. Affected males also often develop cognitive impairment.

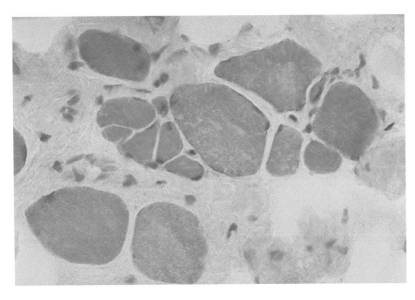

FIGURE 18–21 Becker muscular dystrophy, microscopic

This immunohistochemical stain reveals only small amounts of dystrophin, typical of Becker muscular dystrophy (BMD), which is less common than Duchenne muscular dystrophy. The same *dystrophin* gene is involved in BMD, but with a different mutation than in Duchenne. Some dystrophin is made in BMD, but not normal amounts. Patients with BMD have an onset of muscular weakness in adolescence to young adulthood, and have a less severe course than those with Duchenne muscular dystrophy.

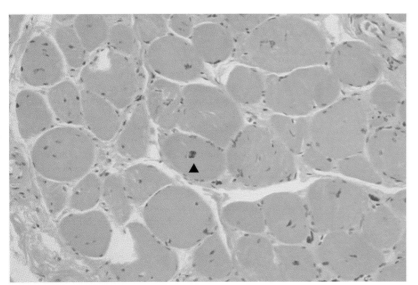

FIGURE 18–22 Myotonic dystrophy, microscopic

Note the central nuclei (▲) in these muscle fibers in cross-section, along with variation in fiber size and fibrosis, typical of myotonic dystrophy, the most common form of adult-onset muscular dystrophy, affecting 1 in 8000 people. There are three forms of the disease: congenital, symptomatic at birth or in the first year of life; classic, with onset between 10 and 60 years; and minimal, with onset after 50 years and only manifesting myotonia and a mild degree of muscle weakness. In the classic form, there may also be cataracts, intellectual changes, hypersomnia, gonadal atrophy, insulin resistance, decreased esophageal and colonic motility, and cardiomyopathy. Frontal balding is a common phenotypic feature.

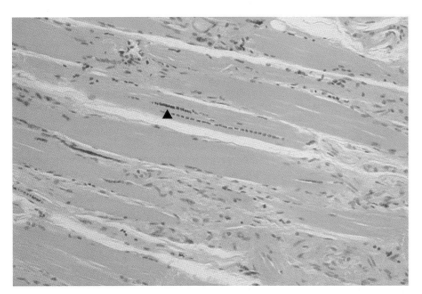

FIGURE 18–23 Myotonic dystrophy, microscopic

In these myofibers in longitudinal section with myotonic dystrophy, note long strings (▲) of nuclei. The gene defect is an expanded CTG trinucleotide repeat sequence (tandem repeats) within the noncoding portion of the *DM-1* gene on chromosome 19 that codes for the dystrophia myotonica protein kinase (*DMPK*) gene. Repeats may accumulate in successive generations. There is a reduction in transcripts of this gene. Skeletal muscle, liver, and brain can be affected. Muscular weakness is apparent early in the neck muscles (such as sternocleidomastoids) and distal limb muscles. The palate, tongue, and pharyngeal muscles also become involved, producing dysarthric speech and swallowing problems.

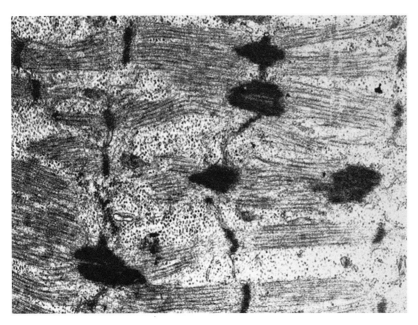

FIGURE 18–24 Nemaline myopathy, electron microscopy

Some "floppy infants" have a congenital myopathy. Clinical findings include hypotonia, muscle weakness, joint contractures (arthrogryposis), and a nonprogressive to slowly progressive course. Some of these myopathies have been described by their characteristic histologic features. The dark rod-shaped subsarcolemmal inclusions seen here in this electron micrograph are known as *nemaline rods*. The "rods" appear to arise from Z bands and are composed of a protein (α-actinin) found in the Z bands.

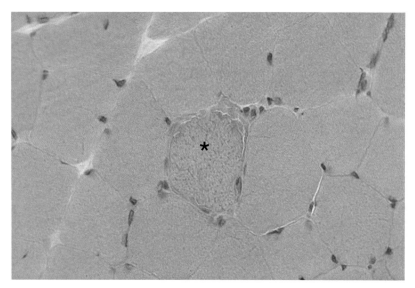

FIGURE 18–25 Mitochondrial myopathy, microscopic

Mitochondrial myopathies are rare diseases marked by "ragged red fibers" containing aggregates of abnormal mitochondria that appear subsarcolemmally and scattered through some muscle fibers. They appear as granular red areas (∗) on H+E staining. Mitochondrial proteins are necessary for oxidative metabolism to maintain normal skeletal muscular, cardiac, and nervous system function. Synthesis of these proteins is directed either by nuclear DNA or mitochondrial DNA. With the latter, the inheritance pattern is maternal; one example is the disorder known as *mitochondrial encephalomyopathy with lactic acidosis and strokelike episodes* (MELAS).

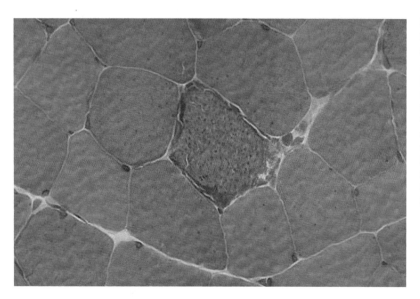

FIGURE 18–26 Mitochondrial myopathy, microscopic

With the modified Gomori trichrome stain, the abnormal mitochondrial deposits here appear as reddish granular deposits, the so-called ragged red fibers. Mitochondrial myopathy may present clinically in several ways: proximal muscular weakness, ophthalmoplegia, encephalopathy, and cardiomyopathy. The onset of these diseases often occurs in childhood or young adulthood, but can also occur in infancy. The increased numbers of mitochondria have an abnormal shape and size. By electron microscopy, some mitochondria can have "parking lot" inclusions.

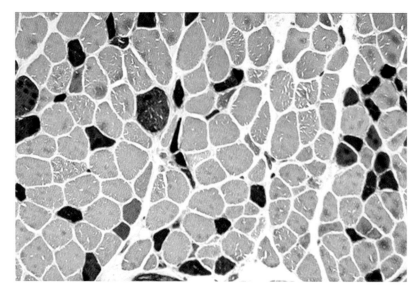

FIGURE 18–27 Type II atrophy, microscopic

There is atrophy of type II muscle fibers as shown with this ATPase stain of skeletal muscle. The darker type II fibers are smaller and not as numerous as the paler type I fibers. This can be a feature of corticosteroid-induced myopathy. The same findings are seen with Cushing syndrome.

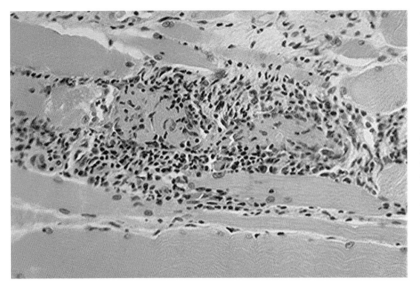

FIGURE 18–28 Polymyositis, microscopic

Shown are marked chronic inflammatory cell infiltrates with degeneration of muscle fibers as part of this autoimmune disease. Polymyositis results from the cytotoxic effects of CD8+ lymphocytes recognizing HLA class 1 major histocompatibility complex molecules on myofiber sarcolemmal membranes. Of the autoantibodies, anti-Jo1 is probably the most common with this disorder. In contrast, dermatomyositis is mainly mediated through a vasculitis affecting small capillaries leading to focal hypoperfusion and muscle fiber atrophy; the myositis is accompanied by a skin rash (typically the violaceous "heliotrope" rash of eyelids) and an increased risk for visceral cancers.

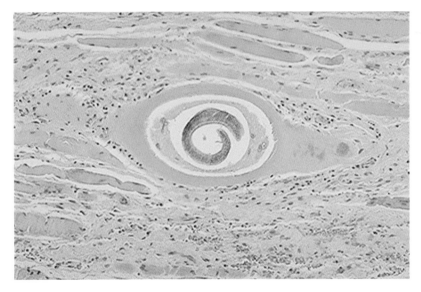

FIGURE 18–29 Trichinosis, microscopic

An encysted *Trichinella spiralis* larva is seen here within skeletal muscle. Humans act as an intermediate host when larvae are ingested while eating poorly cooked or uncooked meat from an infected animal, such as a pig. These larvae mature into adults in the gastrointestinal tract, releasing larvae that penetrate tissues and spread hematogenously to striated muscle. The early phase of infection is marked by fever, muscle pain, and peripheral blood eosinophilia with a T_H2 immune response. A heavy infestation of larvae can even lead to death. However, most cases go unnoticed, and the encysted larvae undergo dystrophic calcification over months to years.

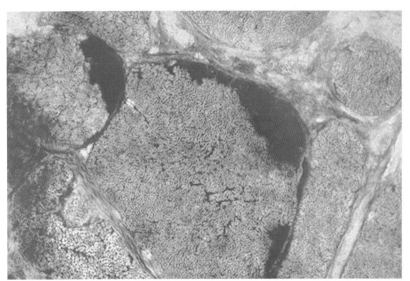

FIGURE 18–30 McArdle disease, microscopic

This is type 5 glycogen storage disease. The onset can be in childhood or adulthood. The myophosphorylase enzyme (part of glycolytic metabolism) is deficient, and excess glycogen becomes deposited within muscle, seen here as the red subsarcolemmal deposits highlighted with PAS stain. This myopathic disease results in muscular weakness, muscle cramps after exercise, myoglobinuria, and lack of an exercise-induced rise in blood lactate. Although the serum creatine kinase can be elevated, there is little or no muscle fiber degeneration or inflammation.

CHAPTER 19

The Central Nervous System

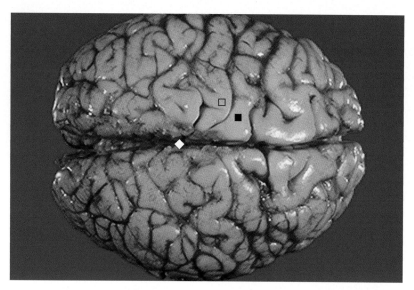

FIGURE 19–1 Normal brain, gross

The superior aspect at the vertex of an adult brain is shown here with the central sulcus (◆) between the right and left hemispheres. Note the pattern of gyri and sulci beneath the thin, filmy meninges (pia and arachnoid layers; the overlying dura has been removed). The Rolandic fissure with the precentral gyrus (■) (motor cortex) and the postcentral gyrus (□) (somesthetic cortex) are seen here. The normal adult brain weighs 1100 to 1700 gm.

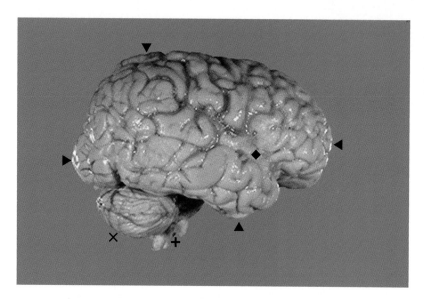

FIGURE 19–2 Normal brain, gross

The lateral view of the brain reveals the frontal lobe (◄), parietal lobe (▼), temporal lobe (▲), occipital lobe (►), cerebellum (×), and brain stem (+). Note the sylvian fissure (◆) separating the frontal lobe from the temporal lobe.

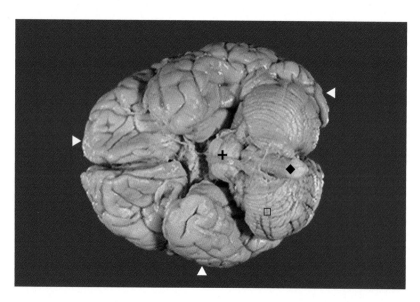

FIGURE 19–3 Normal brain, gross

At the base of the brain can be seen the inferior frontal lobes (►), temporal lobes (▲), pons (+), medulla oblongata (◆), cerebellar hemispheres (□), and occipital lobes (◄).

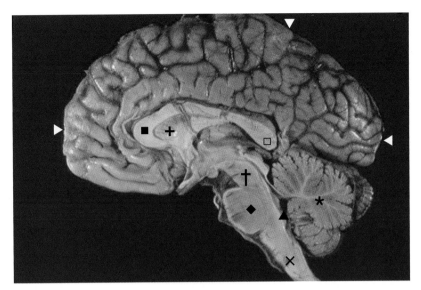

FIGURE 19–4 Normal brain, gross

A sagittal section through the midline of the brain reveals the frontal lobe (▶), parietal lobe (▼), and occipital lobe (◀). The genu (■) and the splenium (□) of the corpus callosum appear above the third ventricle, divided by the thin membrane, the septum pellucidum (+). The midbrain (†), pons (◆), and medulla oblongata (×) form the brain stem. The aqueduct of Sylvius connects the third ventricle to the fourth ventricle (▲). The fourth ventricle lies below the cerebellum (*) and above the medulla.

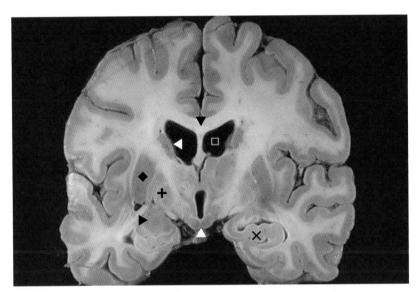

FIGURE 19–5 Normal brain, gross

This coronal section through the center of the brain reveals the mamillary bodies (▲), globus pallidus (+), putamen (◆), caudate nucleus (◀), lateral ventricles (□), corpus callosum (▼), and hippocampus (×). This section is not completely symmetric (as is the case with many CTs and MRIs), so the amygdala (▶) appears on just one side.

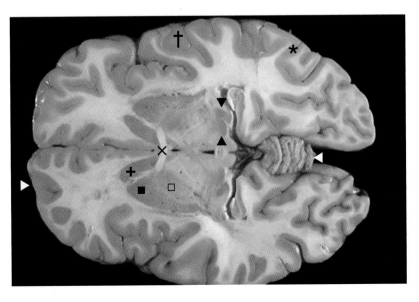

FIGURE 19–6 Normal brain, gross

This axial (transverse) section through the brain reveals the frontal lobe (▶), caudate nucleus (+), anterior commissure (×), putamen (■), globus pallidus (□), medial (▲) and lateral (▼) geniculate nuclei, temporal lobe (†), parietal lobe (*), and anterior vermis (◀) of the cerebellum.

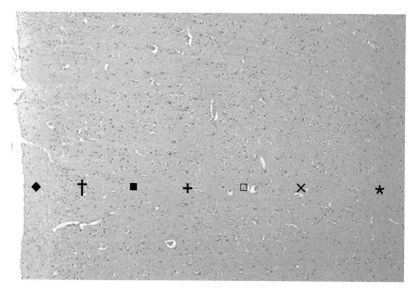

FIGURE 19–7 Normal brain, microscopic

The neocortex (gray matter) of the cerebral hemispheres has six layers that are microscopically indistinct with H+E staining. Beneath the pia-arachnoid at the far left there is an outer plexiform (◆) layer with nerve cells arranged horizontally. Next is the outer granular layer (†) containing small pyramidal neurons. Next is the outer pyramidal cell layer (■) with medium-sized pyramidal neurons. Below this is the inner granular layer (+) of larger pyramidal neurons. Beneath this is the inner pyramidal layer (□) of larger pyramidal neurons. The innermost cortical layer is the polymorphous layer (×) that lacks pyramidal cells. Beneath the cortex is the white matter (*).

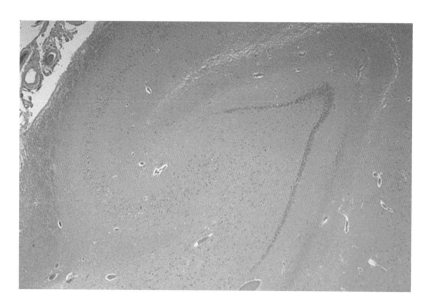

FIGURE 19–8 Normal brain, microscopic

The normal appearance of the hippocampus is seen here at low magnification. Hippocampus consists of "paleocortex" with three layers.

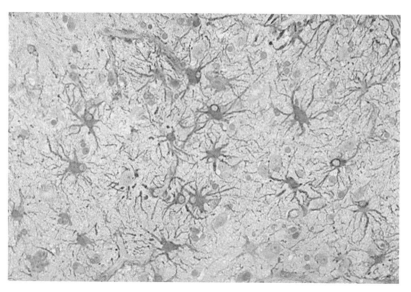

FIGURE 19–9 Normal brain, microscopic

This immunohistochemical stain for intermediate filaments known as *glial fibrillary acidic protein* (GFAP) highlights astrocytes with their prominent processes that extend between neurons. At least one process either extends to the overlying pia or surrounds a capillary to form the blood-brain barrier (BBB) along with endothelial cells and pericytes, a diffusion barrier that prevents the influx of most compounds from blood to brain. Pericytes encircle endothelial cells, providing structural support and aiding in controlling blood flow. Tight junctions (Tjs) between endothelial cells form the selective diffusion barrier. Astrocytic foot processes closely adherent to small vessels aid in the induction and maintenance of the Tj barrier.

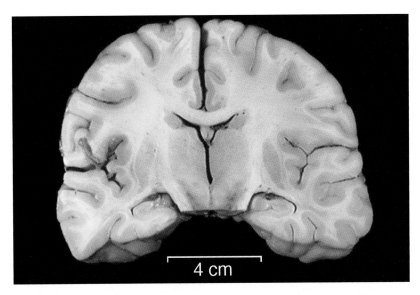

FIGURE 19–10 Cerebral edema, gross

This coronal section of cerebrum demonstrates marked compression of the lateral ventricles and flattening of gyri from extensive bilateral cerebral edema. This patient was climbing a 5000--meter mountain peak and ignored the warning sign of a persistent, worsening headache. The hypoxia leads to endothelial damage with an increase in intracellular edema (cytotoxic edema). In contrast, vasogenic edema results from disruption of the blood-brain barrier by inflammation or neoplasia. In either case, edema increases intracranial pressure, leading to herniation. Normally, the intracranial pressure is less than 200 mm H_2O.

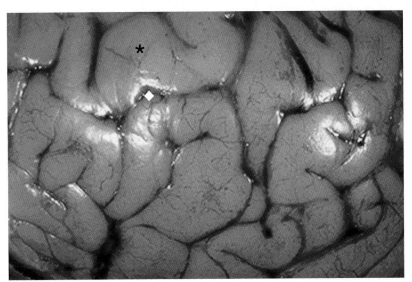

FIGURE 19–11 Cerebral edema, gross

The surface beneath the meninges of the brain with cerebral edema shows widened, flattened gyri (∗) with narrowed sulci (◆). When the blood-brain barrier is disrupted by inflammation or neoplasms, vasogenic edema results from fluid leakage into intracellular spaces. Ischemia results in cytotoxic edema from direct cell injury and an increase in intracellular fluid. Both these conditions can be localized. When there is extensive edema, generally both injury patterns are present.

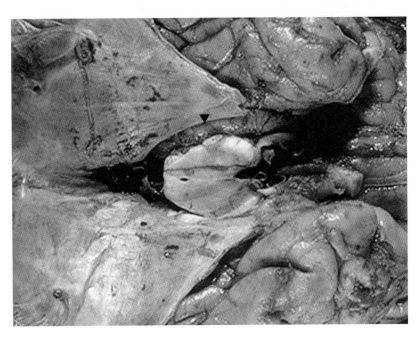

FIGURE 19–12 Herniation, gross

This brain shows medial temporal lobe (uncal) herniation. The medial temporal lobe tissue is pushed beneath the tentorium (▼) and down into the posterior fossa. This can occur either by a mass effect or from edema on the ipsilateral side of the brain. Note the resulting compression of the left side of the midbrain.

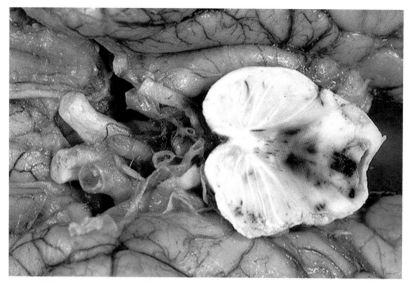

FIGURE 19–13 Herniation with Duret hemorrhages, gross

Medial temporal lobe (uncal) herniation has caused bleeding into the pons, known as *Duret hemorrhage*. When the herniated tissue pushes the brain stem further down into the posterior fossa and stretches and tears the perforating vessels of the pons and midbrain, this type of secondary brain stem bleeding occurs. Note the deep groove on the right medial temporal lobe (uncus) caused by pressure against the tentorium. When the degree of herniation is pronounced, hemiparesis ipsilateral to the side of the herniation may be caused by compression of the contralateral cerebral peduncle.

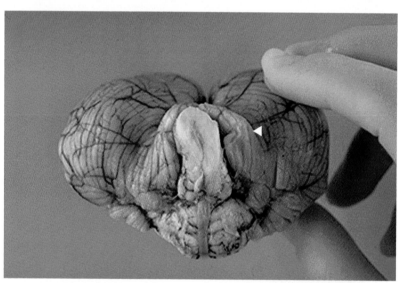

FIGURE 19–14 Cerebellar tonsillar herniation, gross

Acute brain swelling above the tentorium or within the posterior fossa can force posterior fossa contents toward the foramen magnum, and this can often produce herniation of the cerebellar tonsils into the foramen magnum. Note the cone shape of the cerebellar tonsils (◄) around the medulla seen here. Compression of the medulla compromises brain stem centers controlling respiration and cardiac activity, leading to death from herniation.

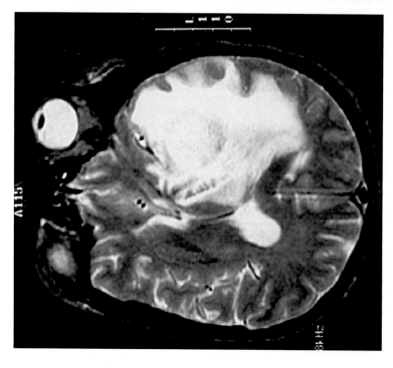

FIGURE 19–15 Cerebral edema, MRI

Seen here is an abscess with inflammation that compromises the blood-brain barrier to produce surrounding edema that appears bright in this T2-weighted axial MRI of the brain at the level of the orbits. Note that fluid appears bright, as in the globe of the eye and in the lateral ventricles compressed by the mass effect of the edema, with shift of the midline to the right. The brain tissue with edema therefore appears brighter as well. This edema is most pronounced in the white matter.

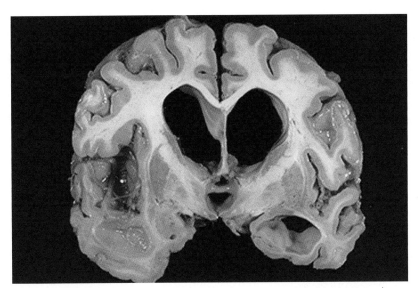

FIGURE 19–16 Hydrocephalus, gross

Note the marked dilation of these cerebral ventricles from hydrocephalus. Hydrocephalus can be due to a lack of absorption of cerebrospinal fluid (CSF), called *communicating hydrocephalus*, or to an obstruction to flow of CSF, called *noncommunicating hydrocephalus*. Hydrocephalus can be a long-term complication of infection, such as a basilar meningitis that leads to scarring that obstructs CSF outflow through the foramina of Luschka and Magendie. Inflammation with scarring of arachnoid granulations at the vertex may diminish CSF absorption.

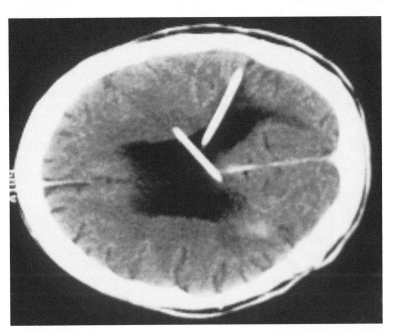

FIGURE 19–17 Hydrocephalus, CT image

In axial view are seen enlarged lateral ventricles in a patient with hydrocephalus. This condition has been treated by placing two shunts (the linear bright objects). Ventricular shunts can be placed acutely to relieve hydrocephalus, or a permanent shunt can be placed with routing of the fluid to the peritoneum, where it is resorbed and recycled. The choroid plexuses normally produce about 0.5 to 1.5 L of CSF per day. This CSF is an ultrafiltrate of plasma that provides a "shock absorber" function for the brain. The CSF circulates through the ventricles and spinal canal. At any time, about 150 mL of CSF fills the ventricular system. CSF is normally reabsorbed at the arachnoid granulations at the vertex of the brain.

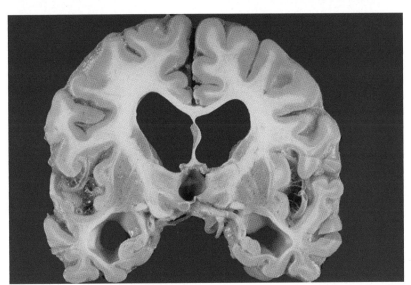

FIGURE 19–18 Hydrocephalus *ex vacuo*, gross

The condition known as *hydrocephalus ex vacuo* results from enough loss of brain parenchyma (as with atrophy) to cause compensatory ventricular enlargement. This coronal section shows a moderate degree of cerebral atrophy, which is more severe in the temporal lobe regions. The sylvian fissures appear enlarged. Note the moderate dilation of the cerebral ventricles, including the temporal horns, secondary to parenchymal loss. There is no intrinsic abnormality of CSF production, flow, or absorption. This patient had Alzheimer disease, which led to the cerebral atrophy.

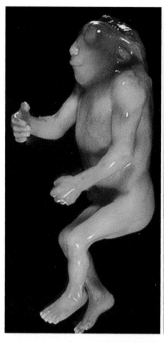
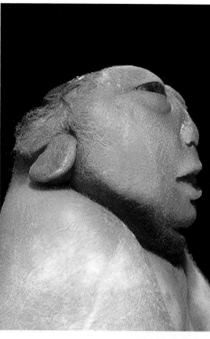

FIGURE 19–19 Anencephaly, gross

The most dramatic form of neural tube defect (NTD) is anencephaly. This condition occurs when there is malformation of the anterior end of the neural tube with failure of formation of the fetal cranial vault. The unprotected brain cannot form when exposed to amniotic fluid. The eyes appear proptotic because of the lack of a forehead for perspective. The reddish tissue at the base of the brain represents the area cerebrovasculosa, a disorganized mass of glial, meningeal, and vascular tissue. A small amount of brain-stem tissue may be spared, providing for short survival after birth. The open defect predisposes to infection. Supplementing the maternal diet with folate before and during early pregnancy can help to reduce the risk for NTD, which otherwise occurs at a rate of about 1 to 5 of 1000 live births.

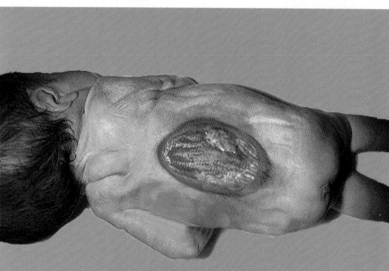

FIGURE 19–20 Meningomyelocele, gross

NTDs are one of the more common congenital anomalies to occur. Such defects result from improper embryonic neural tube closure. The most minimal defect is called spina bifida, with failure of the posterior arch of a vertebral body to completely form, but the defect is not open to the skin. Open NTDs with lack of a skin covering can include meningocele with just meninges protruding through the defect. The meningomyelocele seen here is large enough to allow meninges and a portion of spinal cord to protrude through the defect. Open defects predispose to CNS infection. Such defects can be suspected prenatally by laboratory determination of an elevated maternal serum α-fetoprotein.

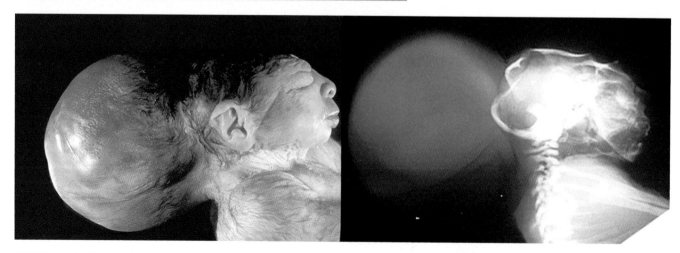

FIGURE 19–21 Encephalocele, gross

This an occipital encephalocele with brain tissue extending through a posterior skull defect that is covered by skin. The cranial vault is present but appears flattened because there is less brain tissue in the cranial cavity.

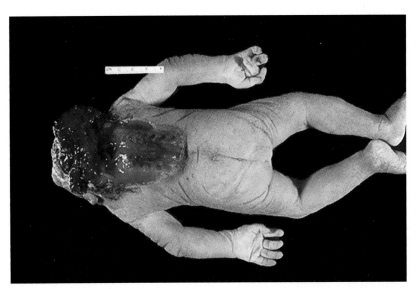

FIGURE 19–22 Rachischisis, gross

The most common form of NTD is a failure of closure of the posterior (caudal) neural tube, leading to spinal dysraphism, or spina bifida. This condition may not be severe, with only a portion of the vertebral arches missing (spina bifida occulta), but with an overlying skin covering, evidenced by a small skin dimple that may contain a tuft of hair over the site of the defect. A more severe form, known as *rachischisis*, is shown here with a large open defect involving the upper thoracic and cervical vertebrae, along with absence of the occipital bone. Since the cranial vault also appears to be absent, the condition seen here is best termed *craniorachischisis*.

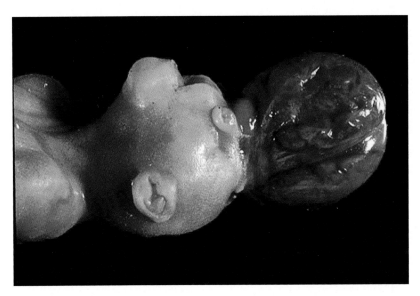

FIGURE 19–23 Exencephaly, gross

This is the rarest form of NTD, known as *exencephaly*. Note here the absence of the cranial vault, but the presence of brain tissue covered by meninges. In this condition, all or part of the fetal cranial vault may be missing, but there is still enough tissue covering the brain to allow its development *in utero*. Exencephaly is most likely to occur in conjunction with an early amnion disruption sequence, or limb–body wall complex, often with amnionic bands involving the head.

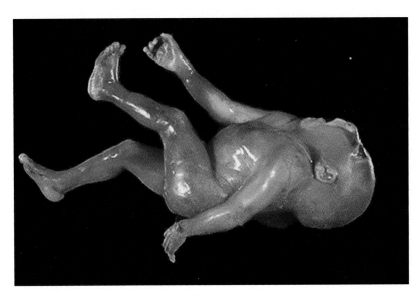

FIGURE 19–24 Iniencephaly, gross

This variation of NTD, known as *iniencephaly*, results from lack of proper formation of occipital bones, along with a short neck and defect of the upper cord. The head is tilted back (giving the appellation "stargazer" to those with this rare condition). An encephalocele or rachischisis typically accompanies iniencephaly. In any form of NTD, the amount of CNS tissue that fails to form or is disrupted or secondarily affected by infection or trauma determines the extent of neurologic deficits, including motor and sensory loss. Bowel and bladder function can be lost. High NTDs involving the spinal cord can lead to quadriplegia, while those in the thoracic or lumbar regions may lead to paraplegia.

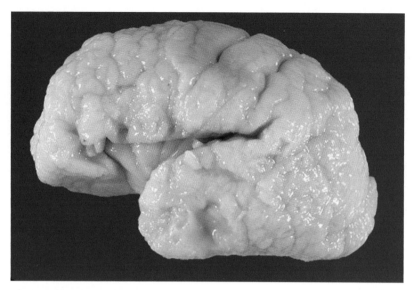

FIGURE 19–25 Polymicrogyria, gross

The developmental abnormality in this newborn brain seen from the left lateral aspect, with loss of normal contours of the cerebral hemispheric convolutions, is called *polymicrogyria*. Note the numerous small gyral bumps over the lateral surface of this left hemisphere. However, these are not separated by sulci microscopically. In this anomaly, the gyri are abnormally fused together, with entrapment of meningeal tissue, and there are no more than four layers of neocortex instead of the normal six-layered neocortex.

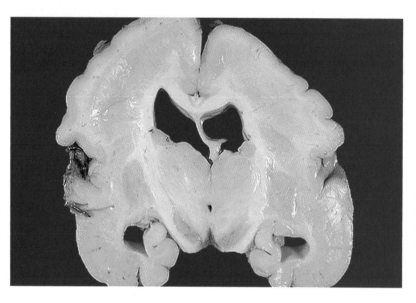

FIGURE 19–26 Lissencephaly, gross

This coronal section of a child's brain shows markedly diminished gyral development, along with marked thickening of the underlying cerebral cortex. This child with lissencephaly (agyria) had severe developmental delay and was confined to a chronic care hospital. Note that the hippocampi and the deep gray matter structures appear normal. Deletion of chromosome 17p13.3 with loss of the *LIS1* gene occurs in the rare Miller-Dieker syndrome with agyria, seizures, and mental retardation. In normal fetal brain development, gyri first become visible at about 20 weeks' gestation, so lissencephaly before 20 weeks is considered normal. After 20 weeks, gyral development normally continues to term in an orderly manner.

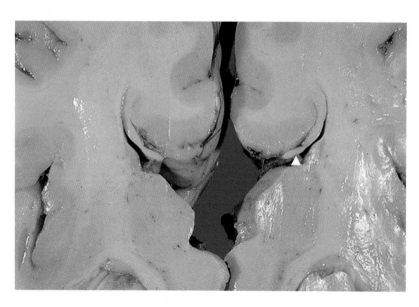

FIGURE 19–27 Agenesis of the corpus callosum, gross

In this coronal section of brain, there is agenesis of the corpus callosum with only Probst bundles (▲) remaining. A Probst bundle is the small bundle of callosal fibers seen laterally. The cingulate gyrus appears displaced downward bilaterally. Agenesis of the corpus callosum, which is one of the most common anomalies seen in the CNS, may occur as an isolated event or in association with other anomalies. It may be complete or partial. It may be completely asymptomatic and detectable only with specialized testing. It may accompany other malformations. The much smaller but adaptable anterior commissure can assume the duties of the missing corpus callosum.

Assoc. c̄ lipomas

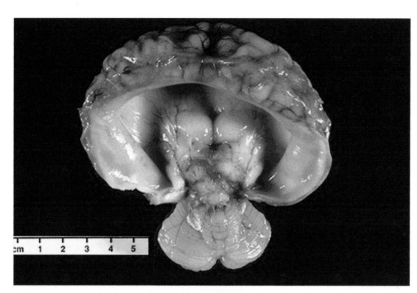

FIGURE 19–28 Alobar holoprosencephaly, gross

Holoprosencephaly is often accompanied by the failure of fetal facial midline structures to form properly, with midline facial defects such as cleft lip, cleft palate, and cyclopia, typically with a chromosomal abnormality such as trisomy 13. It can be seen with maternal diabetes mellitus or occur sporadically. Some cases are associated with mutation of the human *Sonic Hedgehog* gene. The "alobar" form of holoprosencephaly seen here has only a single large ventricle and no attempt at formation of separate cerebral hemispheres.

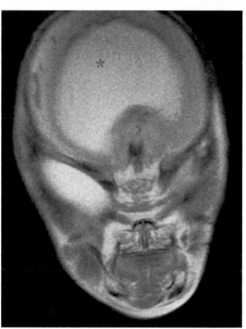

FIGURE 19–29 Holoprosencephaly, MRI

This T1-weighted MRI in coronal view demonstrates a single ventricle (∗) with a surrounding poorly developed rim of cerebral cortex and, at the base of this abnormal ventricle, central fused thalami (◆). These are characteristics of alobar holoprosencephaly. This condition results from failure of development of two cerebral hemispheres from the telencephalon, along with failure of complete thalamic development from the diencephalon. The telencephalon and diencephalon are components of the embryonic prosencephalon.

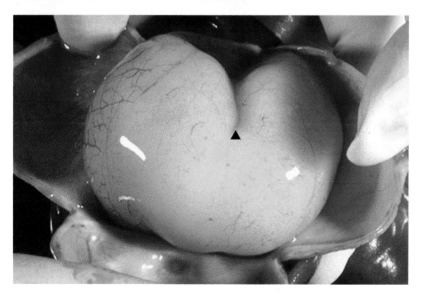

FIGURE 19–30 Semilobar holoprosencephaly, gross

The fetal skull is opened here at autopsy to reveal the semilobar form of holoprosencephaly, so named because there is a small cleft (▲) representing an attempt to separate the hemispheres. There is no apparent gyral pattern here because this stillborn fetus was less than 20 weeks' gestation, and thus the lissencephaly is appropriate for this gestational age. Holoprosencephaly is a grave condition with little or no brain function.

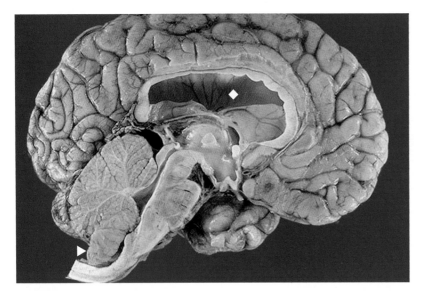

FIGURE 19–31 Arnold-Chiari I malformation, gross

This sagittal section shows the cerebellar tonsils (▶) herniated downward over the cervical spinal cord. There is hydrocephalus (◆), thought to be secondary to poor flow of CSF out the foramina of Luschka and Magendie, owing to the compression of brain tissue within the posterior fossa. Neurosurgical repair can be performed.

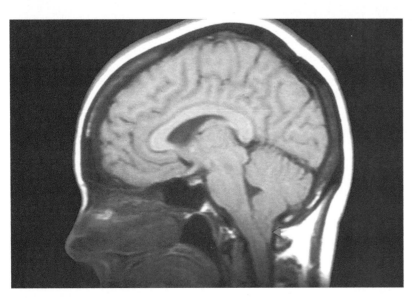

FIGURE 19–32 Arnold-Chiari I malformation, MRI

This MRI of brain in a sagittal view shows the Arnold-Chiari type I malformation. In this malformation, the posterior fossa is small, and the cerebellar tonsils (◀) herniate through the foramen magnum. The lateral ventricles may be enlarged. This is the milder form of the malformation, and many patients will not have any symptoms.

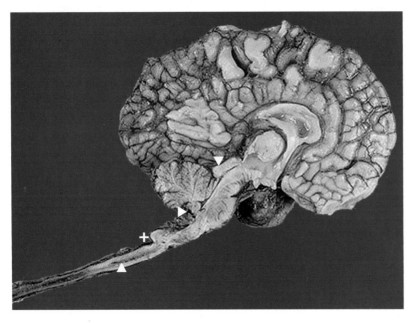

FIGURE 19–33 Arnold-Chiari II malformation, gross

In the Arnold-Chiari type II malformation, there is also a small posterior fossa with tonsillar herniation (▶). This more severe form of the Chiari malformation shows kinking (+) of the medulla over the cervical cord, and there is a syrinx (▲) in the cervical cord as well. The collicular plate (▼) is pulled up (called *tenting*), and there is invariably an associated hydrocephalus. Most children affected by this anomaly also have a lumbar meningomyelocele.

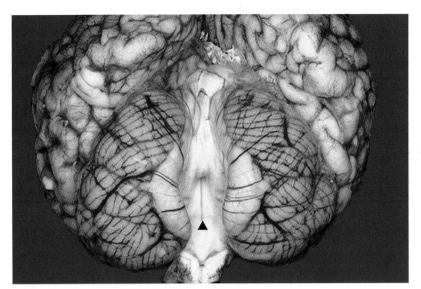

FIGURE 19–34 Dandy-Walker malformation, gross

In Dandy-Walker syndrome, there is enlargement of the posterior fossa beneath the tentorium, accompanied by agenesis of the vermis of the cerebellum. There is replacement of the vermis by a midline cyst lined by ependyma and contiguous with leptomeninges, forming a roofless fourth ventricle. Seen here is the cerebellum with the floor (▲) of the enlarged fourth ventricle. There may be dysplasias of brain-stem nuclei as well.

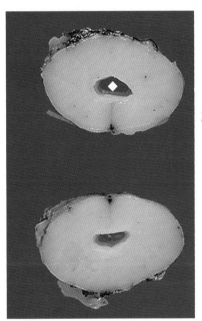

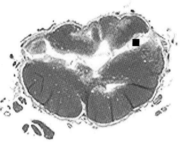

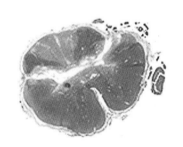

FIGURE 19–35 Hydromyelia, gross, compared with syringomyelia, microscopic

The cross-sections of spinal cord in the left panel demonstrate a prominent dilation (◆) of the central canal known as *hydromyelia*. This cavity most often forms in the cervical cord and is lined by ependyma. With syringomyelia in the right panel, there is a slitlike cavity (■) extending across the spinal cord, which cuts across the pain fibers, leading to loss of upper extremity pain and temperature sensation. Extension of the lesion superiorly into the medulla is termed *syringobulbia*. This lesion is most often associated with the Chiari I malformation. Other associations include cord trauma or intraspinal tumors. If the cavity continues to enlarge, a drain can be placed to relieve the symptoms.

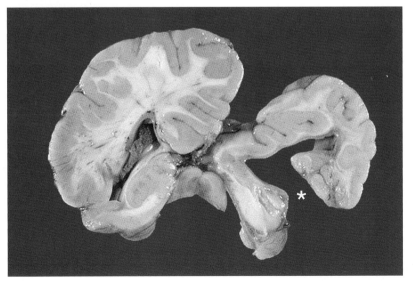

FIGURE 19–36 Porencephaly, gross

Shown here is a large defect (*) involving the left cerebral hemisphere of a child. Porencephaly is defined by an abnormal opening through the cerebral hemisphere between the ventricular system and the subarachnoid space. This condition can be developmental or secondary to an insult, thought to be vascular, early *in utero* that destroys the tissue and produces the defect.

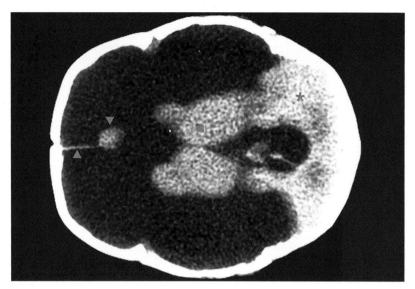

FIGURE 19–37 Hydranencephaly, CT image

All that remains of this fetal brain in the supratentorial compartment are the basal ganglia (■), the inferior occipital lobes (∗), and a small remnant of frontal lobe (▼) adjacent to the falx cerebri (▲). This is a more dramatic example of the result of a developmental or secondary insult *in utero* in which a large portion of the brain is destroyed and never develops. Affected babies are missing most of their cerebral hemispheres. The consequence is a fluid-filled space covered by meninges, mimicking hydrocephalus, but the size of the head is not increased.

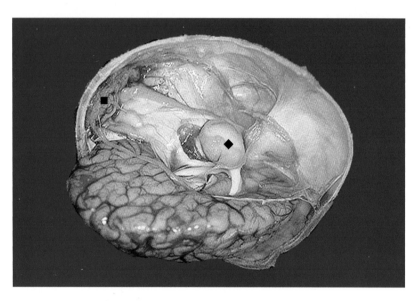

FIGURE 19–38 Hydranencephaly, gross

This is an example of unilateral hydranencephaly, observed at autopsy of a child, with the cranial cavity opened superiorly. The cranial cavity is almost empty on the left. There is a small remnant of the left occipital lobe (■), and there is a bump representing the basal ganglia (◆). The right cerebral hemisphere is formed properly.

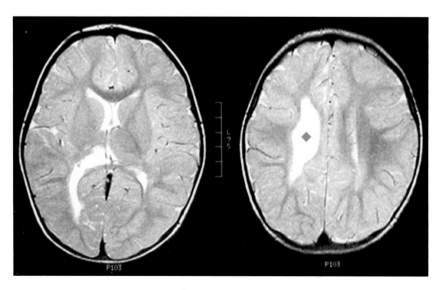

FIGURE 19–39 Cerebral palsy, MRIs

Cerebral palsy is a developmental disorder of motor function present from infancy or early childhood, probably the result of a vascular accident with localized infarction occurring prenatally or intrapartum. The actual event often goes unrecognized until a motor problem such as spastic diplegia or hemiplegia is noted early in development. In this case, the child had impaired motion, particularly of extensor muscles, on the left. Seen here is mild loss of white matter, basal ganglia, and thalamus on the right with ventricular *ex vacuo* dilation (◆). Cerebral palsy is nonprogressive, and the childhood brain has an amazing plasticity with ability to "rewire" itself, minimizing the deficit.

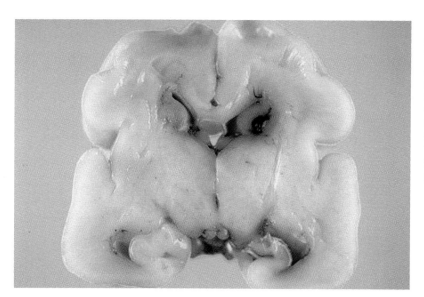

◄ FIGURE 19–40 Germinal matrix hemorrhage, gross

This coronal section of the brain of a 25-week gestational age premature infant displays a left germinal matrix hemorrhage that occurred shortly after birth. The germinal matrix is a highly vascularized area bordering the caudate nucleus and thalamus that is very sensitive to injury from variations in blood pressure as well as hypoxia. The risk for hemorrhage is greatest for premature babies born at 22 to 32 weeks' gestation, with a peak at 28 weeks' gestation.

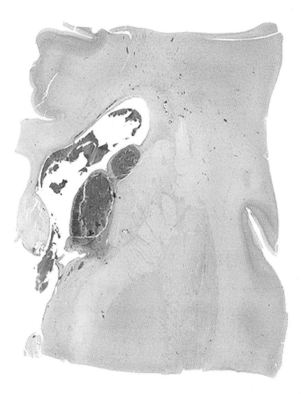

◄ FIGURE 19–41 Germinal matrix hemorrhage, microscopic

This transverse section of fetal brain shows a subependymal hemorrhage in the darker blue, highly cellular germinal matrix composed of developing glia adjacent to the head of the caudate. This hemorrhage can rupture into the adjacent lateral ventricle to produce intraventricular hemorrhage (IVH), which is a feared complication of prematurity.

FIGURE 19–42 Intraventricular hemorrhage, gross ►

This coronal section of a newborn brain shows a very large subependymal hemorrhage extending into and dilating the ventricular system. IVH can be severe, as shown here with blood filling and distending all the lateral ventricles, extending into brain parenchyma, and extending down the third ventricle and out into the subarachnoid space. The prognosis with this extent of hemorrhage is grim. If the infant survives, resolution of the hemorrhage with scarring can lead to obstructive hydrocephalus.

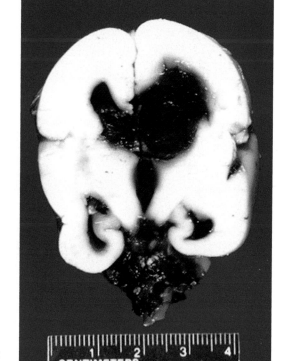

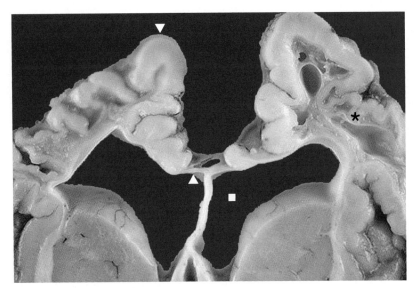

FIGURE 19–43 Leukomalacia, gross

Shown here in the brain of a child is severe leukomalacia in which the white matter has become cystic and markedly shrunken (∗). Note that the corpus callosum (▲) has become only a thin band of tissue, and there is marked *ex vacuo* ventricular dilation (■) from loss of the hemispheric parenchyma. The overlying gray matter (▼) appears better preserved, although there is loss in the cortex as well. Affected patients usually suffer from an anoxic insult around the time of birth and are severely impaired neurologically. Periventricular leukomalacia may be marked by radiographic appearance of bright dystrophic calcifications in addition to the necrosis.

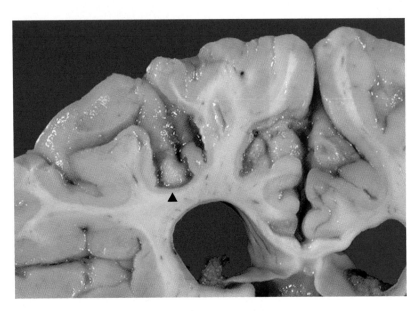

FIGURE 19–44 Ulegyria, gross

In this brain of a child, note the extensive loss of the cortical gray matter (▲) at the depths of these sulci. The remaining thin gyri become gliotic. Ulegyria is usually the result of an anoxic-ischemic event at or around the time of birth. The injury is most pronounced at the depths of the sulci.

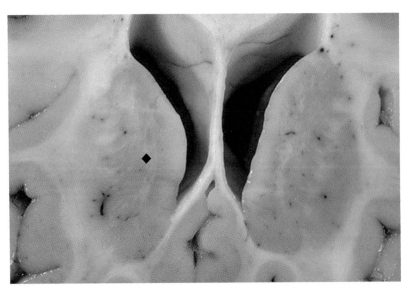

FIGURE 19–45 Status marmoratus, gross

This coronal section of brain through the basal ganglia with caudate and putamen demonstrates an increased irregular white color (♦) of the basal ganglia. This is status marmoratus or "marbled state" due to anoxia, which causes malfunction of the myelinating cells, the oligodendroglia, leading to abnormal myelination and thus the abnormal white areas seen here within the basal ganglia. There is also neuronal loss and gliosis, which also adds to the increased white color. These patients can have severe extrapyramidal movement problems, such as choreoathetosis.

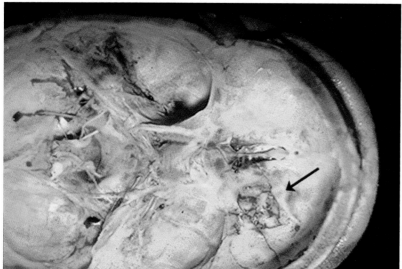

FIGURE 19–46 Skull fracture, gross

Blunt force trauma to the head can lead to skull fracture. The right orbital plate at the base of this skull shows multiple fractures (*arrow*) in an older patient who fell backward. The force of the blow was transmitted forward, resulting in a contrecoup injury pattern. Such basilar skull fractures may also occur with a blow to the side of the stationary head (coup injury pattern). A basal skull fracture may be suspected in a patient with a periorbital hematoma or CSF rhinorrhea or otorrhea.

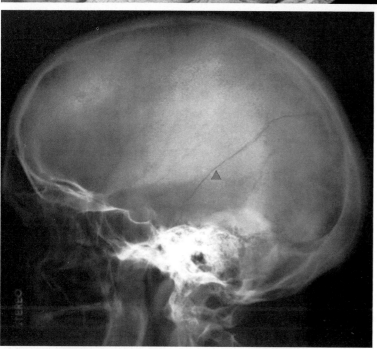

FIGURE 19–47 Skull fracture, radiograph

After a fall, this patient incurred a linear skull fracture, seen here as the long dark line (▲) in this lateral skull x-ray. The fainter branching gray lines represent the normal cranial vascular pattern along the inner skull surface.

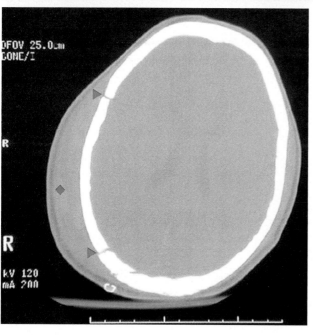

FIGURE 19–48 Skull fracture, CT image

This head CT scan in "bone window" demonstrates a skull fracture (▶) on the right with diastasis of the sutures. However, this is not a depressed skull fracture, and it is not displaced; a displaced fracture results in skull bone extending into the cranial cavity for a distance greater than the skull thickness. A fracture in this location could result from a coup injury as a consequence of a direct blow to that portion of skull. Note the marked overlying soft tissue swelling (♦) in the scalp and that a small overlying skin laceration has been closed with a staple.

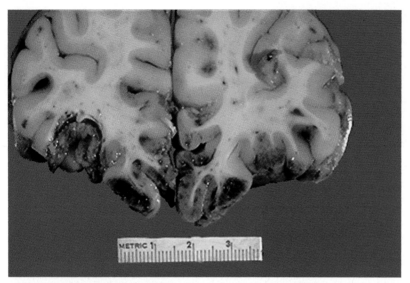

FIGURE 19–49 Cerebral contusions, gross

A coronal section through the frontal lobes of the brain reveals extensive recent contusions (bruises) with superficial gyral hemorrhages. The injury is most pronounced at the crests of the gyri, with relative sparing of cortex in the sulci. More severe lesions have extension of hemorrhage to underlying white matter. This was a contrecoup injury from a fall backward in which the victim struck the occiput, so that the force was transmitted anteriorly to produce the inferior frontal lobe contusions seen here. In contrast, a coup type of brain injury occurs with a direct blow to the head and force delivered to the region of the brain adjacent to the site of impact. There can be edema in cortex in the region of contusion, producing a local mass effect.

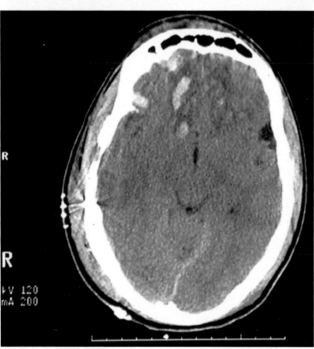

FIGURE 19–50 Cerebral contusions, CT image

The brighter areas of attenuation seen here in the cerebral parenchyma represent subfrontal contusions resulting from a contrecoup injury sustained in a fall backward. This patient also had a subdural hemorrhage that was drained through a burr hole marked by the starburst artefact, with overlying sutures as seen on the right. There is more hemorrhage and edema on the right, with a midline shift to the left and narrowing of ventricles.

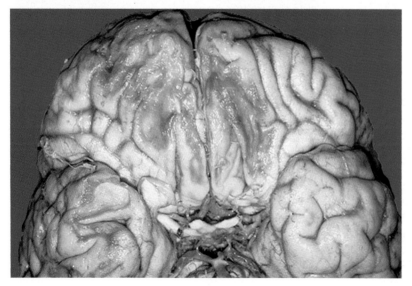

FIGURE 19–51 Cerebral contusions, gross

The inferior surfaces of these frontal lobes and the right inferior temporal lobe tip display old hemosiderin-stained contusions. They are slightly depressed from removal of necrotic cortex by macrophages and subsequent gliosis. These old lesions have been called *plaques jaunes* because of the yellow-to-brown discoloration from the accumulation of the hemosiderin derived from the breakdown of the blood in the superficial cortical hemorrhages. Patients with such contusions may develop a focal or partial seizure disorder years after the accident. There may be loss of smell (anosmia) if the olfactory bulbs are involved.

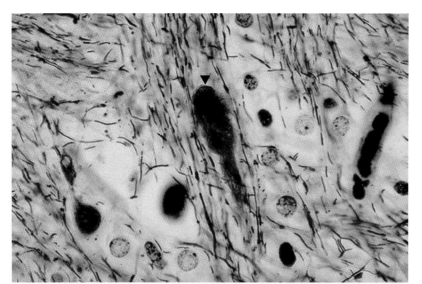

FIGURE 19–52 Diffuse axonal injury, microscopic

This silver stain of the centrum semiovale shows axonal retraction balls (▼) within cerebral white matter. These retraction balls can be formed after shearing force injuries. Such injuries can occur with rotational forces (angular acceleration or deceleration) or with violent shaking, as in "shaken baby" syndrome, or in people ejected from motor vehicles at high speed. The axons are stretched and broken at nodes of Ranvier, then undergo retraction, causing the axoplasm to compress into an enlarged ball. Such involved axonal fibers eventually degenerate. Focal hemorrhages may accompany these lesions. Up to half of patients in coma after trauma have these lesions.

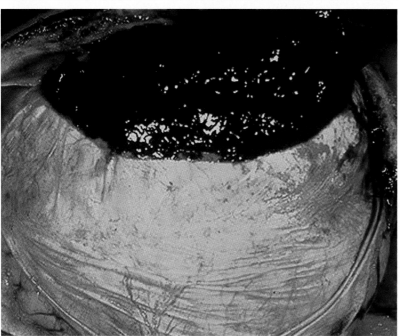

FIGURE 19–53 Epidural hematoma, gross

Blunt force head trauma causing a tear in the middle meningeal artery leads to a collection of blood in the epidural space. This acute arterial bleeding occurs between the dura and the skull and quickly leads to hematoma formation, seen here on the right after opening the cranial vault at autopsy. There is often a skull fracture accompanying this lesion. Since the bleeding from the artery is brisk, these patients may have a short lucid interval after the injury but will quickly lapse into coma because of the brain compression by the expanding hematoma. If not emergently evacuated, the expanding mass of blood will lead to herniation and death.

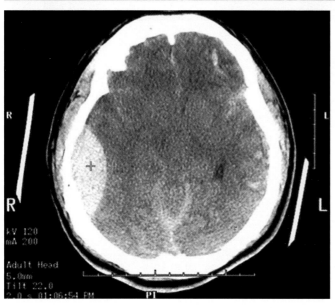

FIGURE 19–54 Epidural hematoma, CT image

Note the large right epidural hematoma with a lens-shaped outline (+), as the smooth dura becomes indented against the underlying cortex on the right lateral aspect of the cerebrum. The epidural hematoma is confined within an area bounded by cranial sutures where the dura is firmly adherent to the skull. This acute blood collection appears bright with CT imaging. Note the mass effect with effacement of the lateral ventricles and the shift of midline to the left. In this case, the patient fell from a height and struck the right side of his head, severing the middle meningeal artery. This epidural hematoma collected within hours.

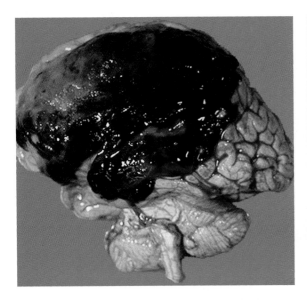
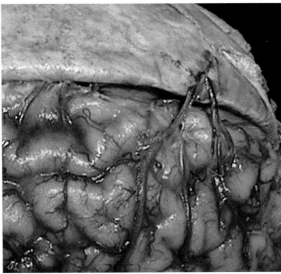

FIGURES 19–55 and 19–56 Subdural hematoma, gross, and bridging veins, gross

A large subdural hematoma is seen in the left panel overlying the left frontal-parietal region. A subdural hematoma forms after head trauma that severs the bridging veins from dura to brain, shown in the right panel where the dura has been reflected to reveal the normal appearance of the bridging veins that extend across to the superior aspect of the cerebral hemispheres. Elderly patients and the very young are at greater risk because their cerebral veins are more vulnerable to injury. Since the bleeding is venous, blood collects over hours to weeks, with variable onset of symptoms. Since the blood collects beneath the dura, a subdural hematoma can be seen to cross the region of cranial sutures.

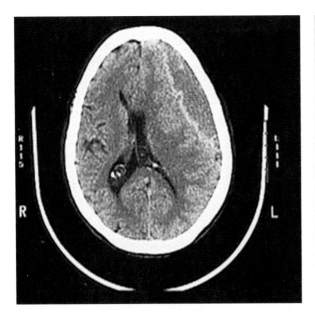
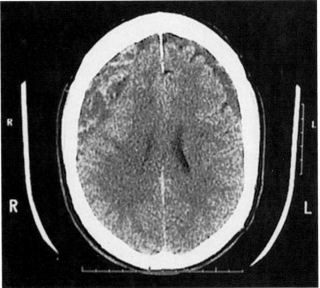

FIGURES 19–57 and 19–58 Subdural hematomas, gross

Shown in the left panel is a large left subdural hematoma (+) with left-to-right shift (◄) and ventricular narrowing. This subdural hematoma interdigitates with the adjacent gyri and sulci but compresses the brain. In the right panel can be seen bilateral subdural hematomas, the right one (+) greater in size than the left (×). There are irregular bright areas within these subdurals, indicating that the hemorrhage was relatively recent, but is not completely bright, so some organization of the hematoma has begun. Clot lysis generally occurs a week after hematoma formation, with granulation tissue, including fibroblastic proliferation from the dura, occurring over the next week, and formation of a neomembrane of connective tissue within 1 to 3 months after the original injury. Symptoms of subdural hematoma have a variable onset from hours to weeks, depending on the amount of bleeding. Rebleeding from delicate vessels within the granulation tissue is common, leading to chronic subdural hematoma.

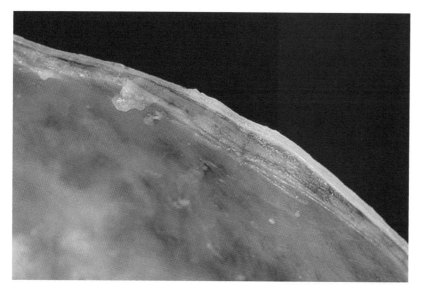

◄ **FIGURE 19–59 Organizing subdural hematoma, gross**

A subdural hematoma gradually organizes with granulation tissue formation and forms a membrane of reactive connective tissue. There may be rebleeding or fluid collection within this membrane, producing a mass effect that impinges on the brain. Note the brownish discoloration of the chronic subdural membrane seen here. These old membranes are only loosely attached to the dura and can be easily peeled away.

FIGURE 19–60 Subarachnoid hemorrhage, gross ►

Acute subarachnoid hemorrhage may follow trauma. Many of these areas of subarachnoid hemorrhage shown here are associated with underlying contusions. Simple subarachnoid hemorrhage without contusions can also occur from superficial damage to vessels over the surface of the brain.

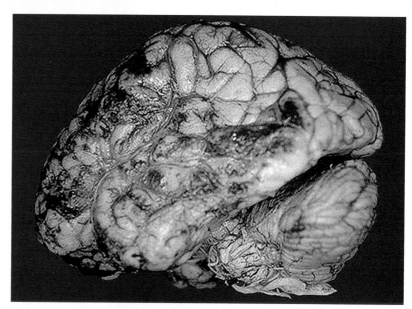

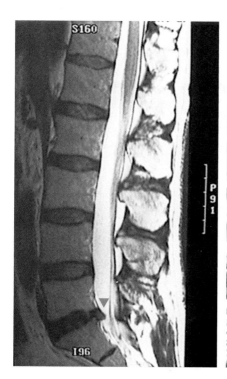

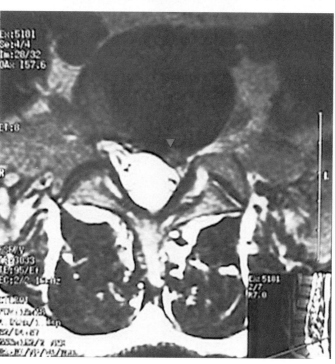

◄ **FIGURES 19–61 and 19–62 Herniated intervertebral disc, MRIs**

In the left panel in sagittal view is shown herniation of the nucleus pulposis of the intervertebral disc between L5 and S1, with compression (▼) of the lumbar spinal cord. Such a herniated disc can compress spinal nerve roots to produce pain and motor weakness. In the right panel, an axial view at L4 shows herniation and compression (▼) of the nerve roots on the left.

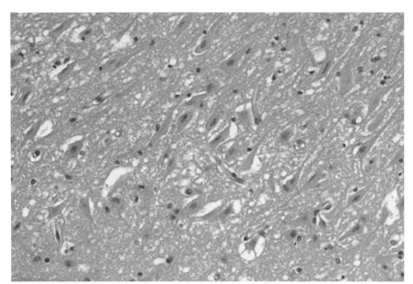

◄ **FIGURE 19–63 Hypoxic encephalopathy, microscopic**

Neurons are highly differentiated cells that are dependent on glucose for continued function, and they are very sensitive to hypoxic injury. Seen here are red neurons in cortex, which are dying 12 to 24 hours after onset of hypoxia. One of the most sensitive areas in the brain to hypoxic injury is the hippocampus. Cerebellar Purkinje cells and neocortical pyramidal neurons are also very sensitive to ischemic events. A global hypoxic encephalopathy occurs with reduction of all cerebral perfusion with reduced cardiac output and with hypotension. Intracranial vascular diseases may reduce blood flow focally to the brain, and the extent of injury depends on collateral circulation.

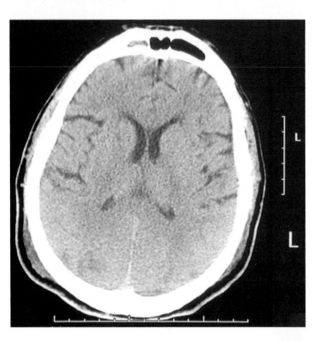

◄ **FIGURE 19–64 Acute cerebral ischemia, CT image**

Shown here are occipital lobe acute infarctions that developed as a result of focal ischemic injury, characterized by loss of gyral distinction, along with decreased attenuation (a darker appearance) of the white matter, compared with the uninfarcted frontal lobes.

FIGURE 19–65 Watershed infarction, gross ►

The bilaterally symmetric dark discolored areas seen here superiorly and just lateral to the midline in this coronal section of the brain at autopsy represent areas of recent infarction in the watershed (border) zone between distal regions of the anterior and middle cerebral arterial circulations. Such watershed infarctions can occur with relative or absolute hypoperfusion of the brain. Hypoperfusion can occur with a drop in cardiac output from cardiac diseases.

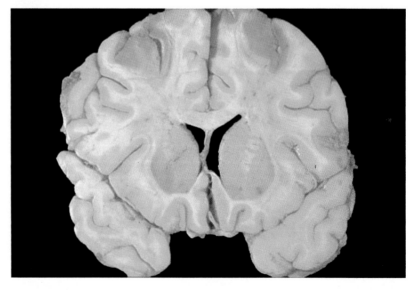

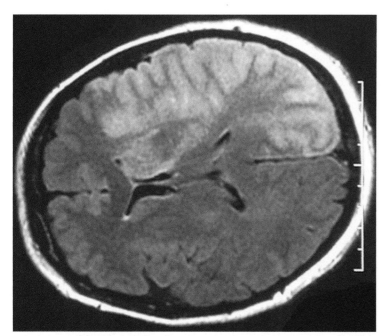

FIGURE 19–66 Cerebral acute infarction, MRI

This FLAIR-mode MRI reveals an area of massive infarction in the left cerebral hemisphere, mostly involving the left middle cerebral arterial distribution, but also in the left posterior cerebral distribution. This infarct is of recent formation, with brain swelling and a slight midline shift to the right causing compression of the ventricular system. Cerebral infarction is most often due to embolic occlusion of a cerebral arterial branch, but thrombotic occlusion can also occur, typically in an area of marked cerebral arterial atherosclerosis. Embolic infarcts are more likely to appear hemorrhagic from reperfusion of the damaged vessels and tissue, either from collateral circulation or after dissolution with breakup of the embolus.

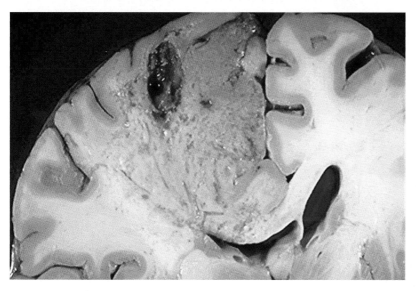

FIGURE 19–67 Cerebral subacute infarction, gross

In this coronal section of brain, a subacute infarct of the frontal lobe shows liquefactive necrosis with beginning formation of cystic spaces as resolution occurs from 10 days to 2 weeks after the initial ischemic event. The initial subacute changes begin 24 hours after the initial ischemic injury with influx of macrophages to remove the necrotic tissue, followed by increasing vascular proliferation and reactive gliosis.

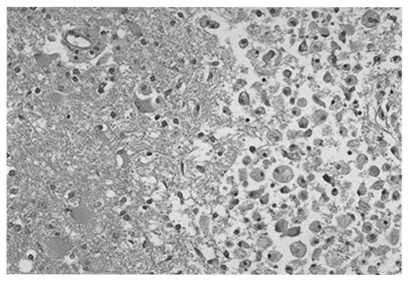

FIGURE 19–68 Subacute infarction, microscopic

At the right are many macrophages that are present in this subacute infarct to phagocytize lipid debris from the liquefactive necrosis. Gliosis is beginning at the left. Ischemic injury leads to infarction. Focal infarction (a "stroke") can result from either arterial thrombosis or embolism. The location and extent of the infarction determine the clinical findings and resulting neurologic dysfunction.

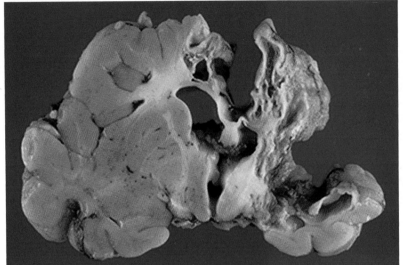

FIGURE 19–69 Cerebral remote infarction, gross

This coronal section of brain shows that most of one cerebral hemisphere and a small part of the other hemisphere have been destroyed. This remote infarction has occurred in the distribution of the right and left anterior cerebral arteries and the right middle cerebral artery. Resolution of liquefactive necrosis leads to formation of a cystic space surrounded by remaining brain tissue. This repair reaction begins 2 weeks after the ischemic injury and proceeds for months.

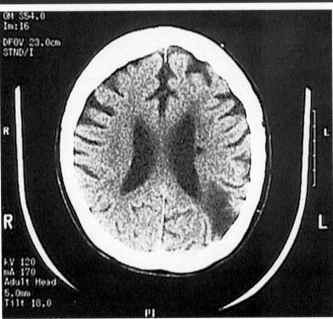

FIGURE 19–70 Cerebral remote infarction, CT image

The decreased area of attenuation seen here in the region of the left occipital lobe is a cystic area from healing of a remote cerebral infarction as a consequence of a thromboembolus to the left posterior cerebral artery. Resolution of the liquefactive necrosis leaves a cystic space. The neurologic deficits following infarction depend on the location and size of the infarct. Patients may be left with motor and sensory deficits. Over time, there may be partial recovery of some lost functions, but this is inconstant and unpredictable. In this case, the patient was left with visual field defects.

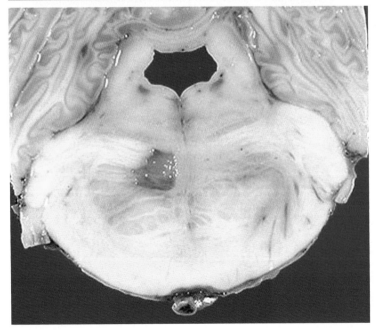

FIGURE 19–71 Lacunar infarction, gross

The arteriolar sclerosis that results from chronic hypertension leads to small lacunar infarcts, or "lacunes," one of which is seen here within the pons. Such lesions are most common in the lenticular nuclei, thalamus, internal capsule, deep white matter, caudate nucleus, and pons. Although these infarcts are typically smaller than 15 mm, and many result in no clinical findings, they can sometimes be strategically located where they damage important tracts, especially the descending corticospinal tracts, leading to hemiparesis.

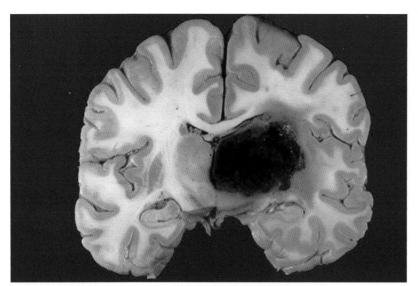

FIGURE 19–72 Cerebral hypertensive hemorrhage, gross

Hypertension is the most common cause of intraparenchymal brain hemorrhage, accounting for more than half of all such bleeds. An intracerebral hemorrhage is another form of "stroke." Hemorrhages involving the basal ganglia area (the putamen in particular) tend to be nontraumatic and caused by chronic hypertension, which damages and weakens the small penetrating arteries. A mass effect from the blood with midline shift, often with secondary edema, may lead to herniation. Hypertensive cerebral hemorrhages originate in the putamen in 50% to 60% of cases, but the thalamus, pons, and cerebellar hemispheres can also be sites of involvement.

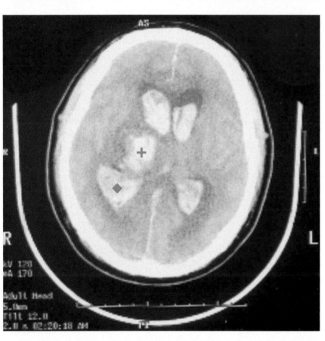

FIGURE 19–73 Cerebral hypertensive hemorrhage, CT image

A hypertensive hemorrhage is present here in the right thalamic region (+). In a minority of such cases, the hemorrhage may extend into the ventricular system (◆), as seen here. Hemorrhages involving the basal ganglia, thalamus, and brain stem are not generally amenable to surgical intervention with removal of the blood. The arteriosclerosis that accompanies chronic hypertension predisposes the small arterial vessels to rupture and produce the hemorrhage. Chronic hypertension is also associated with the development of minute aneurysms, less than 300 μm in diameter, termed *Charcot-Bouchard microaneurysms*, which can also rupture.

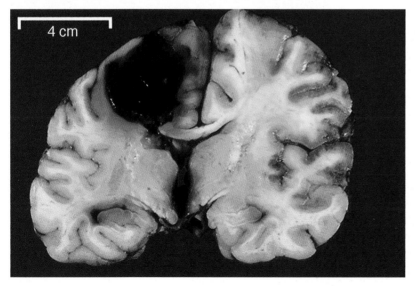

FIGURE 19–74 Lobar hemorrhage, gross

Cerebral intraparenchymal hemorrhages involving the lobes of the cerebral hemispheres may be due to many different etiologies, including a neoplasm, a coagulopathy, infections, vasculitis, amyloid angiopathy, and drug abuse (such as cocaine ingestion). Resolution of a large hemorrhage may leave a cystic region similar to an infarct.

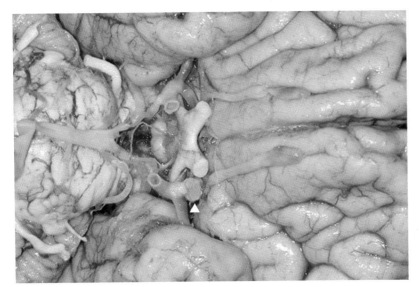

FIGURE 19–75 Berry aneurysm, gross

This nonruptured saccular (berry) aneurysm (▲) is located at the bifurcation of the left middle cerebral and anterior communicating arteries of the circle of Willis at the base of the brain. These aneurysms form at points where there is a developmental weakness in the arterial wall, most commonly at the bifurcation of the anterior communicating, middle cerebral, or internal carotid arteries. These aneurysms occur sporadically and may be present in 1% of people. Saccular aneurysms are more frequent with some genetic conditions such as autosomal dominant polycystic kidney disease, vascular-type Ehlers-Danlos syndrome (type IV), neurofibromatosis type 1, and Marfan syndrome. Half of people with a berry aneurysm have hypertension and are smokers.

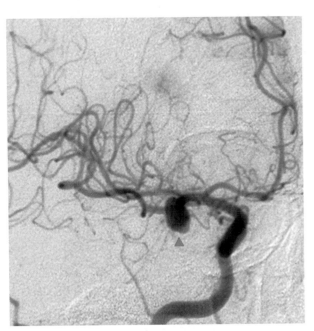

FIGURE 19–76 Berry aneurysm, angiogram

In this lateral view with contrast filling a portion of the cerebral arterial circulation can be seen a berry aneurysm (▲) involving the middle cerebral artery of the circle of Willis at the base of the brain. As the weak wall of the artery, which lacks an internal elastic lamina and a media, expands to form the aneurysm, there may initially be leakage of blood that produces headaches, but there is risk for sudden rupture to produce a severe headache. A sudden increase in intracranial pressure may predispose to rupture. The blood irritates the arteries to produce vasospasm and promote cerebral ischemia. A later consequence of this bleeding is organization with fibrosis at the base of the brain to block outflow of CSF through the foramina of Luschka and Magendie, leading to an obstructive hydrocephalus.

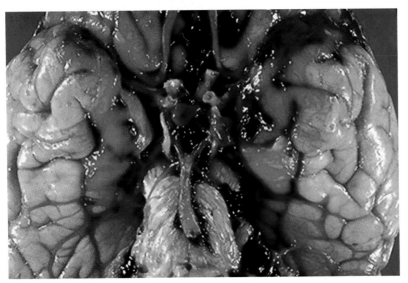

FIGURE 19–77 Subarachnoid hemorrhage, gross

Berry aneurysms take years to increase in size, and larger aneurysms are more prone to rupture, particularly those reaching 1 cm in diameter, so that rupture is most likely to occur in young to middle-age adults. Neurosurgery can be performed with clipping of the aneurysm at its base to prevent bleeding or rebleeding. The subarachnoid hemorrhage from a ruptured aneurysm is more of an irritant producing vasospasm than a mass lesion. In some cases, this arterial blood under pressure may dissect upward into the brain parenchyma. The result is often a sudden, severe headache followed by loss of consciousness.

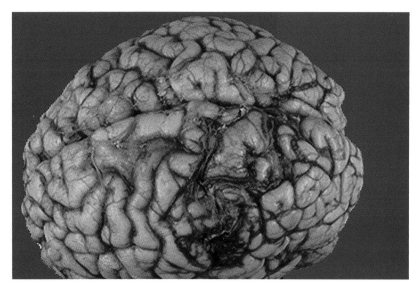

FIGURE 19–78 Vascular malformation, gross

Another cause of intracranial hemorrhage, particularly in people aged 10 to 30, more often in males, is a vascular malformation. Most occur in a cerebral hemisphere in the distribution of the middle cerebral artery. Seen here is a mass of irregular, tortuous vessels over the left posterior parietal region of the brain. Depending on the nature of the vessels composing the lesion, it may be termed an *arteriovenous malformation, cavernous hemangioma, capillary telangiectasia,* or *venous angioma*. These abnormal vascular lesions are prone to bleed. Localized lesions can be resected.

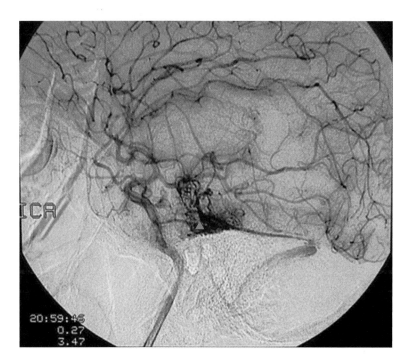

FIGURE 19–79 Vascular malformation, angiogram

Shown is contrast media filling a tortuous collection of irregular small vessels (▲) in the temporal region of the brain. A vascular malformation may bleed, resulting in symptoms that may range from new-onset seizures or headache to sudden loss of consciousness. The bleeding is most often intraparenchymal, but may extend to the overlying subarachnoid space.

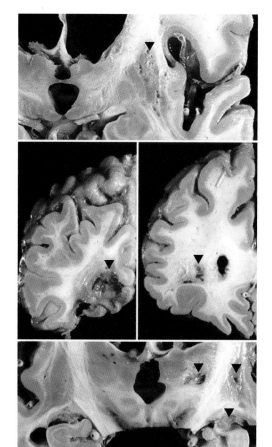

FIGURE 19–80 Vascular (multi-infarct) dementia, gross ▶

Multiple vascular events, including embolic arterial occlusion, atherosclerosis with vascular narrowing and thrombosis, and hypertensive arteriolar sclerosis, may lead to focal but additive loss of cerebral tissue. The cumulative effect of multiple small areas of infarction (▼) may result in clinical findings equivalent to Alzheimer disease, as well as focal neurologic deficits or gait disturbances. However, vascular dementia is marked by the loss of higher mental function in a stepwise, not continuous, fashion. Shown is a collage of cerebral coronal sections in which variably sized remote infarcts are present. Another variation of this process is Binswanger disease, characterized by extensive subcortical white matter loss.

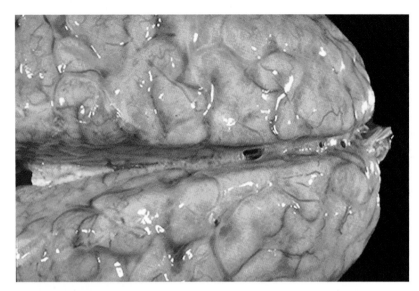

FIGURE 19–81 Acute meningitis, gross

The yellow-tan clouding of the meninges seen here, which obscures the sulci, is due to an inflammatory exudate from acute meningitis. This is most often the result of a bacterial (pyogenic) infection. Routes for intracranial infection include hematogenous dissemination (the most common cause), extension from an adjacent paranasal sinus or mastoid air cells, retrograde flow through facial veins into the cavernous sinus, and trauma with direct implantation by a penetrating injury through the skull. Lumbar puncture will reveal increased intracranial pressure and CSF showing a marked leukocytosis with a preponderance of neutrophils. Patients often present with headache, nuchal rigidity, and changes in mental status.

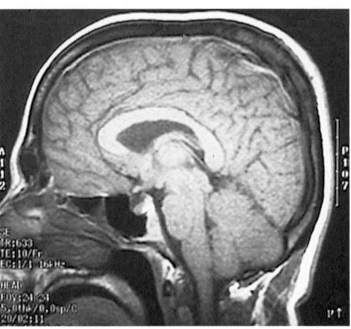

FIGURE 19–82 Acute meningitis, MRI

Seen in sagittal view is bright meningeal enhancement (▶) as a consequence of formation of an exudate covering the meninges in a case of acute bacterial meningitis from *Streptococcus pneumoniae*. The inflammation leads to dilation of meningeal vessels, causing the bright enhancement seen here. The most likely organism causing such a meningitis is age related, with *Escherichia coli* and group B streptococci seen in neonates, *Haemophilus influenzae* in children, *Neisseria meningitidis* in adolescents and young adults, and *Streptococcus pneumoniae* in older adults. Immunization has markedly reduced the incidence of *H. influenzae* and *S. pneumoniae* meningitis.

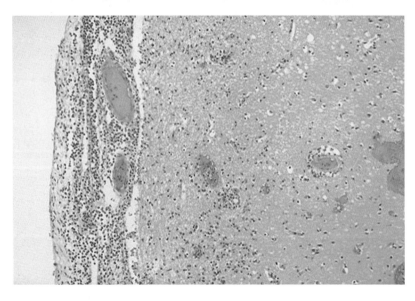

FIGURE 19–83 Acute meningitis, microscopic

A neutrophilic exudate is seen involving the meninges at the left, with prominent dilated vessels. There is edema and focal inflammation (extending down into superficial brain parenchyma through the Virchow-Robin space) in the cortex to the right. This acute meningitis is typical of a bacterial infection. This edema can lead to brain swelling with herniation and death. Resolution of infection may be followed by adhesive arachnoiditis with obliteration of the subarachnoid space leading to obstructive hydrocephalus. Diagnosis is aided by performing lumbar puncture to obtain CSF that typically shows increased leukocytes, mainly neutrophils, decreased glucose, and increased protein. Gram stain and culture can help identify specific microorganisms.

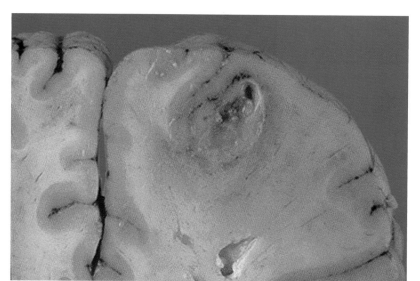

FIGURE 19–84 Cerebral abscess, gross

Here is a coronal section through superior parietal lobe showing a focal lesion with a liquefactive center containing yellow pus and surrounded by a thin wall. Cerebral abscesses usually result from hematogenous spread of a bacterial infection, typically from infective endocarditis or from pneumonitis, but may also occur from direct penetrating trauma or extension from adjacent infection in paranasal sinuses or mastoid. Patients may develop a fever along with focal but progressive neurologic deficits. The mass effect with surrounding edema can increase the intracranial pressure, with risk for herniation.

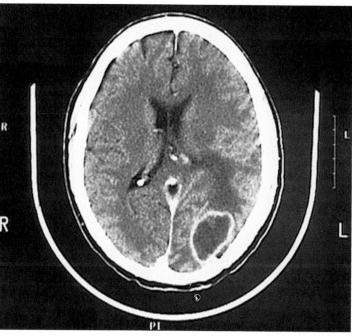

FIGURE 19–85 Cerebral abscess, CT image

This abscess of the left occipital lobe displays prominent "ring enhancement" with a bright border due to the surrounding highly vascular granulation tissue that contains many small vessels at the periphery of the abscess. Most of these cases result from staphylococcal or streptococcal infections. In addition to being destructive of brain tissue, an abscess is a mass lesion, often with surrounding edema, that can increase intracranial pressure and cause herniation. The elevated intracranial pressure may be manifested by papilledema observed on funduscopy. If safe to perform a lumbar puncture, there is usually observed an increased intracranial pressure, and examination of the CSF may show leukocytosis with neutrophilia, along with elevated protein, but often without a decrease in glucose. The abscess may be complicated by rupture and spread to cause ventriculitis, meningitis, or cerebral venous sinus thrombosis.

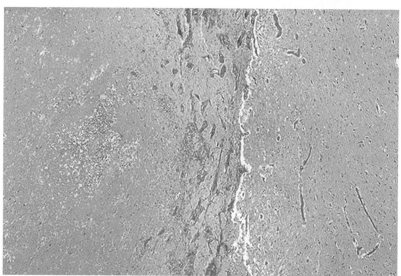

FIGURE 19–86 Cerebral abscess, microscopic

A key microscopic feature of a brain abscess, seen here with trichrome stain, is the organizing wall that contains collagenous fibrosis (the blue staining tissue) in addition to adjacent gliosis in brain. The necrotic center of the abscess is at the left and the adjacent surrounding brain at the right, with the granulation tissue in between. Patients with such an abscess can present with progressive neurologic deficits, headache, and seizures days to weeks after the initial infection. Antibiotic therapy and surgical drainage can be effective treatment options.

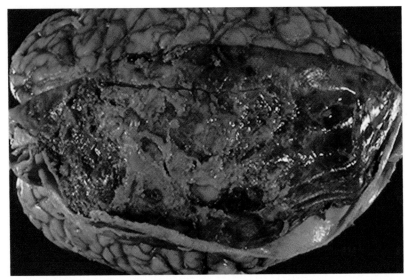

FIGURE 19–87 Subdural empyema, gross

Spread of infection to the subdural space from adjacent bone or paranasal sinuses can occur. In this case, a preexisting subdural hematoma became infected by hematogenous seeding from a pneumonia. The infection tends to remain localized, without extending to involve the meninges. However, vascular structures, including bridging cerebral veins, may be involved with thrombophlebitis, leading to venous infarction. The collection of purulent exudate or blood produces a mass effect with increased intracranial pressure. If unilateral, then papilledema may be evident on funduscopy on that side. Further clinical findings include fever, headache, and nuchal rigidity.

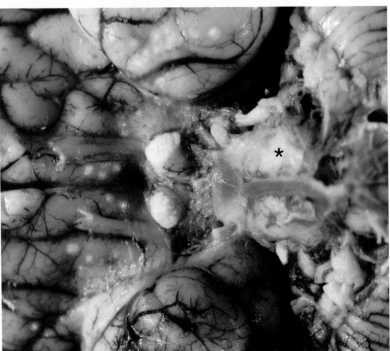

FIGURE 19–88 Tuberculous meningitis, gross

This is the typical basilar meningitis seen with tuberculous meningitis. Note the thickening of the meninges (*) over the pons. *Mycobacterium tuberculosis* infection involving the brain most often produces a meningoencephalitis, or chronic meningitis, that can lead to headache, malaise, mental confusion, and emesis. Examination of CSF obtained by lumbar puncture may show a pleocytosis marked by mononuclear cells with or without neutrophils, an elevated protein, and normal to reduced glucose. The inflammation can lead to scarring that blocks the flow of CSF through foramina of Luschka and Magendie, resulting in obstructive hydrocephalus. An obliterative endarteritis can lead to focal infarction.

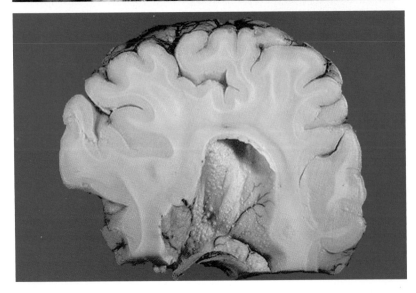

FIGURE 19–89 Neurosyphilis, gross

Note the ventricular surface studded with many ependymal granulations secondary to chronic *Treponema pallidum* infection. This nonspecific finding is seen in other infections or can be caused by chronic pressure hydrocephalus. The perivascular inflammation with abundant plasma cells and lymphocytes can cause focal ischemia with infarction. This granular ependymitis can lead to obstructive hydrocephalus. Gummatous necrosis may be seen. Affected patients may have progressive dementia (general paresis). Involvement of dorsal sensory spinal roots leads to tabes dorsalis with loss of position and pain sense, leading to ataxia and increased risk for trauma (Charcot joint).

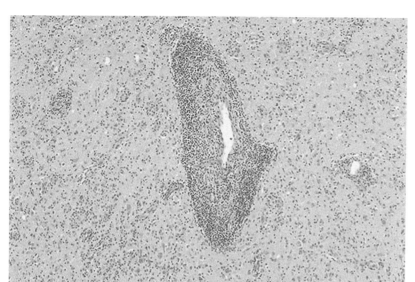

FIGURE 19–90 Viral encephalitis, microscopic

Viral infections of the brain typically involve the cortex (encephalitis), sometimes with meningeal involvement as well (meningoencephalitis). There are many viral infections that can involve the brain. Some, such as rabies virus, involve very specific areas, while others, such as echovirus, coxsackievirus, or West Nile virus, have more general involvement. Seen here are the characteristic lymphocytic infiltrates in the cortical parenchyma as well as around cerebral vessels. Patients may present with fever and altered mental status that can persist for days to weeks. Examination of CSF may show a lymphocytic pleocytosis, moderately increased protein, and normal glucose, while the Gram stain is negative.

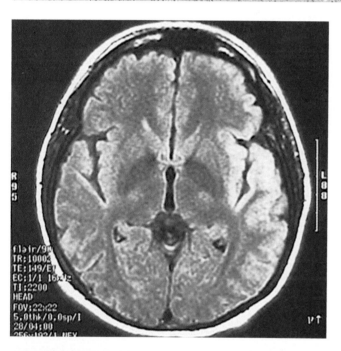

FIGURE 19–91 Viral meningoencephalitis, MRI

In this axial view, there is markedly abnormal signal hyperintensity, mainly in the left temporal lobe and adjacent insular cortex, extending to the meninges. This is consistent with a diffuse viral meningoencephalitis. A condition often called *aseptic meningitis* because bacterial organisms are not demonstrated by routine Gram stain and culture can have an acute onset, similar to a pyogenic bacterial meningitis, it is often caused by viral organisms. Some drugs, such as NSAIDs and antibiotics, may produce similar findings, termed *drug-induced aseptic meningitis*. The CSF shows a leukocytic pleocytosis, elevated protein, and normal glucose.

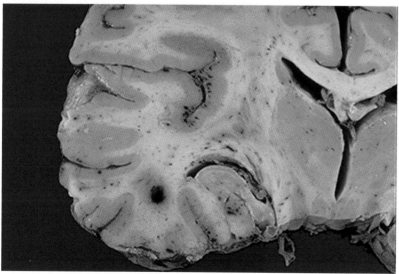

FIGURE 19–92 Herpes simplex encephalitis, gross

Herpes simplex virus (HSV) encephalitis is uncommon but distinctive. Most cases are sporadic and can even occur in immunocompetent people. A prior history of HSV infection is elicited in only 10% of patients. HSV infection of the brain often produces hemorrhages within the temporal lobe, as seen here. Like other viral infections, there are mononuclear cell infiltrates, sometimes with necrosis. Either HSV-1 or HSV-2 can produce these findings in adults, as well as in newborns as a congenital infection. Most cases of adult HSV encephalitis are caused by HSV-1, and the course may extend over 4 to 6 weeks. HSV-2 causes most perinatal cases.

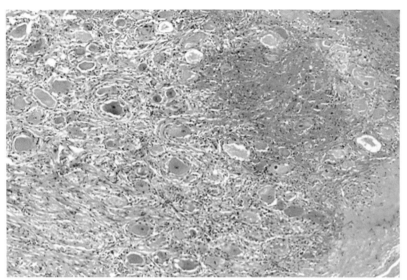

FIGURE 19–93 Varicella-zoster virus infection, microscopic

Chickenpox, a common childhood infection, is caused by the varicella-zoster virus (VZV). It is typically self-limited, but the virus persists and becomes latent in dorsal root ganglia. A postherpetic neuralgia syndrome persists in about 10% of infected people. In some patients, later in life, activation of the virus can produce the painful condition known as "shingles," seen as a vesicular eruption in a dermatome innervated by an infected ganglion in adults who have become immunocompromised. Reactivated VZV produces hemorrhagic lesions of these ganglia, as shown here. In some immunocompromised patients, acute encephalitis can occur.

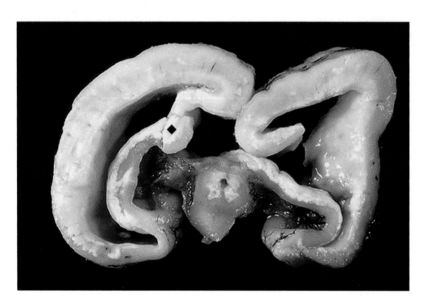

FIGURE 19–94 Congenital cytomegalovirus, gross

Cytomegalovirus (CMV) infection can be a congenital infection that may cause marked destruction of the brain by hemorrhagic necrotizing ventriculoencephalitis. Shown here at autopsy after neonatal death are many chalky white (◆) periventricular calcifications. This infant was infected with CMV *in utero*. In adults *who* are immunocompromised, such as those with HIV infection, CMV may produce a widespread encephalitis, primarily in a subependymal or periventricular distribution.

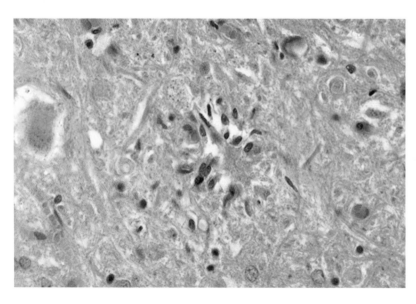

FIGURE 19–95 Poliomyelitis, microscopic

Poliovirus infection produces destruction of motor neurons along with groups of inflammatory cells in the gray matter of the cord. Neuronophagia occurs during acute poliomyelitis, seen here with a small group of inflammatory cells surrounding the remnants of an anterior horn cell. Poliomyelitis is an enterovirus that can lead to anterior horn cell loss or bulbar lower motor neuron loss during the acute stage of the disease. This results in flaccid paralysis with muscle wasting in the distribution of the affected neurons. The severity of the infection determines the degree of impairment. A postpolio syndrome with progressive weakness may occur decades after initial infection.

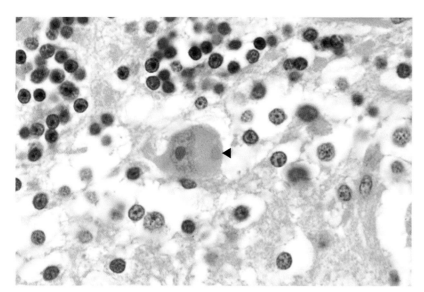

FIGURE 19–96 Rabies, microscopic

Rabies is still prevalent in parts of the world with animal reservoirs. Seen here is a Negri body (◄) within Purkinje cell cytoplasm, the most common site, but Negri bodies can also be identified within the pyramidal cells of the hippocampus. This virus travels intra-axonally from the site of the animal bite, taking 1 to 3 months to travel from peripheral sites to the CNS. Virus then spreads within the CNS to initially cause symptoms of malaise, headache, and fever, while paresthesias may persist at the site of the bite. This is followed by hyperexcitability with convulsions, pharyngeal spasm, and meningismus. Eventually, a flaccid paralysis occurs, followed by coma and death.

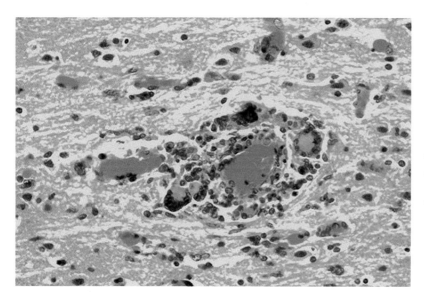

FIGURE 19–97 HIV encephalitis, microscopic

HIV infection often involves the brain through macrophages that are carried there from reservoirs of infection within lymphoid tissues. Shown here is an HIV encephalitis with a focal lesion (microglial nodule) showing perivascular multinucleated cells, which can be infected by HIV. There are few lymphocytes because of the markedly reduced number of CD4 (helper) lymphocytes with progression of HIV infection. The encephalitis can lead to progressive loss of cognitive and motor function, termed *AIDS dementia*. An aseptic meningitis may occur with acute HIV infection.

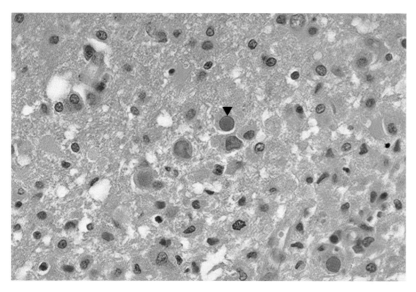

FIGURE 19–98 Progressive multifocal leukoencephalopathy, microscopic

The JC papovavirus (polyomavirus) causes progressive multifocal leukoencephalopathy (PML) in immunocompromised patients, such as those with AIDS, probably from reactivation of virus. PML appears grossly as irregular, multifocal areas of granularity in white matter, similar to the demyelinating plaques of multiple sclerosis. Microscopically, PML lesions have perivascular monocyte infiltrates, astrocytosis with bizarre or enlarged astrocytes (with occasional mitotic figures), and central lipid-laden macrophages. Seen here at the periphery of the lesions are large "ballooned" oligodendrocytes infected with JC virus that have enlarged dark pink "ground-glass" nuclei (▼) containing viral antigen.

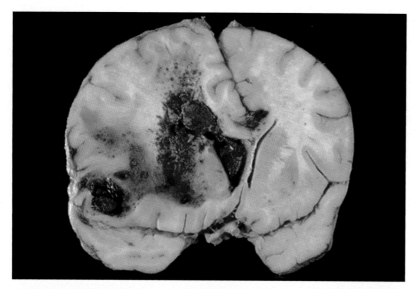

FIGURE 19–99 Aspergillosis, gross

Shown here in this coronal section of brain are focal areas of hemorrhage with prominent brain swelling and a midline shift. This resulted from a disseminated *Aspergillus* infection in an immunocompromised patient who was markedly neutropenic. The postmortem green discoloration has resulted from bile pigments (oxidized to biliverdin by formalin fixation) leaking past a blood-brain barrier destroyed by the invasive fungal hyphae. The branching, septate hyphae of *Aspergillus* are prone to cause vascular invasion with thrombosis and subsequent infarction.

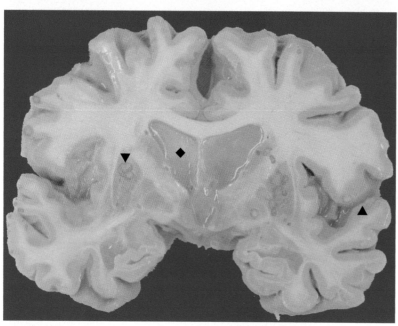

FIGURE 19–100 Cryptococcal meningitis, gross and microscopic

The coronal section shows a thick mucoid exudate within the subarachnoid space (▲), ventricles (◆), and brain parenchyma (▼) in an immunocompromised patient with *Cryptococcus neoformans* meningitis. Perivascular collections of the organisms can cause small cystic spaces within the brain. In the right panel, an India ink stain of CSF reveals the thick, clear capsule of these organisms surrounding these yeasts. The CSF may have a mild to moderate leukocytosis, an elevated protein, but decreased glucose.

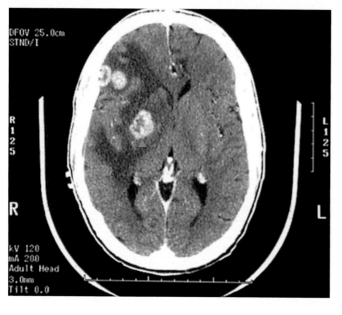

FIGURE 19–101 Toxoplasma encephalitis, CT image

Toxoplasma gondii infection can be congenital in neonates or an opportunistic infection of immunocompromised adults. This CT scan shows several ring-enhancing lesions (▲) with darker areas of surrounding edema that are typical of toxoplasmosis producing multiple abscesses in adults. The vascularity in the organizing wall of an abscess leads to the observed bright ring enhancement with CT and MRI. Congenital *Toxoplasma* infections can produce a cerebritis with multifocal cerebral necrotizing lesions that may calcify. Microscopic examination may reveal *Toxoplasma* pseudocysts containing bradyzoites, but immunohistochemical staining may be needed to identify the small free tachyzoites within the tissues.

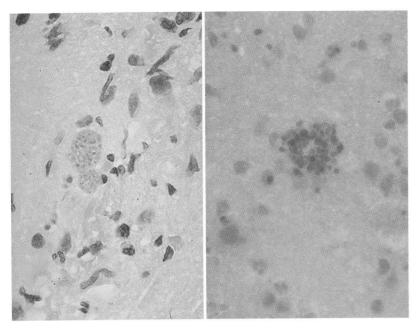

FIGURE 19–102 Toxoplasmosis, microscopic

Toxoplasma gondii infection can result in the formation of pseudocysts, which occur within an infected cell, with the cell membrane forming the cyst wall. Pseudocysts are seen here in the left panel within the cerebrum in a microglial nodule of a patient with AIDS. In the right panel, the immunohistochemical staining with antibody to *T. gondii* highlights the bradyzoites within the pseudocyst as well as adjacent free tachyzoites. The organisms become progressively harder to detect as the lesions become more chronic and organized.

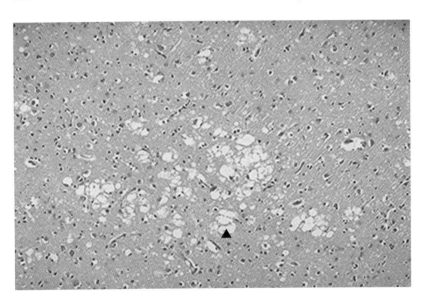

FIGURE 19–103 Creutzfeldt-Jakob disease, microscopic

The vacuoles in the cerebral cortical gray matter seen here represent a spongiform encephalopathy with Creutzfeldt-Jakob disease (CJD). As CJD progresses and neurons drop out, there is marked gliosis in response to the neuronal loss. CJD is a form of rapidly progressive dementia. It has potential for infectious spread, but cases appear sporadically. The agent of CJD is a prion protein (PrP), a neuronal cell surface sialoglycoprotein. The normal prion protein, PrP^c, can undergo conformational change to an abnormal PrP^{Sc}, which is protease resistant (PrP^{res}) and can accumulate and lead to loss of neuronal cell function, vacuolization, and death.

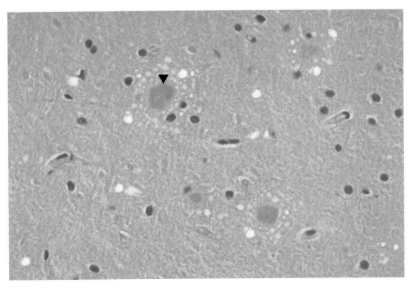

FIGURE 19–104 Variant Creutzfeldt-Jakob disease, microscopic

The relationship of bovine spongiform encephalopathy (BSE), also called *mad cow disease*, to human spongiform encephalopathy is not entirely clear. An outbreak of BSE among cattle in England in the 1980s was followed by the appearance in the 1990s of rare cases of a CJD-like illness characterized by younger age of onset, lack of characteristic EEG findings, longer course of disease, and more extensive spongiform change with plaques (▼) (seen here) compared with typical cases of CJD. These cases, known as *variant Creutzfeldt-Jakob disease* (vCJD), suggest the possibility of a relationship, and cases of vCJD continue to appear in regions where BSE was prevalent.

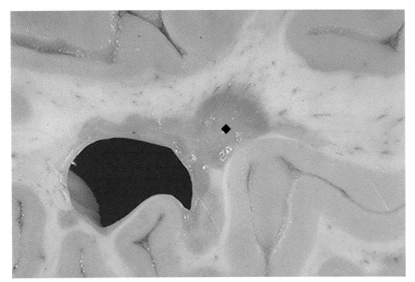

FIGURE 19–105 Multiple sclerosis, gross

Seen here in periventricular white matter is a large "plaque" (◆) of demyelination that has a sharp border with adjacent normal white matter. Such plaques have a gray-tan appearance and are typically associated with the clinical appearance of transient or progressive loss of neurologic function in multiple sclerosis (MS). Since MS is often multifocal, and the lesions appear in various white matter locations in the CNS over time, the clinical course and findings can be quite varied. The finding of chronic inflammation around MS plaques suggests an immune mechanism, and CD4+ T_H1 lymphocytes reacting against myelin antigens, with secretion of cytokines such as interferon-γ that activate macrophages, can be demonstrated.

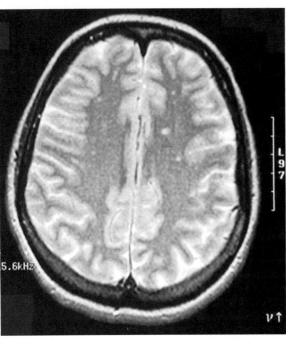

FIGURE 19–106 Multiple sclerosis, MRI

This T2-weighted MRI in axial view shows multiple bilateral small bright foci (▲) that represent areas of demyelinating plaque formation in a patient with an exacerbation of MS. White matter anywhere within the brain and spinal cord can be involved. The appearance in the CSF of an increased protein, mainly from immunoglobulin G that demonstrates oligoclonal bands on electrophoresis, is very consistent with this diagnosis. Myelin basic protein may also be present in the CSF with active demyelination. A moderate CSF pleocytosis is found in one third of cases. A common clinical finding is visual disturbance from optic neuritis. The prevalence of MS is about 1 per 1000 population in the United States and Europe. Most cases occur after adolescence and before age 50, with a female-to-male ratio of 2:1. Most patients have a relapsing and remitting course, with eventual neurologic deterioration and sensory and motor impairments.

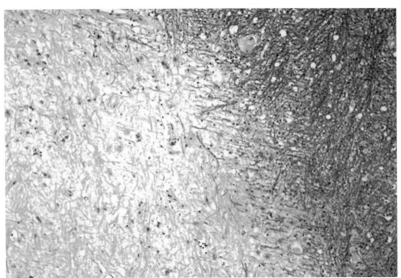

FIGURE 19–107 Multiple sclerosis, microscopic

This Luxol fast blue (LFB) stain for myelin shows lack of staining with demyelination at the left in a sharply demarcated multiple sclerosis plaque. Note the individual myelinated axons still remaining at the edge of the plaque. Axons remain relatively preserved. As the plaque becomes quiescent and inflammation decreases, astrocytes will be found in the lesion responding to the loss of myelin, and oligodendrocytes are decreased. The pale thin strands within the lesion shown here represent the remaining axons.

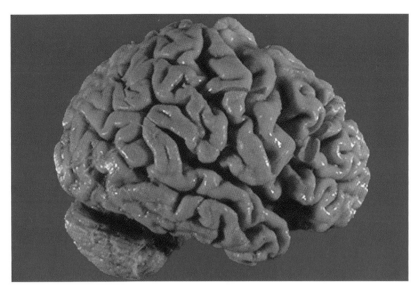

FIGURE 19–108 Alzheimer disease, gross

After removal of the meninges at autopsy, the cerebral atrophy seen here mainly involves the frontal and parietal regions, but also temporal, with relative sparing of the occipital region. This atrophy is characterized by narrowed gyri and widened sulci. This atrophy is due to Alzheimer disease (AD), the most common form of dementia in elderly people. There is a progressive decline in cognition with memory loss and eventual aphasia and immobility. The prevalence of AD increases with age, and more than 40% of people past age 85 are affected. AD is rarely symptomatic before the age of 50, except in people with Down syndrome. Up to 5% to 10% of cases are familial. The typical course from onset to death is 5 to 10 years.

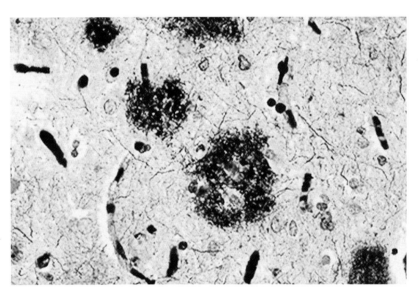

FIGURE 19–109 Alzheimer disease, microscopic

The neocortical neuritic plaques of AD are seen here with a silver stain. There are extracellular deposits of amyloid β-protein (Aβ), a peptide derived from amyloid precursor protein (APP). In the more numerous, smaller diffuse plaques, this Aβ alone is present as filamentous masses. However, the diagnostic neuritic plaques also have dystrophic dilated and tortuous neurites, microglia, and surrounding reactive astrocytes. Such plaques are most numerous in the cerebral neocortex and in the hippocampus, but the diagnosis of AD is made upon finding increased numbers of neocortical plaques for age. This form of dementia is marked mainly by progressive memory loss with increasing inability to perform activities of daily living.

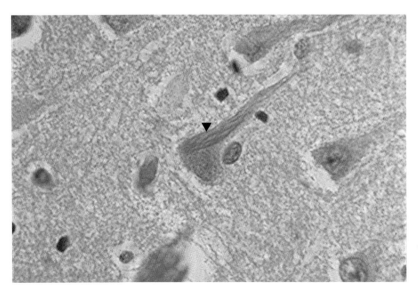

FIGURE 19–110 Alzheimer disease, microscopic

This is a neurofibrillary "tangle" of AD. The tangle (▼) appears as long pink filaments within the neuronal cytoplasm. Neurofibrillary tangles are composed of cytoskeletal intermediate filaments in the form of hyperphosphorylated microtubule-associated proteins known as tau and MAP2. Ubiquitin is also present. The major biochemical defect in AD is a loss of acetylcholine as a neurotransmitter in the cerebral cortex. Genetic defects associated with AD include mutations involving the *APP* gene on chromosome 21, the *presenilin 1* and *2* genes on chromosomes 14 and 1, respectively, and the 4 allele of the a*polipoprotein E* gene on chromosome 19.

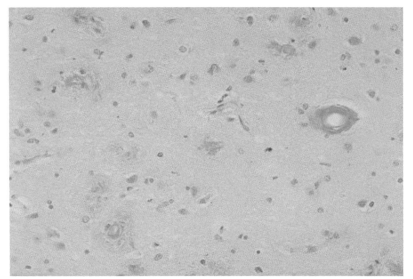

FIGURE 19–111 Alzheimer disease, microscopic

Neuritic plaques with an amyloid core in AD are seen here with Congo red stain. A small peripheral cerebral artery also shows amyloid deposition. The Aβ of AD may be deposited in cortical vessels, principally small arteries and arterioles, leading to an amyloid angiopathy. These small vessels are prone to bleed into cerebral cortex, often extending to the subarachnoid space. It is interesting to note that the gene coding for cerebral amyloid precursor protein (APP) is on chromosome 21, and people with trisomy 21 living past age 40 invariably develop AD.

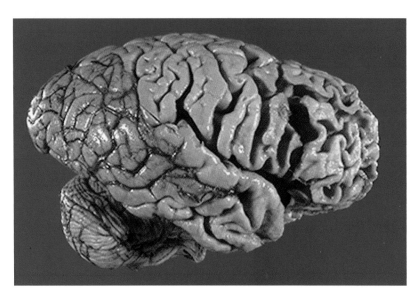

FIGURE 19–112 Pick disease, gross

The very marked frontal and temporal lobe (lobar) atrophy with knifelike thinning of the gyri seen here in a sagittal view of the brain is due to another much less common form of dementia known as *Pick disease*. Cerebral atrophy may be asymmetric. The clinical features are similar to those of Alzheimer disease, but with more pronounced behavioral changes and language disturbances. Microscopically, there is marked loss of cortical neurons with gliosis. Pick bodies, cytoplasmic inclusions that are highlighted by silver stain, are present in the neocortex. Mutations can be found in the *tau* gene, which codes for a microtubular protein associated with the Pick bodies.

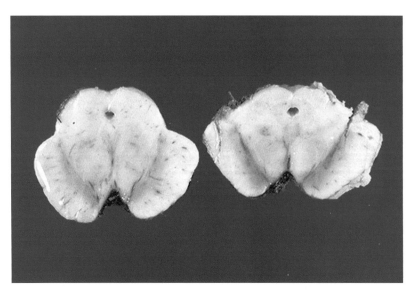

FIGURE 19–113 Parkinson disease, gross

Parkinson disease (PD) includes several conditions of different etiologies that affect primarily pigmented neuronal groups, including dopaminergic neurons within the substantia nigra. Patients usually present with movement problems such as a festinating gait, cogwheel rigidity of the limbs, poverty of voluntary movement, masklike facies, and a pill-rolling tremor at rest. Mental deterioration does not often occur, but some patients may become demented as the disease progresses. Idiopathic PD commonly begins in late middle age, and the course is slowly progressive. Note the loss of dark pigmentation in substantia nigra of the midbrain on the left, compared with normal at the right.

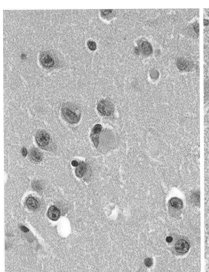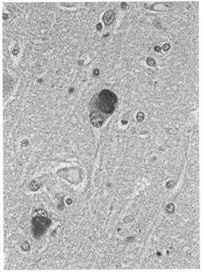

FIGURE 19–114 Lewy body disease, microscopic

About 10% to 15% of patients with parkinsonian symptoms also develop dementia, and in these patients, Lewy bodies appear in the cerebral cortex, as well as within the cytoplasm of pigmented neurons of the substantia nigra. When dementia is the primary feature, the disease can be termed *dementia with Lewy bodies* (DLB), with clinical findings similar to those of AD. For a diagnosis of DLB, the Lewy bodies must be found in the neocortex. They are homogeneous pink bodies on H+E stain, with a surrounding halo. Immunohistochemical staining with antibody to ubiquitin, as seen here, or to α-synuclein is positive in these Lewy bodies.

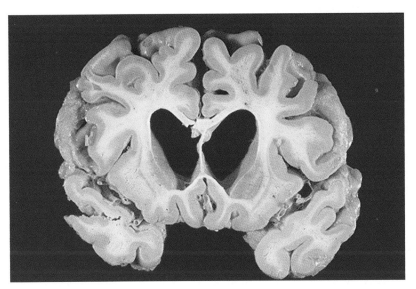

FIGURE 19–115 Huntington disease, gross

A dominant mutation in a gene on chromosome 4 encoding for a protein called huntingtin leads to a patient presentation between the ages of 20 and 50 years with choreiform movements, character change, or psychotic behavior. The abnormal gene contains increased trinucleotide CAG repeat sequences. The greater the number of repeats, the earlier the onset of the disease. Spontaneous new mutations are uncommon. There is severe loss of small neurons in caudate and putamen with reactive astrocytosis. The head of the caudate shown here has become shrunken with *ex vacuo* dilation of lateral ventricles. There is a loss of γ-aminobutyric acid (GABA), enkephalin, and substance P.

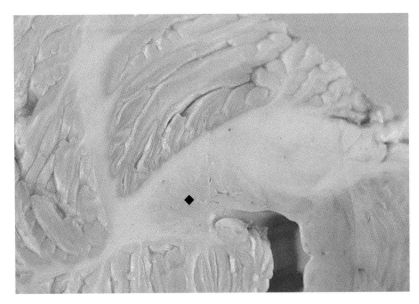

FIGURE 19–116 Friedreich ataxia, gross

This rare autosomal recessive disease has expansions of GAA trinucleotide repeats in the *frataxin* gene on chromosome 9q. Seen here is atrophy of the dentate nucleus (◆) in the cerebellum and thinning of the outflow tract. Patients also have sensory symptoms along with ataxia from loss of spinal cord posterior columns and spinocerebellar tracts. The trinucleotide repeats appear to disrupt production of the frataxin protein involved in the normal processing of iron through cellular mitochondria. Many patients die from cardiac arrhythmias or from congestive heart failure due to cardiomyopathy with inflammation and fibrosis involving cardiac muscle fibers.

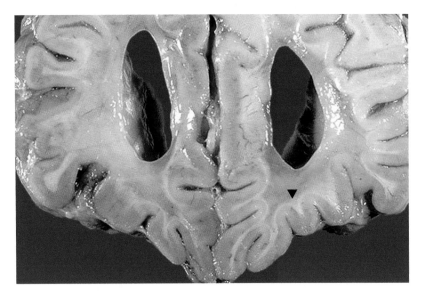

FIGURE 19–117 Metachromatic leukodystrophy, gross

Metachromatic leukodystrophy is a rare autosomal recessive white matter storage disorder caused by the deficiency of arylsulfatase A, resulting in macrophage lysosomal storage of the sphingolipid cerebroside sulfate as sulfatides that impart the metachromasia with toluidine blue stain. This lipid is abundant in myelin, and increased storage mainly affects white matter. Patients suffer from progressive demyelination causing various neurologic symptoms. The disease is fatal, and treatment is not available. In this coronal section of the frontal lobes, note the marked thinning and discoloration (▼) of the white matter, with sparing of the U fibers at the depths of sulci.

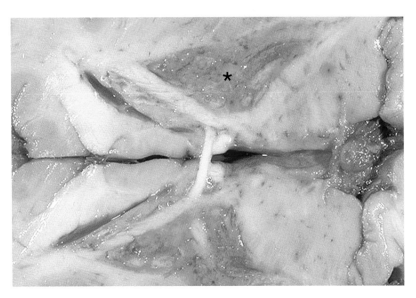

FIGURE 19–118 Leigh disease, gross

Leigh disease is a form of subacute necrotizing encephalopathy characterized by clinical findings in children of lactic acidosis, psychomotor retardation, feeding difficulties, hypotonia or weakness, and ataxia. Dystonias, tremor, chorea, and even myoclonus are also frequently found. This disorder results from abnormalities in mitochondrial oxidative phosphorylation. Both autosomal recessive and mitochondrial pattern inheritance forms of the disease occur. This axial section shows necrotic-appearing lesions (∗) in the putamen bilaterally that correspond to areas of increased signal intensity on T2-weighted MRI.

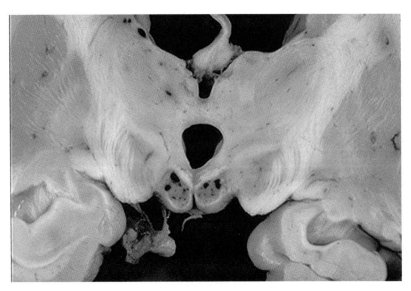

FIGURE 19–119 Wernicke disease, gross

In this coronal section of brain, the small petechial hemorrhages seen in the mammillary bodies (and also found throughout the nuclear groups of the brain stem) are characteristic of Wernicke disease, a complication of thiamine deficiency, most often seen in patients with a history of chronic alcohol abuse. The ophthalmoplegia observed in these patients can be reversed with thiamine replacement. In the chronic form of the disease, called *Korsakoff psychosis*, the mamillary bodies are atrophic. The entire spectrum of this disease is usually referred to as *Wernicke-Korsakoff syndrome*.

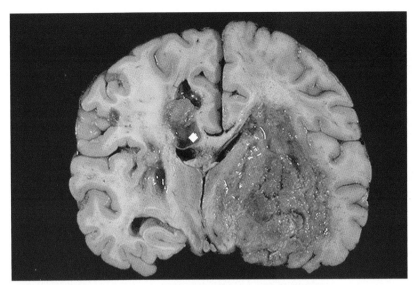

FIGURE 19–120 Glioblastoma multiforme, gross

Gliomas account for more than 80% of all primary brain tumors in adults. Most are located above the tentorium and within the cerebral hemispheres. They are poorly circumscribed. Seen here is the worst form of glioma—a glioblastoma multiforme (GBM). Note in this coronal section that this large mass has extensive necrosis and extends across the cerebral midline (◆) to the opposite hemisphere. Patients may initially present with a new-onset seizure disorder, with headaches, or with focal neurologic deficits. Although this neoplasm is highly aggressive within the brain, metastases outside the CNS are rare.

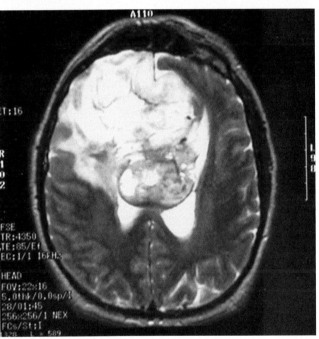

FIGURE 19–121 Glioblastoma multiforme, MRI

This T2-weighted MRI in axial view demonstrates a large GBM involving much of the right anterior cerebral hemisphere. The brightly enhancing tumor is variegated and has central necrosis, edema, and an irregular border. It crosses the midline by the corpus callosum and extends into the opposite cerebral hemisphere. Such a tumor is not resectable, although radiation and chemotherapy may add months to patient survival. Gliomas may begin as low-grade neoplasms that often have *p53* tumor suppressor gene inactivating mutations, and as they progress to higher-grade lesions such as GBM, there is *PDGF-A* amplification, a pattern termed *secondary glioblastoma*, most likely to occur in younger patients. In contrast, the primary glioblastoma pattern in older individuals does not arise in a lower-grade glioma and is characterized by genetic defects, including *EGFR* gene amplification, *MDM2* overexpression, *p16* deletion, or *PTEN* mutation.

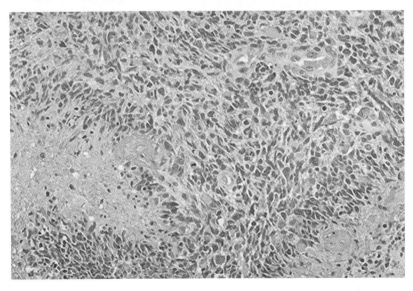

FIGURE 19–122 Glioblastoma multiforme, microscopic

This GBM is highly cellular with marked hyperchromatism and pleomorphism. Note the prominent vascularity as well as the area of necrosis at the left, with neoplastic cells palisading around it. This pseudopalisading necrosis is characteristic of GBM. The cells of a GBM can infiltrate widely, particularly along white matter tracts, and even through the CSF.

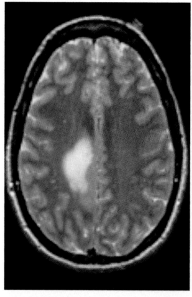
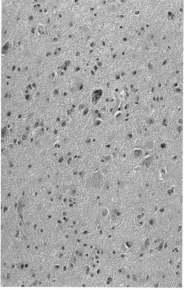

FIGURE 19–123 Astrocytoma, MRI and microscopic

A diffuse fibrillary astrocytoma is a form of glioma that is lower grade and not as extensively invasive as a GBM, but it is still not a discrete mass, as seen in the T2-weighted axial MRI in the left panel. These gliomas tend to enhance brightly because of their abnormal vascularity. In the right panel, this astrocytoma demonstrates increased cellularity and pleomorphism, as compared with normal brain, but far less than a GBM. Note the very pleomorphic cell at the top center. The clinical course may be slowly progressive for years, but astrocytomas have a tendency to become more anaplastic with time as genetic alterations accumulate within the neoplastic cells, and then more rapid deterioration ensues.

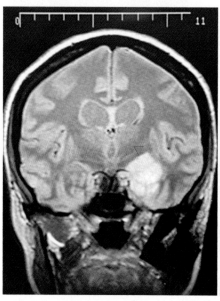
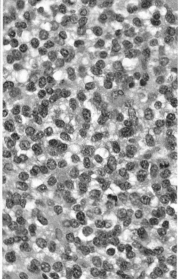

FIGURE 19–124 Oligodendroglioma, MRI and microscopic

This enhanced MRI in coronal view shows an oligodendroglioma (▼) within the left temporal lobe. This type of glioma tends to be well circumscribed, with cystic areas and focal calcification. It enhances as a result of the rich vascular network of anastomosing capillaries within the tumor. Oligodendrogliomas constitute about 5% to 15% of all gliomas; they typically occur within the cerebral hemispheres, usually in white matter, of adults in their 30s and 40s. Typical oligodendrogliomas have round blue nuclei with clear cytoplasm. Most have cytogenetic abnormalities involving chromosomes 1p and 19q. They tend to be slowly progressive over years and can have a better prognosis than other gliomas.

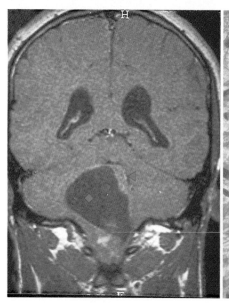
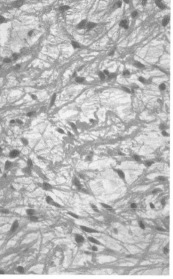

FIGURE 19–125 Juvenile pilocytic astrocytoma, MRI and microscopic

The coronal MRI in the left panel shows a large cerebellar cyst (♦) with a small mural nodule (◄). This is the typical appearance of a juvenile pilocytic astrocytoma, which most often occurs in children below the tentorium in sites such as the cerebellum. It may also occur in optic nerves, floor of the third ventricle, or cerebral hemispheres. These are low-grade astrocytic tumors that are slow growing, are minimally infiltrative, and have a very good prognosis after surgical removal. Seen in the right panel are microcystic change and pilocytic cells with long thin processes that stain immunohistochemically, like those of other gliomas, with glial fibrillary acidic protein (GFAP).

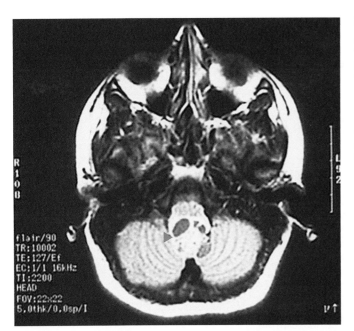

FIGURE 19–126 Ependymoma, CT image

A discrete, bright mass (▶) with cystic areas fills the fourth ventricle in this CT scan of the head. This is the most common site of an ependymoma in children. This neoplasm arises from the ependymal lining cells. Enlargement of the tumor with blockage of the CSF flow in the fourth ventricle may produce hydrocephalus. Although ependymomas tend not to be invasive, they can spread into the CSF and can be difficult to eradicate. In adults, most ependymomas are found within the spinal cord, and some are associated with neurofibromatosis type 2.

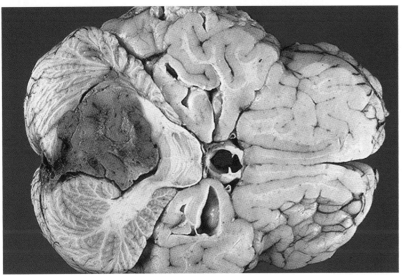

FIGURE 19–127 Ependymoma, gross

This horizontal (axial) section of the brain reveals a large reddish ependymoma with discrete borders that is filling and expanding the fourth ventricle. Ependymomas are usually slow-growing neoplasms, but their location within the fourth ventricle makes complete removal difficult, so the overall prognosis at this location is poor.

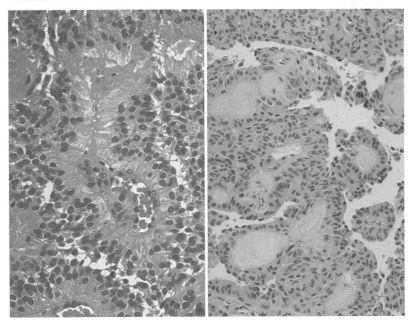

FIGURE 19–128 Ependymoma, microscopic

The microscopic appearance in the left panel of an ependymoma from the fourth ventricle reveals a rosette pattern with the tumor cells arranged around a central vascular space (perivascular pseudorosette). The ependymal processes will stain positively for GFAP. In the right panel is a myxopapillary ependymoma that typically arises in the filum terminale of the spinal cord of an adult. Note that the cuboidal tumor cells are arranged around papillations that have a myxoid connective tissue core.

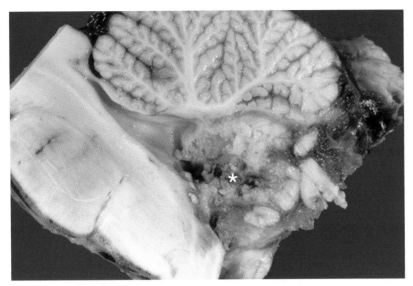

FIGURE 19–129 Medulloblastoma, gross

This sagittal section shows an irregular posterior fossa mass (∗) arising near the midline of the cerebellum and extending into the fourth ventricle above the brain stem. A medulloblastoma is one of the "small round blue cell" tumors, and it most often occurs in children. These highly malignant tumors commonly spread into the subarachnoid space and seed by the CSF into the spinal canal. Cytogenetic alterations involving chromosome 17 are common in this tumor.

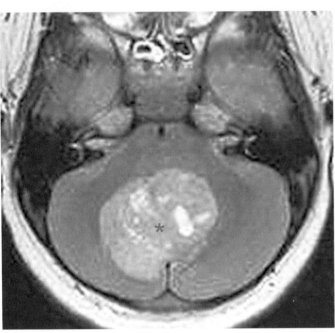

FIGURE 19–130 Medulloblastoma, CT image

This axial MRI through the posterior fossa shows an irregular, variegated mass (∗) with some enhancement arising within the cerebellum. Medulloblastomas occur in the cerebellar vermis in children, where they can occlude the fourth ventricle to cause hydrocephalus. In older patients, these tumors more commonly arise within the cerebellar hemispheres. About 30% of medulloblastomas occur in patients between the age of 15 and 35. Two thirds are found in patients younger than 15 years.

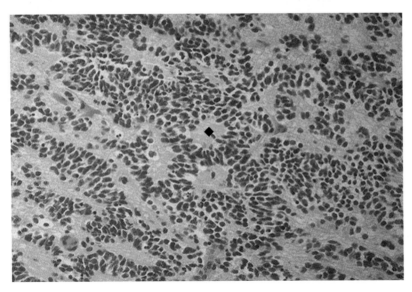

FIGURE 19–131 Medulloblastoma, microscopic

There are poorly differentiated small round blue cells with scant cytoplasm and hyperchromatic nuclei. These cells form rosettes (◆) (called *Homer Wright rosettes*). This is a histologically malignant neoplasm, and mitotic figures are often present in abundance. The location often makes it difficult to resect completely. Although aggressive, this tumor is radiosensitive.

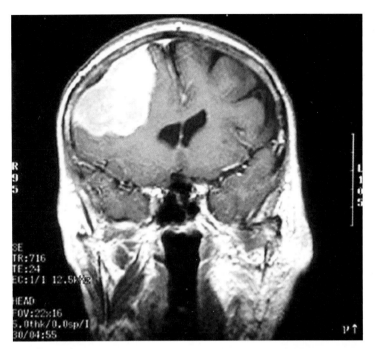

◄ **FIGURE 19–132 Meningioma, MRI**

This MRI in coronal view demonstrates bright enhancement of a meningioma arising in the parasagittal region over the right frontal lobe. Meningiomas often act in a benign manner, growing very slowly, and thus are rarely associated with herniation. The most common locations for a meningioma are parasagittal convexity, lateral convexity, sphenoid wing, olfactory groove beneath the frontal lobe, sella turcica, and foramen magnum. Less commonly, they arise within the ventricular system.

▼ **FIGURES 19–133 and 19–134 Meningioma, gross**

Note how each of these meningiomas beneath the dura has compressed the underlying cerebral hemisphere. These neoplasms, which arise from arachnoid cap cells, are typically well-circumscribed masses that are amenable to resection. Rarely, meningiomas can be more aggressive and invade the underlying brain.

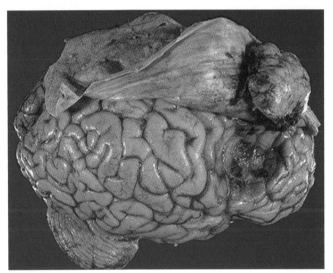

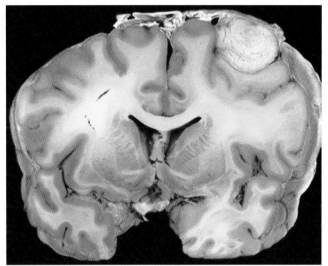

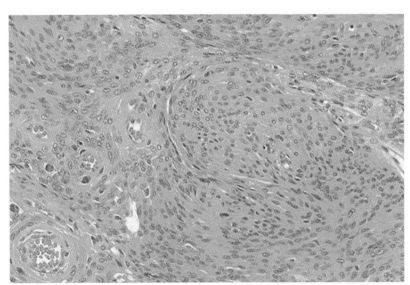

◄ **FIGURE 19–135 Meningioma, microscopic**

Meningiomas exhibit many different microscopic patterns. Here the cells are arranged in a tight, whorled pattern, with oval nuclei containing dispersed chromatin, giving them an open and vesicular appearance. Meningiomas may also contain psammoma bodies or fibroblastic elements. Some meningiomas, particularly when multiple, occur with neurofibromatosis type 2, and sporadic meningiomas often have a mutation involving the *NF2* gene on the 22q chromosome. Atypical meningiomas have a higher mitotic index, increased cellularity, and increased nuclear/cytoplasmic ratio; they are associated with local invasion and increased risk for recurrence after resection. Meningiomas are uncommon in children. The female-to-male ratio is 3 : 2.

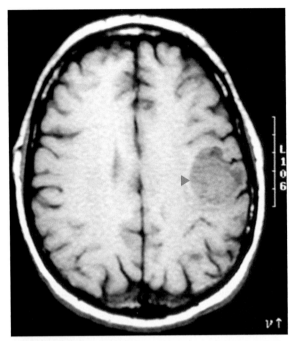

FIGURE 19–136 Metastasis, MRI

This axial T1-weighted MRI shows a solitary peripheral brain mass (▶) with minimal adjacent edema located in the cortex near the gray-white junction. This lesion in a middle-aged man proved to be a metastasis from a pulmonary bronchogenic carcinoma, the most common primary site of brain metastases. Lung, breast, melanoma, kidney, and gastrointestinal tract primaries account for 80% of all metastases to the brain. In some cases, more specific patterns are observed, such as meningeal carcinomatosis. In some cases, the metastases become clinically apparent before the primary site is discovered.

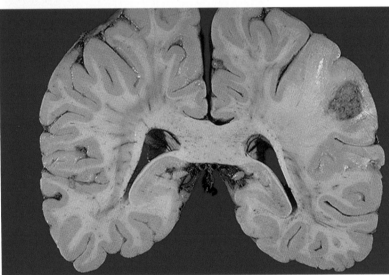

FIGURE 19–137 Metastasis, gross

In this coronal section of brain, there is a red-brown mass located at the gray-white junction. This proved to be a metastasis from a renal cell carcinoma of the kidney. A solitary brain mass in an adult can be either primary or metastatic. The borders of a metastasis tend to be more discrete than those of a primary glioma. A biopsy may be required to tell the difference.

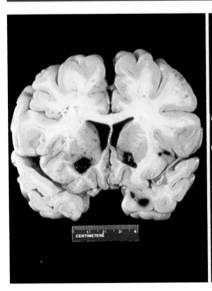
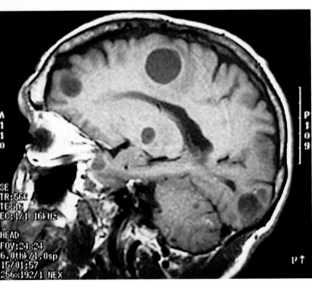

FIGURE 19–138 Metastases, gross and MRI

Multiple tumor masses, as shown here, suggest metastases, rather than a primary neoplasm. In the left panel are darkly pigmented metastases from a malignant melanoma, with the corresponding sagittal MRI showing multiple cerebral masses in the right panel.

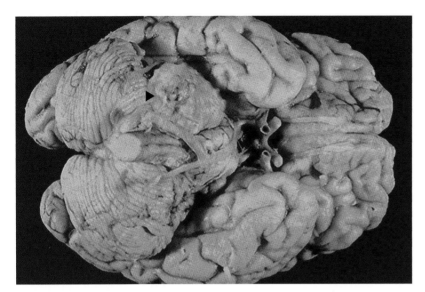

FIGURE 19–139 Schwannoma, gross

In this view of the base of the brain, there is a mass lesion (▶) arising in the vestibular branch of the eighth cranial nerve at the cerebellopontine angle on the right. This is best termed a *schwannoma* (a so-called acoustic neuroma). Patients often present with hearing loss or tinnitus. Other intracranial sites of involvement can include branches of the trigeminal nerve and dorsal roots. These benign neoplasms can be removed. Extradural schwannomas tend to arise in large peripheral nerve trunks. Some cases are associated with neurofibromatosis type 2.

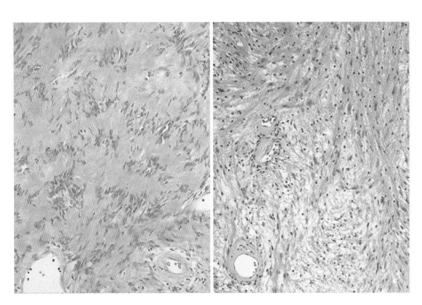

FIGURE 19–140 Schwannoma, microscopic

These are the classic microscopic appearances of a benign schwannoma. Note the more cellular "Antoni A" pattern in the left panel with palisading nuclei surrounding pink areas (Verocay bodies). Shown in the right panel is the "Antoni B" pattern with a looser stroma, fewer cells, and myxoid change. *NF2* gene mutations are typically present in the sporadic occurrences of this neoplasm. Immunohistochemical staining for S100 protein is usually positive in these cells.

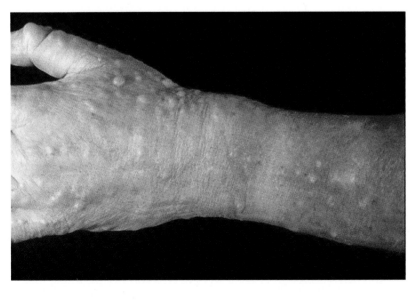

FIGURE 19–141 Neurofibromatosis, gross

Seen here are multiple nodules on the skin surface of the forearm and hand of a patient with neurofibromatosis type I (NF1). There is loss of function of the *NF1* tumor suppressor gene and its protein product neurofibromin, which has a guanosine triphosphatase-activating protein function. The yellow-orange staining of the skin is povidone-iodine (Betadine) solution applied in surgery (this is an amputation specimen) because a neurofibrosarcoma was present in the deep soft tissue of the wrist. The presence of pale brown macules on the skin, known as *café-au-lait spots*, particularly when there are six or more of these spots that are 1.5 cm or larger, is highly indicative of NF1.

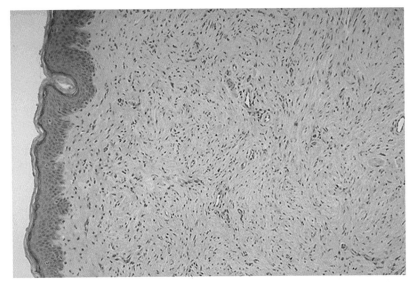

FIGURE 19–142 Neurofibroma, microscopic

The skin overlying a cutaneous neurofibroma may show some hyperpigmentation, but the actual lesion is in the dermis. This most common type of neurofibroma consists of bundles of wavy, elongated spindle cells with small, dark, oblong nuclei and a lot of intervening pink collagen. This lesion is benign and may occur sporadically or in association with NF1. Patients with NF1 may develop the plexiform type of neurofibroma in large nerve trunks. With NF1, there is an increased risk for development of malignant neoplasms, including malignant degeneration of neurofibromas, malignant peripheral nerve sheath tumors, and gliomas.

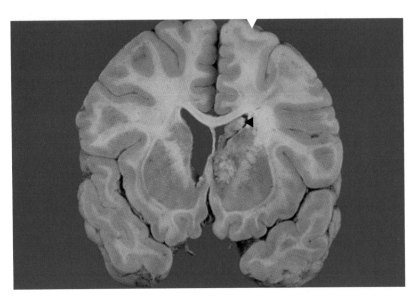

FIGURE 19–143 Tuberous sclerosis, gross

Tuberous sclerosis (TS), or Bourneville disease, is an autosomal dominant condition with an estimated frequency of 1 in 10,000. Neoplasms seen with TS include hamartomatous growths and low-grade neoplasms in a variety of organs, including facial angiofibromas, cerebral cortical tubers, subependymal nodules, giant cell astrocytomas, retinal glial hamartomas and astrocytomas, cardiac rhabdomyomas, renal angiomyolipomas, and subungual fibromas. This coronal section of brain from a patient with TS shows a superior cortical tuber (▼). Note the grayish discoloration in the area of the tuber. There are calcified subependymal glial nodules (◄) seen by the lateral ventricle.

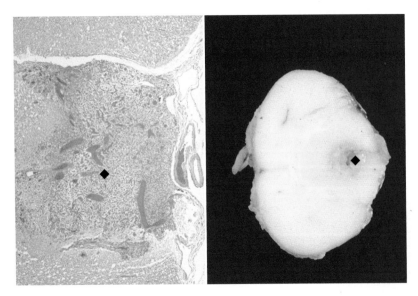

FIGURE 19–144 Hemangioblastoma, microscopic and gross

The axial section of cervical spinal cord in the right panel shows a small dorsal mass (♦) that in the left panel consists of abundant capillaries with intervening stromal cells. Hemangioblastomas may occur sporadically (usually in the cerebellum) or as part of von Hippel–Lindau (VHL) disease, an autosomal dominant condition with a frequency of 1 in 40,000. About 10% of hemangioblastomas are associated with polycythemia. The *VHL* gene acts as a tumor suppressor. The typical neoplasms developing in association with VHL disease are hemangioblastomas, pheochromocytomas, retinal angiomas (often similar histologically to hemangioblastomas), cystadenomas, and renal cell carcinomas.

CHAPTER 20

The Eye

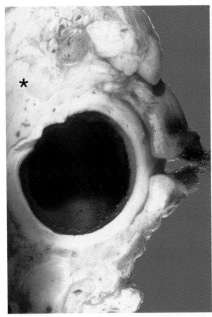
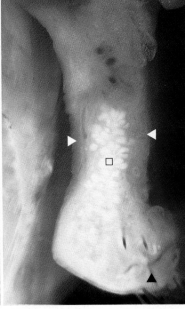

FIGURE 20–1 Normal eye, gross

A sagittal section through the orbit is seen in the left panel, with the relationship of the eyeball to the eyelid apparatus. Note that the orbit in which the eyeball is located contains adipose tissue (*). In the right panel is a closer sagittal view of the upper eyelid. The outer squamous epithelial covering of skin (◄) is at the right. Beneath this are connective tissue and the palpebral part of the orbicularis oculi muscle. Then there is a dense plate of connective tissue called the *tarsus* (□), beneath which to the left are the meibomian glands (►), which secrete fluids forming the tear film. Eyelashes (▲) are seen at the lower right margin of the eyelid.

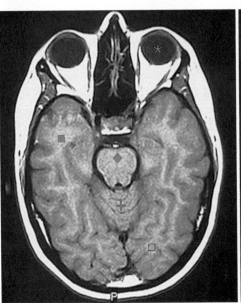
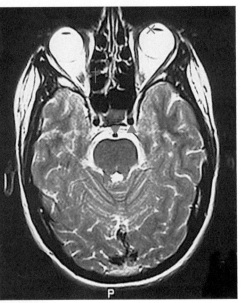

FIGURE 20–2 Normal eyes and orbits, MRIs

Normal axial MRIs (T1 in the left panel, with fat having the brightest attenuation, and T2 in the right panel, with fluid the brightest) demonstrate the temporal lobe (■) and occipital lobe (□), basilar artery (▼), internal carotid artery (▲), basis pontis (◆), aqueduct of Sylvius (►), cerebellar vermis (+), ethmoid sinus (†), pituitary (◄), globe of eye (*), and lens of eye (×).

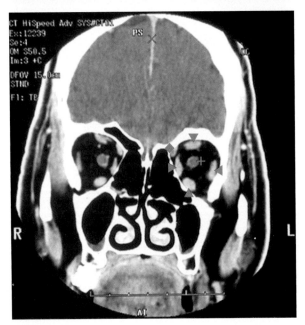

FIGURE 20–3 Normal eye, CT image

This is a normal sinus CT image demonstrating structures in the orbit, including optic nerve (+), superior rectus muscle (▼), superior oblique muscle (◆), medial rectus muscle (►), inferior rectus and inferior oblique muscles (▲), and lateral rectus muscle (◄) in the anterior skull. Within the cranial cavity above are the right and left frontal lobes divided by the falx cerebri (×).

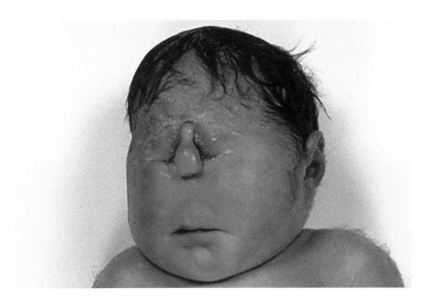

FIGURE 20–4 Cyclopia, gross

This infant with trisomy 13 (Patau syndrome) has cyclopia (single eye) with a proboscis (the projecting tissue just above the eye). The "eye" often consists of nothing more than a slitlike space without a globe. Other ocular anomalies with trisomy 13 when a globe is present may include colobomas, cataracts, persistent hyperplastic primary vitreous, and retinal dysplasia.

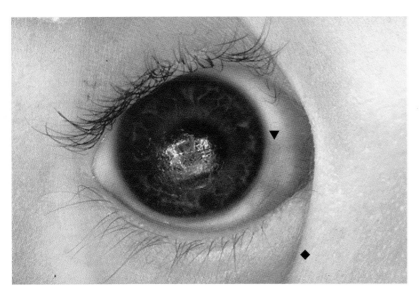

FIGURE 20–5 Trisomy 21, gross

This is a prominent epicanthal fold (◆) adjacent to the eye. Also present is a Brushfield spot (▼). Other ocular findings that can be present with Down syndrome (trisomy 21) include hypertelorism, keratoconus, and oblique palpebral fissures.

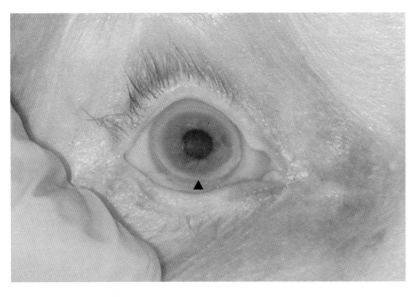

FIGURE 20–6 Arcus senilis, gross

The thin white ring (▲) around the periphery of the cornea seen here is a condition known as *arcus senilis*, or *arcus lipoides*. This is a finding seen with aging in some people and has no pathologic significance. It is due to increased lipid deposition in the periphery of the cornea and thus may appear with hyperlipidemia.

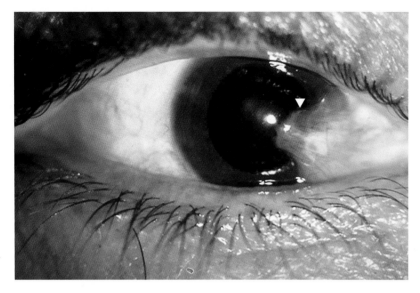

FIGURE 20–7 Pterygium, gross

A pterygium is composed of fibrovascular connective tissue encroaching (▼) onto the cornea, which can interfere somewhat with vision, but does not cause blindness, since the process does not cross the midline. In contrast, a pinguecula would be found only on the conjunctiva. The appearance of this raised, whitish yellow lesion is associated with advancing age and is thought to be the result of environmental or solar exposure with solar elastosis over a lifetime. Inflammation induced within a pinguecula by a foreign body in the eye can produce an actinic granuloma.

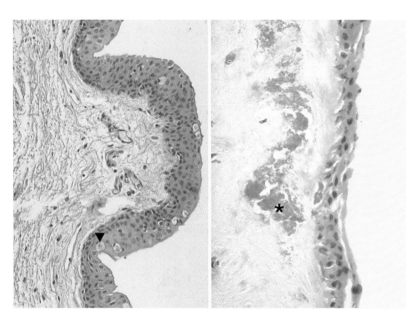

FIGURE 20–8 Normal conjunctiva and pterygium, microscopic

The appearance of normal conjunctival epithelium is shown in the left panel. The conjunctiva forms the mucus membrane of the eyelid, extending posteriorly to the tarsal plate and around the fornix to form the bulbar conjunctiva that extends to the cornea. Note the scattered goblet cells (▼) in this stratified epithelium. At the right is a pterygium. Beneath the thinned conjunctival epithelium is an area of elastosis (*) with basophilic degeneration of the substantia propria collagen.

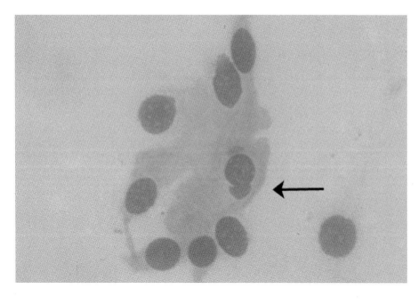

FIGURE 20–9 Trachoma, microscopic

This conjunctival scraping from the eye, with Giemsa stain, reveals an intracytoplasmic elementary body of *Chlamydia trachomatis*. This finding is typical of trachoma, which is a chronic, progressive infection of the upper tarsal plate that produces scarring of the conjunctiva and cornea through inversion of the upper eyelid to direct the eyelashes inward (trichiasis), a process that eventually may lead to partial or complete blindness. In contrast, chlamydial infection acquired by passage through the birth canal can produce a purulent conjunctivitis known as *inclusion blennorrhea*. In children and adults, inclusion conjunctivitis results from limited conjunctival inflammation with *C. trachomatis*.

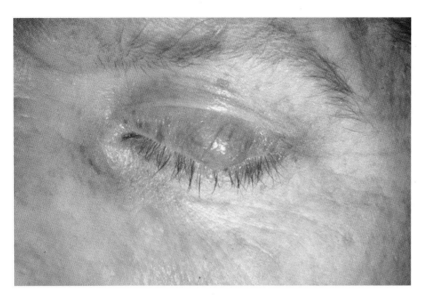

FIGURE 20–10 Chalazion, gross

This localized swelling involves the upper eyelid. A chalazion forms when plugging of a duct from meibomian glands leads to chronic lipogranulomatous inflammation. This is an irritating, but benign, process. A recurrent chalazion should undergo biopsy to rule out the possibility of a sebaceous carcinoma.

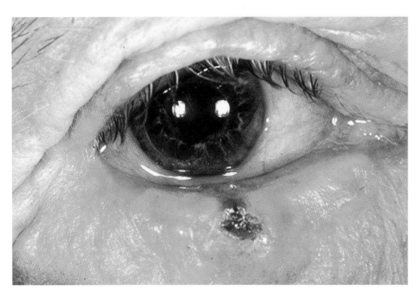

FIGURE 20–11 Basal cell carcinoma, gross

There is a small nodule with central ulceration at the edge of the lower eyelid. This is the most common malignant neoplasm of the eyelid, and it arises in the setting of sun damage from chronic ultraviolet light exposure. The nodule has a central rounded ulceration and raised pink margins. A basal cell carcinoma is slow growing, but in this location, it presents a problem in removal because adequate margins are needed to prevent recurrence, while enough eyelid must be preserved to be functional.

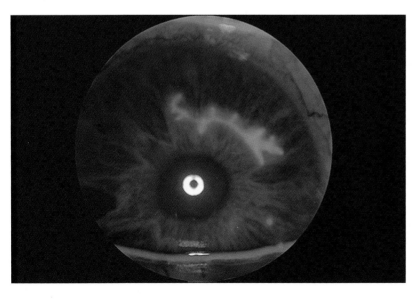

FIGURE 20–12 Herpetic keratitis, gross

Fluorescein dye has been placed onto the surface of the eye, and this is the appearance of the cornea seen by slit-lamp examination under fluorescent light. The dye is collecting at the top and bottom conjunctival margins. The lesion seen is a dendritic ulceration of the corneal epithelium, which is a coalescence of smaller punctate ulcerations. Such a dendritic ulcer is characteristic of infection with herpes simplex virus. Herpetic keratitis is a serious infection because it can be recurrent and can penetrate through the cornea to involve the stroma.

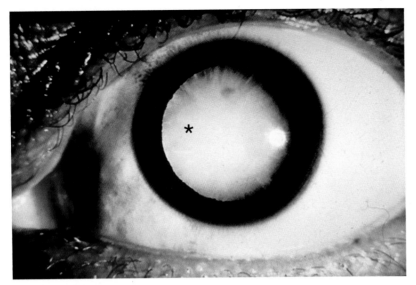

FIGURE 20–13 Cataract, gross

An opacification (∗) of the crystalline lens results from a series of events starting in the lens cortex with rarefaction, then liquefaction, of cortical cells. This leads to fragmentation of lens fibers and extracellular globule formation. In the lens nucleus, there is a progressive increase in the amount of insoluble proteins, which leads to hardening (sclerosis) and brownish discoloration (brunescence). Cataracts are more common in elderly people and those with diabetes mellitus. Such cataracts can be removed and replaced by a lens implant.

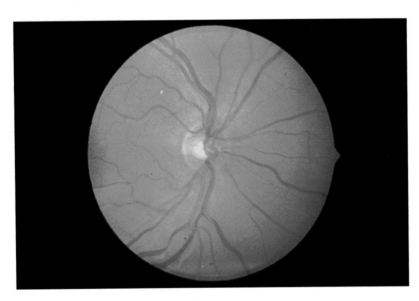

FIGURE 20–14 Normal retina, funduscopy

Here is the normal funduscopic appearance of the retina. Note the arteries (brighter red) emanating from the central optic disk. The larger-caliber and darker retinal veins extend back to the optic disc. These vessels are evenly distributed. Note that the margins of the optic disc are sharp and clear. The normal posterior chamber vitreous is avascular. With aging, liquefaction and collapse of the vitreous can lead to "floaters" in the field of vision.

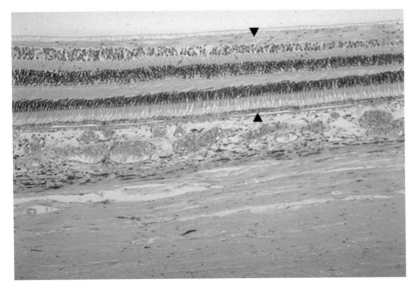

FIGURE 20–15 Normal retina, microscopic

The normal histologic appearance of the retina shows many layers. The lowest layer just above the retinal pigment (▲) epithelium (RPE) and supporting connective tissue is the layer of rods and cones (photoreceptors). Above this are layers of external and internal plexiform and nuclear lamina. The nerve fibers (▼) are at the top and collect together to enter the optic nerve at the optic disc. The RPE aids in maintenance of the photoreceptors, and disturbances of this interface may occur with inherited forms of retinitis pigmentosa.

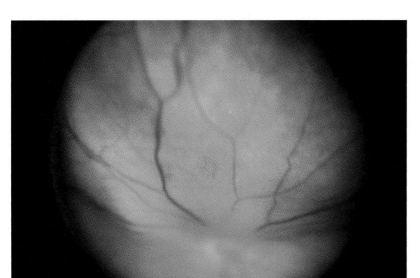

FIGURE 20–16 Ocular melanoma, funduscopy

Bearing a passing resemblance to Jupiter's moon Io is this funduscopic view with an intraocular melanoma that is producing discoloration and bulging underneath the retina on funduscopy. An ocular melanoma usually arises within the pigmented choroidal layer. Melanoma is the most common intraocular neoplasm of adulthood.

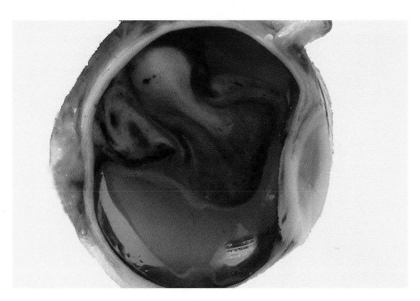

FIGURE 20–17 Ocular melanoma, gross

This cross-section of an enucleated eye shows a darkly pigmented mass extending into the vitreous. This is a choroidal melanoma. Most noncutaneous melanomas arise in the eye. The melanoma may sometimes breach the sclera and invade into orbital soft tissues. The expansion of the melanoma may lead to retinal detachment with sudden visual loss.

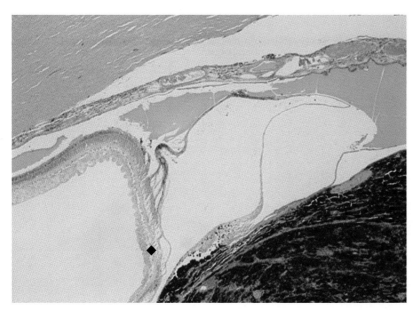

FIGURE 20–18 Ocular melanoma, microscopic

A darkly pigmented mass, a choroidal melanoma, is seen at the lower right, beneath the detached retina (◆). In the eye, unlike the skin, it is the lateral extent of growth, not the depth, that is the greatest factor determining prognosis. Since there are no intraocular lymphatic channels, the spread of this neoplasm from the eye typically occurs initially through the scleral vascular channels, and hematogenous metastases can then occur. The liver is the most common site of distant metastases.

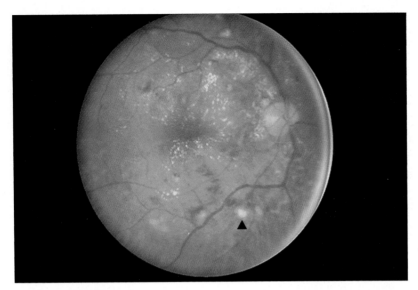

FIGURE 20–19 Diabetic retinopathy, funduscopy

Note the extensive hard exudates (▲), typical of the "background retinopathy" of diabetes mellitus. The microangiopathy that occurs with diabetes mellitus is associated with edema and retinal exudates that are "soft" microinfarcts or "hard" yellowish waxy exudates, which are deposits of plasma proteins and lipids. These hard exudates are more a feature of older people with type II diabetes mellitus. Additional findings with background retinopathy include capillary microaneurysms, dot and blot hemorrhages, flame-shaped hemorrhages, and cotton-wool spots (soft exudates).

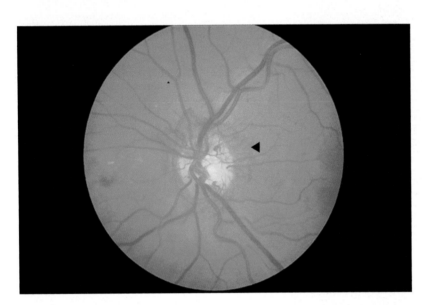

FIGURE 20–20 Diabetic retinopathy, funduscopy

Neovascularization with diabetic "proliferative retinopathy" is shown here. Note the proliferation (◄) of small vessels near the optic disc. These delicate new vessels grow toward the vitreous humor. They are prone to bleed, producing vitreal hemorrhages that obscure vision. A proliferation of fibrovascular and glial tissue ensues, and when this abnormal tissue contracts, there is a risk for retinal detachment. Involvement of the macula by this process markedly diminishes vision. Diabetic proliferative retinopathy may appear after more than 10 years of poorly or uncontrolled hyperglycemia.

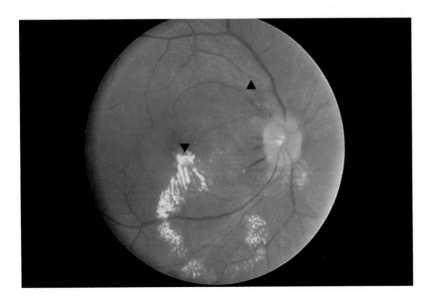

FIGURE 20–21 Hypertensive retinopathy, funduscopy

Seen here is retinal arteriolar narrowing (▲). There are also cotton-wool spots (▼), which represent microinfarcts of the nerve fiber layer. Additional findings with hypertension can include flame-shaped hemorrhages into the retinal nerve fiber layer and papilledema. Other findings may include hard (waxy) exudates.

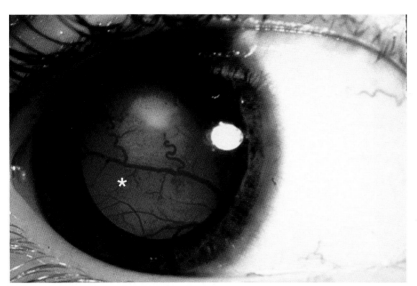

FIGURE 20–22 Retinoblastoma, funduscopy

This is leukocoria, or "white pupil," (∗) caused by the presence of a mass lesion—a retinoblastoma. This is the most common intraocular neoplasm of childhood. Retinoblastomas arise as a consequence of mutations in the Rb tumor suppressor gene and are a classic example of a neoplasm arising from a "two-hit" genetic defect. If the patient inherits one mutated allele (the Rb gene on chromosome 13), either by a point mutation or by deletion of the locus q14 on chromosome 13, then the other allele is typically lost in childhood and a retinoblastoma develops. Such people are at risk for retinoblastoma arising in the other eye as well as additional neoplasms, such as osteosarcoma.

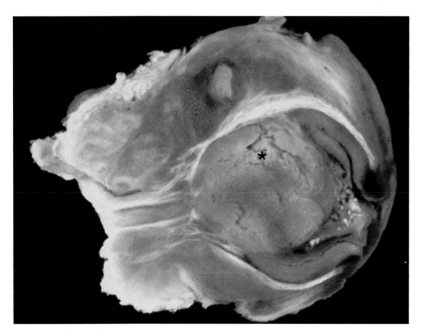

FIGURE 20–23 Retinoblastoma, gross

This sagittal section of an enucleated eye demonstrates a large white mass (∗) pushing into the vitreous and filling most of the globe. This produces the appearance known as "white pupil" (leukocoria) on funduscopic examination. Sporadic, nonfamilial cases represent about 30% to 40% of retinoblastomas, and these patients are not at risk for bilateral retinoblastoma or other neoplasms. In familial cases, there is inheritance of an abnormal *Rb* tumor suppressor gene.

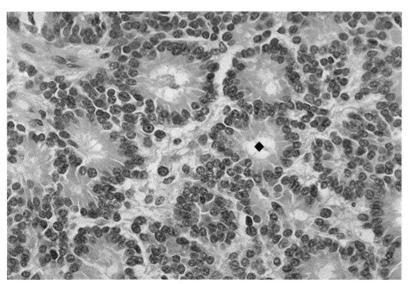

FIGURE 20–24 Retinoblastoma, microscopic

Retinoblastoma is one of the "small blue cell tumors" of childhood. The characteristic microscopic pattern is the circular arrangement of the small blue cells into Flexner-Wintersteiner "rosettes" (◆) as shown here. The spread of this neoplasm from the eye typically occurs through the optic nerve, but hematogenous metastases, often to bone marrow, may occur.

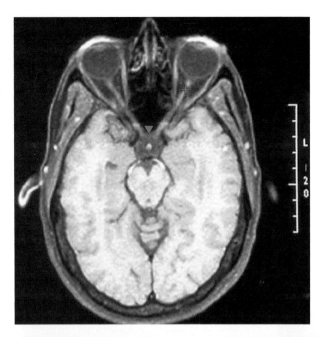

FIGURE 20–25 Optic nerves, MRI

The location of the optic nerves (+) extending to the optic chiasm (▼) is shown in this axial FLAIR MRI. Since the optic nerve is surrounded by meninges, it is affected by changes in cerebrospinal fluid pressure.

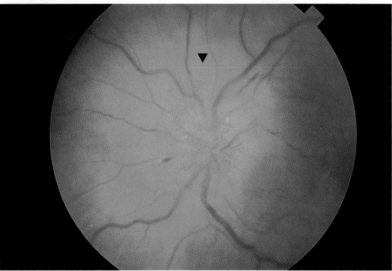

FIGURE 20–26 Papilledema, funduscopy

Note that the margins (▼) of the optic disc are indistinct with blurring because there is swelling with elevation of the optic nerve head. Any condition that increases intracranial pressure (e.g., edema, hemorrhage, mass lesions) may produce papilledema. The presence of papilledema suggests that cerebrospinal fluid pressure has exceeded 200 mm H_2O and that a lumbar puncture should not be performed, or removal of cerebrospinal fluid may be followed by herniation.

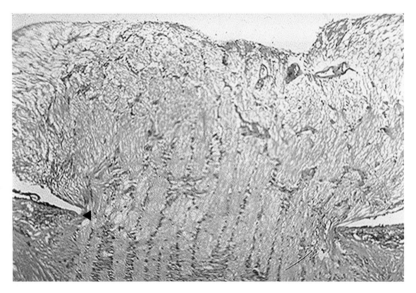

FIGURE 20–27 Papilledema, microscopic

This microscopic section through the head of the optic nerve displays papilledema. Note the bulging of the nerve head above the level (◄) of the surrounding retina, with forward bowing of the lamina cribrosa. The intracranial pressure causing this effect must be relieved, or the patient may suffer herniation (at locations such as the cerebellar tonsils, uncus of hippocampus, cingulate gyrus).

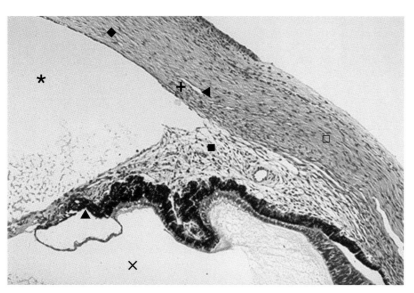

FIGURE 20–28 Normal eye, microscopic

The structures of a fetal eye (small enough to put key structures in close proximity) are seen here at low magnification, including the cornea (◆), the anterior chamber (∗), the posterior chamber (×) the trabecular meshwork (+), the canal of Schlemm (◀), the iris (▲), the ciliary body (■), and the sclera (□). In primary angle closure glaucoma, most likely to occur in small, hyperopic eyes, the angle between the iris and the trabecular meshwork is narrowed, impeding absorption of aqueous humor. Most case of glaucoma are of the primary open angle type, in which there is no obvious point of obstruction, but the mechanism for aqueous absorption malfunctions.

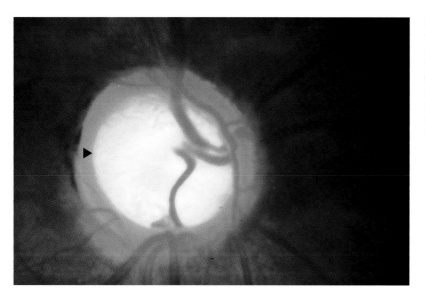

FIGURE 20–29 Glaucoma, funduscopy

This is marked cupping of the optic disc, indicative of glaucoma. Glaucoma results from increased intraocular pressure with damage to the ganglion cells and their axons. This increased ocular pressure over time leads to deepening (▶) of the optic cup with excavation. The vessels shown here appear to "fall into" the deepened optic cup.

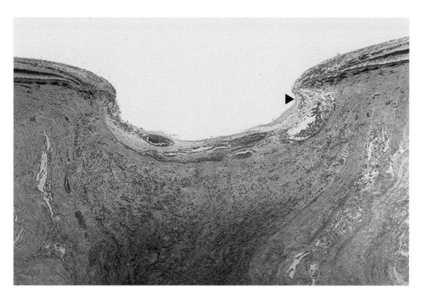

FIGURE 20–30 Glaucoma, microscopic

There is deepening of the optic cup with excavation (▶). The atrophy of the optic nerve leads to progressive loss of vision, regardless of the cause for the increased intraocular pressure.

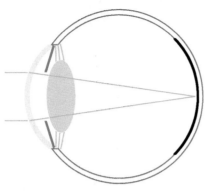

FIGURE 20–31 Normal vision, diagram

Light passes through the cornea and is refracted. The iris can increase or decrease the pupillary diameter to determine the amount of light that enters the eye. The light is further refracted by the crystalline lens, which can be adjusted in shape by the smooth muscle of the ciliary body that tugs on the suspensory ligaments. The aqueous humor in the anterior chamber and the posterior chamber has minimal impact on refraction of light. Ideally, the light is focused precisely on the retina.

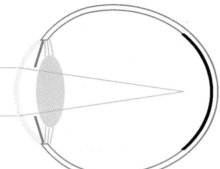

FIGURE 20–32 Myopia, diagram

When the shape of the eye is too long, the light entering the eye becomes focused in front of the retina, and vision is blurred. The crystalline lens can partly adjust for this situation at near distances, so myopia is also known as *nearsightedness*. However, vision at far distances remains blurred. Glasses or contact lenses help to adjust for myopia. About one fourth of all people have some degree of myopia.

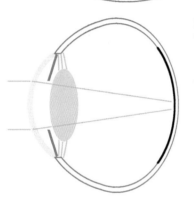

FIGURE 20–33 Hyperopia, diagram

When the shape of the eye is too short, then the focal point for light entering the eye falls behind the retina, and vision is blurred. The crystalline lens can help somewhat to focus the light forward, but once presbyopia occurs, far vision will be better than near vision. Glasses or contact lenses help to adjust for hyperopia.

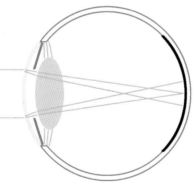

FIGURE 20–34 Astigmatism, diagram

When the shape of the corneal curvature is ovoid, more like a rugby ball than a basketball, then light entering the eye is distorted as it is refracted unevenly. Vision is blurred at all distances. Glasses have traditionally been the only choice for correction, but contact lenses are now able to correct some cases as well. About half of people with myopia also have some degree of astigmatism.

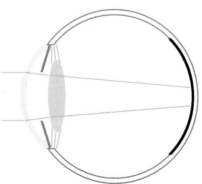

FIGURE 20–35 Presbyopia, diagram

With aging, the crystalline lens loses its flexibility and cannot accommodate focusing, particularly at near distances. By the fifth decade, nearly everyone experiences some degree of presbyopia. Objects must be held farther away to see clearly. People who never had corrective lenses will require them for viewing close objects (reading), while people who have corrective lenses will need bifocals. People with myopia may not need corrective lenses for close distances with the onset of presbyopia.

Figure Credits

Chapter 1

Figure 1–17 Courtesy of Dr. M. Elizabeth H. Hammond, University of Utah; **Figure 1–20** Courtesy of Department of Pathology, The University of Hong Kong; **Figure 1–36** Courtesy of Dr. Walter H. Henricks, The Cleveland Clinic Foundation; **Figure 1–51** Courtesy of Department of Pathology, The University of Hong Kong; **Figure 1–67** Courtesy of Dr. Richard Conran, Uniformed Services University.

Chapter 2

Figure 2–11 Courtesy of Dr. Mary Ann Sens, University of North Dakota; **Figures 2–44, 2–45, and 2–48** Courtesy of Department of Pathology, The University of Hong Kong.

Chapter 4

Figures 4–10 and 4–12 Courtesy of Dr. Sherrie L. Perkins, University of Utah; **Figures 4–30, 4–31, and 4–32** Courtesy of Dr. Carl R. Kjeldsberg, University of Utah; **Figures 4–35, 4–36, and 4–49** Courtesy of Dr. Sherrie L. Perkins, University of Utah; **Figure 4–51** Courtesy of Dr. Carl R. Kjeldsberg, University of Utah; **Figure 4–77** Courtesy of Department of Pathology, The University of Hong Kong.

Chapter 5

Figure 5–90 Courtesy of Dr. Mary Ann Sens, University of North Dakota.

Chapter 6

Figure 6–9 Courtesy of Department of Pathology, The University of Hong Kong.

Chapter 7

Figure 7–11 Courtesy of Department of Pathology, The University of Hong Kong; **Figures 7–62 and 7–63** Courtesy of Dr. Richard Conran, Uniformed Services University; **Figure 7–71** Courtesy of Department of Pathology, The University of Hong Kong.

Chapter 8

Figures 8–9 and 8–21 Courtesy of Dr. Jeannette J. Townsend, University of Utah; **Figure 8–30** Courtesy of Dr. Morton Levitt, Florida State University.

Chapter 10

Figure 10–6 Courtesy of Dr. Morton Levitt, Florida State University; **Figure 10–67 and 10–77** Courtesy of Department of Pathology, The University of Hong Kong; **Figure 10–79** Courtesy of Arthur J. Belanger, Yale University; **Figures 10–94 and** **10–99** Courtesy of Department of Pathology, The University of Hong Kong; **Figure 10–102** Courtesy of Dr. Richard Conran, Uniformed Services University; **Figure 10–103** Courtesy of Arthur J. Belanger, Yale University.

Chapter 11

Figure 11–14 Courtesy of Dr. Mary Ann Sens, University of North Dakota; **Figure 11–16** Courtesy of Dr. Richard Conran, Uniformed Services University; **Figures 11–20 and 11–22** Courtesy of Dr. David Cohen, Tel Aviv University; **Figure** **11–24** Courtesy of Dr. Richard Conran, Uniformed Services University; **Figure 11–25** Courtesy of Arthur J. Belanger, Yale University; **Figure 11–26** Courtesy of Dr. Ilan Hammel, Tel Aviv University.

Chapter 12

Figure 12–28 Courtesy of Dr. Ofer Ben-Itzhak, Technion-Israel Institute of Technology, Haifa, Israel.

Chapter 13

Figure 13–8 Courtesy of Dr. David Cohen, Tel Aviv University; **Figure 13–13** Courtesy of Dr. Richard Conran, Uniformed Services University; **Figures 13–14, 13–27, 13–28, and 13–44** Courtesy of Dr. David Cohen, Tel Aviv University; **Figures 13–57, 13–61, and 13–62** Courtesy of Dr. Hiroyuki Takahashi, Jikei University School of Medicine; **Figure 13–69** Courtesy of Dr. David Cohen, Tel Aviv University; **Figure** **13–86** Courtesy of Dr. Hiroyuki Takahashi, Jikei University School of Medicine; **Figure 13–88** Courtesy of Dr. David Cohen, Tel Aviv University; **Figure 13–91** Courtesy of Department of Pathology, The University of Hong Kong; **Figures 13–92, 13–93, 13–99, and 13–100** Courtesy of Dr. Hiroyuki Takahashi, Jikei University School of Medicine; **Figure 13–122** Courtesy of Dr. Morton Levitt, Florida State University.

Chapter 14

Figure 14–22 Courtesy of Dr. David Cohen, Tel Aviv University.

Chapter 15

Figure 15–27 Courtesy of Department of Pathology, The University of Hong Kong; **Figure 15–58** Courtesy of Dr. Jeannette J. Townsend, University of Utah.

Chapter 16

Figure 16–22 Courtesy of Dr. Sate Hamza, University of Manitoba; **Figure 16–24** Courtesy of Dr. David Cohen, Tel Aviv University; **Figure 16–26** Courtesy of Dr. Lauren Hughey, University of Alabama-Birmingham; **Figure 16–27** Courtesy of Dr. Sate Hamza, University of Manitoba; **Figure 16–28** Courtesy of Dr. Morton Levitt, Florida State University;

Figure 16–29 Courtesy of Dr. Sate Hamza, University of Manitoba; **Figure 16–30** Courtesy of Dr. Ilan Hammel, Tel Aviv University; **Figure 16–37** Courtesy of Dr. Morton Levitt, Florida State University; **Figures 16–40 and 16–42** Courtesy of Dr. Ilan Hammel, Tel Aviv University; **Figure 16–43** Courtesy of Dr. Morton Levitt, Florida State University; **Figure 16–46** Courtesy of Arthur J. Belanger, Yale University; **Figures 16–47 and 16–48** Courtesy of Dr. Sate Hamza, University of Manitoba; **Figure 16–49** Courtesy of Dr. Amy Theos, University of Alabama-Birmingham; **Figures 16–50, 16–52, 16–53, 16–55, and 16–57** Courtesy of Dr. Sate Hamza, University of Manitoba; **Figures 16–58, 16–64, and 16–65** Courtesy of Dr. Morton Levitt, Florida State University; **Figure 16–66** Courtesy of Dr. Sate Hamza, University of Manitoba; **Figures 16–67 and 16–68** Courtesy of Dr. M. Elizabeth H. Hammond, University of Utah; **Figures 16–70, 16–71, 16–72, and 16–73** Courtesy of Dr. Morton Levitt, Florida State University; **Figures 16–75, 16–76, 16–77, and 16–78** Courtesy of Dr. Sate Hamza, University of Manitoba; **Figure 16–83** Courtesy of Dr. Morton Levitt, Florida State University; **Figures 16–88 and 16–89** Courtesy of Dr. Sate Hamza, University of Manitoba.

Chapter 17

Figures 17–19, 17–26, 17–60, and 17–74 Courtesy of Department of Pathology, The University of Hong Kong; **Figure 17–89** Courtesy of Dr. David Cohen, Tel Aviv University.

Chapter 18

Figures 18–1, 18–2, 18–8, 18–11, 18–13, 18–14, 18–15, 18–24, 18–28, and 18–30 Courtesy of Dr. Jeannette J. Townsend, University of Utah.

Chapter 19

Figures 19–14, 19–31, 19–33, 19–34, 19–35, and 19–36 Courtesy of Dr. Jeannette J. Townsend, University of Utah; **Figure 19–38** Courtesy of Dr. Todd C. Grey, University of Utah; **Figures 19–41 19–43, 19–44, and 19–45** Courtesy of Dr. Jeannette J. Townsend, University of Utah; **Figure 19–46** Courtesy of Dr. Todd C. Grey, University of Utah; **Figures 19–59, 19–60, 19–69, 19–71, 19–77, 19–78, 19–84, 19–88, 19–89, 19–92, 19–93, 19–94, 19–95, 19–96, 19–97, 19–116, 19–117, 19–118, 19–119, 19–127, and 19–134** Courtesy of Dr. Jeannette J. Townsend, University of Utah.

Chapter 20

Figures 20–1, 20–4, 20–7, 20–8, 20–10 through 20–17, 20–19 through 20–23, 20–26, 20–27, 20–29, and 20–30 Courtesy of Dr. Nick Mamalis, University of Utah.

Index